3. $Cl + O_2 \rightarrow ClO_2$; ClO_2 + organic chem... chloramines.
see ~~TOR~~TORTORA, 6th. ed. & this book, p...

ic

products.

function, recall.

Chemical Brain Injury

Chemical Brain Injury

Kaye H. Kilburn, M.D.

VNR VAN NOSTRAND REINHOLD
I(T)P® A Division of International Thomson Publishing Inc.

New York • Albany • Bonn • Boston • Detroit • London • Madrid • Melbourne
Mexico City • Paris • San Francisco • Singapore • Tokyo • Toronto

Cover photo: ''Neotoxicosis,'' sculpture by Jabe C. Jackson
Cover design: Jon Herder

I(T)P® An Internationl Thomson Publishing Company
The ITP logo is a registered trademark used herein under license

Printed in the United States of America

For more information, contact:

Van Nostrand Reinhold
115 Fifth Avenue
New York, NY 10003

Chapman & Hall
2–6 Boundary Row
London
SE1 8HN
United Kingdom

Thomas Nelson Australia
102 Dodds Street
South Melbourne, 3205
Victoria, Australia

Nelson Canada
1120 Birchmount Road
Scarborough, Ontario
Canada M1K 5G4

Chapman & Hall GmbH
Pappelallee 3
69469 Weinheim
Germany

International Thomason Publishing Asia
221 Henderson Road #05–10
Henderson Building
Singapore 0315

International Thomson Publishing Japan
Hirakawacho Kyowa Building, 3F
2-2-1 Hirakawacho
Chiyoda-ku, 102 Tokyo
Japan

International Thomson Editores
Seneca 53
Col. Polanco
11560 Mexico D.F. Mexico

1 2 3 4 5 6 7 8 9 10 BBI 01 00 99 98 97

Library of Congress Cataloging-in-Publication Data

Kilburn, Kaye H.
Chemical brain injury / Kaye H. Kilburn.
p. cm.
Includes bibliographical references and index.
ISBN 0-442-02427-4
1. Neurotoxicology. I. Title.
[DNLM: 1. Brain Diseases—chemically induced. 2. Brain Diseases—epidemiology. 3. Hazardous Substances—adverse effects. 4. Environmental Pollutants—adverse effects. WL 348 K48c 1997]
RC347.5.K55 1997
616.8′0471—dc21 97-24105
CIP

http://www.vnr.com
product discounts · free email newsletters
software demos · online resources

email: info@vnr.com

a service of I(T)P®

To my patients who helped me into their brains to see how chemicals injured them.

To my wife Gerrie, who shared this venture and many earlier ones.

Contents

Preface xi

Acknowledgments xix

1 *Introduction: The Brain's New Chemical Plagues* *1*

Key Points 1
Objectives 4
The Audience 4
Messages and Conclusions 5

2 *Neurobehavioral Effects and Exposure Epidemiology* *6*

Choosing Paradigms to Relate Effects to Chemical Exposure 6
Environmental Toxicology 12
Epidemiology 16

3 *Methods for Measuring Neurobehavioral Function: Deriving Prediction Equations for Tests in People Unexposed vs. Those Exposed to Chemicals* *21*

Introduction 21
Physiological Methods 22
Neuropsychological Tests 29
Data Analysis 31
Children's Prediction Equations 44
Unexposed Groups and Prediction Equations 49
Aging, A Perspective on Dementia and Chemical Encephalopathy 49
Appendix 57

4 *Chemically Exposed Patients* *62*

Introduction 62
Objective 1: Associating Patterns of Dysfunction to Chemicals 63
Objective 2: Testing to Detect Impairment 74
Objective 3: New Tests for Other Functions 78
Objective 4: Understanding the Central Nervous System 85
Conclusions 90

5 *Hydrogen Sulfide Exposure from Refineries in Cities* *92*

The 16 Patients 93
A Disastrous Incident in Torrance, California 96
The Unocal Refinery Exposure 104
Casper and Houston Subjects 114
Balance Function and Reaction Times in Refinery Workers Exposed to H_2S 123
Discussion 125
Conclusions 127

6 *Chlorine and Cresylate from a Train Derailment* *129*

Testing of Subjects 129
Discussion 137

7 *Adverse Effects from Hydrogen Chloride* *139*

The Release 140
Testing of Subjects 140
Discussion 145

8 *Effects of Airborne Arsenic at Bryan/College Station, Texas* *152*

Testing of Subjects 153
Discussion 162

9 *Neurobehavioral Effects of Residential Chlordane* *166*

Testing of Subjects 167
Discussion 176

10 *Visual and Neurobehavioral Impairment Associated with Polychlorinated Biphenyls (PCBS)* *180*

The Exposure 181
Testing of Subjects 182
Discussion 187

11 *Exposures to Chemical Mixtures Rich in Trichloroethylene (TCE): Residential and Occupational* *195*

Absorption and Toxicology of TCE 195
Study 1: The Northeastern Phoenix, Arizona Community 196

Study 2: Southwestern Tucson, Arizona Community 217
Study 3: Occupational Exposure at Tinker Air Force Base and Environs Near Oklahoma City, Oklahoma 227
Study 4: Community in the Muscle Shoals, Alabama Environs 235
Trichloroethylene: Summary and General Conclusions 247

12 Combustion—Toluene-Rich Vapor Exposure 254

Exposure and Exposure Surrogates 254
Testing of Subjects 257
Discussion 275

13 Aluminum Recycling: Vinyl Chloride and Other Contaminants 284

Testing of Subjects 285
Discussion 291

14 Diesel Exhaust 296

Background 296
Testing of Subjects 297
Discussion 303

15 Pervasiveness of Impaired Brains: Implications from ''Controls'' Being Abnormal 306

16 Mechanisms of Brain Damage from Chemicals 310

A Speculative Overview 310
Entry of Chemicals into the CNS 311
Lessons from Traumatic Brain Damage 316
Theories for Chemical Brain Damage 319

17 Prognosis and Therapy 334

Prognosis of Chemical Encephalopathy 334
Possible Therapeutic Interventions 340

18 The Future of Neurotoxicology: Needs and Responsibilities 347

Issues in Testing 347
Recommendations 350

19 Legal Proceedings 352

The Cases 356
Conclusions 362
Author's Note 363

20 *Social Changes Needed to Help Brains Survive* *364*

Introduction 364
Immediate Measures for Reversing the Descent into Darkness 365
Strategies for Change 367
What We Must Do in Shaping Human Attitudes 371
Global Issues 375

Suggested Reading 377

Index 379

Chemical Brain Damage: (CBD)
[Clock age of 40 when CBD = brain age 8

Preface

Upton Sinclair's The Jungle *published in book form in 1906 . . . is remembered as a stomach turning exposé of unsanitary conditions and deceitful practices in the meat-packing industry; as such it aroused the ire of a whole nation, from President Theodore Roosevelt on down, and it contributed enormously to the landmark passage of the Pure Food and Drug Act of 1906. (The book is said to have decreased America's meat consumption for decades.)*

—Morris Dickstein's Introduction to *The Jungle*

The thesis of this book is that the brain and the central nervous system, including the affective or emotional centers, such as those manifesting a major depression and progressive degenerative dementia, are targets for chemicals. Brain cell incapacity and/or death reduces function, an effect sometimes interpreted as Alzheimer's disease. Other organ systems, especially the lung, may also be affected but in exposed individuals multiple health complaints frequently arise from the brain.

The reader may doubt that chemical brain damage exists, that it is generalized in the human species, or that key brain functions can be measured accurately. In fact, the aggregate of the observed impairments establishes that chemical brain damage closely resembles aging (as in clock age 40, brain age 80), and that it is a dementia akin to Alzheimer's. Convinced that it cannot be "cured" in most cases, I believe that it must be *prevented* for the survival of the species.

Time is always a precious resource, but it is especially so at deadline time for the brain. The problems that chemical brain injury presents need immediate attention. It took me a decade to learn what I wish to teach you in a few hundred pages. In the hope of saving the human brain, I invite you—in fact, I invite all people "involved in mankind'' (John Donne, 1616)—to share scientific evidence that has been collected since 1987.

Epidemiology, the science that deals with the incidence, distribution, and control of disease in a population, is the approach (see Chapter 2) I have taken to compile persuasive evidence for the existence of chemical brain injury in large populations. The methods of measurement used are crucial in determining brain function, and data analysis is critical in adjusting for aging, level of education, and other factors (see Chapter 3). Particularly striking are the cruel hard facts of collective brain impairment in 269 patients (see Chapter 4) and in over 3,000 people measured since 1987 in 14 neighborhoods and 2 workplaces (Chapters 5 to 14). Possible mechanisms for brain injury, of remarkable variety, are considered (Chapter 16), and some are quite compelling. The plasticity of the brain and converging information about toxic mechanisms of damage define prognosis and treatment (see Chapter 17). Chapter 18 discusses the future of neurotoxicology as science. A chapter on legal proceedings considers the legal history of redress for this form of personal injury in affected populations (Chapter 19). Finally, challenges to think ''big enough'' to solve chemical exposure problems are laid out in Chapter 20.

Chapters 2 through 15 weave together evaluations of single patients and associated clinical findings with epidemiological observations of large numbers of Americans. All were studied by using sensitive methods of measurement gathered from established medical texts. These techniques improved upon measurements originated by Hippocrates, Galen, Paracelsus (toxicology), Ramazzini (occupational medicine), Romberg (balance), Gower (visual fields), William James (psychology), Harriett Hardy (workplace diseases), William Huebner (occupational cancer), Frank Fankhauser (visual field, Octopus), Leonard Goldberg (balance measurement), David Wechsler, Ward Halstead, Richard Cattell, Douglas McNair (POMS test), Russell Brain, Helen Hanninen, Anna Maria Seppalainen, Juhani Juntunen, Peter Arlien-Søborg, and numerous other investigators.

The thoughtful clinician may feel uneasy in that for each patient all possible or appropriate neurological diagnostic tests were not done. How can the author put aside the need for careful, differential diagnosis? How can he avoid not considering all possible spontaneous neurological diseases for each patient? To be specific, why were there no reported electroencephalographs, or quantitative EEGs, skull films, computer augmented tomograms (CT scans), magnetic resonance images (MRI scans), positron-emission tomograms (PET scans) or SPEC scans, no visual or auditory evoked potentials, no cerebral angiography, and no spinal taps and fluid analysis? The answer is that each of these tests has a place, usually well established in clinical diagnosis. For example, EEGs in seizures, CT scans for strokes, angiographs for aneurysm, and spinal fluid analysis for infection. However, none of them alone, nor the aggregate of several or all of them, is sensitive to generalized brain injury unless or until it is gross. These tests mainly localize. They find discrete lesions. In the extensive evaluation of chronic painter's syndrome the single positive test in the most severely functionally-impaired spray painters after 20 to 30 years of exposure was cerebral atrophy shown by brain MRI. Other tests yielded nothing.

Thus, when I confirmed these observations repeatedly in patients exposed to various chemicals, usually by testing patients who have already had various localizing procedures (EEG, MRI, visual evoked potentials, and spinal taps), I moved onward to *destructive differential diagnosis* as advocated by cardiologist Sam Levine late of Boston.

When signs of generalized brain damage were present by neurobehavioral testing, it was concluded the tests for localization would be negative and clinical judgment was applied to omit endless and fruitless inappropriate studies. Studies of chemical brain injury and of cerebral lupus erythematosus have shown blood flow is altered in these situations when the brain is working, doing arithmetic, or juggling concepts in a recall task. These observations suggest that one mechanism of generalized brain injury is altered distribution of blood flow, but this does not mean these are diagnostic or confirmatory tests of the physiological or functional measurements used in the patients and populations who are the subjects of this book.

Some years ago, I found myself attempting to explain to patient after patient with impaired brain function what had happened to them. Reviewing their symptoms and their history, I was forced to consider that exposures to chemicals were the most plausible explanations for disordered balance, constricted visual fields, impaired color discrimination, loss of hearing, of recall, and of the cognitive (problem-solving) functions, and of delays in blink reflex and visual reaction time. For some time, I was encumbered by my own acceptance of the status quo, incredulity at the unexpected, and self-doubt. Although highly skeptical, I was fortunate to be unencumbered by excessive belief in idiopathic psychiatric disorders; but I also was mindful of the current widespread epidemics of dementia and depression.

I have integrated my observations, made deductions, and shared the results of constructive differential diagnosis to consider all possible causes. I have also relied on destructive differential diagnosis, making decisions at the branch points of logic trees—a method used by clinical diagnosticians but one that is rarely acknowledged, perhaps because it repeatedly requires conscious effort. This method was characterized by the late cardiologist Samuel Levine, to eliminate less likely diagnoses and causes by using clinical judgment without exhaustive laboratory investigation. When I applied this method to attributing causes in patients and populations I studied, the elimination of all other causes left a chemical or a mixture of chemicals as the cause of the observed impairment. The hardest preconception for me to overcome was the idea that chemicals generally are beneficial and benign. Admitting the possibility that some—for example, chlorine, hydrogen, sulfide, formaldehyde, ammonia, trichloroethylene, chlordane, polychlorinated biphenyls, and epoxy resins—are adverse, indeed harmful, is the essential step as the diagnostic process is extended to causal attribution.

The concepts of chemical brain damage and its corollary, premature aging of the brain, are at once threatening and frightening. I examined other possible explanations, both conventional and novel, and I made every effort to disprove or invalidate the brain injury hypothesis statistically, logically, and by repeated observation, before presenting it as the main theory. As new examples appeared (sometimes labeled ''nature's experiments'' but in reality *unscheduled human toxicity testing*), they served to strengthen this hypothesis. Even reanalysis of what had been considered unexposed comparison groups showed that eight of these populations had lower test scores and were nearer to sites of possible chemical exposure than the standard four unexposed groups (in Wickenburg, Arizona; Springfield, Louisiana; San Luis Obispo, California; and central Tennessee).

During the past ten years I have analyzed, studied, and considered each patient and exposed population to gain a perspective, to test statistical methods and hypotheses, and to try to come to terms with alarming, saddening facts. The dilemma was a cruel one, as I sought at once to escape from but also to work within conventional thinking. This process is comparable to building added thrust into a rocket or a space shuttle to escape the earth's gravitational field. As frequently happens, the downward pull was from entrenched ideas. As Maynard Keynes put it so well in the preface to his *General Theory*, "The difficulty lies, not in the new ideas but in escaping from the old ones, which ramify, in every corner of our minds." Paraphrasing another of Keynes's observations, the ideas that have been laboriously assembled and presented in this monograph are not complex. Many, when recognized, seem so apparent they may even appear obvious to some readers.

Two conclusions have been drawn from the assembled data. First, we have witnessed a century of proliferation of synthetic chemicals, and during the same time period humans have experienced great increases in cancers, brain damage, asthma, and other epidemic degenerative diseases such as arthritis and coronary heart disease. Second, there is considerable evidence that human reproductive processes have been severely disrupted by chemical exposure. Humans are experiencing malformations and infertility, just as fish and birds are in the Great Lakes ecosystem, in Florida, and elsewhere. Many other species share humans' inability to adapt rapidly to chemicals; on the other hand, insects are the most adaptive animals. Their nervous systems, although targets of several classes of chemicals, avoid eradication and thrive with the newest level of or addition to the world's chemical/pesticide burden. Thus for half a century insects (and their nervous systems) have adapted to pesticides despite escalation of chemical warfare against them. This situation is analogous to bacteria acquiring resistance to antibiotics.

For generations people have been led to believe that chemicals basically are good for them, that better things for better living are made through chemistry. Corporations have portrayed themselves as responding to human needs for shelter, food, and clothing. In the early decades of the twentieth century, while "no apparent harm" was recognized from chemicals, cancer rates mushroomed and new illnesses developed, with astonishing increases in cancer, asthma, connective tissue disease, tight building syndrome, arthritis, end stage renal disease, and many other diseases and illnesses. Chemical pollution of water, air, and land in pesticide poisonings and mass chemical disasters have claimed attention so that tales of Selveso, Love Canal, Michigan's polybrominated biphenyls (PBBs), Times Beach, Minamata, Yusho, Yentang (PCBs), and Bhopal (methyl isocyanate) literally have become household horror stories.

What has happened? Surely we must conclude from the multiple associations between chemicals and disease that something is wrong. New products of human ingenuity and chemical engineering have become integral parts of modern life, from food containers to sprays that "clean," deodorize, and kill insects and bacteria. At the same time, chemicals have seriously degraded our environment; and now they are destroying our most valuable asset, human brains. Although some try to excuse these multiple associations as coincidence, the observations form a coherent pattern, in space and time.

Evidence surrounds us of chemical infiltration in our lives and in our brains. Eighty-two percent of U.S. households use pesticides solubolized in toxic organic chemicals, and 75% use them inside the home, from the 1.1 billion-pound supply used each year of the last decade (USEPA 1988-230-07-88-033). Nearly everyone has clothing cleaned with organic chemical solvents, or, if not, uses an abundance of chemical detergents. We microwave foods in plastic covered by plastic (thus ensuring heat degradation and leaching of toxic monomers). We herd automobiles burning gasoline and diesel into vast derbies. We live in buildings tacked and pasted together with adhesives, fibers, and particle board. Our civilization reeks with chemicals. Yet we do have a choice, and we are responsible for changing the world we now live in. A safer way of living is an option; we must avoid or minimize our contact with these harmful chemicals. Reminders that the earth's ecosystem is being destroyed abound: the Aral Sea is dead, the Black Sea is dying, and the Amazon rain forest diminishes daily; air conditioning chlorofluorocarbons release chlorine to the stratosphere, removing the protective ozone filter so that dangerous ultraviolet light causes more cancers to occur, and solar radiation heats the earth; greater fuel combustion increases carbon dioxide production, and the ''greenhouse effect'' further enhances global warming. The earth's once vast and pristine detoxification systems are now severely damaged, and some, such as air and water, are nearly overwhelmed.

Rachel Carson's *Silent Spring,* published some 35 years ago, was met with grave misgivings by many in the scientific and medical communities. Some of her conclusions about real and potential dangers to human health seemed exaggerated and overly dramatic. Carson's plea for stronger regulatory guidelines for pesticides was thought to have overlooked ''the considerable tightening that's taken place in the past few years,'' commented Dexter Masters, president of Consumers Union, in his introduction to their (CU's) edition of *Silent Spring* in 1962. Unfortunately, in large measure, Rachel Carson's timely warnings have been trivialized, ignored, even debased. Despite the fact that Carson's work resulted in new environmental legislation, regulations, and banning of DDT, her message has been diluted and even cast aside by most of the chemical industry. Human health has been sacrificed to economic growth and profits, the twin idols of our time.

The evidence presented in this book will show that bold new solutions to global health problems are needed, as chemicals are costing us dearly in new and dreadful ways, including eroded brains and degeneration. Programmed cell death (apoptosis) is out of control. The slow destruction of our brains is an oozing lesion that, if not stopped, threatens to destroy our civilization. We must be responsible to those who come after us, our children and their children. The prevention of chemical brain injury must be a top international priority. Investigators must rapidly assemble further evidence before much more damage is done. We must adopt a philosophy to save the brain, and raise people's consciousness of their own health. Extreme measures may be needed to end the production of the chemicals and their wastes that harm the brain, and corporations must be held accountable for this injury. To rescue human intelligence and to save ourselves, we as citizens, unwitting users of chemical poisons, must abandon some comforts and conveniences that we have come to take for granted; otherwise, we will fade into the enveloping night of premature senility and the possible destruction of our species. A new order must be created in which new chemicals are viewed as dangerous until proven safe. Corporations that make chemicals must prove their safety by sponsoring experiments in independent laboratories comparable to those of the U.S. Bureau of Standards and the U.S. Food and Drug Administration. The toxicity assays must no longer be experiments on human populations.

A native of Utah and graduate of its College of Medicine, who had postdoctoral education at Western Reserve, Duke, and London universities as well as Utah, and served on the faculties at Colorado University and University (St. Louis), I moved to Durham and Duke University in 1962 as chief of medicine of the Durham Veterans Hospital. Teaching at Duke and supervising a 200-bed academic medical service, I compressed a veritable lifetime of medical experience into five years of service. I concluded then that *medicine is the diagnosis of advanced degenerative diseases and their palliation in incurable patients.* Finding the causes of some of these incurable degenerative diseases or susceptible chinks in pathogenesis so they could be prevented became my obvious goal.

To test this approach, I began investigating the opportunities for prevention of lung disease when I left the chief of medicine post and created one of the first environmental medicine divisions, at the Duke University Medical Center. Its aim was to prevent byssinosis, cotton dust disease. I soon had developed a staff of 18 faculty excited by this idea, who were trained in epidemiology, immunopathology, ultrastructure, and biochemistry. I was given the freedom to do this by my boss, Eugene A. Stead (chairman of internal medicine at Duke) and a career development award from the National Institute of Environmental Health Sciences (NIEHS). The support for trainees came from an NIEHS training grant, and direct targeted money for byssinosis came from one of the first National Institute of Occupational Safety and Health program project grants. This support was augmented by that of the North Carolina State Board of Health (Occupational Health). Burlington Industries, the textile giant headquartered in North Carolina, provided financial aid and access to cotton mills and workers. Thus instant bridges were built to the academic and the scientific communities, enabling us to coordinate resources from industry, government, and public health to solve a problem called ''Monday morning asthma,'' which was occupational chronic bronchitis. We studied a sample of nearly 4,000 textile workers from a 250,000-worker industry. The dust levels in 12 plants were compared to airways obstruction, prevalence of chronic bronchitis, and byssinosis to produce a dose–response curve for cotton dust; and our chemists isolated several lung-bioactive chemicals from the dust. The reduction of dust levels was federally mandated in 1972; and as the standards were enforced, byssinosis disappeared in the United States, and the textile industry prospered. Following this experience, in the early 1980s I studied workers for effects of asbestos, welding fumes, and fiberglass. These studies highlighted occupational asthma as a growing health problem; but our investigators also discovered that, although the lung was the target organ for some chemicals, it often was the organ of entry, the conduit through which chemicals passed, like anesthetic ethyl ether, to the brain.

Early measurements showed that fiberglass batt makers and laboratory workers exposed to formaldehyde fixatives for tissues shared brain impairment. The tests used were from Wechsler's adult intelligence scale and from the Halstead-Reitan battery. The disadvantages were that these tests were not precise enough and were, in part, subjective. I searched for objective measurements for the brain similar to spirometric volume and flow for the lung. Candidates for the ''brain test'' were visual simple and two-choice reaction time, balance measured by tracking sway, color discrimination, and grip strength. The tests needed to distinguish between groups of chemically exposed and unexposed people. As we gained experience with clinic patients, we added vision testing, contrast sensitivity, and visual fields, borrowed from ophthalmology, and audiometry to quantify hearing. Beginning in 1982, we repeatedly evaluated brain function tests critically, as used to measure unwitting chemical ''experiments'' occurring as accidents or because of residence near factory or Superfund sites. By the end of 1996, some 269 patients had been examined (one to three weekly in clinic), as had over 3,000 chemically exposed and over 600 unexposed referents from 22 population samples. It became clear that the brain was the primary and the ultimate organ damaged by many chemicals.

Chemical brain damage is a global problem. It is so important and demanding of quick and lasting solutions that it should be the long-sought unifying force to federate world governments. Our fellow inhabitants of the earth must heed this call to arms. Scientists throughout the world, in Sweden, Finland, and Denmark and elsewhere, have paved the way in showing that workers are brain-damaged from occupational chemicals. But outside the workplace vastly greater exposure zones are chemically laden air, soil, and water. Chernobyl serves as a powerful example of the internationality of pollution by radiation, which even engulfed the logical and cautious people of Sweden. We must not ignore its harsh lesson. The danger of ignoring this call is to sink further into a chemically induced slumber from which there will be no awakening.

Strategies for change can be cooperative or adversarial. I find both approaches to be possibilities as I endeavor to treat the brain disorder that has been diagnosed. The adversarial one is reactive and thus promises to be too slow, except in emphasizing the situation (Chapter 18). It appears that a cooperative strategy is sounder and may give us some hope (see Chapter 19); clearly it would be faster and less wasteful than so-called legal remedies that have not yet prevented brain damage from chemicals. However, criminal punishment may be needed to reinforce society's mandate to recalcitrant corporate officials.

An example of a cooperative approach was the governmental incentives given to industry to find renewable sources of energy in the 1970s, with seed money and tax breaks that brought many practical solutions to the pilot plant stage. Some of the developments included hydrogen fuel for vehicles, photovoltaic cells, and wind-powered electrical generators; some were already well accepted, whereas others were novel. At the same time, conservation, in fuel-efficient transportation and space heating, eased demand or the growth of need. Unfortunately, to prevent loss of market share, the oil companies took over the energy companies as the crisis eased, and their political maneuvers killed the applications of the innovations, particularly in the conservation of fuel. All the earth-saving solutions lacked the enormous profitability of petroleum. These corporate takeovers could have been prevented by an alert government directed toward public interest by a concerned (knowledgeable) citizenry.

Is the threat of chemical harm to human brains massive enough to change world political-economics? Can this threat, the specter of the loss of brain power, change energy and materials cycles from unbridled consumption to a conservative use of resources—to husband creative humans rather than brainless consumers? A new revolution in thought is required to bridge the gaps between the scientific community, public health professionals, environmentalists, corporations, and the world's governments. Surely nothing could instill more fear and spur more changes in humankind than the loss of the brain, that complex organ that makes us truly human.

Each day in clinic and field studies I collect more evidence of chemicals that damage the brain. This work may have its critics: persons skeptical about the mounting evidence and secure in the status quo of intuition, treasured proverbs, profit sharing, stock options, and a belief in the benevolence of chemical companies. Some may attempt to trivialize the findings, or deny them, and pretend to themselves and others that the chemical brain injury reported herein did not hit scores on patients and over 3,000 fellow humans in exposed groups. It seemed unlikely to me too at first, but the concept that all chemicals are good "ain't necessarily so." Our only hope lies in mobilizing human coalitions of doctors, nurses, victims, and lawyers united by the idea of saving the brain. This book gives concerned citizens an important tool. Our compassion for the humans who have been irrevocably damaged must force the changes needed to rescue the human brain.

It is critical that product users show corporations how their behavior must change. A changeover to closed loop industrial economics, which regards waste as an aberration, is a critical step. It will provide us the opportunity to create useful products from dangerous by-products. The effort will be spurred by user boycotts and by criminal proceedings against CEOs of the offending corporations and companies. The crime of chemical injury is as indictable as are other personal assaults.

The patients studied, victims in a chemical world, have made their personal contribution. Their increasingly frequent tragedies need to be studied as examples of chemical injury, not just by health professionals and others in the vanguard but by society's members. Society's leaders must be made to insist that chemical production be regulated and the production of questionable unsafe chemicals be prohibited.

If not reversed, brain erosion, a direct result of chemical exposure, will dwarf the epidemics of Alzheimer's disease and AIDS as mere blips on the path to early death. It is almost impossible to imagine the effects of premature senility on a society. The picture is one of disaster, a future without hope of rescue that is made more ominous by the findings of Chapter 15, which show only four of thirteen comparison groups of the chemically exposed were not impaired. Nine groups had signs of chemical brain injury.

These changes are your responsibility. Today's generations need you, the informed recipients of this warning, as teachers and leaders to take the message painted boldly here and integrate it into actions designed to prevent chemical brain damage. This danger appears “white hot,” compelling a solution. I cannot picture a more general or massive threat to humankind and the earth than widespread progressive brain damage. Not only “religious” and internecine warfare (as in Bosnia, Chechnya, Northern Ireland, Iraq, Afghanistan, and Cambodia), but abortion, AIDS, the Ebola virus, crime, poverty, and family collapse pale by comparison to brain loss. Brain loss may even be contributing to most social problems. Enactment of regulations to stop the use of asbestos, remove lead from gasoline, reduce cotton dust in textile mills, lower benzene levels in gasoline, and stop production and use of chlorinated pesticides and polychlorinated biphenyls has taken a generation. But this has been a generation in which exceptions to these “rules” are the rule; a generation of transportation of toxic technology “overseas”; a generation of repeated rediscovery of toxicity; and, sadly, a generation of increasing brain damage.

This world problem needs strong medicine, using as a model the U.S. Food and Drug Administration, the FDA, a world-renowned model of effectiveness and integrity in government regulation of chemicals. Its Delaney clause, which prohibits carcinogenic substances in food, should be amended to include neurotoxic chemicals. Putative economic interests must not prevent the outright prohibition of brain-damaging pesticides and other harmful chemicals.

The other key to solving this problem is education. An open-minded and compassionate citizenry, concerned enough about these chemicals to boycott them, will tell the chemical industry that it must make safe chemicals from production loops without toxic wastes. Let us all work together to save the dearest part of our humanity, the human brain.

Acknowledgments

I gratefully acknowledge the contributions of the following individuals:

Bradford E. Hanscom for skills in measurement and management of data. He translated my streams of consciousness into flows of electrons.

John C. Thornton for evolving sound statistical strategies and applying them to these data.

Alice Avila, whose word processing talents made possible the writing of this book's many drafts.

Many colleagues who have wondered with me about brain injury, and particularly four who saw earlier drafts and suggested ways to simplify and clarify these findings and their plausible mechanisms: Iris R. Bell, M.D. of Tucson, Arizona; William S. Lynn, M.D. of Smithville, Texas; John Chapman, M.D. of Dallas, Texas; and John F. (Jack) Finklea, M.D. of Myrtle Beach, South Carolina.

Attorneys for the plaintiffs, who encouraged these studies by their support, moral and financial; and their adversaries, who have challenged these methods and the conclusions and thereby helped me to refine the argument.

1

Introduction: The Brain's New Chemical Plagues

God may forgive your sins of omission, but your nervous system won't.

—Alfred Korzybski

KEY POINTS

Several key points must be emphasized before we examine the particulars of our studies. The following paragraphs summarize our organizing principles.

1. The brain is the most sensitive organ for injury from chemicals.

2. Major symptoms of toxic chemical exposure to the brain include memory loss, headache, irritability, lack of concentration, and insomnia.

3. For the objective demonstration of brain impairment, a paradigm is needed like that applied to the respiratory system 30 years ago in subjects exposed to air pollution. Forced expiration in one second provided the best objective confirmation for chest tightness, and shortness of breath and midflow was an even more sensitive measure. To objectively confirm chemical brain injury, a rich assortment of possible tests have been collected for over a century; but only a few of these time-honored tests, which helped psychologists to solve school assignment and social maladjustment problems, can detect the effects of chemicals. The best of the new measurements have come from performance testing, their results paralleling the recognition of the effects of air pollution by testing pulmonary function.

4. In order to generalize the experience, observations of the functional effects of the same chemical on different populations are essential.

5. It is critical that tests show the absence of effects as well as the presence of effects. Truth is not often found easily or without travail, just as the path of discovery is seldom straight. The only way the author found to assuage his own skepticism and change his beliefs was to repeatedly analyze a growing, indeed multiplying, experience. Thus, repetition is the price one pays for reproducible results. When one must depend upon human subjects in "circumstantial" exposure incidents or "catastrophes," the elements of choice, flexibility, and control are absent. One is a hunter-gatherer, not a farmer. The entire paradigm at first seems random and unweighty, alien to the scientist who performs experiments. However, if one is committed to understanding the phenomena and is utterly without other choices, one can do what was done here: *squeeze meaning out of man-made disaster experiments, whether performed on persons or on populations.*

6. *What the nightmare is:* Human brains have been injured, and more are endangered every day by chemicals that saturate the world. Evidence abounds that chemical brain injury is common and generally misdiagnosed. Imagine a plague so generalized, so devastating, yet so insidious, that a majority of humankind becomes dysfunctional. Suppose further that this dysfunction affects the brain so that perception and memory gradually fade, disorganizing behavior and thrusting its victims into a world of diminishing prospects and individual (social) disorganization. Should such individual dysfunction rise above a trivial frequency, the collective costs to society could be enormous.

7. *Why and how we sympathize with the chemically injured:* Consider the victim's view of brain damage. Ponder having your own brain function rendered erratic and prone to error. Contemplate living without recall, living in a fog of amnesia. Further, place yourself in the impaired person's shoes; consider the frustration and fear flowing from unusual symptoms, including sensitivity to odors, holes in the memory, an inability to recall, feeling lost in familiar places, an inability to concentrate thoughts or sustain intelligent effort. It is almost impossible to imagine having perceptions and judgments that cannot be trusted; but if we can imagine this at all, we must sympathize with the chemically injured.

To appreciate and be sympathetic to patients exposed to chemicals, one must at least entertain the thought that some chemicals can injure people. Those diagnosticians whom patients confront are annoyed by baffling symptoms and presentations that seem unnatural as they are novel in their intensity, diversity, and persistence. These observations frustrate physicians, who thrust such patients into generally accepted pigeonholes of medical and/or psychiatric diagnosis. If doctors are confused by seeing symptoms beyond their experience, how can they reassure patients that they are not crazy, and help them avoid by label or implication the stigma of mental illness? It wants insight. We can start by putting ourselves in their position, considering their feelings, their observations, and the possible causes.

8. *What myths must be abandoned:* The biggest myth to abandon is that humans resist chemicals. Human effects imitate and magnify the effects of chemicals demonstrated in subcellular preparations, cells, and other animals. Humans, even those over 25 years old, hate to abandon the comfortable myth of their own permanence, their invulnerability. We think that chemicals can do no evil; they have revolutionized our way of life—what we eat, wear, drive, work at, use and consume, and live in. The earth's dominance by humans is believed to be risk-free. But recall that dwelling in cities brought plagues in the Middle Ages.

9. *Why this book was written:* People's burdens of chemicals continue to increase behind such misleading slogans as ''World's Best Exterminator'' (best exterminator of the world?). Our overutilized and overpopulated world is saturated with chemicals. Most abundant are the petrochemicals, and perhaps the most toxic are those laced with chlorine. Are the Alzheimer's epidemic and other modern plagues of asthma, cancer, and failure to reproduce related to chlorinated chemicals and other harmful substances? Nearly 300 patients unfolded to us their tragic stories of disturbed function and lack of understanding, and of being misunderstood. Then came evidence from exposed populations that supported these patients' singular experiences. Environmental epidemiological observations gave us clinical insights. Measurements on 3,000 Americans exposed at home to chemicals and over 600 unexposed referents were the key. This book is really their story, a collective biography of patients and a collection of hometown incidents. Describing these cases, cataloging them, organizing the episodes, the physiological testing, and the statistical paradigms broadened our arguments. The length and the complexity of these stories precluded the publication of a series of journal papers. At best, scattered journal articles are not linked together by most readers. For coherence and completeness, a book was the necessary and appropriate vehicle.

10. *What testing the brain's performance can yield:* From 1982 to the present, the functions of the brain have been found by our investigators to be impaired in symptomatic chemically exposed subjects. Most of these sick people were massively exposed, often precipitously and without warning. The evidence of the neurotoxicity of these chemicals slowly produced patterns, reinforced by the findings in 14 populations studied similarly. Most members of these populations have had frequent and multiple adverse health complaints, which they have associated with living near chemicals, that is, near refining, manufacturing, processing, or disposal operations. Accompanying their complaints have been ''clusters'' of leukemia and brain and kidney cancers and excesses of birth defects and of lupus erythematosus and scleroderma, the serious disseminated diseases of connective tissue. Adverse effects on the brain affect most exposed subjects and appear much earlier than do cancers and birth defects, which rarely affect more than a few subjects after long latent periods. The defining measurements apparently become abnormal at an undefined interval after exposure, often within a year or two of the exposure. Sometimes birth defects and cancers have appeared in concurrent clusters.

11. Our hypothesis has become: *the brain is the prime target for chemicals.* This possibility makes sense because inhaled chemical vapors diffuse across the lung's extensive surface area (80 square meters or one third the area of a tennis court), which is paved with an amazingly thin (0.5 μm) alveolar membrane, to enter the bloodstream, going to the heart and then to the brain. The brain evolved for eons the ability to detect sights, sounds, smells, vibrations, pains, and thumps from the environment. Logically, it retains in the rhinencephalon (smell brain) a sensitivity–vulnerability to chemicals from the environment, which enter by the olfactory stalks that perforate the cribriform plate of the nose. However, the lungs facilitate the diffusion into the blood of large quantities of chemicals, the brain's Achilles' heel. Timed measurements of brain function objectively verify impairments of balance, recall memory, and cognition perceived by patients as symptoms. Thus, neurological dysfunctions, recorded numerically, can be compared across intervals of time.

OBJECTIVES

The book has several objectives:

1. To survey and describe human brain injury from chemicals, that is, chemical encephalopathy, from two sources of data: (1) 269 patients examined in consultation and (2) 14 populations tested after "chance exposure" to environmental chemicals. Both patients and populations were compared statistically to similarly tested unexposed subjects.
2. To examine methods for measuring nervous system dysfunction from chemicals in 269 patients, to contrast and compare their sensitivity and efficiency. The statistical analysis of effects of exposure was adjusted for known and demonstrated influences of age, sex, educational attainment, height, and other factors to help isolate the effects of exposure from other factors.
3. To show that the concepts derived herein may extend beyond chemical brain injury, providing possible causes for dementia and depression, attention deficit disorder, post-traumatic stress, chemical sensitivity, chronic fatigue, and "degenerative brain diseases," which are current epidemics.
4. To help physicians and others share the feelings of and have empathy with these patients, as individuals and as populations. To open the eyes, ears, and minds of the less afflicted to the chemically brain injured.
5. To integrate new information on chemical effects into the previous context of brain damage and to propose coherent interpretations of the information.
6. To review evidence that the human brain is a major target for chemicals, which turn its evolutionary sensitivity to environmental chemical stimuli to vulnerability.
7. To show that precise measurements help to quantify brain impairment.
8. To propose some strategies that may help prevent further brain destruction, for personal and societal application.

THE AUDIENCE

The book is primarily intended for those physicians who are annoyed by patients' unusual symptoms and presentations. Such patients lie outside the "usual diagnoses." Nearly all clinically active physicians see such patients, but people with such problems gravitate to internists, family practitioners, and those physicians working in occupational health, in environmental medicine, in emergency rooms, and as consultants to those doing primary care. However, this book is also intended for the people who suffer from chemical brain injury, and the health workers who are trying to help them. It is meant also for city planners and their regional counterparts; for just as chemically exposed patients have annoying and vexatious problems, so do cities, towns, and neighborhoods, their habitats. Medical solutions to these problems are unlikely, and at this point appear to be impossible; the solutions are social and political. Finally, this book is intended for patients who may find understanding and comfort in the realization that work on their chemical brain disease is under way, which promises to improve our understanding of the brain and its neurophysiology, as well as the epidemiology of its contemporary diseases.

The science & study when & where disease occurs, & how it is transmitted

MESSAGES AND CONCLUSIONS

The book's major messages are:

1. The number, variety, and metric tons of chemicals used per year have increased exponentially in the twentieth century, eclipsing all past usage. An example is chlorine; some 13 million tons are used in the United States every year.
2. An increasing number of chemicals slow and disorder brain function prematurely, imitating aging or accelerating it.
3. Synthetic chemicals are ubiquitous in the world, including its oceans, making direct and unwitting human exposure increasingly probable and practically unavoidable.
4. A test battery for brain function has evolved. Findings in fourteen exposed populations and four nonexposed populations are described.

That only four of thirteen populations studied for comparison to chemically exposed groups had no impairment bodes ill for this nations' brain function (Chapter 15).

Age was found to be the most powerful and important modifier of brain function, as shown by coefficients for age and its quadratic (age squared) in the linear regression models of most tests. The magnitude of the factor of chemical exposure status sometimes equaled or exceeded the age factor. Exposure often interacted with age and other factors, including gender, educational attainment (school grade completed), and race. Less often, urban vs. rural class, income level, occupational and other specific exposures (such as pesticide use), and affective (emotional) status were important. Educational attainment in years of school completed (ed level) was the practical surrogate for intellectual endowment, and thus was an important predictor of both cognitive "fluid" performance tests and long-term memory and verbal skills.

Major conclusions about chemicals are:

1. Chemicals permeate modern life.
2. Airborne chemicals have been the major source of chemical exposure in the twentieth century.
3. Home, residential, and neighborhood exposures are by airborne, downwind, or concentrically spread chemicals. (Workplaces are relatively less important as sources of exposure.)
4. The lung is the major entry organ for chemicals.
5. Inhaled gases that are irritant and deadly, such as hydrogen sulfide, chlorine, and hydrochloric acid, damage the brain.
6. Pesticides absorbed by inhalation, which kill insects by harming their brains, also damage the brains of larger species, including humans. These substances include arsenic, chlordane (chlorinated cyclodienes), organophosphates, and synthetic pyrethrins.
7. Trichloroethylene (TCE) and toluene, nearly ubiquitous solvents, cause general brain impairment; and TCE also causes specific blink dysfunction (via the trigeminal nerve-pons-facial nerve).

The key conclusions of our investigations are:

- Many chemicals impair brain function.
- The pattern of functional loss resembles accelerated aging.

2

Neurobehavioral Effects and Exposure Epidemiology

CHOOSING PARADIGMS TO RELATE EFFECTS TO CHEMICAL EXPOSURE

Physicians solve problems of human disease by fitting a patient's symptoms, physical signs, and laboratory abnormalities to the template of a known disease or disorder. Such differential diagnosis is a pattern-fitting problem and depends on a hierarchy of similarities and differences. This procedure was perfected largely with the infectious illnesses, those due to living agents. But it also worked for diseases of unknown etiology and for the classic poisons—lead, mercury, and arsenic—and for microbial, plant, and animal toxins.

Except for acute infectious diseases and trauma, health problems frequently come to light after months, years, or decades of incubation or latency. Asbestosis, mesothelioma, and lung cancer are good examples of diseases with long latencies, which are recognized decades after asbestos exposure. Leukemia and lymphoma due to benzene exposure have shorter latent periods (5–7 years). One difficulty in attributing cause when latent periods are long (lasting for years) is that by the time a disease is recognized, exposure conditions and opportunities for their measurement have changed or even disappeared. Modification of industrial processing operations may have occurred a decade or more after exposure; or there may have been changes in raw materials, intermediates, and end products. Often economic forces, such as markets, labor costs, prices of raw materials, foreign exchange rates, and governmental regulations, are responsible for processing changes.

Public health and environmental agencies tend to be ''exposure-driven''; they usually start with exposure in investigating human health hazards, in contrast to physicians, who are disease-oriented. Unfortunately, one reason for this is that statutes and rules enforced by the Occupational Safety and Health Administration of the Labor Department or by the U.S. Environmental Protection Agency and complementary state agencies focus on chemical agents and established ''permissible exposure limits.'' In this

TABLE 2.1 Hierarchy of exposure data or surrogates (Environ Epi)*

Types of Data	Approximation to Actual Exposure
1. Quantified personal measurements of dose	Best
2. Quantified area or ambient measurements in the vicinity of the residence or other sites of activity	|
3. Quantified surrogates of exposure (e.g., estimates of drinking water use)	|
4. Distance from site and duration of residence	|
5. Distance or duration of residence	|
6. Residence or employment in geographic area in reasonable proximity to site where exposure can be assumed	|
7. Residence or employment in defined geographic area (e.g., a county) of the site	Poorest

* Caveat: Effects are manifest in a human population whose members have a wide range of sensitivity, which may be one or more orders of magnitude.

paradigm, effects on highly sensitive humans, functioning like the canaries in coal mines, are examined only *after* evaluation of the exposure evidence. For ongoing exposures, as in standard industrial operations, this approach works. However, it frequently cannot be applied to environmental exposures, which vary even more than those of intermediate variability, such as construction site exposures. Furthermore, following this traditional approach does away with the obligation to define the human hazard if the exposure cannot be measured because it is history, a convenient administrative escape from the problem.

Many real-world health problems have resulted from past exposures that were not measured at the time of exposure, cannot be measured now, and are not easily modeled (Table 2.1). For example, air concentrations (fiber counts) of asbestos are rarely measurable when asbestosis is diagnosed 20 or more years after exposure. Conditions have changed greatly in shipbuilding and construction, where, even before asbestos use was prohibited, exposures were highly variable and difficult to sample or duplicate. Doses of chemicals have not been measured in eco-disasters from Minamata Bay to Chernobyl and Bhopal. Rapid response measurements, though possible, are exceptional. Under the best of circumstances, relevant measurements are rare, are often accidental, and incompletely characterize individuals within the population. Furthermore, estimates of dose based on the available data must rely on only a few measurements of chemical residues sampled from soil or water. Historical reconstructions of the nature and the concentration of these chemicals fail because of missing data; so dose estimates are usually no better than guesses. They are not improved by additional refining, simply because the data are seriously flawed. This situation undermines and often defeats the traditional approach. A strategy of characterizing exposure first prevents progress in problem solving. The resulting delays, often endless, are victories for the polluter and scuttle the process. If there have been no measurements, an endless pursuit of the impossible ensues.

Fortunately, there is another way. It is more fruitful to study health effects first, rather than exposure, and to measure or model exposures only if adverse effects are shown. One begins with the widely accepted assumption that human health problems have causes. The next logical assumption is that the brain is the most sensitive target of harmful agents, developed as it is for environmental sensing, making associations via

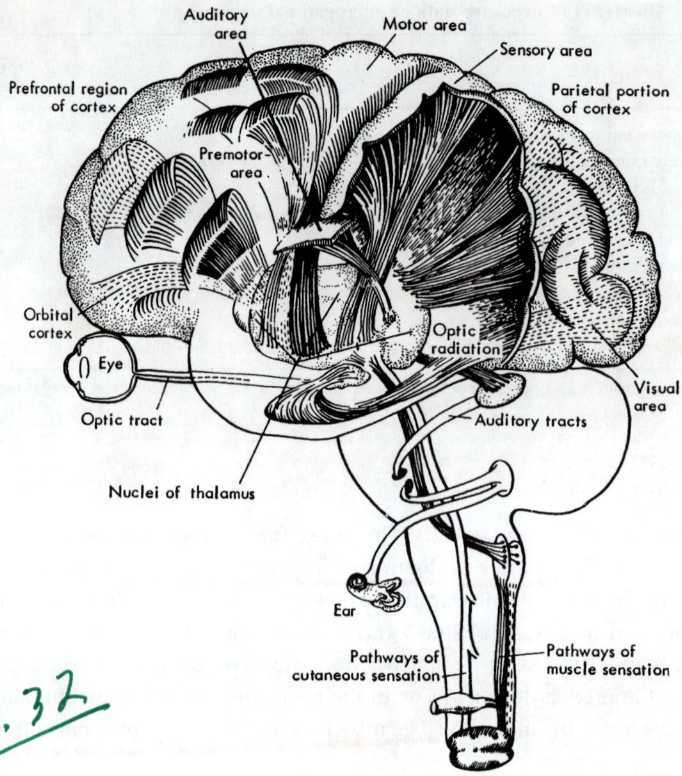

FIGURE 2.1. A human brain is portrayed with the major cortical zones. The eye's visual receptors radiate to the occipital cortex; likewise the ear to the auditory area of the temporal lobe, and the cutaneous and muscle sensation to areas of the parietal cortex. (Adapted from J.W. Papez, A proposed mechanism of emotion, *Arch Neurol Psychiat,* 1937;38:725–743.)

memory, and decision making (Figure 2.1). Our investigations indicate that performance impairments, symptoms, and disturbed mood states such as depression, confusion, and anxiety are probably caused by chemicals from our *chemical world.* For the central nervous system, the performances measured are balance, reaction time, vision, hearing, odor perception, and so on. Furthermore, chemicals that cause CNS effects may act on the lung, liver, immune system, kidney, bone marrow, and other organs as well.

Until recently, reports of adverse effects from chemicals have focused on cancer, birth defects, or excessive numbers of many irritative and nervous system symptoms, not on disorders of the brain or of multiple systems controlled by the brain. However, disorders of the human brain and the central nervous system, including mood status or affective functions, are the most disconcerting ones and impair essential brain-governed functions. Most investigators (1–6) have analyzed symptoms from the populations surrounding or downwind of oil refineries or chemical manufacturing, Superfund, abandoned, or ghost sites. Frequent symptoms include excessive fatigue, headache, dizziness and disorders of balance, and diminished recent and sometimes long-term memory. Less common are difficulty in concentrating, sleep disorders, irritability, shifts of mood, nausea, indigestion, bloating, intolerance to alcohol, and loss of sexual interest (1–6). As seen in Chapters 4 through 14 of this book, high symptom frequencies in populations should be considered as distress signals analogous to an individual's fever, rapid pulse, and rapid breathing.

These complaints do not disappear by labeling them as annoyances (1); attributing them to excessive environmental concerns, worry, or “outrage” (2–5); or regarding them as stress-related illnesses triggered by odors (5). Investigators who have simply interviewed people with complaints who live around malodorous industrial plants, oil refineries, and waste dumps have coined the phrase “environmental worry” to excuse the residents' concerns. This is done by using answers to questions about concerns such as odor to discount, that is, “correct,” the prevalences of other symptoms. Thus, a neighborhood's concern for exposure from chemicals “adjusts” the symptom prevalences downward and “factors away” disorder-signaling symptoms. Focusing on distress associated with odors has even led to “corrections” of other symptoms for odor perception or sensitivity. “Crowd disease” or epidemic hysteria is a similar apologetic construct, developed from occupational and tight building investigations, used to explain adverse symptoms associated with odors (6). “Mass psychogenic illness” (7) is another ingenious construct invoked to explain responses to chemicals such as hydrogen sulfide (8, 9). Such exercises in apologetics contrast sharply with the direct approach, which is objective testing of neurobehavioral functions.

These ingenious apologies are similar to the four so-called diagnostic myths applied to pain—myths that also are used to explain the symptoms in subjects exposed to chemicals: (1) continual pain (distress) after multiple surgical (societal) procedures is either psychogenic or an undesirable side effect; (2) a high analgesic (medication) intake is for addiction not pain; (3) a lawsuit combined with undiagnosable pain (problems) is a psychogenic action; and (4) negative findings in repeated tests combined with bizarre complaints signal a psychogenic origin (10).

Investigators of the vexatious problems arising from exposure to toxic environmental chemicals regard them as difficult, unimportant, unknowable, or psychiatric. Perhaps this is so because the problems are outside their professional comfort zone. Furthermore, it has been nearly impossible to bury the archaic notion that psychiatric illnesses are “functional,” with fundamentally different causes from those of organic illness. This idea is illogical because emotional and behavioral symptoms are mediated by the central nervous system, which is the common pathway for many different pathological processes due to diverse causes. The point here is that a clean admission of uncertainty or of ignorance stimulates problem solving, whereas mislabeling problems with untestable constructs such as psychiatric disorders, “odor-worry-symptoms,” and “environmental worry” impairs it. These prejudicial and adversarial labels suggest lack of empathy, artful deception, or arrogant cleverness.

The effects of environmental chemical exposure are most inexpensively sampled by measuring complaint frequencies and profile of mood states (POMS) scores. In our investigations, high symptom frequencies and high POMS scores were strongly associated in chemically exposed populations with impaired function (11–14) (Chapters 4–14). Both complaint frequencies and POMS scores were low in unexposed populations, in which objective testing was also normal. Additional comparisons, which we strongly recommend, should verify that a symptom frequencies questionnaire and a POMS score can provide quick and economical initial evaluations. If not, then testing of balance and reaction time may be the screening methods of choice.

Clusters of neoplastic diseases of a few years' latency, such as leukemia and lymphoma (15, 16), and of longer latency (20+ years), such as lung, breast, and bladder cancers, in residents near some chemical sites have aroused community concern just as asbestos-related lung cancers and mesotheliomas worried shipyard and construction workers one or two decades ago. Bladder cancers in western New York State have been attributed to cumulative effects of low doses of trihalomethanes absorbed over protracted periods from chlorinated water supplies (17). Leukemia and bladder cancer were associated with tetrachloroethylene leaching from water pipe lining materials in northern Cape Cod, Massachusetts (18), causing cumulative low-dose residential exposures. Many occupational and environmental cancers (19, 20) were observed earlier, the first by London surgeon Percevil Pott, who found scrotal cancer in chimney sweeps 200 years ago. Late in the nineteenth century bladder cancers were seen in aniline dye workers, and lung cancers developed in radon-exposed miners; and into the twentieth century hepatic angiosarcomas were found in vinyl chloride workers, and kidney and brain tumors occurred in excess in plastics and rubber workers. Also in the twentieth century, many other examples have been added to this list. Identifying environmental chemical hazards by causation of cancer is relatively slow and laborious, even for sentinel tumors such as mesothelioma. Large numbers of patients must be studied because of a low incidence of deaths from specific cancers. The greatest difficulty has been thought to lie in the time offsets, which make hazard identification from cancer nearly useless for warning residents, concerned citizens, investigators, or regulators soon enough for them to intervene in exposed communities. Interactions of multiple chemicals in causing common cancers may be even more vexing.

Clusters of birth defects concern, and even frighten, the public more than cancer. Ideas that birth defects may be due to environmental exposures to chemicals also have increasingly troubled investigators. Analyses have ranged from the speculations of Richard Doll's (21) classic paper ''Hazards of the first nine months: an epidemiologist's nightmare'' through Roberts and Lowe (22), who were properly inclusive in asking ''Where have all the conceptions gone?'' Lauren Saxen's essay from Finland (23) concluded that obtaining reliable data on pregnancy and its outcome is nearly impossible, even in Finland with its excellent social records, unless they are collected prospectively. Although prospective studies are clearly superior to them (24–26), historical and retrospective studies showed cardiovascular and renal birth defects in excess at Woburn, Massachusetts (27) and Tucson, Arizona (28), where trichloroethylene from industrial operations contaminated groundwater at concentrations over the EPA action level of 5 ppb.

Other systems besides the reproductive organs respond to environmental chemicals. Chemically induced disorders of porphyrin metabolism, enhanced by sunlight, cause the phototrophic skin disorders. The lung responds to sulfur dioxide, nitrogen oxides, phosgene, chlorine, cigarette smoke, asbestos, cotton dust, ammonia, diisocyanates, and a long list of natural and synthetic chemicals with obstruction of small airways with mucus and cellular infiltrations, and then by necrosis and fibrosis. These changes in small airways cause oppressive chest tightness, wheezing and shortness of breath, and asthma. The cardiovascular system is less well studied than the lung, but trinitrotoluene (TNT), carbon monoxide, carbon disulfide, and 1,1,1-trichloroethane and trichloroethylene cause arrhythmias and sudden death (29, 30). Similarly the renal system is adversely affected by lead, cadmium, phenacetin and other analgesic drugs, and solvents.

Brain effects start with the first cranial nerve. Anosmia and hyposmia have been attributed to cadmium (31) and parosmia and cacosmia to solvents (32). Controversy surrounds human perception of odor, which is a key finding at many toxic sites and is accompanied by a high frequency of varied symptoms (33). Odor also appears to trigger

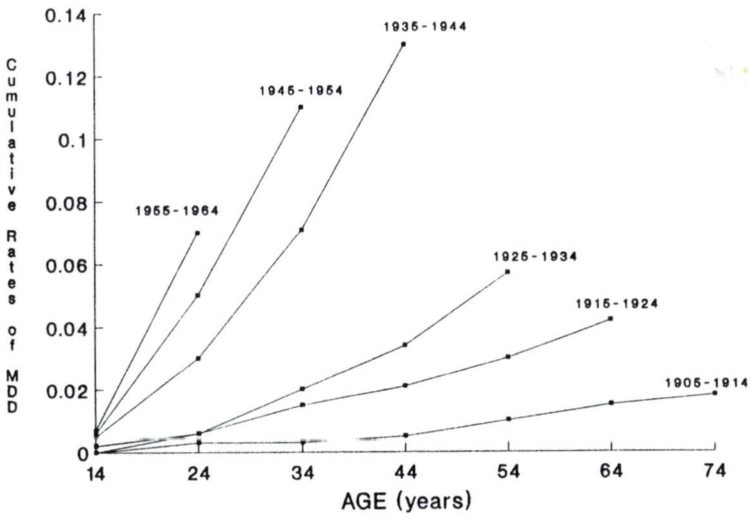

FIGURE 2.2. The rates as percentage for major depressive disease (MDD) as lifetime prevalences are graphed for the five Epidemiology Catchment Areas (ECA) of New Haven, Baltimore, St. Louis, Durham, and Los Angeles collectively by decades for birth cohorts (whites only). The rate of increase for subjects born in the twentieth century's first 50 years is rising steeply without overlap. (From M.M. Weissman and G.L. Klerman, Depression: current understanding and changing trends. With permission from the *Annual Review of Public Health.* Copyright © 1992 by Annual Reviews Inc.)

limbic kindling (34) although some investigators consider this to be odor-behavioral sensitization—an odor–worry–stress process that is trivial (6).

It is the thesis of this book that the brain and the central nervous system, including the affective or emotional centers, such as those manifesting major depression (Figure 2.2) and progressive degenerative dementia (Figure 2.3), are targets for chemicals. Thus, brain cell death, as neuron loss (Figure 2.4), reduces function, an effect that in some circles is interpreted as an epidemic of Alzheimer's disease (Figure 2.5). The limbic system mediates enhanced toxicity for the immune and endocrine systems via the hypothalamus and the pituitary, and these CNS amplifiers are powerful in influencing or controlling other organ systems. CNS defenses now appear to be breached more often and in more ways than was once thought. Thus, single high-dose exposures to hydrogen sulfide, chlorine, or ammonia for only a few seconds (35) or low-dose exposures to hydrogen sulfide (12), trichloroethylene (11), or toluene (13) over many years impair brain function (see Chapters 5, 11, and 12).

Although multi-organ systemic diseases could arise via endocrine or immune end-organ mechanisms coincidentally, it is plausible to consider them orchestrated by signals transmitted through the limbic system to the hypothalamus and the pituitary (34, 36). Thus in some patients chemicals acting primarily on the brain will disorder cardiovascular control and regulation of muscle response and breathing to cause physical deconditioning. "Total body" pain is a frequent symptom in some patients. Chemicals disrupt sexual function, altering control of the limbic system's reproductive and maternal and husbandry functions (as demonstrated in animals). Chemicals also cause thyroid and adrenal hypofunction through the hypothalamic–pituitary axis (36).

A number of individuals exposed to chemicals have developed progressive multi-system dysfunction with: pain; impaired balance, vision, and performance; defective

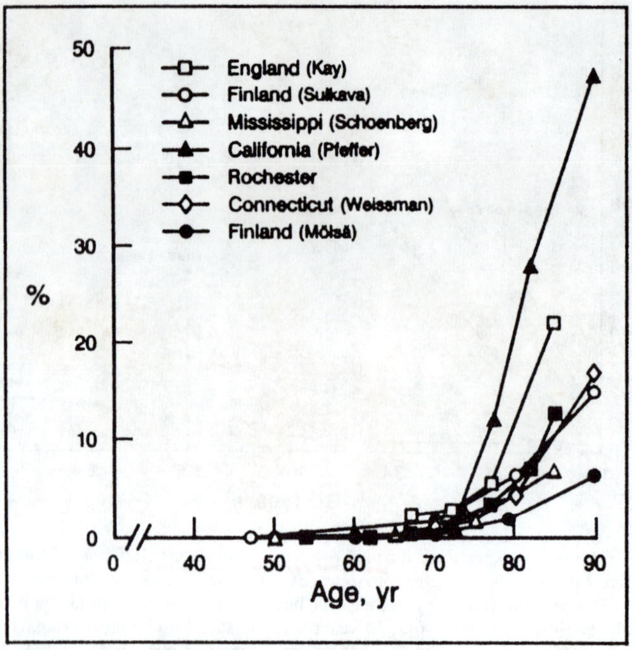

FIGURE 2.3. The age-specific rate of dementia (primary progressive degenerative) rises rapidly after age 70 in all seven cohorts studied but most rapidly in California and in England. (From E. Kokmen et al., Prevalence of medically diagnosed dementia in a defined United States population: Rochester, MN, January 1, 1975, *Neurology,* 1989;39:773–776. Copyright © 1989 American Academy of Neurology.)

cardiovascular and blood pressure regulation with orthostatic hypotension and exercise deconditioning; impotency and failure of erection; immune dysfunction, both cellular and humoral; and endocrine deficits, especially of the thyroid and the pancreas. Detailed descriptions of these patients are a complex undertaking that is beyond the scope of this book.

ENVIRONMENTAL TOXICOLOGY

Useful Generalizations

First, adverse human health effects frequently have long latent periods; so the effects of exposure may need to cumulate for years for investigators to detect impairments.

Second, such periods have implicit problems for researchers measuring exposure doses of chemicals. Monitoring has rarely been in place in such exposure, but even so doses are moving targets. Their evaluation depends on methods of detection used, rates of chemical exposure (involving such factors as chemical purity, mixing, containment, and leakage), and ecologic factors (wind direction and velocity, heat, humidity and water drainage, aquifers, soil porosity, distance to bedrock, etc.).

Third, rarely can environmental chemical exposures be characterized by historical reconstruction or modeling. Relatively precise or realistic time sequences have been much more difficult to reconstruct historically in these cases than for occupational exposures such as exposure to asbestos fibers (37).

Fourth, more than a decade of attempts to characterize the human health risk from

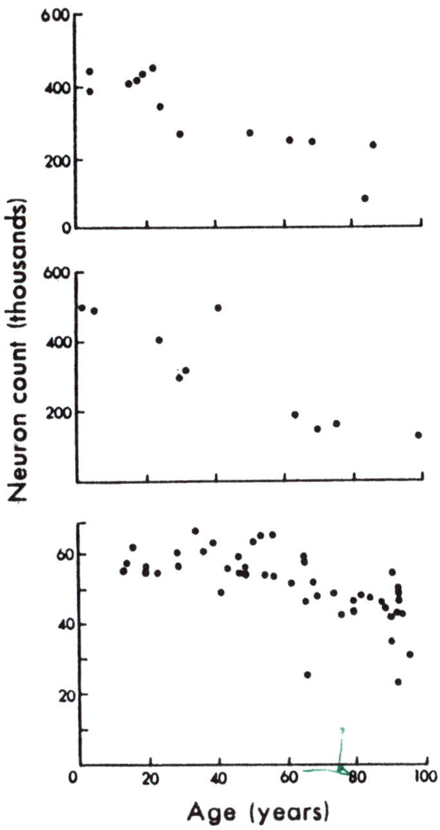

FIGURE 2.4. Falling numbers of neurons with age, counted in fixed human brain preparations from substantia nigra (top), medial basal forebrain (middle), and motor neuron area of lumbosacral spinal cord (bottom). (From K. Brizzee, On aging of the brain, in *Neurobiology of Aging,* Plenum Publishing Corporation, 1975. With permission.)

chemicals at manufacturing or waste dump sites show that contemporary air, water, and soil measurements are related imperfectly, if at all, to conditions of human exposure. Modeling using numerous assumptions has limited use.

Fifth, although limited models do exist, their ability to predict human risk is largely untested. A first step would be to correlate the dose estimates with adverse health effects. End-points or outcome effect measurements have a hierarchy of sensitivity. Questionnaires asking patients to remember previously diagnosed or characterized clinical, medical, and neurological disorders are not only insensitive but biased by impaired recall due to aging, educational level, acculturation, and intelligence. Current symptoms are more reliable than memories but may not match defined illnesses. To avoid these limitations, investigators focus on current symptoms in the following way. Both published and anecdotal experience indicates three groups of symptoms in subjects with environmental chemical exposures: (1) The respiratory group includes: dryness and irritation of eye, nose, and throat; reduced sense of smell; cough, chest tightness, burning or chest pain, shortness of breath, and palpitations. (2) The central nervous system group includes: headache, unsteadiness or dizziness, difficulty in concentrating, easy distraction, memory loss, emotional liability, unstable moods, sleep disturbances, in-

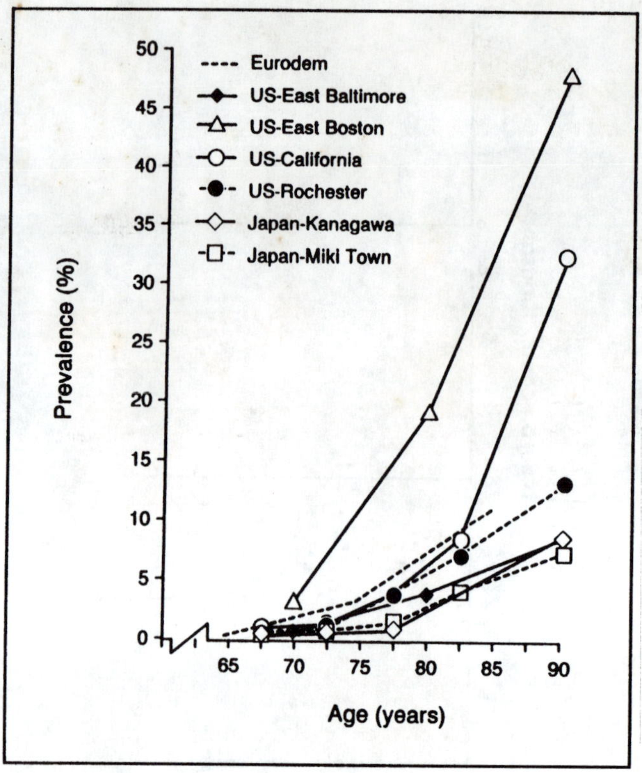

FIGURE 2.5. The age-specific prevalence rates for Alzheimer's disease are similar across seven studies in Europe, Asia, and the United States. The higher rates (earlier onsets) in Boston and California are attributed to retirement village sites but raise questions. (From M.M. Breteler et al., Epidemiology of Alzheimer's disease, *Epidemiol Rev* 1992;14:59–82. With permission from Johns Hopkins University School of Hygiene and Public Health.)

somnia, and somnolence. (3) The vegetative group encompasses: indigestion, nausea, decreased appetite, bloating, decreased sex drive, decreased alcohol tolerance, and fatigue.

Accompanying these symptoms are perceived clusters of birth defects or cancer, including leukemia and lymphoma, in the residential area. High prevalence populations, confirmed by epidemiologic studies showing such results as birth defects in Tucson (28) and leukemia at Woburn (38, 39), frequently show additional health disturbances, from respiratory infections to excessive systemic lupus erythematosus or scleroderma. These observations led our investigators to the conclusion that chemical effects in a population are rarely localized to one organ system. The human brain, with its mood or emotional sector, blink reflex (40), and balance, reaction time, and other cognitive-psychomotor functions and visual fields (41), has emerged as a major chemical target and thus an area for investigation.

Why do dose–response estimates based on occupational groups not apply to the general population? This question has teased and perplexed occupational and environmental physicians and epidemiologists alike. It is helpful to recount the differences between occupational and environmental groups. Environmentally exposed groups are subjects ''chosen at random'' from the general population with the full range of human

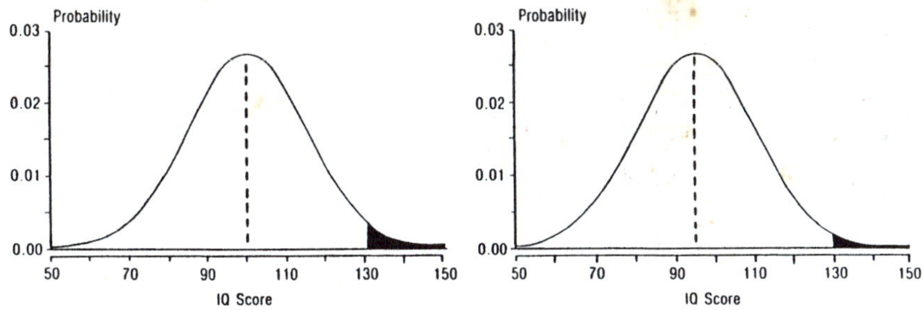

A Distributions of intelligence test scores. Left: standardized mean 100; standard deviation 15. Right: mean 95.

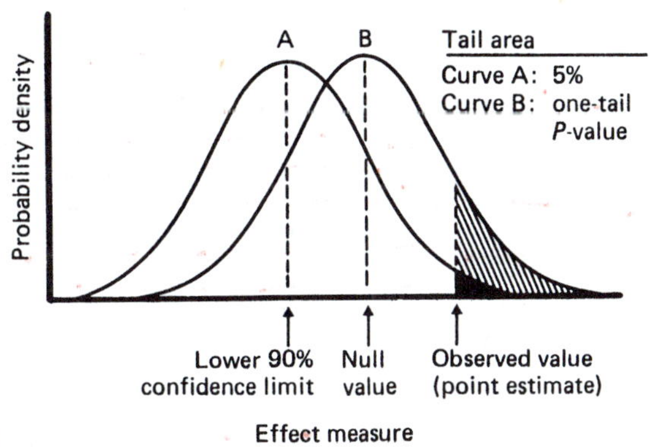

B

FIGURES 2.6.a and 2.6.b Compare the symmetrical distribution of intelligence as a standardized average with a mean of 100 on the left to that produced by shifting the mean 5 points to the left (Figure 2.6a). If there were 2.3 million subjects originally above IQ 130, the shift of mean to 95 would reduce the number to 1 million, a reduction of 1.3 million. This illustrates the major social problem originally envisioned for lead exposure. Other neurotoxic chemicals would have similar distributions of effect. Such examples help us to visualize how an environmentally exposed population's sensitivity to adverse chemicals is distributed across a wide range, compared to occupational groups who have been preselected for lack of sensitivity and then attenuated by dropout to accentuate resistance to adverse effects. Figure 2.6b overlays standard distribution curves so that they overlap, making obvious the magnitude of the effect on brain function in a population, that is normally distributed. (Modified from B. Weiss, Neurobehavioral toxicity as a basis for risk assessment, *Trends Pharm Sci* 1988;9:59–62.)

sensitivity (Figure 2.6a,b). In contrast, most workers are healthy "survivors," who have endured exposures that eliminated their sensitive or reactive colleagues who left work and so escaped study. This was well illustrated during studies of the cotton dust disease, byssinosis. In North Carolina in 1970, not a single worker in ten cotton textile mills had asthma. The clear implication was that cotton dust triggered asthma, and as asthmatics could not endure the exposure, they left employment early, often on their first day. Currently, the mills have effective means of dust control, and asthmatic workers are working safely in them. This model may apply to chemically exposed workers and to symptoms in other organ systems. Workers who develop unpleasant or distressful symptoms tend to self-select out of further exposure. Continuing this logic, after those subjects in the sensitive and reactive "tail" remove themselves from the Gaussian distribution curve, the dose needed for an average effect will be greater by a few percent to an order of magnitude, depending on the portion of the original dose–response curve that remains (42).

Transportation

Hauling of hazardous chemicals by water, rail, and highway spreads risk to the general population, police, and fire fighters, as well as to transport workers. Members of the public who live near transport links, particularly interstate highways, are at risk, as are dwellers in trailer and mobile home parks. One and one-half billion tons of hazardous material traveled 784 billion miles in 1982 (43). Only 2,400 substances are classified as hazardous by the Code of Federal Regulations, but more than 60,000 other chemicals await review for possible inclusion in the list. Trucks haul half of all hazardous material, mostly petroleum products and chemicals. Rails carry 73 million tons of hazardous material per year, and coastal and inland waterways 549 million tons per year.

Transport-related chemical exposures occur almost daily; the following four examples illustrate their potential for mischief. In 1992, a spill of metham sodium (a soil fumigant and pesticide) above Dunsmuir, California sterilized the Shasta River and poisoned neighbors and cleanup workers. A trainload of butyl alcohol and vinyl chloride derailed near Austin, Texas in 1987, and three tank cars caught fire, forcing the evacuation of 5,000 residents. The derailment of 43 railroad tank cars at Livingston, Louisiana in 1982 spilled phosphoric acid, perchloroethylene, and hydrofluorosilicic acid, and burned vinyl chloride monomer, styrene monomer, plastic pellets, and lubricating oil. Also, a car containing tetraethyl lead exploded, and carloads of toluene diisocyanate and sodium hydroxide leaked. This particular wreck illustrated that chemicals with the potential for explosive combination, vaporization, and incineration may be sharing a train, ready to combine during a wreck. CNS and multiple-organ system disorders and deaths occurred in the emergency response team, in drivers of cleanup trucks, and among the neighbors of the derailment site. In April 1996, a derailed train spilled tank car loads of chlorine and potassium cresylate (phenolic acid) near Alberton, Montana, creating on scene a green cloud of chlorine that burned pine needles and the lungs of people, dogs, and horses. Thereafter polychlorinated phenols produced at the site persisted to render the town noxious and uninhabitable for months (see Chapter 6).

EPIDEMIOLOGY

A major impediment to studying the effects of chemicals on the human brain is that conducting scientific experiments involving exposure of human subjects to known or suspected toxins is unthinkable and unethical. Only ignorant chance has a ''license'' to conduct human exposures, which are labeled ''accidents.'' After adverse health effects are known or strongly suspected, it is not ethical to expose human subjects to harmful agents deliberately. A society's moral prohibition of planned experiments means that chance ''experiments'' must be studied diligently and understood. Opportunistic observations of such ''unknowing experiments'' have produced valuable information, which will continue to flow from them. Among the limitations of this approach, investigators must study an already selected exposed group of subjects, including the affected and the nonaffected, clients and nonclients in lawsuits, volunteers and community advocates. Frequently, people are willing to participate in these studies because they have complaints. Those who are uninterested or unmotivated, perhaps including some individuals who are not seriously affected or are undamaged, are almost impossible to study, even when financial incentives are offered to them (please see in Chapter 11 that exposed nonclients did not differ from exposed clients). Differences of age, sex, educational attainment, income, and some relatively unimportant factors subdivide the original categories further. The investigators' freedom is further limited by a virtual absence of public funds, so that the cohort design must focus on those individuals most likely to be abnormal, vocal clients, complainers, and the immediate downwind neighbors of the site, rather than on choices made from a classic sampling matrix. Some of these factors simply call for maintaining a proper perspective; they do not preclude obtaining reliable information.

Studying "worst cases" first is economical; and if other causes of impairment than the chemical and/or the site in question can be excluded, a crucial distinction has been made. Usually greater care can be exercised in the selection of "unexposed" groups compared to exposed subjects, by focusing on the absence of exposure to the index chemical and to major confounders and sometimes even on random nomination. Nevertheless, it is axiomatic that all groups, both exposed and unexposed, must be *volunteers*. This restriction is not avoidable in a free society; so it cannot be a legitimate criticism of the design. Potential unexposed subjects are recruited from census tracts or voter registration lists, from membership rolls in churches, unions, or lodges, or from their children's schools, which act as contact or access sites. In the absence of any coercion beyond that tolerated in most contemporary societies, all participants will be volunteers; all are ultimately self-appointed. However, the forces modifying their status may differ, including monetary rewards. Unexposed subjects are generally paid to participate, whereas clients in lawsuits look to future compensation for damages.

Longitudinal comparisons are rarely possible; ideally, each subject serves as his or her own (prior to exposure) control, and many uncertainties of the comparisons are eliminated. This situation is rarely attainable, so groups must be heterogeneous and large enough that distributions of age and educational level are similar and gender ratios equal. Adjustments for differences in age and education depend upon prediction equations (see Chapter 3). The time courses of impairments after exposure could be defined by multiple tests and evaluations separated by suitable time intervals, but this approach is rarely possible. Furthermore, the possible bias induced by familiarity and/or learning on test reliability and reproducibility appears insignificant but needs to be assessed. Periodic retesting is mandated for members of occupational groups exposed to hazardous materials, such as fire fighters, chemical spill cleanup teams, and workers in the chemical industry. In such evaluations, three comparisons of test results across time intervals showed stable performance over intervals of a year or less in verbal recall or visual reproduction and in constructional tasks such as block design (44–46).

Cross-sectional studies of exposed groups and local unexposed groups that were cohort-matched provided our investigators with several unexposed and thus referent populations (12, 13, 44, 46–47) with nearly identical test results. This encouraged their combination into a nationally representative unexposed group to define the U.S. population's test performance when unexposed to chemicals. Prediction equations were modeled for these tests, which confirmed the "unexposed status" of subsequent unexposed groups and facilitated decisions about the abnormality of new "exposed" groups in pilot studies. Age was the most important independent variable, and educational level adjusted to a large measure for aptitude or native ability. Most of the other potential confounding factors either "averaged out" or did not influence regression models, as their coefficients were insignificant.

Having greatly elevated mood scores (self-assessed by the profile of mood states) as an independent variable was highly correlated with other abnormalities but was not predictive of performance on any test in regression models; so a group's elevated POMS scores, although correlated with abnormality overall, did not mean that the subjects with the most elevated scores were the most impaired.

The key steps in the epidemiological design are to match the cohorts, collect data about possible confounding factors, and compare performance for the groups. Making adjustments for the effects of age and/or educational level was an appropriate strategy even when matching was close; and covariance analysis, which adjusted for sex, ethnicity, and urban–rural differences, was useful.

Performance on so-called overlearned tasks, such as information, picture completion and similarities from the WAIS, and vocabulary tests, provides a reasonable picture of premorbid (pre-exposure) ability, which like educational attainment is related to intelligence or aptitude; and it confirms the similarity of exposed groups to unexposed groups prior to or in the absence of exposure (48, 49). Observations have confirmed in exposed subjects that the educational level coefficients of overlearned tests are larger than are those for scores on block design performance, digit symbol, and Culture Fair (a test resembling Raven's matrices using visual designs). The premorbid mental performance status can be approximated successfully for comparisons of groups. Scores on constructional and visualization tasks are reduced more by the effects of chemical exposure than is overlearned cultural memory, as evaluated by Wechsler's WAIS subtest of information, picture completion, similarities tasks, and vocabulary scores (13). These tasks ''resist'' chemical damage, and subjects' or patients' scores thus show that they approximate their pre-exposure level of performance.

References

1. Deane M and Sanders G: Annoyance and health reactions to odor from refineries and other industries in Carson, California 1972. *Environ Res* 1978;15:119–132.
2. Neutra RR: Epidemiology for and with a distrustful community. *Environ Health Perspect* 1985;62:393–397.
3. Mendell MJ: Interpretation of self-reported symptom data in settings with likely over-reporting due to environmental worry. *Arch Environ Health* 1991;46:124.
4. Neutra R, Lipscomb JA, Satin KP, and Shusterman D: Factors that might contribute to higher symptom rates sometimes observed around hazardous waste sites. *Arch Environ Health* 1991;46:120.
5. Shusterman D, Lipscomb J, Neutra R, and Satin K: Symptom prevalence and odor–worry interaction near hazardous waste sites. *Arch Environ Health* 1991;46:119.
6. Shusterman D, Lipscomb J, Neutra R, and Satin K: Symptom prevalence and odor–worry interaction near hazardous waste sites. *Environ Health Perspect* 1991;94:25–30.
7. Kerckhoff AC: Analyzing a case of mass psychogenic illness. In: *Mass Psychogenic Illness: A Social Analysis,* MJ Colligan, JN Pennebaker, and LR Murphy (eds.). Hillsdale, NJ: Lawrence Erlbaum Assoc., 1982.
8. Modan B, Swartz TA, Tirosh M, Costin C, Weissenberg E, et al.: The Arjenyattah epidemic a mass phenomenon: spread and triggering factors. *Lancet* 1983;2:1472–1474.
9. Landrigan PJ and Miller B: The Arjenyattah epidemic: home interview data and toxicological aspects. *Lancet* 1983;2:1474–1476.
10. Pincus JH and Tucker GJ: *Behavioral Neurology* (3rd ed.). Oxford: Oxford University Press, 1985, pp. 287–314.
11. Kilburn KH and Warshaw RH: Effects on neurobehavioral performance of chronic exposure to chemically contaminated well water. *Intl J Toxicol Indust Health* 1993;9:391–404.
12. Kilburn KH and Warshaw RH: Neurobehavioral impairment downwind from a petroleum refinery with a desulfurization unit: low dose hydrogen sulfide exposure. *Toxicol Indust Health* 1995;11:185–197.

13. Kilburn KH and Warshaw RH: Neurotoxic effects from residential exposure to chemicals from an oil reprocessing facility and Superfund site. *Neurotox Teratol* 1995;17:89–102.
14. Kilburn KH and Warshaw RH: Neurobehavioral testing of subjects exposed residentially to ground water contaminated from an aluminum die-casting plant and local referents. *J Toxicol Environ Health* 1993;39:483–496.
15. Linos A, Blair A, Gibson R, Everett G, Van Leer S, et al.: Leukemia and non-Hodgkin's lymphoma and residential proximity to industrial plants. *Arch Environ Health* 1991;46: 70–74.
16. Shore DL, Sandler DP, Davey FR, McIntyre OR, and Bloomfield CD: Acute leukemia and residential proximity to potential sources of environmental pollutants. *Arch Environ Health* 1993;48:414–420.
17. Vena JE, Graham S, Freudenheim J, Marshall J, Zielezny M, et al.: Drinking water, fluid intake and bladder cancer in western New York. *Arch Environ Health* 1993;48:191–198.
18. Aschengrau A, Ozonoff D, Paulo C, Coogan P, Vezina R, et al.: Cancer risk and perchloroethylene (PCE) contaminated drinking water in Massachusetts. *Arch Environ Health* 1993; 48:284–292.
19. Hunter D: *The Diseases of Occupations* (4th ed.). Boston: Little, Brown and Company, 1969, pp. 812–835.
20. Symons MJ, Andjelkovich DA, Spirtas R, and Herman DR: Brain and central nervous system. In: *Brain Tumors in the Chemical Industry in U.S. Rubber Workers,* IJ Selikoff and TC Hammond (eds.). *Ann NY Acad Sci* 1982;38:146–159.
21. Doll R: Hazards of the first nine months: an epidemiologist's nightmare. *J Irish Med Assoc* 1973;66:117–126.
22. Roberts CJ and Lowe CR: Where have all the conceptions gone? *Lancet* 1975;1:498–499.
23. Saxen L: Population surveillance for birth defects. In: *Birth Defects,* AG Motulsky and W Lenz (eds.). Amsterdam: Excerpta Medica, 1974.
24. McDonald AD: Maternal health in early pregnancy and congenital defects final report on a prospective inquiry. *Brit J Prev Soc Med* 1961;15:154–166.
25. Klemetti A: Relationship of selected environmental factors to pregnancy outcome and congenital malformations. *Annales Pediatriae Fenniae* Suppl. 26, 1966, Vol. 12.
26. Villumsen AL: *Environmental Factors in Congenital Malformations.* Copenhagen: FADL Forlag, 1970.
27. Lagakos SW, Wessen BJ, and Zelen M: An analysis of contaminated well water and health effects in Woburn, Massachusetts. *J Am Stat Assoc* 1986;81:583–596.
28. Goldberg SJ, Lebowitz MD, Graver EJ, and Hicks S: An association of human congenital cardiac malformations and drinking water contaminants. *JACC* 1990;16:155–164.
29. Kobayashi H, Hobara T, Kawamoto T, and Sakai T: Effect of 1,1,1-trichlorethane inhalation on heart rate and its mechanism: a role of autonomic nervous system. *Arch Environ Health* 1987;42:140–143.
30. Jones RD and Winter DP: Two case reports of deaths on industrial premises attributed to 1,1,1-trichloroethane. *Arch Environ Health* 1983;38:59–61.
31. Amoore JE: Effects of chemical exposure on olfaction in humans. In: *Toxicology of the Nasal Passages,* CS Barrow (ed.). New York: Hemisphere Publishing Corp., McGraw-Hill Book Co., 1986, pp. 155–190.
32. Emmett EA: Parosmia and hyposmia induced by solvent exposure. *Brit J Indust Med* 1976; 33:196–198.
33. Neutra R, Lipscomb J, Satin K, and Shusterman D: Hypotheses to explain the higher symptom rates observed around hazardous waste sites. *Environ Health Perspect* 1991;94:31–38.
34. Bell IR, Miller CS, and Schwartz GE: An olfactory-limbic model of multiple chemical sensitivity syndrome: possible relationships to kindling and affective spectrum disorders. *Biol Psychiatry* 1992;32:218–242.
35. Kilburn KH and Warshaw RH: Profound neurobehavioral deficits in an oil field worker exposed to hydrogen sulfide. *Am J Med Sci* 1993;306:301–305.

36. Brodal P: *The Central Nervous System.* Oxford: Oxford University Press, 1992.
37. Kilburn KH and Warshaw RH: Asbestos disease in construction, refinery and shipyard workers. *Ann NY Acad Sci* 1991;643:301–312.
38. Byers VS, Levin AS, Ozonoff DM, and Baldwin RW: Association between clinical symptoms and lymphocyte abnormalities in a population with chronic domestic exposure to industrial solvent-contaminated domestic water supply and a high incidence of leukemia. *Cancer Immunol Immunother* 1988;27:77–81.
39. Ozonoff D, Colten ME, Cupples A, Heeren T, Schatzkin A, et al.: Health problems reported by residents of a neighborhood contaminated by a hazardous waste facility. *Am J Indust Med* 1987;11:581–597.
40. Feldman RG, Chirico-Post J, and Proctor SP: Blink reflex latency after exposure to trichloroethylene in well water. *Arch Environ Health* 1988;43:143–148.
41. Kilburn KH, Warshaw RH, and Hanscom B: Balance measured by head (and trunk) tracking and a force platform in chemically (PCB and TCE) exposed and referent subjects. *Occup Environ Med* 1994;51:381–384.
42. Weiss B: Neurobehavioral toxicity as a basis for risk assessment. *Trends Pharm Sci* 1988; 9:59–62.
43. List G and Abkowitz M: Estimates of current hazardous materials flow patterns. *Transportation Quarterly* 1986;40:483–502.
44. Kilburn KH and Warshaw RH: Neurobehavioral effects of formaldehyde and solvents on histology technicians: repeated testing across time. *Environ Res* 1992;49:714–720.
45. Kilburn KH and Warshaw RH: Neurotoxicity around a Superfund site: failure of distance, direction and length of residence to predict effects. Submitted.
46. Kilburn KH and Warshaw RH: Neurobehavioral impairment in residents near a solvent source in electronics manufacturing. Submitted.
47. Kilburn KH, Warshaw RH, and Shields MG: Neurobehavioral dysfunction in firemen exposed to polychlorinated biphenyls (PCBs): possible improvement after detoxification. *Arch Environ Health* 1989;44:345–350.
48. Ryan CM, Morrow LA, Bromet EJ, and Parkinson DK: Assessment of neuropsychological dysfunction in the workplace: normative data from the Pittsburgh Occupational Exposures test battery. *J Clin Exper Neuropsych* 1987;9:665–679.
49. Ladd CE: WAIS performance of brain damaged and neurotic patients. *J Clin Psychol* 1964; 20:114–121.
50. Papez JW: A proposed mechanism of emotion. *Arch Neurol Psychiat* 1937;38:725–743.
51. Weissman MM and Klerman GL: Depression: current understanding and changing trends. *Annu Rev Publ Health* 1992;13:319–339.
52. Kokmen E, Beard M, Offord KP, and Kurland LT: Prevalence of medically diagnosed dementia in a defined United States population: Rochester, MN, January 1, 1975. *Neurology* 1989;39:773–776.
53. Breteler MM, Claus JJ, van Duijin CM, Launer LJ, and Hofman A: Epidemiology of Alzheimer's disease. *Epidemiol Rev* 1992;14:59–82.

3

Methods for Measuring Neurobehavioral Function: Deriving Prediction Equations for Tests in People Unexposed vs. Those Exposed to Chemicals

INTRODUCTION

The terms aging and senescing are frequently used synonymously although *aging* may imply the attainment of maturity, whereas *senescing* is the sum of deteriorative processes. Age-related postmaturational changes are usually implied in behavior studies, the caveat being that although developmental events and stem cell pools may be of great importance to the outcome, the term aging is used despite having both natural and deteriorative process meanings (1). Aging in the central nervous system is characterized by selective regional neuronal loss, not by global cell loss.

For the nontechnical reader this chapter provides a general understanding of neurobehavioral function measurement, including an example evaluation of balance function, from unexposed subject data and a simultaneous analysis, using covariance methods, of matched unexposed and exposed groups. Both physiological methods and neuropsychological tests are discussed. For those investigators or students who wish to use the prediction equations clinically or epidemiologically for adults or children, the equations are described in a section on data analysis, in a methods manual, and on a disk.

A final section of the chapter provides a perspective on dementia and chemical encephalopathy. The ideal scientific experiment would measure the performance of unexposed subjects, expose them to a chemical, and remeasure their performance. For such designed experiments, large groups of animals or human subjects frequently are needed. For human subjects this ideal approach can be used for therapeutic chemicals, as in controlled clinical drug trials, but even here moral considerations are reinforced by society's mandates that the benefits must outweigh the risks. Deliberate exposure of fellow humans to chemicals considered toxic is unethical; but "bad luck" and mischance in the real world, in what are called "accidents," periodically provide "incidents of chemical exposure." What was learned from such "experiments of nature" is the substance of this book, using measurement methods discussed in this chapter. Opportunities presented themselves for investigators to observe and measure the outcomes of otherwise impossible experiments, salvaging insights for society's benefit. The data and interpretations reviewed in Chapters 4 to 14 are based on comparisons of exposed and unexposed groups that shared many features, ideally differing only by their chemical exposure.

Exposure is examined here in the context of aging. The logic and statistical analyses of the reference or unexposed group, those persons aging without a specific (known) chemical burden, were made from cross-sectional measurements. This evaluation included adjustments for differences in age, educational achievement, sex, race, body size, and strength. The unexposed populations provided the data needed to isolate and quantify the effect of chemical exposure. Exposure status was examined by dose measurements and such surrogates as exposure gradients reflected by distance, direction, and duration.

The best strategy was analysis of covariance, which adjusted for all the above-described factors contributing to differences between groups before attributing effects to chemical exposure. Prediction equations were calculated (regression-based) for each function or test from data gathered on unexposed populations. The equations were tested for potential modifying and confounding factors by using a third unexposed population. Scores on other tests, including the profile of mood states (POMS), were examined as independent variables and rejected. Applying these equations to the exposed group helped isolate the "exposure effect" on each neurobehavioral test for each subject. Each test was considered in detail to create a "standard strategy."

The prediction equation modeling used 408 subjects, 216 females and 192 males, 337 from Wickenburg, Arizona and 71 from Smithfield, Louisiana. The results for adults who completed each test (e.g., balance), ages 18 to 81 (264 subjects, 143 female and 121 male), are described as Group A (see Table 3.1). Twenty-nine adults recruited from San Luis Obispo, California, 17 male and 12 female (Group B), were used to validate the equations (see Table 3.2). Screening by questionnaire excluded from modeling those persons with possibly confounding chemical exposures and medical conditions. The cohort comparison design for exposure effect had 294 exposure zone subjects (EZS) from Phoenix, compared to 161 adult regional unexposed subjects. All were between the ages of 18 and 83 years, and had lived in these areas for 4 to 25 years. The regional unexposed subjects were recruited from voter registration rolls of Wickenburg, Arizona to match Phoenix exposed subjects for sex, age, and years of educational attainment (highest school grade completed). There was no current or historical evidence of chemical contamination of air or of water in Wickenburg. All protocols were approved by the Human Studies Research Committee of the University of Southern California School of Medicine. All subjects gave their written informed consent for the study and were compensated.

Methods used to test subjects are given in the following pages. An appendix to the chapter gives additional information on methods, including reasons why some of the tests were chosen.

PHYSIOLOGICAL METHODS

Reaction Time

Reaction speeds were timed by using a computerized visual stimulus generator for the letter A for the visual choice and the letters A and S for the two-choice test, as previously described (2, 3), from the appearance of the letter to cancellation. Touching the corre-

TABLE 3.1 Descriptive information on populations used in developing prediction equations (Wickenburg and Springfield, 264)

	Mean	Standard Deviation	Minimum	Maximum
		GROUP A		
Age yrs	44.2	19.7	18	83
Educational Level yrs	12.8	2.2	8	24
Height cm	168.4	9.5	135.9	194.3
Weight kg	75.2	17.2	41.0	127.0
Women				
Grip Strength Right	30.7	7.7	9	53
Left	28.8	6.9	12	49
Weight kg	68.4	15.4	41	125
Men				
Grip Strength Right	52.0	10.6	27	83
Left	49.7	10.6	24	82
Weight kg	82.9	15.0	57	127
Simple Reaction Time	269	52	193	442
Choice Reaction Time	531	97	392	736
Sway Speed Balance				
Eyes Open cm/s	0.80	0.20	0.43	1.47
Eyes Closed cm/s	1.27	0.42	0.56	3.54
Blink Reflex Latency R-1 ms				
Glabellar Right	14.5	1.8	10.0	20.0
Left	14.8	1.9	9.2	19.9
Supraorbital Right	13.1	2.1	7.1	18.3
Left	13.1	2.2	6.9	18.6
Color Score Women	136	30	117	314
Men	151	56	117	378
Culture Fair	27.9	7.6	8	44
Digit Symbol	54.9	13.7	24	90
Vocabulary	23.6	8.5	4	46
Block Design	30.4	9.5	7	51
Verbal Recall	21.9	6.2	5	39
Information	17.8	5.6	4	29
Picture Completion	15.1	2.8	4	20
Similarities	20.4	4.9	6	28
Pegboard Women	72.1	19.9	48	148
Men	79.4	24.4	50	180
Trail Making A	28.5	7.8	18	54
Trail Making B	72.8	37.3	37	180

sponding key on an A and S keypad (Neuro-Test Inc., Pasadena, CA) was the endpoint. Subjects were seated comfortably before a 65-cm-tall table with eye-to-screen and eye-to-keypad distances of 55 and 50 cm in a room at 22°C with subdued lighting (Figure 3.1). The computer clock recorded the time from flashing the letter on the screen until it disappeared. Pseudorandom numbers determined the stimulus order for choice (visual and two-choice) reaction time and the latency between succeeding letters, which varied from 3 to 9 seconds. The 0.8-cm-high 14 × 6 cm keypad instrument yields slightly faster measurements than those obtained from an earlier computer keyboard version (2, 3). "Processing time," which was calculated as CRT − SRT for each subject, was also compared to CRT.

One block of 20 trials for simple reaction time (SRT) allowed the subject to have

TABLE 3.2 Descriptive information on population used in testing prediction equations (San Luis Obispo, 29)

	Mean	Standard Deviation	Minimum	Maximum
	GROUP B			
Age yrs	40.2	9.8	20	61
Educational Level yrs	12.6	2.4	5	19
Height cm	67.7	3.4	60	73
Weight kg	79.0	13.3	52.7	101.8
Grip Strength kg				
Women Right	35.8	4.6	29	45
Left	34.0	6.0	20	42
Men Right	62.6	8.5	52	80
Left	59.3	9.3	47	77
Simple Reaction Time	282	62	168	670
Choice Reaction Time	532	91	305	794
Balance Sway Speed sm/s				
Eyes Open (SO)	0.73	0.16	0.50	1.24
Eyes Closed (SC)	1.05	0.23	0.58	1.63
Blink Reflex Latency R-1 ms				
Glabellar Right	13.9	1.8	11.4	16.7
Left	13.7	1.9	11.0	17.5
Supraorbital Right	12.6	1.9	9.6	16.4
Left	13.4	2.0	10.2	16.5
Culture Fair	30.4	6.8	14	41
Digit Symbol	57.4	13.7	22	71
Vocabulary (not done)				
Block Design	30.0	11.6	0	48
Verbal Recall	22.6	4.3	1	15
Information	18.9	6.2	4	27
Picture Completion	14.7	3.2	9	20
Similarities	20.1	5.8	11	28
Pegboard Women	67.1	11.1	55	100
Men	70.8	6.9	61	89
Trail Making A	33.3	11.9	14	81
Trail Making B	76.8	34.3	21	180

13 practice trials, and then the median of the final 7 trials was scored as the SRT for each subject. After a brief rest, three 20-response trials were made for choice reaction time (CRT), and the median of the final 7 responses was determined for each trial. The lowest median of the last 7 responses from the three trials is reported as the natural logarithm (ln). Thus, irrespective of sequence, the fastest median (minimal time) was chosen.

Balance—Speed of Sway

Balance was tested by a computerized head-tracker (Neuro-Test, Inc., Pasadena, CA), which records the horizontal path and speed of movement of a sound source mounted on the head by using two microphones mounted 36 cm apart on the arm of a tripod 35 cm from the head (4) (Figure 3.2). These sway measurements are equivalent to those obtained from a force platform (5). The minimal sway speed of three consecutive

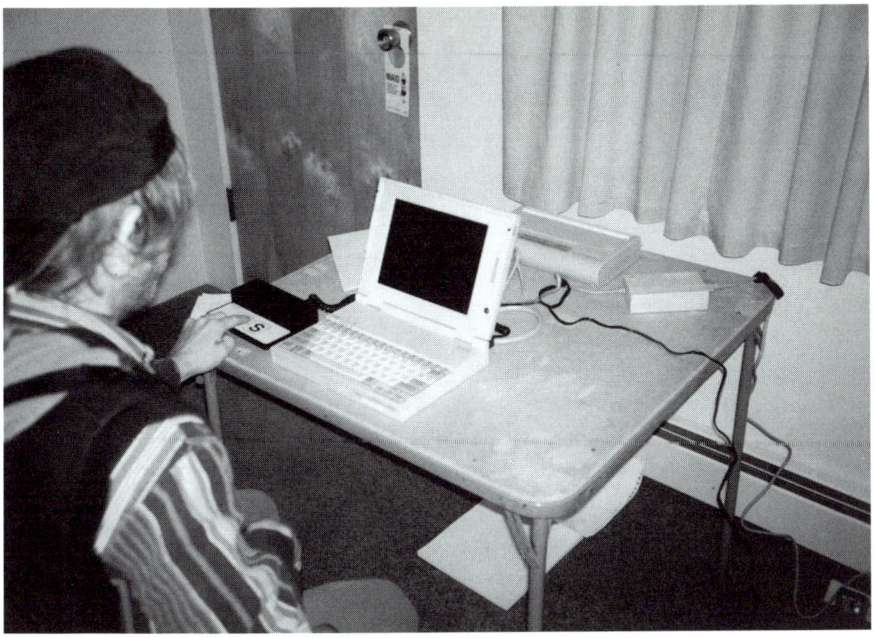

Reaction Time Simple - Choice

FIGURE 3.1. A left-handed subject observing the microcomputer screen for appearance of an A. His index finger is poised over the A of the touch-sensitive keypad for simple reaction time. A position midway between A and S is used for choice reaction time. Results are stored in the computer and printed (printer shown behind the computer).

alternating 20-second trials was recorded with the subject's eyes open in one sequence and with the eyes closed in another sequence (see Figures 3.3a–c).

Blink Reflex Latency R-1 (BRL R-1)

Specially constructed low voltage electromyographic amplifiers connected to a computer were placed on a nonconducting table. The subjects had surface (differential) electrodes attached over the upper and lower orbicularis oculi muscles of both eyes. When needed to reduce electrical interference, a ground electrode was placed initially under the chin but finally on the mid-forehead. The subjects were seated comfortably in a dimly lit room and rested with their eyes gently closed (relaxed). Electromyographic (EMG) recordings were made from the lateral two-thirds of the orbicularis oculi muscles, bilaterally, after tapping of the supraorbital notches on the right and the left. The differential EMG amplifiers permitted low interference recording from electrodes without shielding.

The specially designed low voltage EMG amplifiers permitted electromyographs to be made in ordinary rooms, even those with fluorescent lights, when proximity to major sources of electrical or magnetic fields such as power line transformers was avoided (6). For electrical stimulation, amplifiers were modified so that the electrical stimulus died out within 8 ms; so it did not interfere with the EMG signal. Electrical stimulation was generated by variable current amplitude and duration apparatus, generally at 2.0

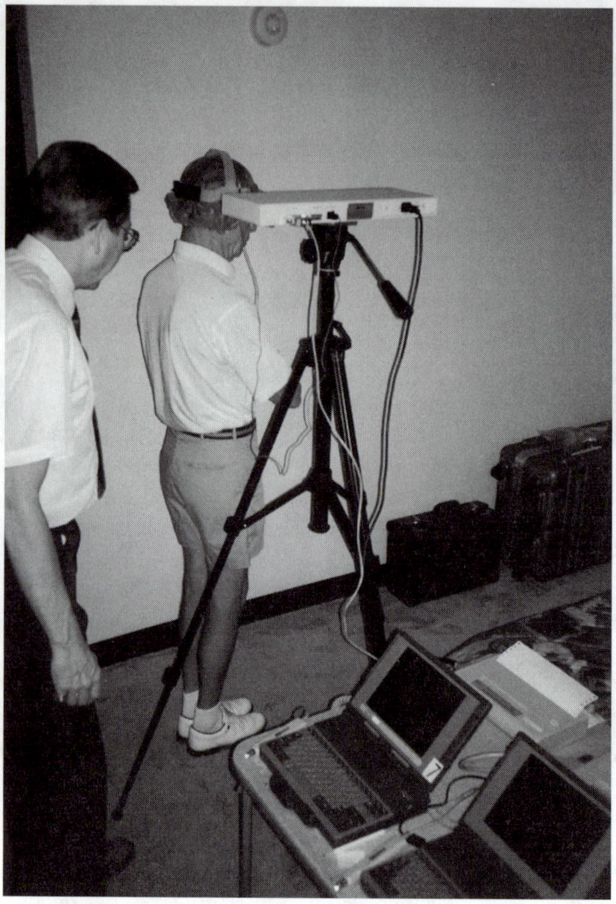

Balance by Body Tracking

FIGURE 3.2. The sound emitter on the head band is seen over the left upper edge of the dual microphone detector, which is 36 cm long. The tripod is adjusted to detector height. A microcomputer, labeled 7, is graphing movement as an interrupted line of 16 dashes per second for each 20-second trial (sway eyes open alternates with eyes closed three times).

microamperes and 2.0 ms. After preliminary testing showed that the order of electrical or mechanical stimulation did not bias the outcome, mechanical stimulation, which caused less pain and habituation, preceded electrical testing in the 19 comparisons. For our earlier studies, glabellar stimulation and bilateral recording had preceded left and right supraorbital stimulation. Blink reflexes elicited by mechanical stimulation caused minimal discomfort to the subjects. A measurement series consisted of ten taps to the supraorbital notch on each side to elicit BRL R-1 right and left (Figures 3.4 and 3.5). Glabellar stimulation by tap (7) produced BRL R-1 less consistently than this and with more delay; so it was abandoned.

Grip Strength and Vibration

Grip strength was measured for both hands by using a dynamometer calibrated in kilograms. The vibration sense of the outstretched index finger and the great toe was

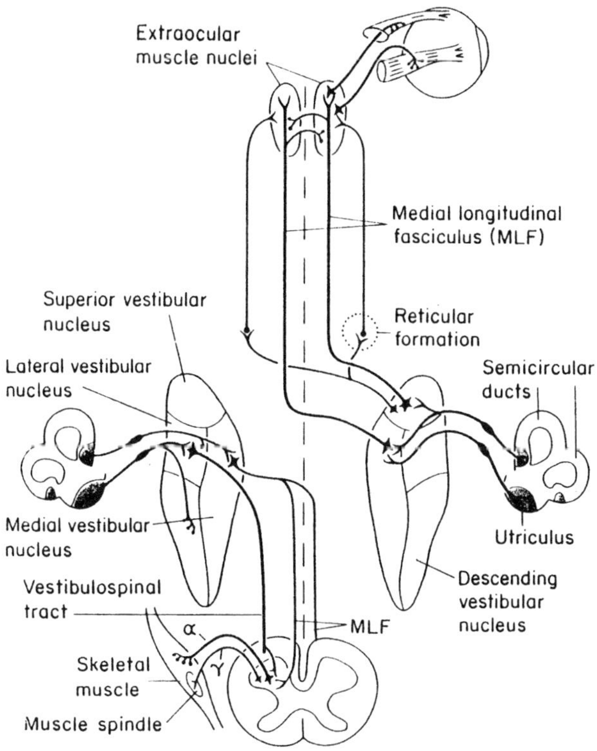

FIGURE 3.3a. The left and right vestibular nuclei are connected to the semicircular canals and the medial longitudinal fasciculus of the spinal cord, which receives input from muscle spindles.

measured to extinction against the author's right index finger and thumb with a 128 Hz tuning fork.

Color Discrimination

Color discrimination was measured with the desaturated Lanthony 15 hue test under constant illumination (8), and was scored by the method of Bowman (9). Contrast sensitivity was measured by using plates of circular photographic grids of variable space separation (Vistech).

Visual Fields

Visual fields were measured by automated perimetry using a computer algorithm (Allergan-Humphrey or BioRad Corp.). The threshold test was used with 350 to 500 light points tested per eye, and took 20 to 30 minutes for both eyes (see Figures 3.6 and 3.7).

Hearing

Hearing was measured at frequencies from 500 to 8,000 Hz by a skilled technician using a standard manual audiometer. Thresholds at each frequency were established

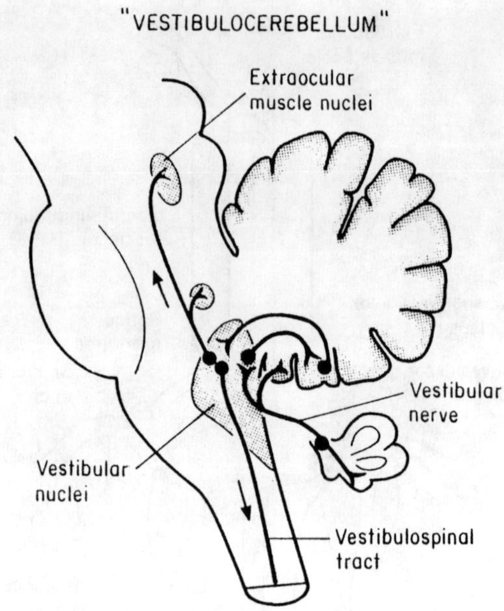

FIGURE 3.3b. The ventral or vestibulocerebellum shown in the sagittal section has input connections from the vestibular nuclei and extraocular muscle nuclei into the cerebellum.

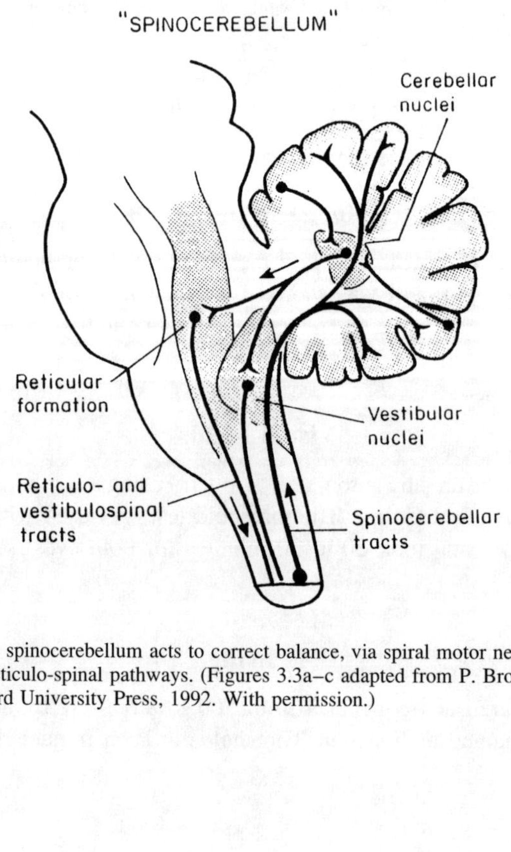

FIGURE 3.3c. The spinocerebellum acts to correct balance, via spiral motor neurons through vestibulo-spinal and reticulo-spinal pathways. (Figures 3.3a–c adapted from P. Brodal, *The Central Nervous System,* Oxford University Press, 1992. With permission.)

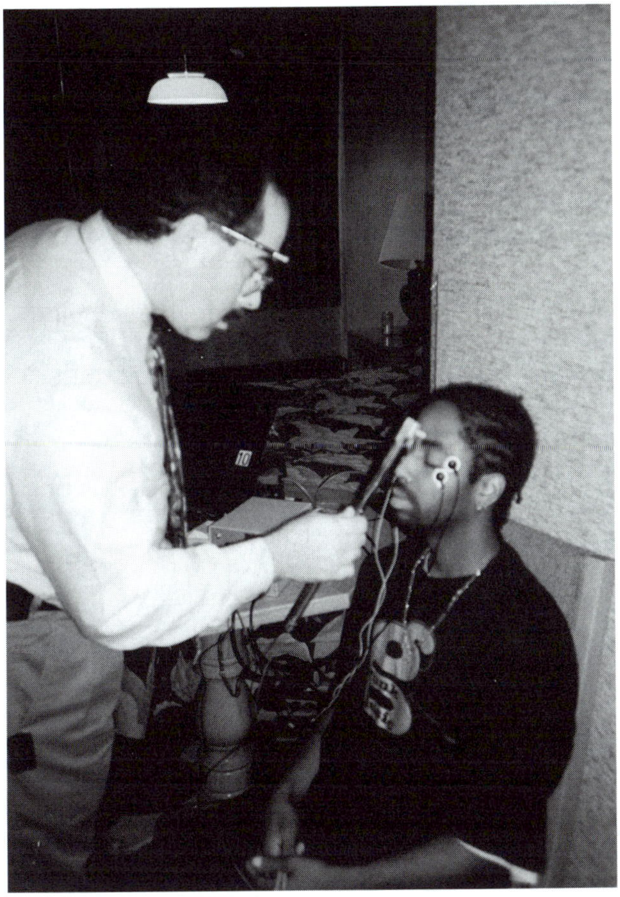

Blink Reflex Latency R-1

FIGURE 3.4. Skin microelectrodes are connected lateral to the upper and lower lids via a special amplifier to a microcomputer. A 3-mm-diameter rubber hammer-contact (for initiation of timing) is used to strike sharply the supraorbital branch of the trigeminal nerve when the eyes are resting closed. The initial signal BRL R-1 is recorded.

by using a bracketing steps approximation algorithm. The results were expressed as the sum of percentages of hearing loss at each frequency for each ear.

Spirometry

For spirometry, the subject stood, took in a maximal breath with a nose clip, and expired fully for at least 10 seconds, otherwise following ATS recommendations (10) (Figure 3.8). Comparisons were made to spirometry results from a Michigan unexposed population (11).

NEUROPSYCHOLOGICAL TESTS

Immediate memory or recall was measured by verbal and visual recall and by digits forward and backward from Wechsler's Memory Scale (12). The Culture Fair (battery

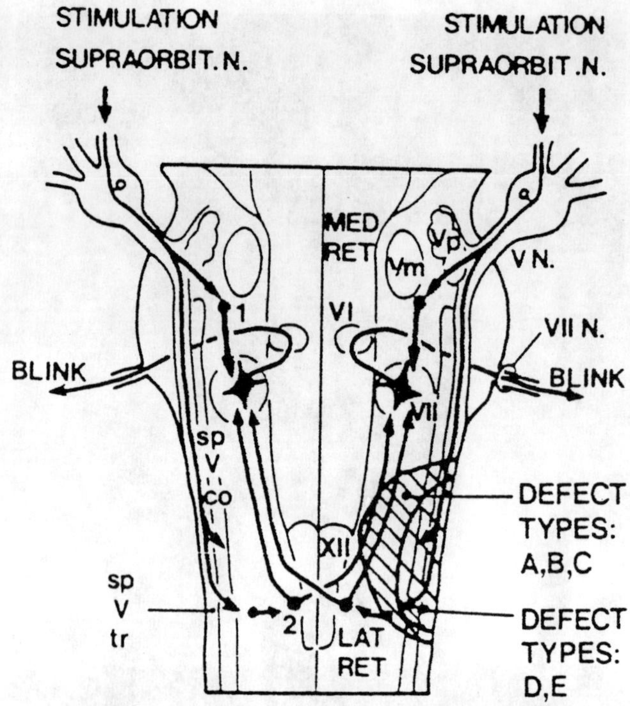

FIGURE 3.5. Inputs (as down-pointing arrows) from the supraorbital nerve run to the nucleus of the trigeminal V cranial nerve and hence to the nucleus of the facial VII cranial nerve, and are conducted to the eyelids (lateral arrows). Impulses also cross to the opposite 7th nerve, inferior to the nucleus of cranial nerve XII, for contralateral blink R-1. (From B. W. Ongenboer de Visser, Comparative study of corneal and blink reflex, in *Motor Control Mechanisms in Health and Disease,* J. E. Desmedt, ed., Raven Press, 1983. With permission from Lippincott-Raven Publishers.)

2A) and vocabulary tests were done in groups (Figure 3.9). Culture Fair tested nonverbal, nonarithmetical intelligence based on the selection of designs for similarity, difference, completion, and pattern recognition and transfer (13, 14) Culture Fair resembles Raven's progressive matrices (15). The vocabulary test came from the multidimensional aptitude battery (16). Block designs from the Wechsler Adult Intelligence Scale (WAIS-R) (17), the Knox blocks, were used to test constructional, interpretative, and integrative capacity (Figure 3.10). The digit symbol test, also from the WAIS, measured attention and integrative capacity. The grooved pegboard (18) from the Lafayette battery was used. Three tests—trail making A and B and fingertip number writing, which measure dexterity, coordination, decision making, and peripheral sensation and discrimination—were taken from the Halstead-Reitan battery (19, 20). Long-term memory was assessed by using information, picture completion, and similarities from the WAIS-R. Subjects self-appraised their emotional status during the preceding week by using the profile of mood states (POMS) (21, 22), which consisted of 65 words describing tension, anxiety, depression, anger, vigor, fatigue, and confusion. The choice of tests and their conceptual domains are available in a methods manual and a disk.*

* Available from Neurotest Inc., P.O. Box 5374, Pasadena, CA 91107.

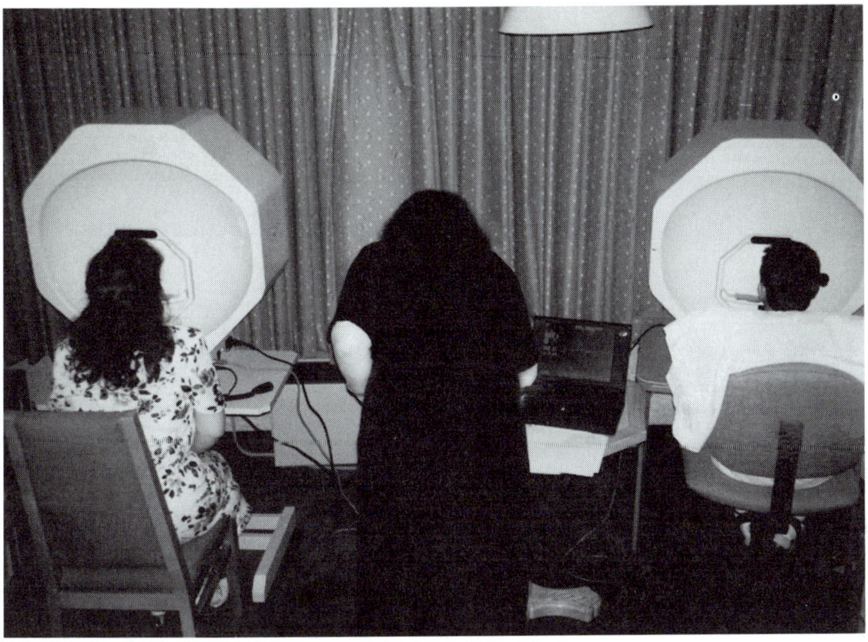

Visual Fields

FIGURE 3.6. An adult and a 10-year-old (right) are doing visual fields on a light-emitting-diode-equipped height-adjustable bowl (Med Lab Technologies, North Wales, PA). A chin rest, eye patch for the eye not being tested, forehead rest, and central focus (red) spot help fix position while 80 central 30° displays are presented. The blind spot is located, and location and brightness required are plotted on the microcomputer screen and stored. The room is in semidarkness.

DATA ANALYSIS

Minor variance of numbers of subjects in different test groups and variance due to missing data were randomly distributed. Analysis of each test yielded equations (i.e., results were modeled). Adults (age 18 years and above) and children (age 17 and under) were modeled separately. (See Tables 3.1 and 3.2 for information on the population studied.)

Stepwise Multiple Regression Techniques

These models were used to develop the regression equations for each test, including retention of variables with significant coefficients, usually as functions of age, gender, and educational level but sometimes height, grip strength, or weight. The Box-Cox transformation was used to study the need to transform the dependent variable (23); thus, transformed variables were used if they better approximated Gaussian distribution than original data.

Transformations of the independent variables, age and height, were also considered. The models were evaluated by using graphical methods to study residual plots (24). An influence analysis was performed to determine if there were any inconsistent data points. Cook's distance statistic was used as a measure of influence (23). A lack of fit test was performed on the final model, using the F-statistic to compare the estimate of

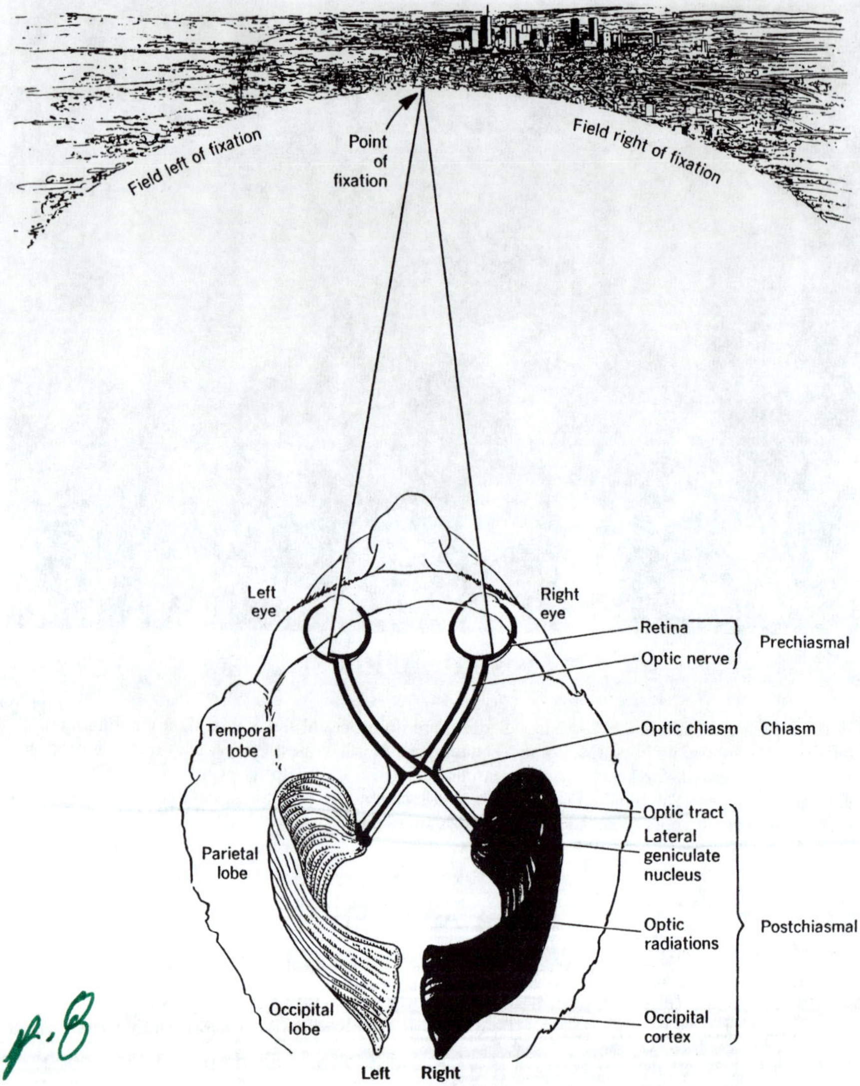

FIGURE 3.7. Illustration of the major central connections from the retina to the occipital cortex, which, with Figure 2.1, indicates the enormous brain substance devoted to vision and its radiation and association. (From D. R. Anderson, *Perimetry with and without Automation,* C. V. Mosby, 1987. With permission from Mosby-Year Book, Inc.)

error obtained from replicates to the lack of fit component of the model's residual sum of squared error.

Validation of Models

The final models were validated by using the data in Group B (Table 3.2). The observed values for verbal recall, information, picture completion, and similarities were compared to the predicted values obtained from the models, using a paired t-test. The Group B

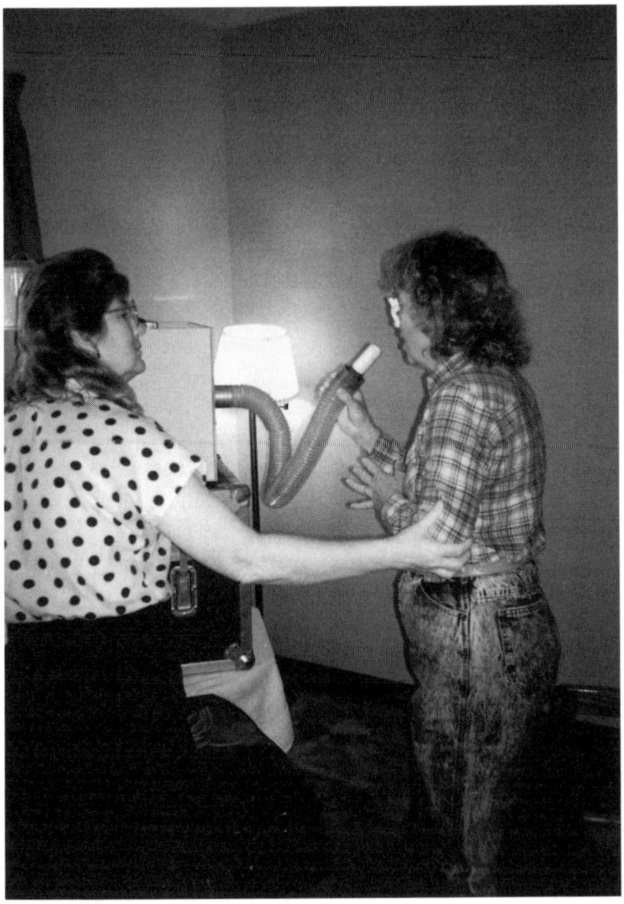

Spirometry

FIGURE 3.8. The patient, with nose occluded, holds the tubing and blows a full inspiration into the spirometer. A mechanical pen mechanism records on a timed (moving) graph.

data were used to estimate the parameters of the models. An F-statistic was used to test the hypothesis that the parameter estimates obtained by using Group B were equal to the parameter estimates of the models.

Failure to Model Visual Reproduction and Profile of Mood States

Visual reproduction, consisting of the recall of four simple line drawings from Wechsler's memory scale, was also measured and analyzed by modeling. None of the factors—age, quadratic of age, educational level, height, weight, gender—were significant coefficients. Therefore, this test and POMS, which also had no significant coefficients, could not be modeled, but the POMS unexposed to exposed difference was significant (Figure 3.11).

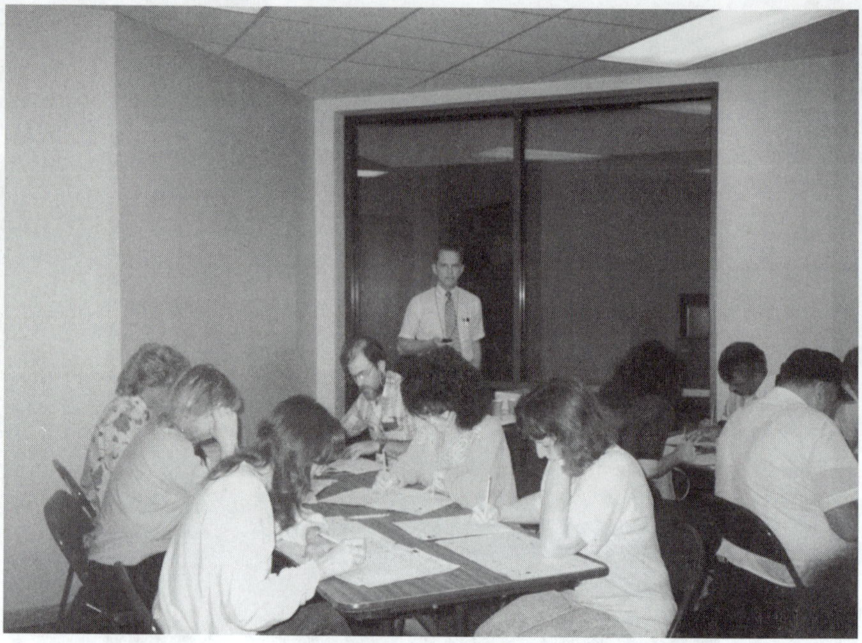

A

Culture Fair

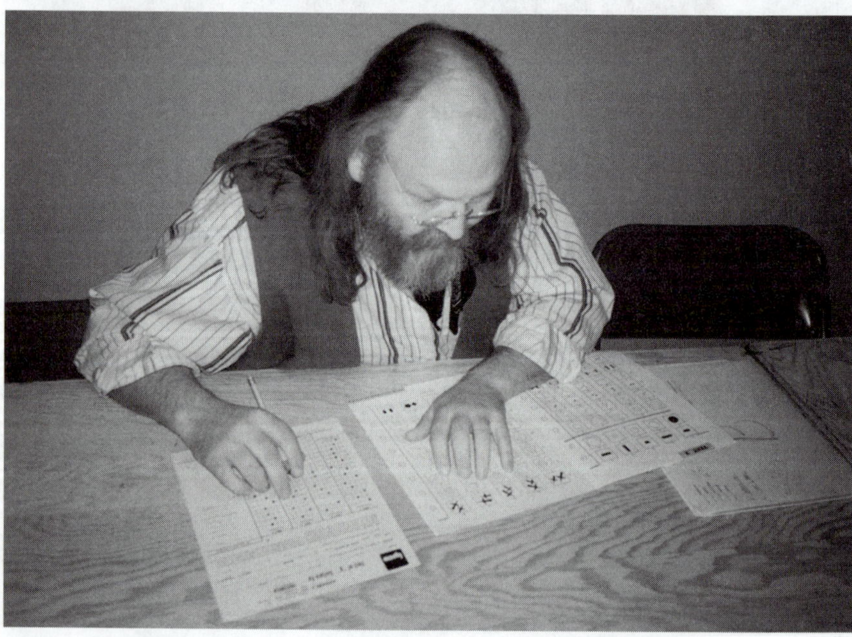

B

FIGURE 3.9. Culture Fair (test 2 is shown in Figure 3.9a) is given in groups that are instructed for each subtest and timed. Vocabulary testing is done similarly, as was the profile of mood states.

(POMS)

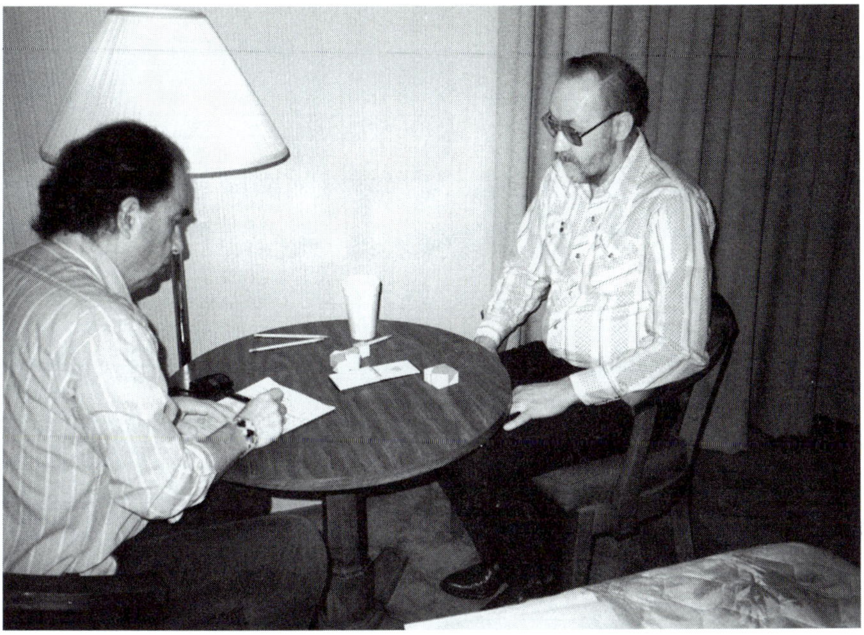

Block Design

FIGURE 3.10. Block design from the WAIS using the Knox blocks is done individually, together with digit symbol, recall, embedded memory, grooved pegboard, and trail making A and B.

Age Effect and Other Factors (Independent Variables)

Age contributes as a significant coefficient to all models but vocabulary, reducing performance and frequently slowing it, as in blink and other physiological measures (Table 3.3) and psychomotor and cognitive tests (Table 3.4). The quadratic of age (age squared) adjusts further for the accelerated rate of decline in most tests and contributes materially to decay slopes when those test results are examined graphically. Height influences speed of sway, a plausible finding. Years of school completed for adults has a major influence on the Culture Fair test of intelligence and digit symbol, block design, verbal recall, information, vocabulary, and picture completion tests. Women performed better than men in BRL R-1 (blink), digit symbol, peg placement, trail making B, and information and picture completion tests (Tables 3.3 and 3.4). Gender differences are not significant in children 5 to 17 years old. There were no explanations for the gender differences in certain functions in adults, but body size (height and weight) and (grip) strength were not responsible for them.

The adjustment of individual tests to correct for mismatching of age and educational level helps investigators avoid being misled, especially in pilot studies.

Predicted Values' Utility for Initial Comparisons

The predicted values can help investigators to recognize that an initial sample of an exposed group is adversely affected, as well as the converse, that an ''unexposed refer-

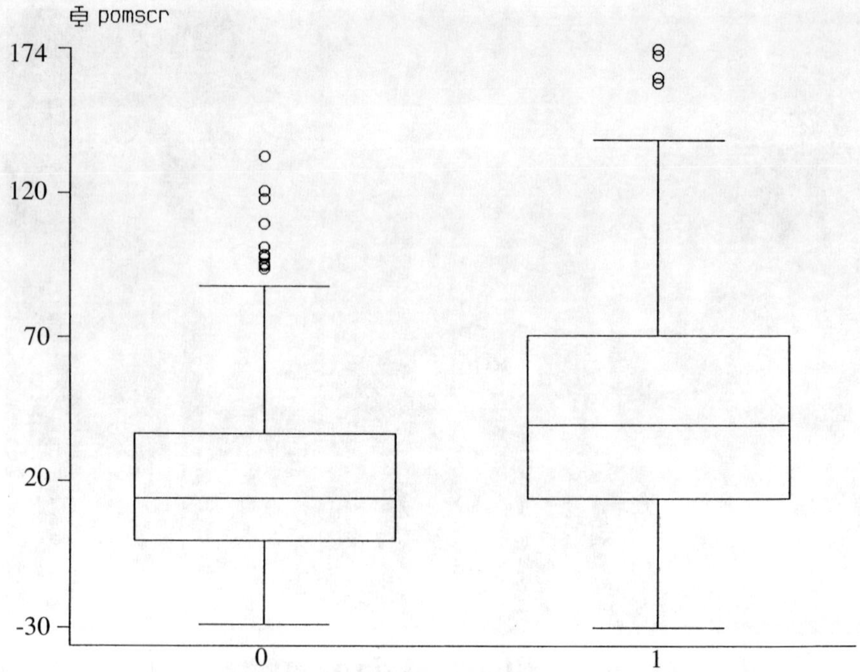

FIGURE 3.11. The box plots with standard deviation, confidence lines, and outliers (circles) are shown for profile of mood state scores for unexposed (left) and exposed (right) groups from Arizona (see Chapter 11).

ent group'' is truly unexposed. For most tests, the mean value plus or minus 1.5 times the standard deviation provided confidence intervals that included 91 to 97% of the normal group. Thus, abnormal performance was found in 3 to 9% of ''normals,'' a value similar to the well-established limits for interpreting pulmonary function tests (25–27) and metabolic (28), cardiovascular (29), and renal functions (30).

Comparison of These Predicted Values to Past Normative Values

These statistically ''robust utilities,'' data drawn from two distinct parts of the United States, were sufficiently large for statistical confidence and were validated by a third population. The equations provide performance ''standards'' for preliminary interpretation. In effect, the challenge of these data to other investigators is to compare the performances of their unexposed groups to these results. For some tests, especially the WAIS-R components and Culture Fair, normative data have been published and are available in manuals (31, 32). However, often such data were compiled and tables prepared on populations residing in just one locality, 40 or 50 years ago, with varying proportions of men and women; and they are not as suitable as these new equations for current applications.

Changing Patterns of Response through Growth and Aging

There appear to be two orderly progressions of change with the change in slope or break-point, from gains of function for 17 or 18 years (of age) and thereafter deteriora-

TABLE 3.3 Regression equations for balance, sway speed with eyes open (SO) and with eyes closed (SC), and simple reaction time (SRT) and choice reaction time (CRT), all transformed to natural logarithms (ln), and for blink reflex latency R-1 (untransformed) and color discrimination as the reciprocal of the measurement of the 4th power $1/m^4$

Variable	Constant	Age	Age^2	Height cm
ln (SO) min =	−0.248333	−0.009634	0.000164(1)	
(r^2 = 0.31, Standard Deviation = 0.196)				
ln (SC) min =	−0.585707	−0.023074	0.000315	0.015156
(r^2 = 0.32, Standard Deviation = 0.251)				
ln (SRT) =	5.620 average ± 0.198 standard deviation			
(No significant coefficients)				
ln (CRT) Coefficient	6.059766	+0.0032495		
(r^2 = 0.16, Standard Deviation = 0.158)				
Supraorbital BRL R-1 Right				
Women	10.1729	+0.0439		
Men	11.6613	+0.0439		
Supraorbital BRL R-1 Left				
Women	10.6683	+0.04035		
Men	12.0082	+0.04035		
SO r r^2 = 0.22, Standard Deviation = 1.890				
SO l r^2 = 0.24, Standard Deviation = 1.892				
Color $1/m^4$				
Women $3.06 \cdot 10^9 - 3.28 \cdot 10^{-11}$ age $+ 7.5 \cdot 10^{-11}$ edl $+ 1.63 \cdot 10^{-11}$ wt kg				
Men $2.34 \cdot 10^9 - 3.28 \cdot 10^{-11}$ age $+ 7.5 \cdot 10^{-11}$ edl $+ 1.63 \cdot 10^{-11}$ wt kg				
r^2 = .16 Standard Deviation = $1.6 \cdot 10^9$				

tion, except for BRL R-1, which shows a single slope from age 5 to 83 years in which females are faster than males, and for vocabulary, which increases with age until 70 years. Pulmonary expiratory flows show a similar change in slope at about 25 years in both sexes (25). For most people neurobehavioral performance declines after age 18, with completion of growth and graduation from high school. Whether declines of vocabulary are delayed when education continues through college and beyond or vocabulary differences simply reflect better endowment requires further measurement and analysis of a stratified sample.

Balance as a Detailed Example

The 264 subjects modeled were between 18 and 82 years of age, and had a mean best sway speed (minimum) with eyes open (SO) of 0.77 cm/sec and with eyes closed (SC) of 1.20 cm/sec (Table 3.1) (Figure 3.12). The 29 Group B subjects were similar, with eyes open speed 0.73 cm/sec and eyes closed speed 1.05 cm/sec (Table 3.2). The regression equation for the natural logarithm of SO depended upon age, which explained 31% of the variance (Table 3.3). The regression equation was ln(SC) min = −0.585707 − 0.023074*age + 0.000315*age^2 + 0.015156* height cm. The coefficients for age, age^2, and height explained 32% of the variance (Table 3.3) (Figure 3.13). Balance (speed of sway) with the eyes open was predicted by a constant and by linear and

TABLE 3.4 **Regression equations for cognitive functions, long-term memory, and perceptual motor speed**

Variable	Constant	Age	Age^2	Ed Level	Gender
COGNITIVE					
Culture Fair =	20.58158	+0.139534	−0.0044115	+0.89799	
(r^2 = 0.55, Standard Deviation = 5.128)					
√Digit Symbol =	6.605874	+0.0040577	−0.0003602	+0.127995	−0.5133185
(r^2 = 0.49, Standard Deviation = 5.675)					
Vocabulary =	−14.27959	+0.496220	−0.004175	+2.019418	
(r^2 = 0.43, Standard Deviation = 6.43)					
Block Design =	17.30686	+0.3796239	−0.0050091	+0.6257439	
(r^2 = 0.08, Standard Deviation = 9.16)					
VERBAL RECALL					
Immediate =	16.86416	−0.1057962		+0.7655161	
Delayed =	17.44594	−0.1088503		+0.4204638	
(Im: r^2 = 0.11, s = 6.8; delay r^2 = 0.08, s = 7.5)					
LONG-TERM MEMORY					
Information[1.5]	−75.17349	+2.269642	−0.0190123	+7.180807	+13.3691
(r^2 = 0.41, Standard Deviation = 26.3)					
Picture Completion[2]	135.3622	+0.986655	−0.0161115	+6.39117	+30.28474
(r^2 = 0.075, Standard Deviation = 76.7)					
Similarities[2]	69.41152			+28.90335	
(r^2 = 0.10, Standard Deviation = 174.7)					
PERCEPTUAL MOTOR SPEED, TRANSFORMED AS SHOWN, INVERSE FOR PEGS, NATURAL LOGARITHM FOR TRAIL MAKING A AND B					
1/Peg Women =	0.0176046	+0.00000451	−0.00000134		
(r^2 = 0.60, Standard Deviation = 0.002)					
1/Peg Men =	0.0144217	+0.0000887	−0.00000206		
(r^2 = 0.56, Standard Deviation = 0.002)					
ln Trails A =	3.28093	+0.010244		−0.0222522	
(r^2 = 0.33, Standard Deviation = 0.28)					
ln Trails B =	4.237346	+0.0128135		−0.0463335	+0.0855713
(r^2 = 0.37, Standard Deviation = 0.33)					

quadratic parameters of age. Height was an added factor for balance with the eyes closed. Gender, weight, strength, and educational level had no significant coefficients.

The predicted values for Group B subjects were compared to their observed values by a Student's paired t-test, and the values showed no significant differences. Also, the coefficients estimated for the model Group A in Tables 3.3 and 3.4 and those calculated for Group B were not significantly different (ln SO $p = 0.67$); ln SC $p = 0.78$). In short, coefficients from Group A worked for Group B.

Balance in adults, sway speed with the eyes open, was transformed as the natural logarithm to improve the distribution of these data; age and age^2 and exposure were significant independent variables, but exposure did not interact with age and age^2 (Figure 3.12). The equation (shown below) explained 25% of the variance (r^2). The equation for sway speed with the eyes closed (given below) had, in addition, coefficients for height and for interactions of exposure with age and exposure with the quadratic of age (age^2), and explained 21% of the variance, r^2.

$$\ln \text{SO min} = -0.0100446\ \text{age} + 0.0001783\ \text{age}^2 + 0.042375\ \text{exposure} - 0.2109417\ \text{constant}$$

Adjusted $r^2 = 0.25$, standard deviation $= 0.28$

(*continued on page 40*)

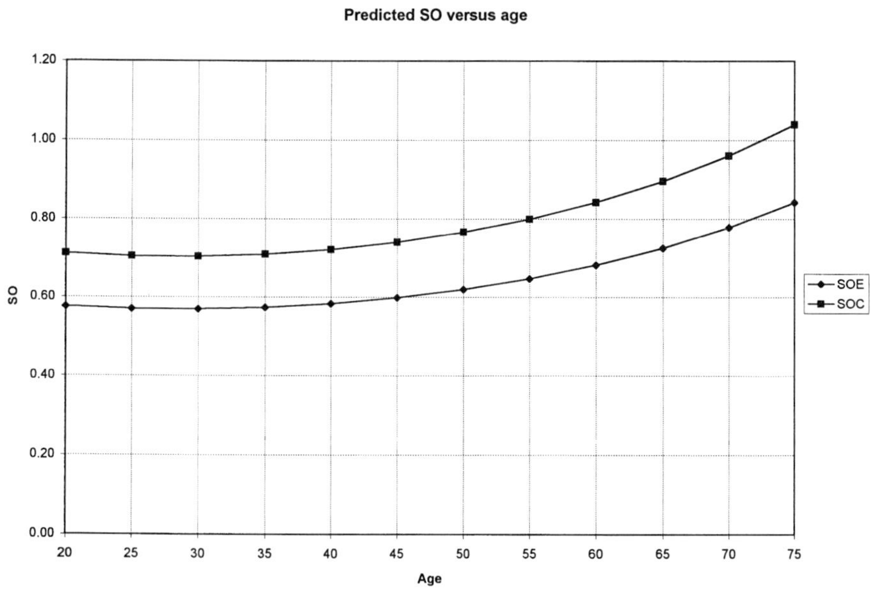

FIGURE 3.12. The sway speed with eyes open (SO) is plotted vs. age for unexposed adults from Wickenburg (SOC) and exposed adults from Phoenix (SOE), showing a parallel relationship from age 20 to 75. Untransformed data are plotted for simplicity.

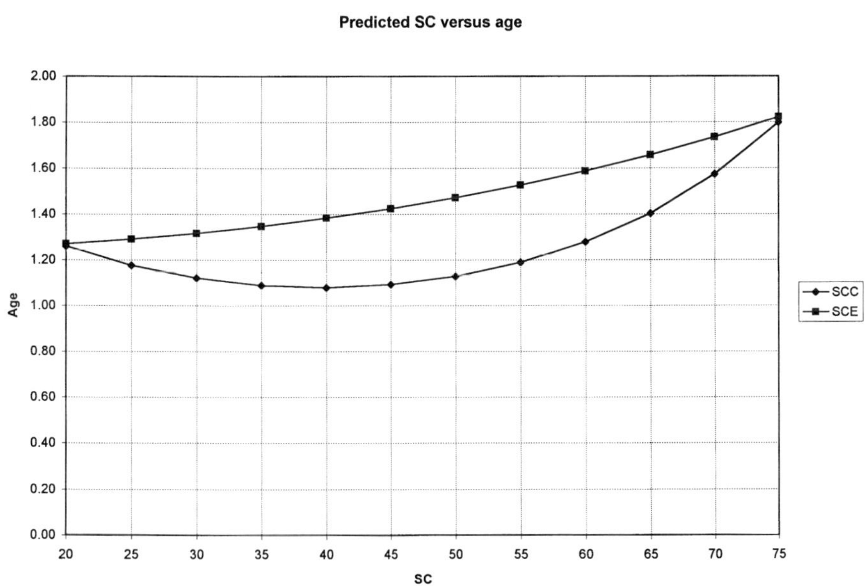

FIGURE 3.13. Plotting the subjects as in Figure 3.12 for sway speed with eyes closed shows initial divergence, as unexposed initially improve with age and cross the origin at age 60, whereas exposed subjects appear to increase sway speed linearly with age, and thus toxicity accrues. Untransformed data have been plotted for simplicity.

TABLE 3.5 Summary of exposure's contribution to aging in adults

No Effect		Difference without a Gradient		Increased Difference with Age	
Information	NP	ln Simple Reaction Time	P	ln Balance SC min	P
Similarities	NP	ln Choice Reaction Time	P	Block Score	NP
		ln Balance SO min	NP	1/Pegboard, Men	P
		Culture Fair A (ed lev)	P	Story Imm	P
		Vocabulary (ed lev)	P	Color4	P
		√Digit Symbol (ed level, sex)	NP	Grip l Women	P
		1/Pegboard, Women	P		
		ln Trails A exp ed lev	P		
		ln Trails B exp ed lev	P		
		Pict Comp^2 exp ed lev	P		
		Blink gt r exp (sex)	P		
		Grip l Men	P		
		Grip r Men	P		
		Grip r Women (wt)	P		
		Blink gt r (sex)	P		
		Blink lt l (sex)	P		

( ) = Interactions.

P = Observed was significantly different from predicted.

NP = Observed was not different from predicted.

$$\begin{aligned}\ln \text{SC min} = & -0.0322527 \text{ age} + 0.0004075 \text{ age}^2 + 0.0203717 \text{ height} \\ & + 0.6185967 \text{ exposure} + 0.0325044 \text{ exp*age} \\ & - 0.0003411 \text{ exp*age}^2 - 0.6415982 \text{ constant}\end{aligned}$$

$$\text{Adjusted } r^2 = 0.21, \text{ standard deviation} = 0.33$$

The sway speed with eyes closed of unexposed subjects improved from age 18 to 45 years and then inflected to slowly deteriorate to age 65 years, after which the decline was more rapid to age 80 (Figure 3.13). Exposed subjects declined progressively from age 20 years and increased their rate of impairment after age 60 years to age 80. For sway with eyes closed, the curves for exposed and unexposed subjects overlap at approximately age 75 years.

Patterns of Exposure–Age Interactions in Prediction Equations

Analysis of the effects of exposure in exposed vs. unexposed groups was examined by simultaneous regression models, which added exposure as a variable to equations that adjusted for age, gender, educational level, and other factors. This analysis produced three patterns, described below.

The No Effect of Exposure Pattern

The simplest pattern was found for two overlearned memory tests, information (Figure 3.14) and similarities (Table 3.5, Column 1). The absence of effects of exposure suggests that these functions were relatively protected from chemical effects on the brain. This is plausible for overlearned memory, which is thought to be retrieved from various sites and by different associations from those of cognitive functions. This result replicates the

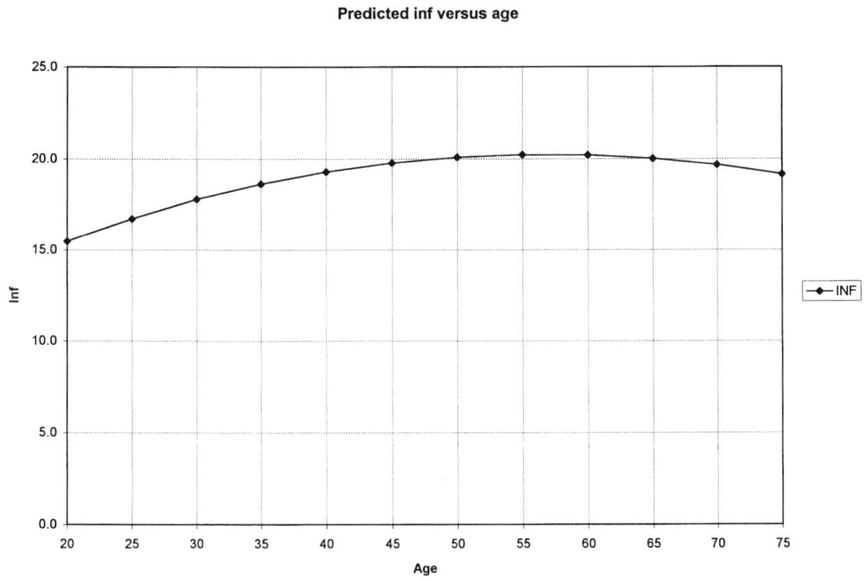

FIGURE 3.14. Information test scores of the WAIS increase with age until they decrease at age 75 in both exposed and unexposed subjects, which have been plotted together. Information is an example of a test resistant to effects of chemical exposure, the no-effects pattern.

Ryan et al. (33) findings that information and similarities scores in solvent-exposed workers were not significantly different from the scores of unexposed subjects.

The Parallel Difference Pattern

The second pattern showed that exposed were worse than unexposed subjects across the adult age range, without an exposure–age gradient. Most tests were included in this pattern (Table 3.5, Column 2; Figure 3.15). Exposure to TCE impaired the SRT and the CRT equally in subjects 17 to 83 years old, in agreement with the postulate that age impairs exposed and unexposed subjects equally. Also the absence of a gradient implies no increased sensitivity to TCE related to aging, or that the exposure effects plateaued with time despite the exposure's continuing for 10 to 38 years. The other interpretation is that for pattern 2 tests, a modest exposure impaired test performance to a given extent, but a somewhat longer exposure (which assumes a greater dose) had no additional effect. This explanation does not explain the recruitment of additional subjects into the affected group or more tests becoming abnormal as doses increased.

A variation of this approach, comparison of observed to predicted test scores for each exposed individual, was summarized for each group's performance on each test as observed/predicted, with significant difference indicated by P and not significant by NP (Table 3.5). Significant differences were seen for all blink measures, both reaction times, perceptual motor speed, picture completion, and three of four grip strengths. The cognitive tests (Culture Fair, vocabulary, block design, and digit symbol scores) had an adjustment for educational level, and digit symbol scores were higher in women than in men. Moreover, by this analysis the exposure difference in balance assisted by vision, which is sway with eyes open, was neither increased with age nor parallel, but disappeared.

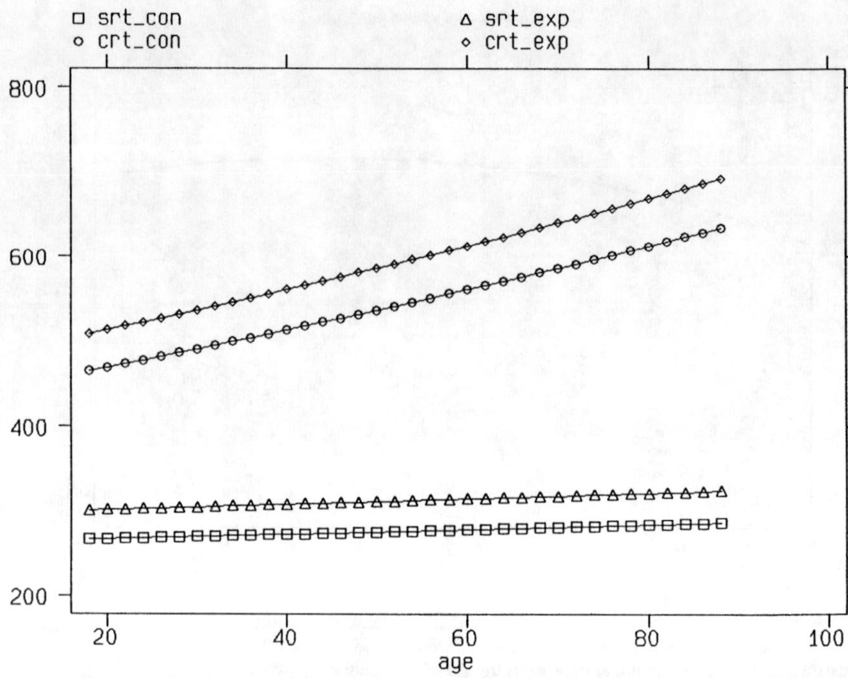

FIGURE 3.15. Simple reaction time (SRT) plotted in the lower pair of lines is parallel but not identical for unexposed (squares) and exposed (triangles) subjects, showing no effect of aging and a step increase from exposure with a parallel difference. The choice reaction time increased with age, but the effect was without an increment from greater durations of exposure, again a parallel difference.

The Increasing Difference or Divergent Pattern

The third pattern, shared by six tests, showed progressively greater differences between exposed and unexposed subjects as they aged (Table 3.5, Column 3). Thus, the six tests in pattern 3, which showed increased difference between the groups with advancing age (Figure 3.16), *are apparently most sensitive to chemical effects on the brain.* Those *impaired progressively* by chemical (TCE) exposure were balance with eyes closed (uncompensated by visual correction) (Figure 3.13), facilitated constructional and decision-driven movements as for making block designs and placing pegs (in men but not women) (Figure 3.16), immediate recall of verbal information, color discrimination, and grip strength of the left hand in women. Scores on none of these tests interacted with educational level. These six tests show progressive or cumulative effects of TCE, with long duration of exposure expressed as aging. Exposed subjects had observed scores that were different from their predicted values except for the block design score.

Cautions in generalizing: An obvious caution is that these *tentative aging patterns* are for human exposure to TCE and related chemicals and were constructed from cross-sectional observations (see Figures 3.17 and 3.18). ''Generational differences'' could be responsible. Greater susceptibility of exposed persons to the effects of TCE in Phoenix, with an age gradient, seems a less likely explanation than the hypothesis that the six tests depend upon brain functions most susceptible to TCE. This ranking should be tested in additional TCE-exposed groups and unexposed subjects.

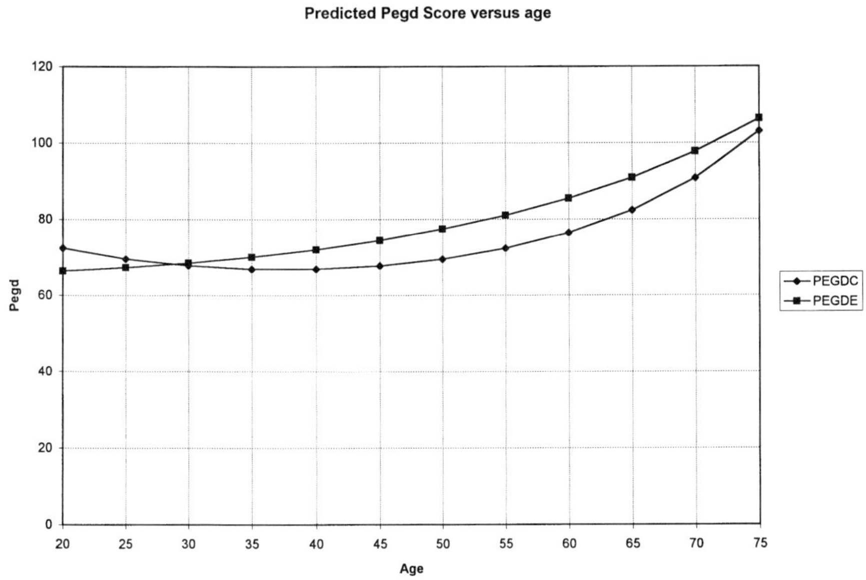

FIGURE 3.16. When peg placement was plotted for unexposed subjects, it resembled sway with eyes closed with consistency of performance across the decades. However, exposure caused an increasing difference, divergence. Note that after 65 or 70 years, advanced aging narrows the difference.

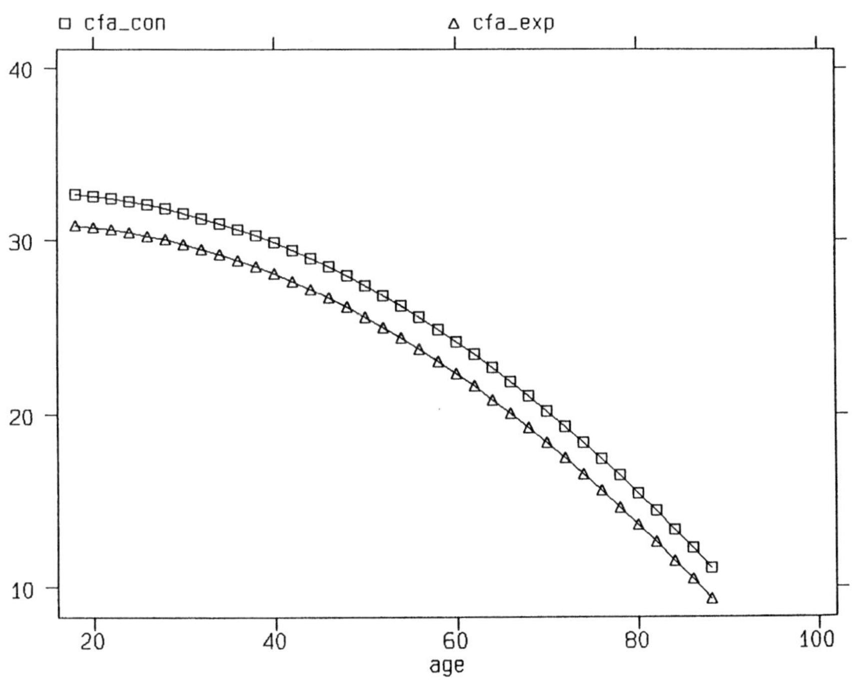

FIGURE 3.17. A Culture Fair problem-solving facility decreased with age in both unexposed and exposed subjects on a parallel path, maintaining the exposure difference after age 18.

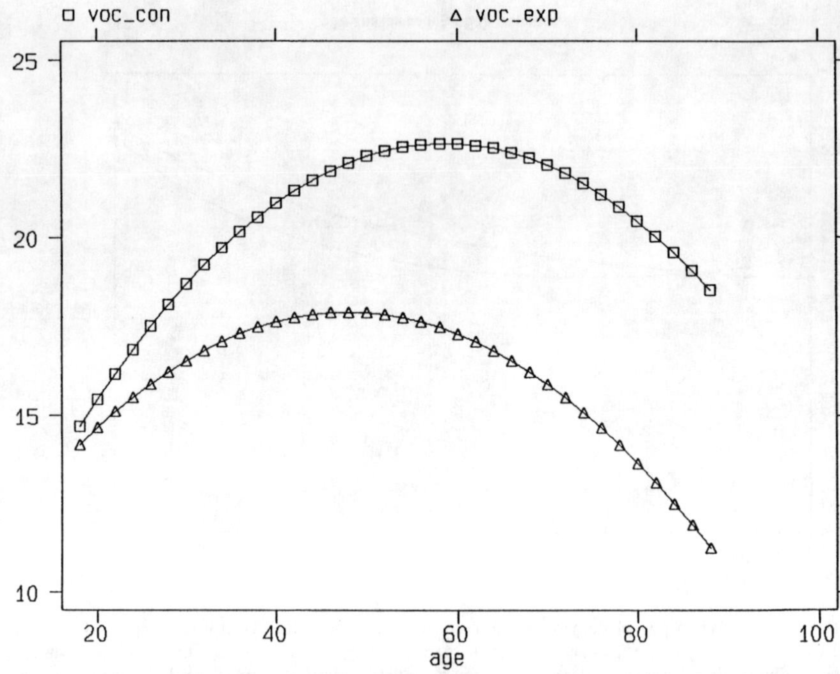

FIGURE 3.18. Vocabulary diverged, as unexposed (squares) improved more from age 18 to 60 than did exposed (triangles) subjects. Improvement with age was shown only by vocabulary and information.

CHILDREN'S PREDICTION EQUATIONS

Recruitment of Children

Children from Wickenburg aged 5 to 17 years were recruited from families participating in the adult unexposed testing and through a direct appeal to the Wickenburg schools (Table 3.6). One hundred forty unexposed children and 50 children in the Phoenix TCE exposure area had demographic variables recorded (Table 3.7) and neurophysiological and neuropsychological functions measured by the same team who measured adults. As shown in Table 3.7 for the blink reflex latencies, children's mean scores were lower and ranges were smaller, and thus blink reflex latencies were faster with tighter ranges than those of adults. In other tests, children had not attained adult levels of function.

Prediction Equations for Children

Prediction equations for children were calculated by using methods identical to those for adults, but the equations differed from those for adults (Tables 3.8 and 3.9). For example, balance in children with their eyes open had the same age-related factors as did eyes open balance in adults, plus a weight coefficient. The equation for balance with eyes closed was simpler in children than in adults, with age, age^2, and age^3 coefficients but no height factor. The logarithm of the Romberg coefficient, which is defined as sway speed eyes closed minus sway speed eyes open, also had these age coefficients.

In children the reciprocal of simple reaction time (1/SRT) was complexly related to age by factors—linear, quadratic, and cubed, for age, age^2, and age^3—assumed to

TABLE 3.6 Demographic factors in Wickenburg Children

		N	Mean	Standard Deviation	Minimum	Maximum
Age yrs	Female	71	11.2	3.5	6	17
	Male	69	11.9	3.0	5	17
Height cm	Female		146.6	17.0	109.2	170.9
	Male		152.6	19.6	118.1	191.3
Weight kg	Female		42.4	16.0	17	82
	Male		47.7	18.1	18	90
Educational Level yrs	Female		6.2	3.3	0	12
	Male		6.0	2.7	0	11

TABLE 3.7 Comparison of neurophysiological and psychological function in exposed and unexposed children

	Unexposed		Exposed		
Group Number	140		50		
Variable	Mean	Sd	Mean	Sd	*p*
Age yrs	11.8	3.6	11.5	3.6	.622
Educational Level yrs	6.4	3.1	5.4	3.4	.085
Simple Reaction ms	339	112	372	109	.068
Choice Reaction ms	610	169	634	177	.404
Sway Balance cm/s					
Eyes Open	1.01	.32	1.05	.37	.500
Eyes Closed	1.58	.47	1.66	.57	.321
Glabellar Tap Rt ms	14.2	1.9	14.4	1.5	.616
Lft ms	14.1	1.7	14.6	1.7	.115
Supraorbital Lft ms	12.4	2.0	13.3	1.6	.005
Rt ms	12.2	1.9	13.5	2.0	.0001
Color Score sc	12.2	7.4	12.6	7.5	.274
Vocabulary sc	11.7	7.1	9.8	5.6	.113
Culture Fair A sc	27.7	8.0	25.9	7.0	.154
Pegboard sc	76.2	16.5	87.4	30.6	.002
Trails A sc	39.6	19.9	57.5	40.3	.0002
Trails B sc	90.3	47.9	105.9	51.6	.064
Story 1 Immed sc	10.7	4.7	7.9	4.4	.003
Delayed sc	8.9	4.9	15		
Story 2 Immed sc	11.7	4.6	9.4	4.72	.005
Delayed sc	10.5	4.7	21		
Visual Immed sc	34.2	5.9	41		
POMS Score sc	26.5	31.3	47.8	40.8	.0003
Recall sc					
Delayed sc	31.1	8.8	41		
Information sc	10.4	5.9	18		
Picture Completion sc	13.6	3.6	12		
Similarities sc	17.1	6.0	23		

cm/s = centimers per second

ms = milliseconds

sc = score

TABLE 3.8 Regression equations for children

$\ln SO = 0.7596114 - 0.1104259{*}a + 0.0025562{*}a^2$

$\ln SC = 1.257265 - 0.1344279a + 0.0039492{*}a^2$

$1/SRT = .0040729 - 0.0007869{*}a + 0.0000991{*}a^2 - 3.19{*}10^{-6}{*}a^3$

$\ln CRT = 7.829683 - 0.1268126{*}a + 0.0033161{*}a^2 + 0.0035915{*}wt - 0.0045782{*}ht$

$\ln (GT\text{-}r) = 2.018447 + 0.0528029{*}a - 0.0017526{*}a^2 - 0.0100668{*}wt + 0.080333{*}ht$

$\ln (GT\text{-}l) = 1.911663 + 0.0681283{*}a - 0.0026597{*}a^2 - 0.0061934{*}wt + 0.0077071{*}ht$

$\ln (SO\text{-}r) = 1.526509 + 0.0606141{*}a - 0.0026003{*}a^2 - 0.0103171{*}wt + 0.0144259{*}ht$

$\ln (SO\text{-}l) = 1.697107 + 0.0871964{*}a - 0.0034333{*}a^2 - 0.005281{*}wt + 0.0068854{*}ht$

1/color

$sc^3 = -3.41{*}10^{-7} + 1.16 \times 10^{-7}{*}a - 4.06 \times 10^{-9}{*}a^2$

Cognitive

$CFA = -15.66124 + 6.229909{*}a - 0.2534487{*}a^2 + 1.421694{*}el$

$\sqrt{voc} = 5.860609 - 1.55846{*}a + 0.1790093{*}a^2 - 0.005516{*}a^3$

$\sqrt{ds}\ f = -1.164025 + 0.6342703{*}a - 0.0229418{*}a^2 + 0.051568{*}ht + 0.1794944{*}el$

$m = -1.688315 + 0.6342703{*}a - 0.0229418{*}a^2 + 0.051568{*}ht + 0.1794944{*}el$

$blk\ sc = -39.05384 + 4.63204{*}a - 0.2002309{*}a^2 + 0.0494275{*}ht + 1.645775{*}el$

Perceptual

$1/peg = -0.0069721 + 0.0027045{*}a - 0.000083{*}a^2$

$\ln TA = 5.558796 - 0.2397209{*}a + 0.0100872{*}a^2 - 0.1006756{*}el$

$\ln TB = 6.839672 - 0.2866691{*}a + 0.0115289{*}a^2 - 0.1208341{*}el$

Verbal Recall

$Immed\ f = -20.45236 + 4.838071{*}a - 0.2694524{*}a^2 + 0.0376995{*}wt + 2.534434{*}el$

$m = -9.28619 + 4.838071{*}a - 0.2694524{*}a^2 + 0.1713615{*}wt + 1.428794{*}el$

$Delay\ f = -30.05675 + 7.370622{*}a - 0.348673{*}a^2 + 1.776773{*}el$

$m = -24.49505 + 7.370622{*}a - 0.348673{*}a^2 + 1.776773{*}el$

Long-Term Memory

$\ln inf\ f = -2.326847 + 0.1822948{*}a - 0.0117412{*}a^2 + 0.0436136{*}ht + 0.2218975{*}el$

$m = -0.094453 + 0.1822948{*}a - 0.0117412{*}a^2 + 0.0095606{*}ht + 0.2218975{*}el$

$PC^{1.5} = -63.91384 + 11.0652{*}a - 0.4923605{*}a^2 + 0.6528867{*}ht + 2.958863{*}el$

$Sim = -25.49114 + 4.043402{*}a - 0.192306{*}a^2 + 0.2653335{*}ht + 1.174325{*}el$

a = age	ht = height cm
a^2 = age squared	wt = weight kg
a^3 = aged cubed	el = educational level
male = 1	

be due to development, as contrasted to adults, in whom ln SRT had no coefficients (see Tables 3.8 and 3.9). For choice reaction time, transformation to the natural logarithm, ln CRT, was preferred for children as for adults; age and age^2 coefficients were found as for 1/SRT, but with an added weight factor.

Children's blink reflex latencies, which, as noted, were faster than those of adults, had different coefficients in the prediction equations (Table 3.8). Here the dependent variables were log transformations, but for adults they were untransformed. Children did not differ in these tests by gender, but adults did. All children's equations for

TABLE 3.9 Children, variance explained (r^2 and standard deviation

Test	r^2	Standard Deviation
ln SO_3	.47	0.200
ln SC_3	.33	0.2417
ln rom	.09	0.18736
1/SRT	.47	0.00059
ln CRT	.68	0.13907
ln (GT-r)	.14	0.122
ln (GT-l)	.17	0.1145
ln (SO-r)	.15	0.1474
ln (SO-l)	.15	0.1426
$\sqrt{voc}$	.51	0.839
cfa	.54	5.076
1/peg	.56	0.0025
ln TA	.54	0.2886
ln TB	.65	0.2859
$\sqrt{ds}$	.80	0.58
blk scr	.48	7.90
Verbal Recall Immed.	.47	6.226
Verbal Recall Delayed	.36	7.089
ln Information	.66	0.3867
$PC^{1.5}$	.40	14.759
Similarities	.50	4.217

supraorbital and glabellar tap had coefficients for age, the quadratic of age, and weight and height, which appear to be developmental (body size) measurements.

The color score equations, 1/color $score^3$, were simpler in children than in adults and related only to age and age squared.

Of the cognitive measures, children's Culture Fair and the square root of vocabulary had linear, quadratic, and cubed coefficients for age, but did not need educational level. In contrast, the square root of children's digit symbol had, in addition to linear and quadratic coefficients for age, coefficients for height, gender, and educational level, like those of the adult equations. The block design score added a height (developmental) factor for children to the age and educational level factors that adults had.

In the perceptual motor domain, the reciprocal of grooved pegs in pegboard (1/GPP) in children, as in adults, had linear and quadratic age coefficients; so there were no differences between them in the form of the equations. Children's ln TA, like that of adults, had a factor for educational level. Trail making ln B had an education coefficient, just as did ln TB in adults, but no gender difference.

Immediate verbal recall had quadratic age, educational level, and weight coefficients in children, but the 30-minute verbal recall delayed lacked the weight coefficient as a ''measure of development'' factor, which is a puzzling finding.

The long-term memory tests had the greatest differences between children and adults, beginning with different transformations. In children, information was logarithmic, and picture completion was a power function at 1.5, but similarities was not transformed. Children's information, as the natural logarithm, added height to age and educational level, whereas $PC^{1.5}$ and similarities had age, height, and educational level coefficients.

TABLE 3.10 Summary of exposure contribution to aging in children

No effect		Difference without a Gradient		Difference Increases with Age	
Grip right	NP	Vocabulary	NP	SRT	P
Grip left	NP	Pegboard	NP	CRT	NP
		Trails B (ed level)	NP	SO (age^2)	NP
		$Color^3$	NP	SC (age^3)	NP
		Story Imm	P	Culture Fair A	NP
		Blink gt left	P	Trails A	P
		Blink gt right	P	Blink so left	P
		Blink so right	P		

( ) = Interactions.
P = Observed was significantly different from predicted.
NP = Observed was not different from predicted.
gt = Glabellar tap.
SO_2 = Balance eyes open.
SC_3 = Balance eyes closed.

Differences Between Adults and Children

Clearly for neurobehavioral functions children, except for blink reflex latency, are not small adults but are progressively attaining function. The equations just reviewed confirm graphic examination of these data. The plots of these functions, direct (linear) or suitably transformed, against age were complex curves with sharp junctions of development and the beginning of decrease or deterioration. Blink reflex latency R-1, the exception, was linear from age 5 to 83 years.

When children exposed to TCE had the expected age effect adjusted by using the unexposed group (Table 3.10), they also presented the three patterns shown by adults: (1) a pattern of no effect; (2) a parallel or level exposure effect across the age range, with no gradient from exposure; and (3) a pattern of increasing difference with age, an exposure–age gradient. Only grip strength had no exposure difference. Blink reflex latency, vocabulary, and pegboard measures in both children and adult women showed a level effect of exposure. However, children had more tests showing increased effect with age and exposure than did adults (Table 3.10), including balance with eyes closed and with eyes open, simple and choice reaction time, Culture Fair, trail making A, and left supraorbital blink latency. The children's list of tests in column 3 is quite different from the adult one. Only balance with eyes closed is common to both. Children had gradients assuming that duration of exposure is reflected by age, despite our finding none in adults. The logical inference is a greater sensitivity to exposure in children, with the most discriminatory tests showing an exposure gradient with cumulation (age). After such observations are confirmed, a shorter battery of tests would be feasible as the key measurements needed for follow-up studies.

Even to be certain that this pattern profiles the effects of TCE on neurobehavioral function, iterations are needed of these tests in other exposed groups. Additional investigations of groups exposed to other chemicals and subjected to these analyses will determine their profiles. From the profiles in Table 3.5 in adults and Table 3.10 in children, comparisons can be made to group responses to other chemicals and to follow-up studies across a number of years to test these predictions. The relative sensitivity of brain functions/processes to chemicals can be compared by using physiological brain imaging.

UNEXPOSED GROUPS AND PREDICTION EQUATIONS

Adults from various parts of the country who have been exposed to chemicals have almost identical performances on the test battery, suggesting that additional "national" samples match those used to produce the prediction equations. In essence, this means that the age decrements of unexposed adults are similar and confirm the practical applications of expressing these data in models. It has been helpful to compare data from each new unexposed group with the models to determine whether values were within expectation or whether, as in a Phoenix group in 1987, they were abnormal—a finding that suggested effects of unknown exposures and triggered further investigation. In Phoenix the probable explanation, chemical exposure, was discovered later. Comparing the functional scores of a new, presumably exposed, group to the prediction formulae based on the national unexposed groups, via prediction equations, makes an initial assessment of pilot inquiries quick and economical.

AGING, A PERSPECTIVE ON DEMENTIA AND CHEMICAL ENCEPHALOPATHY

The intuitive idea that mental and neurological functions slow or decrease after age 25 in humans is supported by much evidence (34–36). Use of age-adjusted test scores aids comparisons of exposed and unexposed groups. The problem of norms is complicated by educational and cultural changes across year-of-birth cohorts, which interact with age (37). There are decreases in intelligence measured by the WAIS-R across the ages and across the year-of-birth cohort such that ability appears to be decreasing, as the "norms" for the 13-test WAIS-R have been one IQ point higher for each 4-year interval since their standardization. These problems, plus questionable comparability of Wechsler's normals to people 50 years after testing, mean that for epidemiological studies contemporary unexposed groups are essential. It is not clear whether the tests become outdated, or group intelligence is slipping. Wechsler (34) showed that the decrease in IQ (intelligence as calculated from his scale) paralleled that for forced vital capacity, but that test component scores from the WAIS-R decreased at different rates with aging (Figure 3.14). Lung volumes measured by spirometry are proportional to height. Flows and vital capacity are reduced progressively after 25 years of age, and flows are reduced further by each year of smoking cigarettes so that cigarette smoking accelerates "lung aging" (38). Aging effects on Culture Fair A and vocabulary were quite different, with Culture Fair exhibiting an inexorable decrease from age 18 to 85 (Figure 3.17), as did Wechsler's IQ. In contrast, vocabulary was cumulative, peaking near age 60 before declining and showing a large exposed (see lower curve) to unexposed difference from age 18 to 85 (Figure 3.18).

Brain Damage

CNS trauma, tumors, cerebrovascular accidents, and alcoholic encephalopathy reduce neurobehavioral performance (39). Batteries of tests in the 1950 to 1980 era attempted to distinguish damage from each of these from normal aging by comparing brain-damaged groups to age-matched "control" subjects (40). Responses to drugs were affected by aging (36). Distinguishing chronic brain disease (41) from the "ordinary effects of aging" has defined Alzheimer's disease, which constitutes a major proportion of all dementia, some 60 to 77% (42). Dementia in the elderly may be caused by vascular disorders (43), drugs (44), anesthetic agents (45), and depression (46). Differentiating ordinary effects of aging from brain damage has been addressed most frequently by making age-matched comparisons.

Longitudinal Studies of Brain Aging

Several careful long interval studies of intellectual function and aging have modified the picture of inexorable decline (47). The Iowa State study (48) examined 363 male college freshmen in 1919, 127 of these individuals who were retested in 1950, and 96 who were retested in 1961, using the Army Alpha test. Eight subtests included: (1) following directions, (2) arithmetical problems, (3) practical judgment, (4) synonym–antonym, (5) disarranged sentences, (6) number series completion, (7) analogies, and (8) information testing. Performance peaked overall, and intellectual function began declining in the fifties, with only small declines until age 60. Schaie (49) confirmed these findings in the 21-year Seattle, Washington study, from 1956 to 1977, using psychometric testing including five of Thurstone's primary mental abilities. The study used a sequential methodology of cross-sectional and longitudinal data analysis, the latter to look, as in the Iowa study, at intrasubject changes. Several abilities improved into midlife and showed aging declines in the late fifties and the sixties, with substantial decline in late seventies and early eighties. Fluid (performance or problem-solving) abilities declined earlier, the "don't hold" category; but crystallized (informational or verbal) abilities, the "hold" ones, declined precipitously only in advanced old age. The Duke studies of aging (50, 51) in healthy individuals found that Wechsler performance scale decrements occurred in the seventies, and verbal scales declined in the early eighties.

A New York State study of 2,000 aging twins began in 1946 when 1,603 who had reached the age of 60 were measured by using Wechsler subtests; and 268 of these subjects were tested, with survivors retested and analyzed, well into their eighties (52). Although nonspeeded (untimed) cognitive functioning was maintained at least until age 75 in healthy survivors, timed (speeded) test scores decreased 12% across the 68 to 75 year span, which was significant. Furthermore, test scores and survival were correlated. Also, the first retest scores increased, though not significantly, from initial scores, a phenomenon attributed to test familiarity.

Chemically Produced Aging Changes in Mice

Weiss (53) suggested that age-related declines in neurobehavioral function could be produced by toxicants such as methylmercury and acrylamide, and further that effects of prenatal exposure of mice to methylmercury may only appear in middle age or senescence, as attrition from aging reduces neuron numbers.

Integrating Human and Animal Data

One challenge is to ascertain whether observations of normal human brain aging by Wechsler (34) and others and Weiss's deductions of age-related declines in the brains of chemically exposed mice (53) can be integrated—for example, in interpreting the larger age coefficients on regression analysis of neurophysiological tests in cohorts of chemically exposed human subjects. Fast functioning is a property of the intact young

CNS. Small delays reflect adverse effects (54). For some neuropsychological functions delay is not so critical (34) as it is for reaction time (42). In fact, Wechsler (34, 55) argued that with aging cognitive performance was slowed, not lost. However, in using other tests a difference emerges. Recall of new pictures of landscapes, animals, and people was significantly worse in aged subjects than in younger ones, and their forgetting rate, as a percentage of correct responses, was greater as well. Also there was a mild defect in acquisition (56).

Differential Effects of Aging

Horn and Cattell (57) found age differences in factors of mental ability by testing 57 variables for 23 mental ability factors in 297 persons, mostly between 15 and 51 years old (mean 27.6 ± 10.6 standard deviation). Fluid abilities (associative memory, figural relations, intellectual speed, induction, and intellectual level) decreased after age 21, whereas crystallized abilities (ideational fluency, associational fluency, experimental evaluation, mechanical knowledge, and verbal comprehension) all increased with age from the younger group ages 14 to 17) into the group 40 to 61 years old.

These findings led these authors to observe that superimposed on the basic structure of heredity "are those (patterns of loss) resulting from injuries, particularly in the central nervous system (CNS), but also other physiological structures." Such injuries occur throughout life and are often irreversible, hence cumulative, both within a given individual and within groups of individuals; so means for intellectual performance can be computed. There are innumerable ways in which small CNS injuries can occur, for example, by carbon monoxide poisoning, lead poisoning, high fever, blows to the head, and anoxia resulting from a variety of causes, as well as vascular occlusion. An individual may accumulate the effects of several such injuries. Effects of large, easily detected injuries, which leave a person viable, are not so clearly seen to accumulate within an individual; but they become statistically more frequent as the average age of subjects increases so that such accumulation is seen more clearly in groups than in individuals.

Adults Perhaps Less Testable

Adults frequently lack the "first, fine careless rapture [with] which children approach competitive tests" (58). Twenty-one percent of general hospital patients refused psychological tests in one study (59), and as many as 50% of adults refused to be tested in another (60). In contrast, younger adult Army recruits in World War I were successfully tested and placed by use of the Army Alpha and Beta test batteries (61, 62), although serious questions have been raised as to bias and to generalizations from these data (63). This has not been a problem in either exposed or unexposed groups in the author's investigations, in which usually 85 to 90% of chemically exposed and unexposed subjects who were scheduled came for testing. This difference suggests, not surprisingly, that hospitalized patients "captured" for psychological testing may be less motivated than are chemically exposed groups and their reference subjects.

Increased Age Coefficient Suggestive of Accelerated Aging

Significantly larger age coefficients (in the prediction equations) in the exposed than in the unexposed population in many of the present studies of neurotoxic effects suggest accelerated aging. These increases are inferred to be effects of chemical exposure after the elimination of confounding factors. The difficulty of attributing these effects to a specific chemical exposure does not diminish the probability of the relationship in these epidemiological studies.

Physiological Tests More Sensitive than Psychological Tests

The psychological tests of cognitive function that were previously shown to have age effects (57, 63) were less sensitive for detecting abnormality in present subjects than were the neurophysiological tests: a balance test, blink reflex latency, visual fields, and simple and choice reaction time. The difference in sensitivity is 1,000 times; these measurements are in milliseconds or centimeters/second, compared to counting errors and measuring time in seconds. Culture Fair test of intelligence (2A) and trail making B were the most sensitive psychological tests. As experience with this testing grows, patterns of age coefficients may suggest specific chemical toxicants. As CNS dysfunction is the toxicological challenge of the 1990s (64), these tests should help describe the effects of exposure to hazardous wastes (65), and public health should benefit as subtle neurologic changes replace cancer and birth defects as end-points for study (66).

Organic Dementia

Organic brain syndrome (67) or senile dementia is a problem of increasing prevalence and concern with aging. Between the ages of 70 and 79, from 1.9% of subjects in Denmark to 4.9% in Japan were so labeled, and above age 80 the percentages rose to 3.2% in Denmark and 22% in England (68). The working definition for dementia is mild cognitive impairment or a decline from a previous higher level of function (69). Lishman's extended definition (70) aptly characterizes the pattern: ''An acquired global impairment of intellect, memory and personality, but without impairment of consciousness.'' Dementia is usually progressive, long-lasting, and often irreversible, but these features are not included in the definition, which is a constellation of symptoms of chronic and widespread brain dysfunction excluding prognosis and etiology.

Causes

Iatrogenic drugs, including anticholinergics, hypnotics, and psychotropics, may cause clouding that exceeds benign senescent forgetfulness. The Geriatric Mental Examination and Comprehensive Assessment and Referral Evaluation may aid in its recognition (69). The latter reports on: decline in memory, use of notes as reminders, forgetting names of acquaintances, destructive or critical memory lapses occurring less than once a month, and errors in cognitive testing.

Prevalence of Dementia Unknown

Formal neuropsychological testing has not been done in large populations, and the sampling in smaller studies has not been random. For example, a pilot study of 61 subjects, 32 demented and 29 not demented, who had been divided by physician assessment in New York (71), applied a brief (1 hour) battery of tests of verbal memory: the Benton visual retention test, a mini-mental state test, the Rosen drawing test, language tests (word association, category naming, and comprehension and similarities) from the Wechsler Adult Intelligence Scale, and identities and oddities from the Mattis dementia rating scale. The testing results agreed with the assessment in all but two cases. Application of the methods to 430 healthy elderly subjects showed 19% of those with less than eight years of education met the dementia criteria, compared to 5% with more than eight years of education. Although adjustment of raw scales for educational level improved the separation, the implication is that *those with less brain capacity, as shown by attainment of education, become demented earlier.*

Time, Socioeconomic, Gender, and Other Factors

A generalization that has evoked controversy is that "time is key"; thus many aged subjects, particularly those with above average educational achievement, perform tests well if they are not timed (72). Again, in most such tests educational attainment is negatively correlated with aging; those with more education (ability) lose it less quickly with aging. Yet even this result is complex, as perceptual–organization (fluid or don't hold) functions decline while verbal ability is preserved.

Studies of children have shown a socioeconomic gradient and differences between ethnic groups (73), which are most plausibly explained by an environmentally based model, impacted by hunger and malnutrition, adverse environmental stimuli, and inadequate obstetrical and pediatric care affecting children and carrying over to adulthood (74). Part of the urban/rural difference observed by this researcher in a northern Alabama study may be due to a convergence of these factors, as a local reference group's mean test scores were below those of national reference groups (74). Finally, there are gender differences (men and women as groups performing differently on some tests) and differences associated with ethnicity that make separate analyses essential.

Causal Hypotheses that Downplay Chemicals

Six hypotheses were proposed in 1980 by Mortimer (67) for causation of dementia, especially senile dementia of the Alzheimer's type: (1) genetic factors (familial patterns and chromosome losses); (2) viral causes (kuru and Creutzfeldt-Jacob disease); (3) immune system factors (rising titers of brain-specific antibodies with age); (4) aluminum; (5) sociopsychologic factors (stress, social isolation, economic status); and (6) multiple insults: subacute damage from head trauma, nutritional status, occupational and environmental factors, alcohol, and drugs. Except for aluminum, chemicals did not receive major emphasis, nor did possible chemical insults to the developing brain or cumulative multiple low-dose chemical insults, although the latter are of concern in occupational exposure (45).

Biomarkers Needed

Aging research is impeded by a paucity of biological markers and suitable models of aging. Models with controlled genomes would permit study of environmental variables in small populations, because of phenotypic variation in human subjects. Ideally, biomarkers should be linear and should be analyzed by noninvasive methods (75).

References

1. Martin GM: Interactions of aging and environmental agents: the gerontological perspective. In: *Environmental Toxicology and the Aging Process,* SR Baker and M Roger (eds.). New York: Alan R. Liss, 1985.

2. Miller JA, Cohen GS, Warshaw R, Thornton JC, and Kilburn KH: Choice (CRT) and simple reaction times (SRT) in laboratory technicians: factors influencing reaction times and a predictive model. *Am J Indust Med* 1989;15:687–697.
3. Kilburn KH, Warshaw RH, and Thornton JC: An examination of factors that could affect choice reaction time in histology technicians. *Am J Indust Med* 1989;15:679–686.
4. Kilburn KH, Warshaw RH, and Hanscom B: Are hearing loss and balance dysfunction linked in construction iron workers? *Brit J Indust Med* 1992;49:138–141.
5. Kilburn KH, Warshaw RH, and Hanscom B: Balance measured by head (and trunk) tracking and a force platform in chemically (PCB and TCE) exposed and reference subjects. *Occup Environ Med* 1994;51:381–385.
6. Kilburn KH, Thornton JC, and Hanscom B: A field method for blink reflex latency R-1 (BRL R-1) and prediction equations for adults and children. *Electromyo Clin Neurophys* 1997 in press.
7. Shahani BT and Young RR: Human orbicularis oculi reflexes. *Neurology (NY)* 1972;22: 149–154.
8. Lanthony P: The desaturated panel D-15. *Doc Ophthalmol* 1978;46:185–189.
9. Bowman KJ: A method for quantitative scoring of the Farnsworth panel D-15. *Acta Ophth* 1982;60:907–916.
10. ATS Statement. Standardization of spirometry—1987 update. *Am Rev Respir Dis* 1987;136: 1285–1298.
11. Miller A, Thornton JC, Warshaw R, Bernstein J, Selikoff J, and Teirstein AS: Mean and instantaneous expiratory flows, FVC and FEV_1: prediction equations from a probability sample of Michigan, a large industrial state. *Bull Eur Physiopathol Resp* 1986;22:589–597.
12. Wechsler D: A standardized memory scale for clinical use. *J Psych* 1945;19:87–95.
13. Cattell RB, Feingold SN, and Sarason SB: A culture free intelligence test. II Evaluation of cultural influences on performance. *J Educ Psych* 1941;32:81–100.
14. Cattell RB: Classical and standard score IQ standardization of the IPAT: culture free intelligence scale 2. *J Consult Psych* 1951;15:154–159.
15. Raven JC, Court JH, and Raven J: *Standard Progressive Matrices.* London: H. K. Lewis and Co, 1988.
16. Jackson DN: *Vocabulary: Multidimensional Aptitude Battery.* Port Huron, MI: Sigma Assessment Systems, Inc., 1985.
17. Wechsler D: *Adult Intelligence Scale Manual* (revised). New York: The Psychological Corporation, 1971/1981.
18. Matthews C, Cleeland CS, and Hopper CL: Neurological patterns in multiple sclerosis. *Dis Nervous Syst* 1970;31:161–170.
19. Reitan RM: A research program on the psychological effects of brain lesions in human beings. In: *International Review of Research in Mental Retardation,* NR Ellis (ed.). New York: Academic Press, 1966.
20. Reitan RM: Validity of the trail-making test as an indicator of organic brain damage. *Percept Motor Skills* 1958;8:271–276.
21. McNair DM and Lorr M. An analysis of mood in neurotics. *J Abnorm Soc Psychol* 1967; 69:620–624.
22. McNair DM, Lorr M, and Droppleman LF. *Profile of Mood States.* San Diego, CA: Educational and Industrial Testing Service, 1971/1981.
23. Stata Corporation: *State Reference Manual,* Release 3.1, Vol. 2. 702 University Drive East, College Station, TX 77840, 1993.
24. Hamilton LC: *Regression with Graphics, a Second Course in Applied Statistics.* Pacific Grove, CA: Brooks/Cole Publishing Co., 1992.
25. Morris JF, Koski A, and Johnson LC: Spirometric standards for healthy nonsmoking adults. *Am Rev Resp Dis* 1972;103:57–67.
26. Schmidt CD, Dickman ML, and Gardner RM: Spirometric standards for healthy elderly men and women: 532 subjects ages 55 through 94 years. *Am Rev Respir Dis* 1973;108:933–939.

27. Kilburn KH, Warshaw RH, Thornton JC, Thornton K, and Miller A: Predictive equations for total lung capacity and residual volume calculated from radiographs in a random sample of the Michigan population. *Thorax* 1992;47:517–523.
28. Bernstein RS, Thornton JC, Yang MU, Wang J, Redmond AM, Pierson RN, et al.: Prediction of the resting metabolic rate in obese patients. *Am J Clin Nutrition* 1983;37:595–602.
29. Jones NL: *Clinical Exercise Testing* (3rd ed.). Philadelphia, PA: W. B. Saunders Company, 1988.
30. Smith HW: *Principles of Renal Physiology.* New York: Oxford University Press, 1956.
31. Cattell RB: Classical and standard score IQ standardization of the IPAT: culture free intelligence scale 2. *J Consulting Psych* 1951;15:154–159.
32. Wechsler D: *Adult Intelligence Scale Manual* (revised). New York: The Psychological Corporation, 1971.
33. Ryan CM, Morrow LA, Bromet EJ, et al.: Assessment of neuropsychological dysfunction in the workplace: normative data from the Pittsburgh Occupational Exposures Test Battery. *J Clin Exp Neuropsychol* 1987;9:665–679.
34. Wechsler D: The problem of mental deterioration. In: *The Measurement of Adult Intelligence* (3rd ed.). Baltimore, MD: Williams & Wilkins Co., 1944, pp. 54–69.
35. Potvin AR, Syndulko K, Tourtellotte WW, Lemmon JA, and Potvin JH: Human neurologic function and the aging process. *J Am Geriatrics Soc* 1980;28:1–9.
36. Potvin AR, Tourtellotte WW, Pew RW, Albers JW, Henderson WG, and Snyder DN: The importance of age effects on performance in the assessment of clinical trials. *J Chron Dis* 1973;26:699–717.
37. Parker KCH: Changes with age, year of birth cohort, age by year of birth cohort interaction, and standardization of the Wechsler intelligence tests. *Hum Dev* 1986;29:209–222.
38. Morris JF and Temple W: Spirometric ''lung age'' estimation for motivating smoking cessation. *Preventive Med* 1985;14:655–662.
39. Russell EW: A multiple scoring method for the assessment of complex memory functions. *J Consult Clin Psych* 1975;43:800–809.
40. Reed HBC and Reitan RM: A comparison of the effects of the normal aging process with the effects of organic brain-damage on adaptive abilities. *J Gerontol* 1963;18:177–179.
41. Wells CE: Chronic brain disease: an overview. *Am J Psychiatry* 1978;135:1–12.
42. Kokmen E, Beard CM, Offord KP, and Kurland LT: Prevalence of medically diagnosed dementia in a defined United States population: Rochester, Minnesota, January 1, 1975. *Neurology* 1989;39:773–776.
43. Hachinski V: Preventable senility: a call for action against the vascular dementias. *Lancet* 1992;340:645–648.
44. Stewart RB and Hale WE: Acute confusional states in older adults and the role of polypharmacy. *Annu Rev Publ Health* 1992;13:415–430.
45. Saurel-Cubizolles MJ, Estryn-Behar M, Maillard MF, Mugnier N, Masson A, and Monod G: Neuropsychological symptoms and occupational exposure to anaesthetics. *Brit J Indust Med* 1992;49:276–281.
46. Robins LN, Helzer JE, Weissman MM, et al.: Lifetime prevalence of specific psychiatric disorders in three sites. *Arch Gen Psychiatry* 1984;41:949–958.
47. Schaie KW: What can we learn from the longitudinal study of adult psychological development? In: *Longitudinal Studies of Adult Psychological Development.* New York: Guilford Press, 1983, pp. 1–39.
48. Cunningham WR and Owens WA: The Iowa State study of the adult development of intellectual abilities. In: *Longitudinal Studies of Adult Psychological Development,* KW Schaie (ed.). New York: Guilford Press, 1983, pp. 20–39.
49. Schaie KW: The Seattle longitudinal study: a 21-year exploration of psychometric intelligence in adulthood. In: *Longitudinal Studies of Adult Psychological Development.* New York: Guilford Press, 1983, pp. 64–135.
50. Palmore E: *Normal Aging.* Durham NC: Duke University Press, 1970.

51. Palmore E: *Normal Aging II.* Durham NC: Duke University Press, 1974.
52. Jarvik LF and Bank L: Aging twins: longitudinal psychometric data. In: *Longitudinal Studies of Adult Psychological Development,* KW Schaie (ed.). New York: Guilford Press, 1983, pp. 40–63.
53. Weiss B: Neurobehavioral toxicity as a basis for risk assessment. *Trends Pharm Sci* 1988; 9:59–62.
54. Talland GA: The effect of warning signals on reaction time in youth and old age. *J Gerontol* 1964;19:31–38.
55. Wechsler D: The measurement and evaluation of intelligence of older persons. In: *Old Age in the Modern World.* Edinburgh and London: E. and S. Livingstone, 1955, pp. 275–279.
56. Huppert FA and Kopelman MD: Rates of forgetting in normal ageing: a comparison with dementia. *Neuropsychologia* 1989;27:849–860.
57. Horn JL and Cattell RB: Age differences in primary mental ability factors. *J Gerontol* 1966; 21:210–220.
58. Cattell RB: The measurement of adult intelligence. *Psychological Bulletin* 1943;40:153–193.
59. Weisenburg T, Roe A, and McBride KE: *Adult-Intelligence: a Psychological Study of Test Performances.* New York: Commonwealth Fund, 1935.
60. Yerkes RM: Psychological examining in the U.S. Army men. *Natl Acad Sci* 1921;15 #2.
61. Wells FL: Army Alpha revised. *Person J* 1932;10:411–417.
62. Gould SJ: *The Mismeasure of Man.* New York: W. W. Norton, 1981.
63. Russell EW: Three patterns of brain damage on the WAIS. *J Clin Psych* 1979;35:611–620.
64. Becker CE and Lash A: Detecting subtle human CNS dysfunction: challenge for toxicologists in the 1990's. *Clin Toxicol* 1990;28:vii–xi.
65. National Research Council. *Environmental Epidemiology,* Vol. 1: *Public Health and Hazardous Wastes.* Washington, DC: National Academy Press, 1991.
66. Kilburn KH: Evidence that the human nervous system is most sensitive to environmental toxins. *Environ Carcinog Rev* (*J Environ Sci Health*) 1990–91;C8(2):327–337.
67. Mortimer JA: Epidemiological aspects of Alzheimer's disease. In: *The Aging Nervous System,* GJ Maletta and FJ Pirozzolo (eds.). New York: Praeger Publishers, 1980, pp. 307–331.
68. Kay DWK: Epidemiological aspects of organic disease in the aged. In: *Aging and the Brain,* CM Gaitz (ed.). New York: Plenum Press, 1972, pp. 13–27.
69. Henderson AS and Huppert FA: The problem of mild dementia. *Psychological Med* 1984; 14:5–11.
70. Lishman WA: *Organic Psychiatry, the Psychological Consequences of Cerebral Disorder.* Oxford: Blackwell Scientific, 1978, pp. 24–27.
71. Stern Y, Andrews H, Pittman, et al.: Diagnosis of dementia in a heterogeneous population. *Arch Neurol* 1992;49:453–460.
72. Pirozzolo FJ and Lawson-Kerr K: Neuropsychological assessment of dementia. In: *The Aging Nervous System,* GJ Maletta and FJ Pirozzolo (eds.). New York: Praeger Publishers, 1980, pp. 307–331.
73. Amante D, VanHouten VW, Grieve JH, Bader CA, and Margules P: Neuropsychological deficit, ethnicity, and socioeconomic status. *J Consult Clin Psych* 1977;45:524–535.
74. Kilburn KH and Warshaw RH: Neurobehavioral testing of subjects exposed residentially to ground water contaminated from an aluminum die-casting plant and local referents. *J Toxicol Environ Health* 1993;39:101–114.
75. Williams JR, Spencer PS, Sahl SM, et al.: Interactions of aging and environmental agents: the toxicological perspective. In: *Environmental Toxicity and the Aging Process,* SR Baker and M Rogul (eds.). New York: Alan R. Liss, 1987.
76. Ongenboer de Visser BW: Comparative study of corneal and blink reflex. In: *Motor Control Mechanisms in Health and Disease,* JE Desmedt (ed.). New York: Raven Press, 1983.
77. Anderson DR: Perimetry with and without Automation (2nd ed.). St. Louis, MO: C. V. Mosby, 1987.

APPENDIX

Reaction Time

The same subjects as tested for balance had a mean SRT of 269 ms and a CRT of 531 ms (Table 3.1). The 29 Group B subjects were similar with SRT of 282 ms and CRT of 532 ms (Table 3.2). The regression equation for the natural logarithm of SRT had no age coefficient (Table 3.3). The regression equation for CRT had an age factor, which explained 16% of the variance (Table 3.3). Using "processing time," derived by subtracting SRT from CRT, was inferior to using CRT alone.

The first validation procedure compared predicted values for Group B subjects with their observed values by a Student's paired t-test and showed no significant differences. A second procedure showed that the coefficients estimated for model Group A and those calculated for Group B were not significantly different: ln SRT ($p = 0.22$) and ln CRT ($p = 0.71$); thus coefficients from Group A worked for Group B.

Blink

The 231 subjects modeled, who were between 18 and 83 years of age, had a mean blink reflex latency R-1 (BRL R-1) after glabellar tap on the right (GT__r) of 14.5 ms and on the left (GT__1) of 14.8 ms, and that elicited by right supraorbital tap (RT__r) was 13.1 ms and left (LT__1) was 13.1 ms (Table 3.1). The 29 Group B subjects were similar for BRL, with GT__r and GT__1 13.9 ms and 13.7 ms and RT__r and Lt__1 12.6 ms and 13.4 ms (Table 3.2). The regression equation for GT__r and GT__l for women differed from that for men, but they had the same age and weight variables (not shown). The coefficients for age, age^2, gender, and weight explained 23% of the variance on the right and 30% on the left. BRL after supraorbital stimulation had a female–male difference for the single age coefficient. The variances explained by the equations were 22% and 24%, respectively (Table 3.3). Thus blink reflex latency was age- and gender-dependent. Height, strength, and educational level were not significant factors.

The validation, which compared predicted values for Group B subjects with their observed values by a Student's paired t-test, showed no significant differences. Results shown in Tables 3.3 and 3.4 and those calculated for Group B were not significantly different. Coefficients derived from Group A worked for Group B.

Color

Color discrimination was tested with both eyes open in 143 women and 117 men with the Lanthony 15 disk desaturated hue test, as calculated by the method of Bowman; and raw scores, not the square root, were used in modeling. Many subjects had perfect scores; so modeling was corrected for this distribution by transforming scores to the reciprocal of the quadratic (4th power) (Table 3.3). The constant was lower for men by 0.720×10^{-9} compared to women, but the coefficients for age, educational level, and weight were identical.

Cognitive Performance

The 260 subjects modeled for Culture Fair were between 18 and 82 years of age, had a mean score of 27.9, a vocabulary score of 23.6 (in 193), a digit symbol score of 54.9, and a block design score of 30.4 (in 253) (Table 3.1). Four subjects found to be outliers were excluded from the models. The 29 Group B subjects were similar, with a Culture Fair score of 30.4 and block design score of 30.0 (Table 3.2). Culture Fair was predicted by age and educational level, which explained 55% of the variance (Table 3.4). The regression equation for the square root of digit symbol differed for women and men and had age level factors. For men the constant was 6.092555 with the coefficients the same as for women. These coefficients explained 49% of the variance. Vocabulary also had coefficients for age and for educational level, which explained 43% of the variance. Block design had the same factors of age and educational level, which explained 8% of the variance.

The validation procedure for each of these tests compared predicted values for Group B subjects with their observed values by a Student's paired t-test, and it showed no significant differences (Table 3.4).

Recall

Verbal recall results, immediate and delayed, were linear with age and educational level, and so were modeled in 197 subjects aged 18 to 83 with mean educational level of 12.9 years. The age and educational level results differed only slightly; the constant was larger and the coefficient for educational level was smaller in delayed compared to immediate verbal recall.

Perceptual Motor Speed (PMS)

The pegboard times for 261 subjects modeled between 18 and 83 years of age were differentiated by gender because for women mean GPP was 72 seconds, whereas for men it was 79 seconds (Table 3.1). The 29 Group B women were 67.1 seconds and men 70.8 seconds (Table 3.2). The regression equations for the inverse of pegboard time (1/peg) in women and men were age-dependent (Table 3.4) with the same coefficients but a smaller constant in men. They explained 60% of the variance for women and 56% for men. In Group B the observed values and those predicted from the equations were not significantly different.

The average performance for 261 Group A subjects for TMA was 28.5 seconds, or natural logarithm (ln) 3.35 (Table 3.1). For the 29 subjects of Group B the mean was 33.3 seconds (ln 3.35 (Table 3.2). The ln (TMA) was age-dependent (Table 3.4). In this equation age explained 33% of the variance. The predicted ln (TMA) for Group B was 3.41, while the observed ln (TMA) was 3.32, values that were not significantly different ($p < 0.108$).

The average time for ln (TMB) in Group A was 72.8 seconds (ln 4.29). For the 29 subjects of Group B it was 76.8 seconds (ln 4.34). The regression equation for ln (TMB) in women was $4.237346 + 0.0128135 \times \text{age} - 0.0463335 \times \text{ed level}$ (Table 3.4). In men the constant was increased slightly to 4.322907. This equation explained 37% of the variance in both men and women. The value predicted for ln (TMB) for Group B was 4.19, which was nearly identical to the observed average of 4.22 ($p = 0.65$).

Thus, for each of the three PMS tests, comparison of predicted values for Group B subjects with their observed values by a Student's paired t-test showed no significant differences. For these tests the elapsed time (penalty) for correcting errors extended performance times. Errors as an independent measure were significant.

Memory

The regression equation for information (to the 1.5 power) had coefficients for age and educational level, differed by gender, and explained 41% of the variance (Table 3.4). The equation for picture completion score (squared) had the same age and educational level factor and differed by gender but explained only 7.5% of the variance. Similarities (squared) had a coefficient only for educational level, which explained 10% of the variance.

The predicted values for Group B subjects, when compared to observed values by a Student's paired t-test, showed no significant differences. Also, the coefficients estimated for model Group A in Table 3.4 and those calculated for Group B were not significantly different. Information, picture completion, and similarities were not administered to all groups; so further comparisons were impossible.

Children

We had three opportunities to use this neurotest battery on school children who were exposed to chemicals. The first study is described in Chapter 11 (TCE); and two studies are discussed here, where we compare the lessons learned.

Biloxi

A group of 27 students were studied, at Biloxi, Mississippi, who had attended classes in a one-story junior high school while a polyurethane roof was being laid. Earlier testing had revealed profound impairment for memory and other psychological functions in their home economics teacher; therefore, children were tested who had been in this teacher's classroom. This pilot study matched cohorts with 14 exposed and 13 comparison children from an unexposed school, aged 16 to 17 years with similar educational levels. The adult test battery was used in this group. The physiologic functions of exposed and unexposed choice reaction time and balance, as speed of sway with eyes open and with eyes closed, were not significantly different (Table 3.11). Exposed and

TABLE 3.11 Neurobehavioral test results in teenage Biloxi, Mississippi children (p values by t-test with minimal level of significance 0.05)

	Exposed	Unexposed		
	14	13		
Number	Mean Sd	Mean Sd	Difference	p
Choice Reaction Time	556 ± 127	509 ± 45	47	NS
Balance Sway Speed				
Eyes Open	1.14 ± .39	1.27 ± .51	0.13	NS
Eyes Closed	1.42 ± .55	1.40 ± .57	0.02	NS
Cognitive				
Culture Fair Total	62.6 ± 6.4	68.2 ± 5.5	3.6	NS
Block Design	29.1 ± 10.0	31.8 ± 6.0	2.7	NS
Perceptual Motor Speed				
Trails A	38.0 ± 23.8	34.1 ± 7.9	3.9	NS
Trails B	71.5 ± 30.1	65.6 ± 14.0	5.9	NS
Profile of Mood				
States Score	58.9	31.7	27.2	.0001
Depression	10.2 ± 7.2	15.2 ± 9.7	5.0	.0001

unexposed cognitive and perceptual motor speed results were also similar. Only POMS score and depression results were significantly different for exposed and unexposed students. Thus, this exposure had no effect on the students' neurobehavioral performance.

Bergholz–Steubenville

The second group of children were from a Bergholz, Ohio, elementary school that was downwind of a metal reclaiming operation where several workers had developed neurotoxic impairment. These men were scrapping dual-layer metal railroad tank cars. These cars had an inner lining that rusted through, allowing the chemical contents to escape into the fiberglass insulation between the steel layers. During metal cutting for scrapping, oxyacetylene welding torches ignited this fiberglass to produce a smoky irritating fume, which was associated with neurobehavioral impairment in the welders.

Children in the adjoining elementary school developed eye, nose, and throat irritation, together with problems of attention and memory that stimulated investigation. Comparison children were studied from the unexposed town of Steubenville, Ohio.

TABLE 3.12 Descriptive and neurobehavioral testing on 13 matched pairs of Ohio children

	Bergholz Exposed	Steubenville Unexposed
Descriptive	Mean Sd	Mean Sd
Age yrs	13.3 ± 0.5	13.2 ± 4.4
Height cm/Weight kg	64.4/139	62.9/123
Education Level	6.6 ± 0.9	6.4 ± 1.0
Grip Strength Right	31.2 ± 7.7	28.6 ± 6.7
Left	27.8 ± 8.8	26.6 ± 8.0
Pulse	72.0 ± 14.3	68.1 ± 10.8
POMS Score	22.5 ± 30.6	26.0 ± 13.0
Cognitive Functions		
Culture Fair	64.1 ± 7.0	57.3 ± 6.8
Block Design	27.5 ± 7.1	26.7 ± 8.6
Digit Symbol	55.9 ± 9.6	55.3 ± 9.7
Embedded Figures	32.0 ± 4.9	30.8 ± 4.3
Memory		
Recall of		
Story 1	12.2 ± 3.8	12.4 ± 3.7
2	8.9 ± 2.5	8.5 ± 2.8
Visual (Pictures)	10.5 ± 2.2	10.8 ± 3.2
Digits Forward	6.2 ± 1.6	6.5 ± 1.8
Backward	3.8 ± 1.1	4.4 ± 1.6
Perceptual Motor Speed		
Pegs Dominant	69.3 ± 5.4	71.3 ± 12.4
Nondominant	79.0 ± 14.5	75.8 ± 12.4
Trails A	32.2 ± 7.0	32.6 ± 10.3
Trails B	67.5 ± 18.4	68.6 ± 20.0
Finger Writing Right	2.0 ± 3.5	2.5 ± 2.1
Left	2.5 ± 3.4	2.6 ± 2.5
Long-Term Memory		
Information	12.8 ± 3.9	10.6 ± 6.0
Picture Completion	13.8 ± 2.8	14.7 ± 1.8
Similarities	19.5 ± 5.4	20.5 ± 3.1

TABLE 3.13 Neurological testing and profile of mood states for 13 matched pairs of Ohio children (no differences statistically significant)

Descriptive	Bergholz Exposed Mean ± Sd	Steubenville Referents Mean ± Sd
Simple Reaction Time 1	334 ± 62	335 ± 73
2	376 ± 88	339 ± 78
3	370 ± 90	366 ± 116
Choice Reaction Time 1	680 ± 177	624 ± 107
2	684 ± 160	628 ± 138
3	692 ± 117	651 ± 145
Body Balance (Distances inches)		
Eyes Open 1	.51 ± .17	.49 ± .12
2	.51 ± .13	.51 ± .11
3	.49 ± .15	.49 ± .14
Eyes Closed 1	.57 ± .18	.49 ± .14
2	.56 ± .17	.52 ± .12
3	.61 ± .22	.59 ± .19
POMS—Affective Status Inventory		
Tension	9.1 ± 7.2	9.7 ± 5.1
Depression	6.6 ± 7.1	9.7 ± 6.5
Anger	10.5 ± 8.0	11.4 ± 5.3
Vigor	17.0 ± 4.7	18.3 ± 5.0
Fatigue	6.3 ± 6.7	6.1 ± 4.1
Confusion	6.9 ± 3.5	7.4 ± 3.2
POMS Score	22.5 ± 30.6	26.0 ± 13.0

The 35 standard symptoms were statistically significantly more frequent in the exposed children. Because the age distributions differed for exposed and comparison children (six were under eight years in the exposed group and were unmatched) and the youngest comparison children were 12 years old, 13 age-matched pairs of 13 to 14 year olds were compared (Table 3.12). These children were cooperative and easily tested. There were no significant differences in neurobehavioral test scores between exposed and comparison children. Simple and choice reaction times and sway speed, with eyes open and closed, were nearly identical for the two groups (Table 3.13). There was no significant difference in the profile of mood states score or for the scores of its six components. Exposed children and unexposed children from the neighboring town had almost identical scores for trail making A and B. Exposed children had slightly higher scores for cognitive tests than unexposed children, but these and other test differences were not statistically significant.

From our experience with a reference group and two groups with symptoms from chemical exposures and matched unexposed subjects, it appears that these tests can be used without modification for teenage children. Subsequent study and modeling of function of the reference group, Wickenburg children, suggested that these tests should be limited to children over age 7 because of wide developmental variation in neurobehavioral function in younger children, which is not adjusted by age coefficients. Also, vocabulary and some other tests require more knowledge and longer attention spans than possessed by many younger children. This problem could be reduced by careful individual matching, by using sizable unexposed groups, or by using data from each child prior to his or her exposure.

4

Chemically Exposed Patients

It is our duty to remember at all times and anew that medicine is not only a science, but also the art of letting our own individuality interact with the individuality of the patient.

—Albert Schweitzer

INTRODUCTION

This chapter describes what has been learned from examining and testing for brain damage 269 chemically exposed subjects, 255 adults and 14 children. It introduces a spectrum of disorders associated with chemicals that, although having symptoms and signs, are mainly detected and described by making sensitive measurements of brain function. Thus, electronic timing of neurological functions in milliseconds and timing of time-tested neurobehavioral functions in seconds serve to quantify differences in performance. This strategy greatly enhances clinical descriptions in the tradition of Sydenham, Heberden, Bright, and Charcot, adding the dimension of timing of performance. Timing is as essential in describing these brain disorders as were those clinicians' elegant descriptions associated with organ abnormalities studied at autopsy, which provided the clinicopathological correlations that distinguished between many clinically confusing disorders in their eras.

Objectives

The prime objective of our investigations was to determine whether a specific test or profile of tests was associated with exposures to a chemical or class of chemicals. The second objective was to find out whether test profiles of effect were related to specific brain disorders, to guide more effective testing. Could the tests be ranked by their capacity to detect impairment, their sensitivity and specificity? A third objective was to use accumulating experience to evolve additional measurements of nervous system function. The fourth objective was to use the chemical effect profiles to enhance our insight into the human central nervous system.

Methods of testing are outlined in Chapter 3, by which a clinical picture of the brain disorders can be elaborated. Investigators must have an understanding of all parts of this medical puzzle to comprehend the argument that many familiar, even commonplace, chemicals generally considered to be safe are damaging the human brain.

OBJECTIVE 1: ASSOCIATING PATTERNS OF DYSFUNCTION TO CHEMICALS

What is new in this investigation is the use of sensitive measurements to detect impairment earlier than previously was possible. Chemical brain damage is not new. Bernardino Ramazzini and Lewis Carroll wrote about madness or devastating brain disease from mercury exposure, and Hippocrates, Benjamin Franklin, Donald Hunter, and others attributed brain damage in workers to exposures to lead, manganese, arsenic, and carbon disulfide. This new age of chemical neurotoxicity is evidenced in people exposed mainly by inhalation at home or as bystanders at work or in the community. Central nervous system (CNS) poisons are everywhere. When they do not kill, these chemicals produce two major patterns: (1) incidents of painful and perplexing brain injuries and disabilities; and (2) the insidious erosion of function, as if aging were hastened, sometimes by decades.

Assembling the Puzzle

In analyzing the ongoing process of chemical impairment, evaluation of the 255 adult patients allows us to make some generalizations; and more patterns have emerged from the encephalopathy associated with specific chemicals and chemical mixtures. As we have attempted to assemble a large mosaic from single facts and clusters of findings and their associations, a picture has emerged. In developing methods for generalizing and learning from these patients' experiences, we have emphasized classification, subdividing the patients by specific chemical exposure and then examining prevalences of test abnormalities. Certain physiological methods discriminated exposed persons from unexposed normal ones the best: balance testing, reaction time, measurements of blink reflex latency, hearing acuity, and mapping visual fields. The impairment needed defining criteria; so associations between sensitive tests were examined by making comparisons of patients' test results to their expected performance. Studies repeated at six months or after longer intervals defined the course of the disorder when possible. We applied clinical judgment consisting of intuition, deduction, guesses, speculation, and what cardiologist Sam Levine called destructive differential diagnosis, a ruling-out based on pivotal exclusions. Often when observations did not fit generally accepted concepts, we recalled George Gershwin's' classic advice that "It ain't necessarily so."

Comparing Chemically Exposed Patients to Populations

Lessons from individual patients were corrected and refined by analyses of populations, groups sharing chemical exposures. The composite wisdom emerged that neurobehavioral dysfunction is caused by chemicals common to contemporary human environments, especially indoors. Such injury from chemical exposure incidents is random, common, not often attributed to chemicals, and frequently misdiagnosed. More often it is labeled with one of the popular tags, old age and stress being probably the most frequent ones. Psychasthenia, hysteria, somatization (disorder), and post-traumatic stress are other worn labels. Curiously, the patient often defies being labeled, and the physician admits as much, but this realization is seldom followed by appropriate inquiry.

An initially perplexing discovery was that several irritant gases—previously considered to be fatal in large doses but only to cause temporary problems at lesser ones—caused permanent injuries. A possible explanation for delayed recognition is that months or years may elapse from exposure to brain damage, as if a pathogen were incubating.

The Group of Clinic Patients

For comparison to chemically exposed populations the 255 diverse adult patients were considered as a group. They were an average of 43.9 years old with 13.1 years of educational achievement (Table 4.1), similar to populations exposed to chemicals (Table 4.2). More men than women were seen as patients (55 45%), whereas the ratio was reversed in the exposed populations. The 14 children were too few and too scattered in the chemical groups for us to determine if they are more sensitive to exposure than adults. Most clinic patients were from California, with 18 from Louisiana, 16 from Nevada, 6 each from Texas and Ohio, 30 from 10 other states, and 5 from foreign countries.

Over the same interval over 3,600 exposed people were studied by using these methods in epidemiological investigations. In four groups of 659 subjects (Table 4.2), impairment was attributed to arsenic trioxide, chlordane, and ''most plausibly causal known neurotoxic agents,'' trichloroethylene and toluene (Figures 4.1a–d). The other six populations were exposed to hydrogen sulfide, chlorine, hydrochloric acid, polychlorinated biphenyls, aluminum remelting, and diesel exhaust. The single-agent studies extended the scope of the known effects of the four chemicals studied, from their role as neurotoxins for insects and experimental animals to their effects on humans.

The 255-member adult patient group averaged one more year of education than other

TABLE 4.1 Descriptive information on 255 adult subjects

			Mean	Standard Deviation	Minimum	Maximum
Age yrs			43.9	11.8	19	77
Educational Level yrs			13.1	3.3	0	24
Women			116			
Men			139			
Women	Height cm		164.6	25.1	141.0	189.0
	Weight kg		72.1	18.9	45.9	159.1
Men	Height cm		174.3	7.7	154.9	193.0
	Weight kg		86.1	18.0	56.8	165.9
Women	Grip kg	Right	27.5	8.0	6	50
		Left	25.2	8.5	7	50
Men	Grip kg	Right	47.2	16.0	3	80
		Left	46.1	14.6	3	84

TABLE 4.2 Comparison of 135 clinic patients exposed to many chemicals and four populations exposed to a predominant chemical

	Clinic Patients		Trichloroethylene Phoenix		Toluene Combustion		Arsenic Bryan		Chlordane Houston	
	255		237		131		75		216	
	Mean	Sd	Mean	Sd	Mean	Sd	Mean	Sd	Mean	Sd
Age yrs	43.9	11.8	51.8	17.6	40.5	14.1	45.3	16.0	32.9	11.4
Ed Level yrs	13.1	3.3	12.2	2.7	11.1	2.3	12.0	3.4	11.5	2.1
Simple Reaction ms	393	186	334	118	328	112	341	124	414	235
Choice Reaction ms	650	209	618	153	575	108	593	177	639	226
Sway Balance cm/sec										
Eyes Open	1.05	0.62	0.87	0.49	0.96	0.31	0.92	0.47	0.95	0.35
Eyes Closed	2.00	1.38	1.59	0.77	1.49	0.57	1.43	0.72	1.48	0.60
Blink Reflex Latency R-1 ms										
Right	13.6	2.0	14.2	2.1	14.7	1.9	13.8	2.3	13.5	2.3
Left	13.4	2.2	13.9	2.1	14.9	1.9	13.7	2.2	13.2	2.3
Culture Fair A	25.6	7.9	23.5	9.0	24.3	8.8	25.0	9.0	25.4	8.1
Block Design	27.4	10.2			31.0	9.4				
Vocabulary	20.7	11.1	19.3	9.4			18.2	11.7	16.0	7.7
Perceptual Motor Speed										
Pegboard sec	86.7	40.4	88.0	29.9	81.0	26.4	79.1	21.3	76.1	20.5
Trails A sec	43.8	30.3	44.3	22.2	38.5	22.8	42.3	23.3	44.7	19.4
Trails B sec	98.7	53.1	99.7	43.5	86.8	38.4	88.7	39.4	93.1	37.1
Verbal Recall	17.0	6.8	17.8	6.5	17.4	6.4	17.5	6.4	16.9	6.4
Stories 1 & 2										
Finger Writing										
Right	3.8	4.0	2.6	3.2	2.4	2.9			2.9	3.5
Left	3.2	3.8	2.2	2.8	2.0	3.2			2.4	3.4
Embedded Memory										
Information	17.3	5.9	17.9	5.6	14.4	4.8	16.7	6.4	13.1	5.9
Picture Completion	14.4	3.6	14.4	3.0	14.9	4.0	14.2	4.1	13.2	3.9
Similarities	20.3	5.1	19.8	4.6	18.8	6.3	18.6	6.6	16.6	5.9
POMS sc	81.7	42.2	50.5	39.3	56.2	39.9	48.0	37.7	72.2	43.6
Depression	20.8	13.1	14.2	11.9	15.5	12.4	14.1	11.7	20.7	14.4

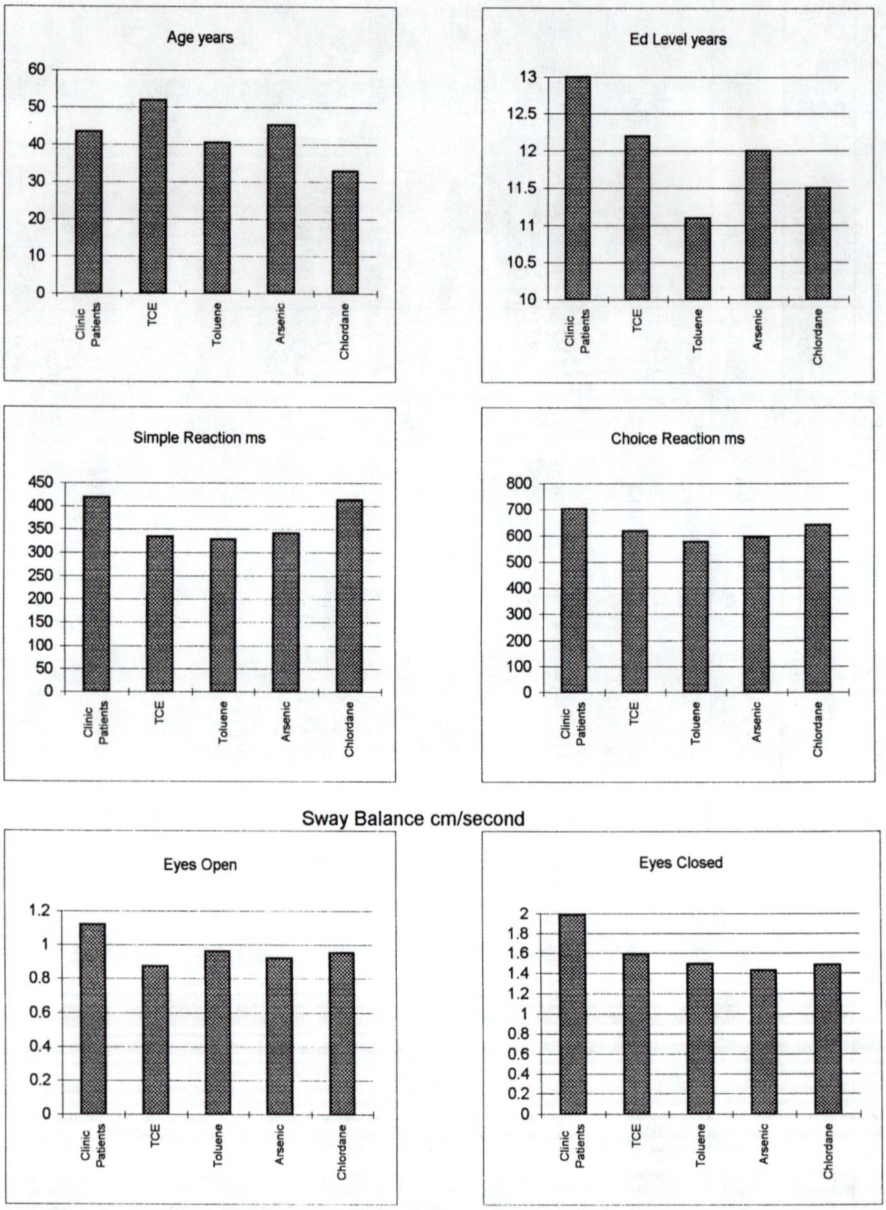

FIGURE 4.1a. Comparison of clinic patients to four populations exposed to a predominant chemical.

groups. They had many different chemical exposures, but their average simple reaction time nearly matched that of the chlordane group, whereas choice reaction time and balance speed of sway, measured with eyes closed and with eyes open, were more abnormal in this group than in the other groups. The patients' blink reflex latency values, delay in the first electromyographic signal for eye closure, were slower than those exposed to toluene but faster than those for the trichloroethylene-exposed groups and those for persons exposed to arsenic, which specifically impairs the trigeminal-

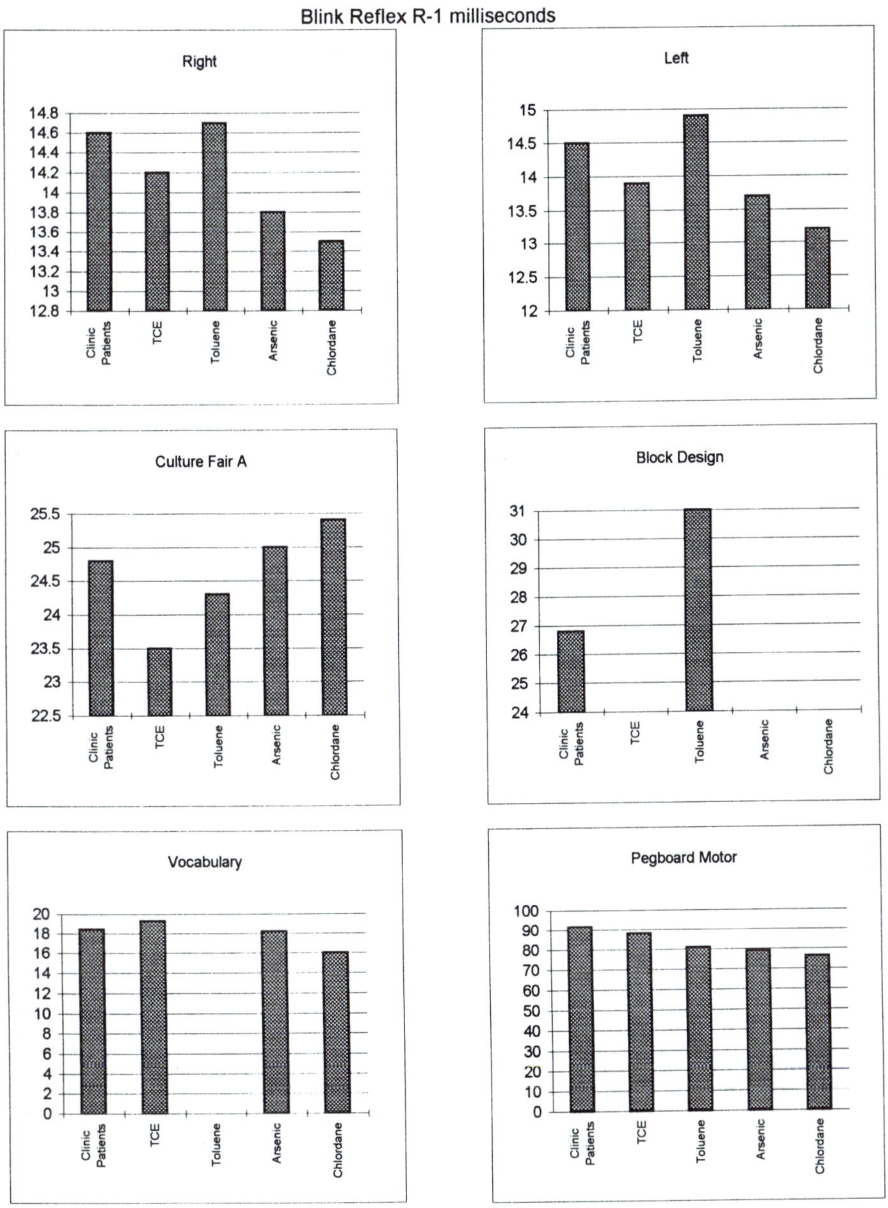

FIGURE 4.1b. Comparison of clinic patients to four populations exposed to a predominant chemical.

pons-facial nerve path as well as peripheral nerves. In contrast, chlordane had no effect on blink. Clinic patients' POMS scores, including the depression score, exceeded those of the population groups, which is best explained by their being self-selected.

Scores on tests in other domains showed that the clinic patients were similar to the four chemically exposed populations. This generalization applies to Culture Fair and vocabulary but not to block design in the cognitive domain, and to the perceptual motor speed domain of pegboard, trails A and trails B, and to finger writing errors. Scores

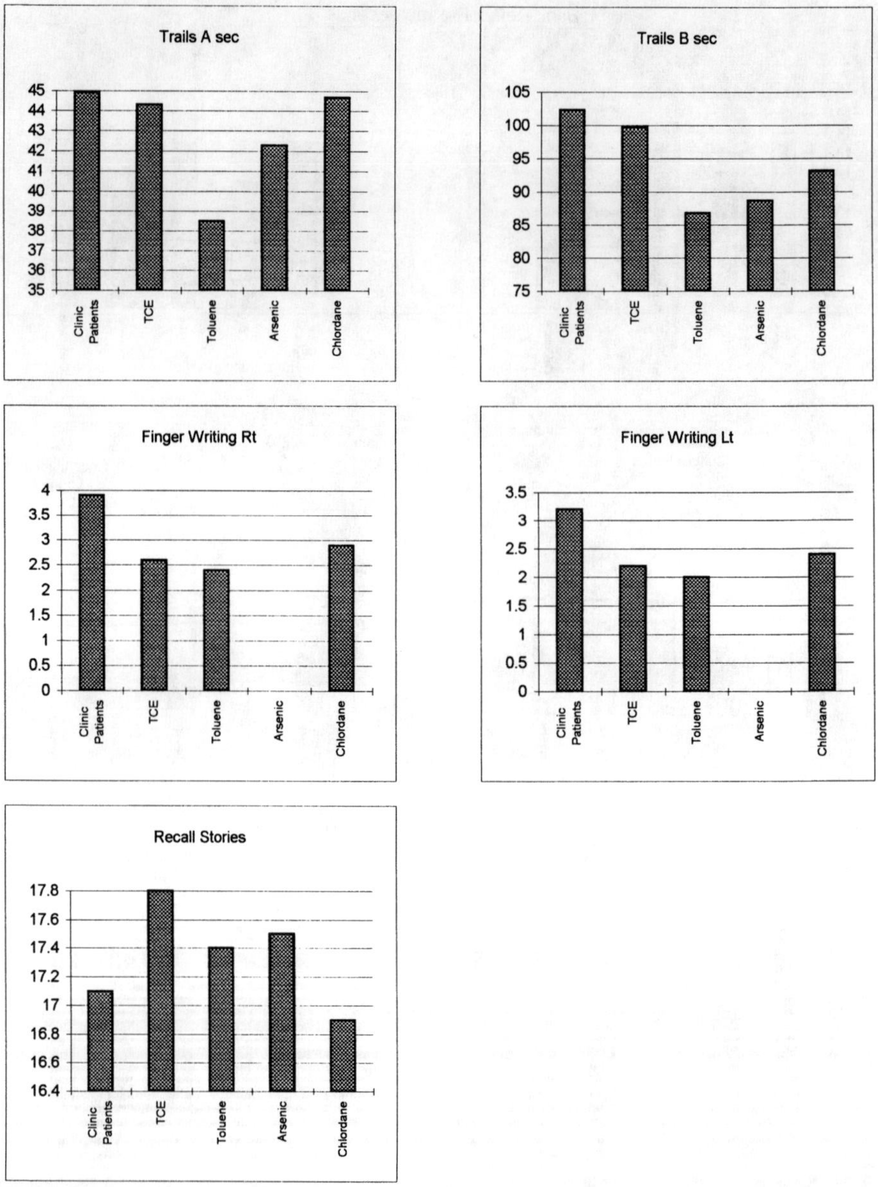

FIGURE 4.1c. Comparison of clinic patients to four populations exposed to a predominant chemical.

for verbal recall of stories were also nearly identical for the five groups. The embedded memory tests were equal to the others' results or slightly higher for the clinic patients with their greater educational attainment, confirming that these most intact, least chemically affected, functions were appropriate for endowment as measured by educational attainment. The distributions of test scores of the clinic patients as a group were bell-shaped, as were the distributions for each exposed population. There was no evidence of chemicals selecting sensitive subjects on one edge of the distribution. These neurotoxic

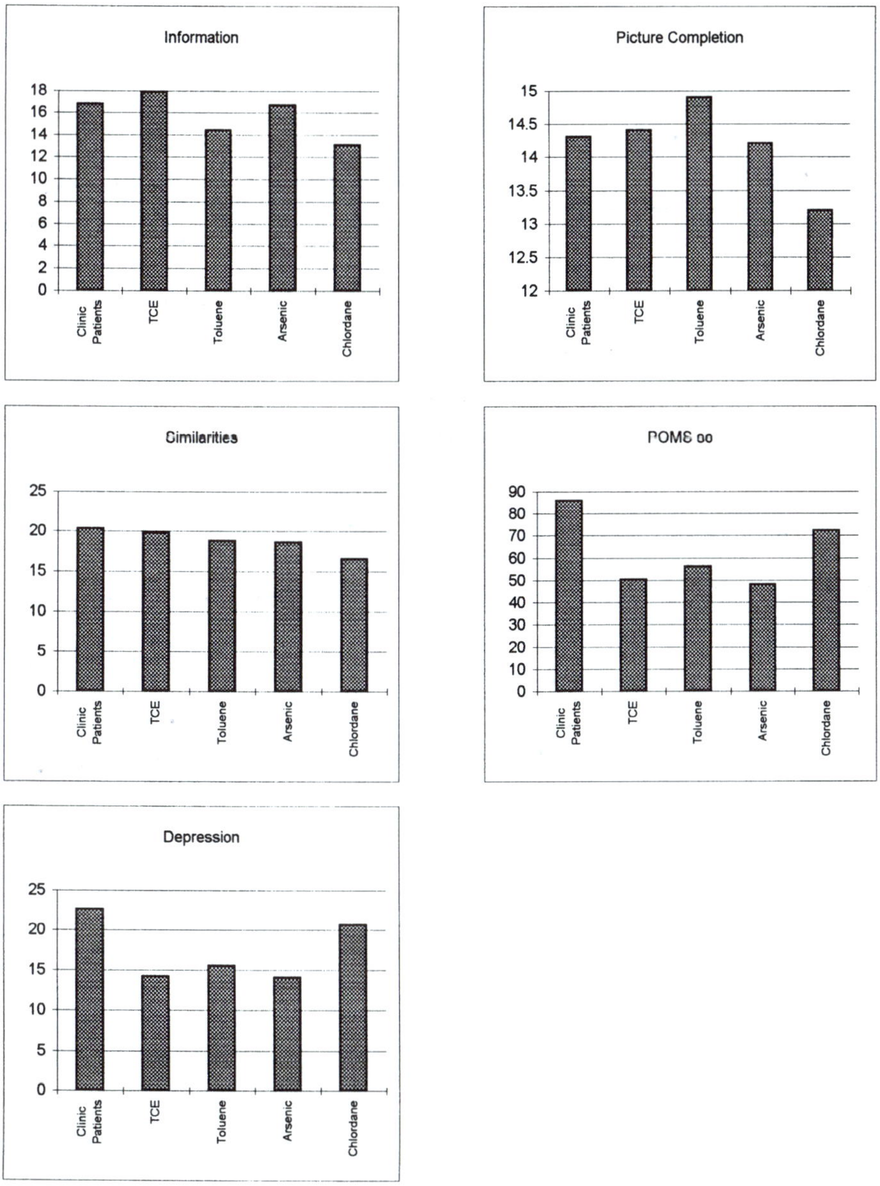

FIGURE 4.1d. Comparison of clinic patients to four populations exposed to a predominant chemical.

chemicals impaired brain function similarly in all groups, as occurs with the aging of "normal" subjects.

Half of these patients were referred for diagnosis by attorneys. The remainder were referred by physicians, other patients, or themselves. Distress from brain damage, when it was recognized by physicians, often was considered to be due to a psychiatric illness. Attributing a patient's brain damage to chemical exposure seemed difficult, for other physicians and, initially, for me.

Clinical Recognition and Attribution to Chemicals

Patients recognized that they had been hurt and often associated their problems with chemical exposures. They had accepted their distress as the flu, ''extreme fatigue,'' or aging. Their feeling badly immediately or quite soon after a chemical exposure incident helped them see or presume a relationship more easily than was possible after months or years of insidious illness, which eroded perception, logical thought, recall, memory, cognitive function, balance, and vision. Delay in recognition of illness as different typically took years. Long gradual deterioration made associations more tenuous and uncertain and connections difficult. Thus, when the temporal linkage is close and the exposure incident is dramatic, it *is* ''the cause,'' especially if competing causes are absent or trivial. ''After, therefore, because of'' attributions to chemical exposure (''post hoc ergo proter hoc''), which are probable in life, are doubted by many medical practitioners. They forget how much detective work was required to relate Legionnaire's disease or Lyme disease or AIDS to their causes. In the absence of ''hot pursuit'' evidence, disorders with longer incubation periods, such as lung cancer from asbestos, radiation, and cigarette smoking, are considered impossible to explain.

Traditional physicians reject an unexpected ''possible cause'' of illness just as a novel antigen is rejected by the immune system. Reflexive denial is an unconscious but time-tested coping method. The spirit of inquiry blesses too few of us, despite our giving lip-service to it. A diagnosis of psychiatric illness, another denial mechanism, invokes the ''brain mystery'' to explain what is un-understandable. Ergo, dismiss the patient with a strange new illness into the sea of ''unfathomable psychiatric illness.''

Exposures to Chemical Mixtures

There were 24 major probable chemicals to which more than one patient of the 269 (including children) was exposed (Table 4.3) and 12 organic chemical mixtures. Twenty-six patients were ''indoor-air''-exposed, fifteen patients were exposed to a massive outdoor diesel fire (a mini–Gulf War), and seven locomotive mechanics and six electricians were exposed to diesel exhaust indoors (considered in detail in Chapter 14). Eight patients had inhaled organic waste chemicals, six exposures were to welding fumes, and five were exposed to evaporating gasoline, five to epoxy systems, and five to photographic chemicals. In only six patients was impairment associated with contaminated water supplies. The major common thread in these exposures was the combustion or vaporization of petroleum products. Unfortunately, exposure to chemical mixtures provided few clues for causation of brain damage or of specific CNS impairment; however, estimating the potential for harm from exposures to mixtures of chemicals is a real-world problem. Clearly, unequivocal causal attribution, even to major chemicals in mixtures, will continue to be difficult; so a ''more likely than not'' attribution is the practical approach. Patients who have had a single-incident exposure to just one chemical provide the strongest basis for causal associations.

Chemicals and Patterns

One hundred fifty-seven patients had a predominant chemical exposure: formaldehyde in 20, hydrogen sulfide in 19, organophosphates in 10, chlordane in 10, chlorine in 14, PCBs in 7, trichloroethylene and 1,1,1-trichloroethane in 7 each. Pyrethrins were in 5,

TABLE 4.3 Major chemicals or mixtures associated with chemical encephalopathy in 266 patients

Major Chemicals	*n*	Major Chemical Mixtures	*n*
Formaldehyde	20	Indoor air	26
Hydrogen sulfide	19	Diesel exhaust	16
Organophosphates (Dursban)	19	Diesel/gasoline fire	15
Chlorine (HCl)	14	Waste chemicals	88
Chlordane	10	Chemicals ignited by welding	6
PCBs	7	Water supply	6
Trichloroethylene	7	Fires	6
1,1,1-Trichloroethane	7	Gasoline	5
Pyrethrins	5	Epoxy	5
Styrene monomer	4	Spray paint	5
Methyl bromide	4	Photographic chemicals	5
Vinyl chloride	4	Benzene, toluene, 1,3 butadiene	5
Ammonia	3	Sodium sulfur battery fire	1
Cadmium	3		
Nitrogen tetroxide	3		
Carbon monoxide	3		
Ethylene dichloride	3		
Thiophene, *n*-hexane	3		
Cyanide	2		
Silane	2		
Polyurethane	2		
Hydrochloric acid	2		
Manganese	2		
Mercury	2		
Sodium azide	1		
Vinyl acetate	1		
Atrazine (herbicide)	1		
Dripolene	1		
n-Hexane	1		

and styrene monomer, methyl bromide, and vinyl chloride each had 4 patients. No subject's examination was characteristic of a ''spontaneous'' neurological disorder (1–3). As experience accrued, the plausibility of associations increased, and randomness decreased so that order emerged, especially for gases—previously classified as irritants—that damage the nervous system: formaldehyde, chlorine, hydrogen chloride, hydrogen sulfide, ammonia, nitrogen tetroxide, and vinyl chloride monomer.

Matches between these chemicals and patterns of test abnormality began when exposed subjects' scores were significantly different from the composite reference group defined in Chapter 3. Patterns emerged for patients exposed to the same chemical so that the generalizations have predictive capacity, which improves with larger groups.

Patterns Observed

Specific patterns of impairment from particular chemicals seemed a plausible expectation. Analysis was started with 10 to 20 patients exposed to hydrogen sulfide, chlordane, chlorine, diesel exhaust-aldehydes, and formaldehyde (Table 4.4; Figures 4.2a–d). Tentative patterns observed extended those patterns described before (1, 4), and some variance between chemicals encouraged these evaluation efforts. Tests were grouped

TABLE 4.4 Comparison of test profiles of patients with five chemical exposures, percentage of subjects in category with abnormality

	Hydrogen Sulfide	Chlordane	Chlorine	Diesel	Formaldehyde
Number	19	10	14	10	20
Age (years)	41.5	44.3	31.6	56.4	50.0
Ed Level	12.7	12.8	11.0	12.9	15.9
Physiological					
Sway Eyes Open	57++	33	60++	20	25
Sway Eyes Closed	79+++	67++	90++++	60++	63++
Simple Reaction	43	33	60++	60++	38
Choice Reaction	57++	44+	60++	70++	63++
Blink Supraorbital Tap					
Right ms	50+	13	40+	75+++	100++++
Left ms	43+	50++	50++	75+++	100++++
Cognitive Function					
Culture Fair	50++	50++	50++	100++++	63++
Block Design	57++	22	40+	ND	75+++
Digit Symbol	50++	20	30	ND	50++
Vocabulary	60++	22	50++	75+++	0
Perceptual Motor					
Pegboard	29	33	10	13	38
Trails A	29	44	10	75+++	38
Trails B	64++	33	30	75+++	63++
Fingerwriting Errors	64++	33	10	100++++	50++
Recall of Stories	64++	56++	60++	75+++	63++
Embedded Memory					
Information	36	13	20	ND	17
Picture Completion	29	0	10	ND	17
Similarities	29	0	0	ND	17
Affective Status					
Symptom Frequency	75+++	56++	80+++	78+++	87+++
POMS Score	57++	88+++	100++++	26	75+++
Depression	79+++	75++	100++++	43+	50++

≤49 = + 75–89 = +++
50–74 = ++ ≥90 = ++++

somewhat arbitrarily into six functional domains: physiological, cognitive, perceptual motor speed, recall, embedded memory, and affective (5). The embedded memory domain was most resistant to the chemicals, as described by Ryan et al. (5, 6).

Hydrogen sulfide's effects were on balance, choice reaction time, and blink, and it did not affect embedded memory; also cognitive (Culture Fair), recall (stories), perceptual motor speed (trail making B and finger writing), and affective (POMS score and frequencies of symptoms) domains were impaired. The formaldehyde pattern was most similar to that of hydrogen sulfide; BRL R-1 (blink) was prolonged in all subjects. Chlorine had greater impact on the physiological measures than psychological ones, particularly balance but little effect on perceptual motor speed. Diesel exhaust contains aldehydes, but there may have been exposure to trichloroethylene in the locomotive mechanics though not in train crewmen; the railroad workers showed impaired balance, reaction time, and BRL R-1 (blink). There also were large reductions in cognitive function, perceptual motor speed, and recall from diesel exposure, but there was little impact on affective status. Chlordane, like hydrogen sulfide, affected principally the physiological domain (balance, reaction time, and blink) plus Culture Fair in the cogni-

⇒ GLYCOSALATION (Sugar binding of Protein)

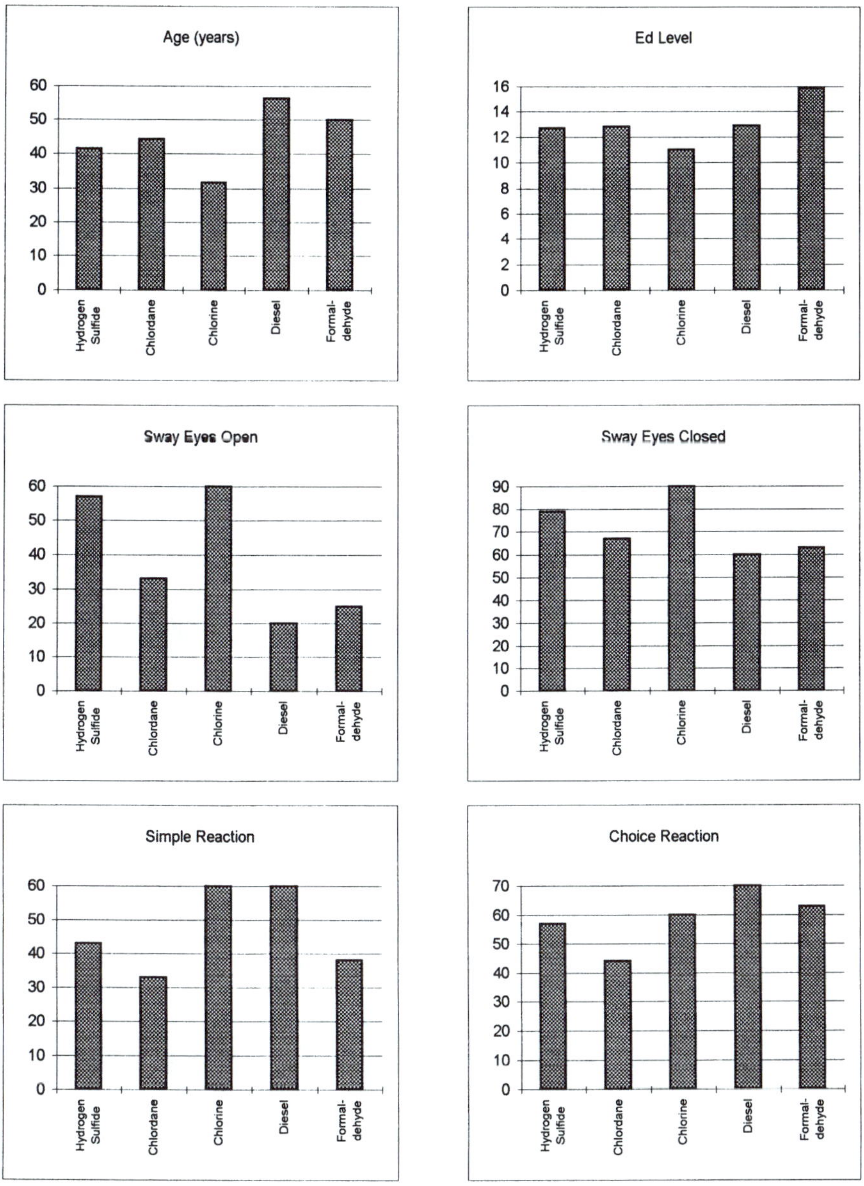

FIGURE 4.2a. Comparison of five chemical exposures in clinic patients by ANOVA. Value is percent abnormal.

tive domain and story in the recall domain, but had a large impact on the affective domain. The pattern of chlordane most resembled that of chlorine except for its minimal effect on blink and visual fields. Whether or not characteristic patterns emerge for such chemicals as ammonia, phenol, sodium azide, cadmium, and others with addition of more patients, the generalization is of a theme with variations rather than distinct patterns.

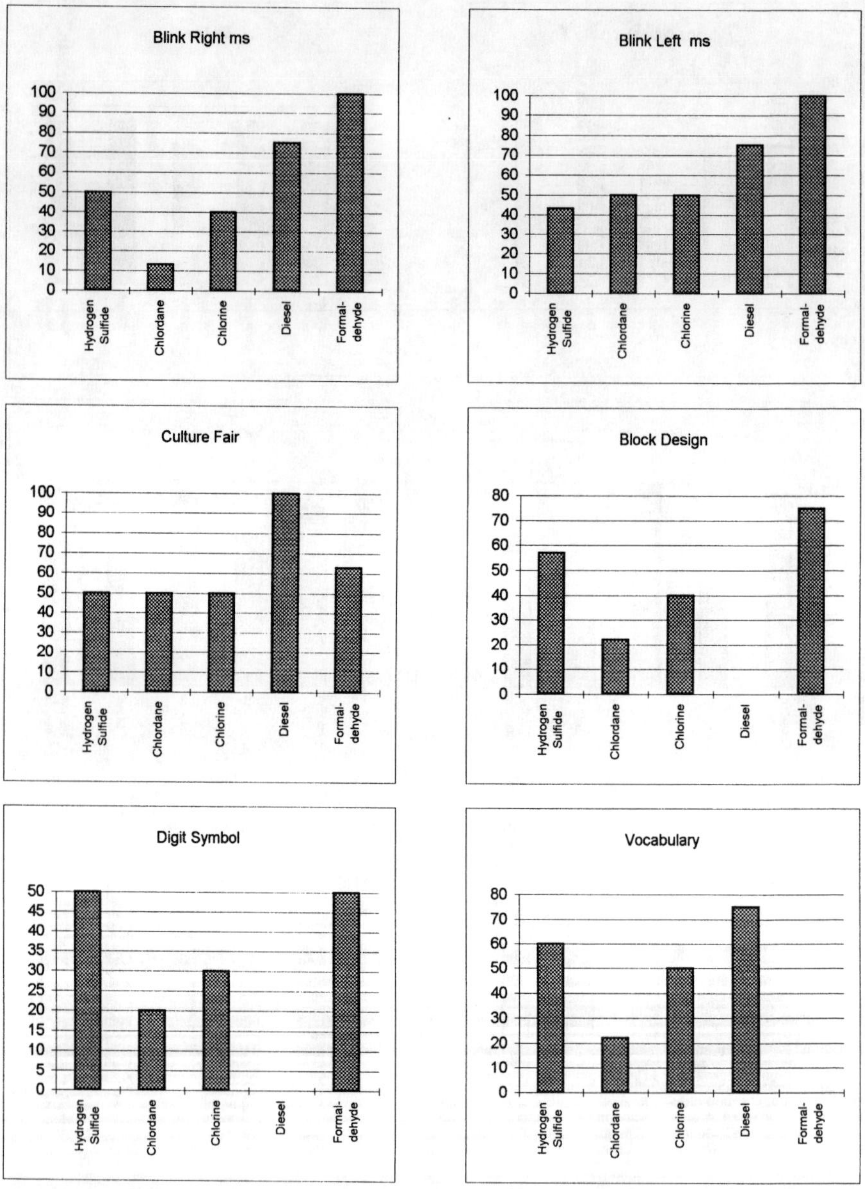

FIGURE 4.2b. Comparison of five chemical exposures in clinic patients by ANOVA. Value is percent abnormal.

OBJECTIVE 2: TESTING TO DETECT IMPAIRMENT

The second objective was to determine the relative sensitivity of these tests. The distribution of people by their numbers of abnormal tests is logarithmic (Table 4.5). Thus, 34 of the 255 consecutive unselected chemically exposed adults had no or one abnormality and were eliminated, leaving 222 patients. The minimal list of the most sensitive

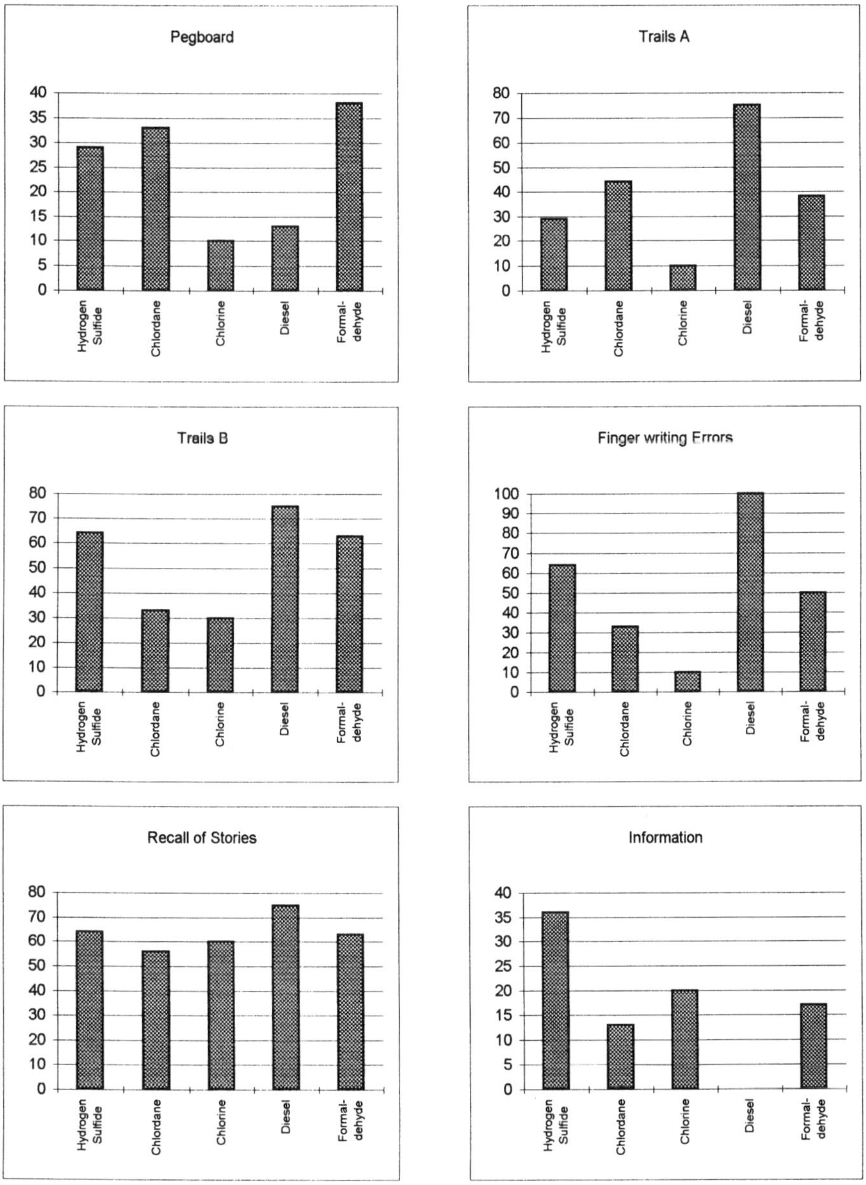

FIGURE 4.2c. Comparison of five chemical exposures in clinic patients by ANOVA. Value is percent abnormal.

tests for ''economical'' recognition of impairment and/or diagnosis compares exposed subjects to unexposed, expressed as percentage of predicted (Table 4.6). Sway with eyes closed heads the list, followed by choice reaction time, sway with eyes open, simple reaction time, digit symbol, visual performance right eye and then left eye, vocabulary, peg placement, grip (strength) left, Culture Fair, trail making A, grip right, hearing right, immediate verbal recall, trail making B and delayed verbal recall, down to 20%.

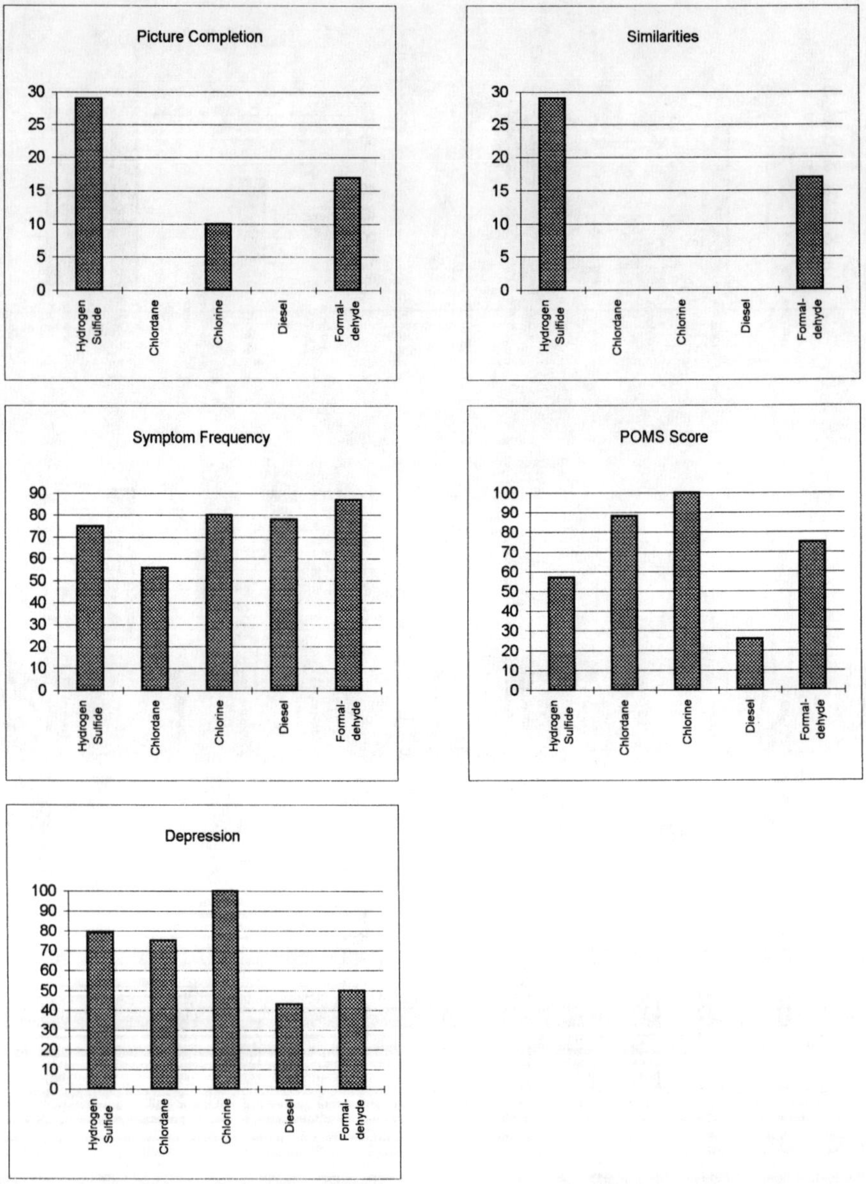

FIGURE 4.2d. Comparison of five chemical exposures in clinic patients by ANOVA. Value is percent abnormal.

The prevalence of each abnormality, defined by values that are more than one and a half standard deviations from the mean of the referent group, provided a second ranking (applied in Table 4.7 to the initial 115) after the 30 patients with no or one abnormality were dropped. For the 115 subjects with at least two abnormal tests, the prevalences, seen in the first column, were simple reaction time (58%), choice reaction time (55%), balance with the eyes open (48%), recall of stories (45%), vocabulary (44%), balance with eyes closed (43%), placing pegs in a pegboard (38%), Culture

TABLE 4.5 Frequency of abnormalities among adults

Number of Abnormalities	Number of Patients	Percent
0	12	4.7
1	22	8.6
2	26	10.2
3	17	6.6
4	20	7.8
5	19	7.4
6	25	9.8
7	11	4.3
8	16	6.3
9	9	3.5
10	13	5.1
11	12	4.7
12	10	3.9
13	8	3.1
14	10	3.9
15	7	2.7
16	5	2.0
17	6	2.3
18	4	1.6
19	1	0.4
20	1	0.4
22	1	0.4
25	1	0.4

Fair score (31%), trail making A (30%), blink reflex latency after left supraorbital tap (29%), and trail making B (27%). Other tests were positive in less than 20% of the patients.

The 96 patients with four abnormalities, seen in the second column, had similar rankings to those in the first column, but rank order changed more. The 23 patients with 10 or more abnormal tests, mainly peg placement, Culture Fair, trail making, and vocabulary, moved upward suggesting that when chemical injury is extensive, these cognitive and perceptual motor speed abnormalities are nearly universally abnormal. Equally important, the abnormalities of embedded memory functions, picture completion, and similarities (information not shown) remain infrequent and consistent with their reflecting preexposure mental capacity as formed by others (5).

A third strategy is to combine two or more tests to pick the abnormality (diagnose), comparing those subjects selected by this combination to those abnormal on a majority of tests. This approach worked best when the selection or key tests were balance with the eyes closed, choice reaction time, and blink reflex latency R-1 (after supraorbital taps). When the three key tests were abnormal—that is, scores of each were outside the mean plus or minus 1.5 standard deviation (see Chapter 3)—patients had three or more additional abnormal tests, and they often had ten or more. Patients with two of three key tests abnormal were definitely impaired and had more abnormalities than this group's average. Substitution of Culture Fair A, trail making B, or fingertip number writing errors for any key test reduced the certainty of selection. The POMS score was always greater than 50 when two key tests were abnormal; so it did not aid selection. The greatest discrepancy from hypothesized rankings was for blink reflex latency,

TABLE 4.6 Tests on clinic adults in order of percentage of group that were abnormal

		Percentage Abnormal
Sway—Balance Eyes Closed		53.8
Choice Reaction Time		42.7
Sway—Balance Eyes Open		39.9
Simple Reaction Time		39.1
Digit Symbol sc		37.8
Visual Performance	Right	37.7
	Left	32.9
Vocabulary sc		30.1
Peg Placement sec		27.7
Grip Strength kg Left		26.9
Culture Fair A sc		25.5
Trail Making A sc		25.3
Grip Strength kg Right		24.2
Hearing Right		23.6
Verbal Recall Immediate sc		23.6
Trail Making B		21.1
Verbal Recall Delayed		20.1
Hearing Left		17.4
Information sc		17.1
Picture Completion sc		15.2
Supraorbital Tap ms Left		11.9
Finger Writing Errors Left		11.7
Supraorbital Tap Right		8.7
Finger Writing Errors Right		8.5
Similarities sc		4.5
Color Discrimination	Left	1.5
	Right	1.0

which required deviations greater the 1.5 times the standard to trigger abnormal, which may be too liberal a criterion. Experience suggests that BRL R-1 may be highly sensitive for particular chemicals, such as TCE and formaldehyde.

OBJECTIVE 3: NEW TESTS FOR OTHER FUNCTIONS

One novel test, blink reflex latency, and two standard tests applied in new ways, visual fields by automated perimetry and hearing by audiometry, appeared to be of great value as experience was gained. As these tests were introduced after the initial 45 patients, the experience with them is less than that with balance or reaction time. Blink reflex latency R-1 (BRL R-1), the delay of electromyographic (EMG) R-1, has been associated with trichloroethylene exposures (7). The BRL R-1 was abnormal in 62% of these consecutive patients after exposure to many different chemicals (Table 4.8; column 2). Also, as described above, this is a sensitive indicator, joining balance and choice reaction time as an ''early'' abnormality detector after a single chemical exposure or after ''relatively light'' prolonged exposures. Blink latency of R-1 after a glabellar tap was

TABLE 4.7 Comparison of rank order by percentage of subjects with each test abnormality grouped as two or more, compared with four or more and with ten or more abnormalities

Number of Abnormalities	2	4	10
Number of Patients	115	96	23
1 Simple Reaction Time	58	65	94
2 Choice Reaction Time	55	57	77
3 Sway Speed Eyes Open	48	53	70
4 Stories	45	49	71
5 Vocabulary	44	50	67
6 Sway Speed Eyes Closed	43	44	63
7 Pegboard	38	46	83
8 Culture Fair A	31	37	77
9 Trail Making A	30	33	78
10 Supraorbital Tap Left	29	35	28
11 Trail Making B	27	32	57
12 Block Design	20	23	36
13 Supraorbital Tap Right	18	20	14
14 Glabellar Tap Left	17	22	25
15 Glabellar Tap Right	15	18	44
16 Picture Completion	12	15	29
17 Similarities	5	6	14
18 Color Score	4	3	—

TABLE 4.8 Blink latency and visual fields abnormality and patterns

	Number Tested	Abnormal Blink RL	Any Abnormality of Visual Fields	Scotoma	Enlarged Blind Spot	Nerve Fiber	Constricted
Chlorine	7	5	5	5	2	1	1
Formaldehyde	5	4	4	2	1		1
Hydrogen sulfide	3	2	2	1	1		
Vinyl chloride	3	2	2			2	
Cadmium	2	2	2				2
Organophosphates	2	2	2	2	1	1	
Methyl bromide	2	2	2	1	1		1
Epoxy	2	0	2		1	1	1
Carbon monoxide	1	1	1				1
Indoor air	1	1	0				
Dripolene	1	1	1				1
Manganese	1	0	1			1	
Hypoxia	1	0	1				1
Ammonia	3	1	1				1
Chlordane	2	0	1	1	1		
Gasoline	3	1	0				
	39	24	27	12	8	6	10

abnormal in 89% of patients with abnormal visual fields. Their mean values were highly abnormal, 16.0 ms right and 16.1 ms left versus 14.5 ms right and 14.6 ms left in unexposed. More chemicals were associated with delay of BRL R-1 than had been suspected earlier, even if there were some errors of attribution in selecting the ''most responsible chemical'' from multiple exposures for some patients. Finally, patients whose blink was unaffected by a given chemical were usually the least exposed, were younger (often in their twenties), and were tested relatively early, weeks or months after exposure, perhaps before the full injury pattern had developed.

Chlorine and the TCE-related chlorine-containing chemicals vinyl chloride and trichloroethane are the major chemicals previously known to delay BRL R-1. Formaldehyde, cadmium fumes, silanes, ammonia and ammonium thiocyanate, and organophosphorus compounds (Dursban and Diazinon) delay blink R-1. Only the organophosphorus compounds are chlorinated. In contrast, gasoline (containing toluene as a major neurotoxicant), manganese, epoxy systems (resins and accelerators), air supply contaminants, and nickel cadmium battery fumes do not lengthen BRL R-1.

Visual Field Defects: Correlations with Chemicals

Visual fields testing to 30° by computerized automated perimetry using Allergan-Humphrey or BioRad devices showed that defects in the central 30° zones of the retina were frequent. They consisted of single and/or multiple scotoma, enlarged blind spots, arcuate scotoma or nerve fiber defects, and constricted fields (Table 4.8; columns 3–7). Visual field defects were found in 71% of the last 38 subjects tested. Blink abnormality frequently accompanied visual field defects; thus of these 38 only 4 had normal visual fields and 4 had normal blink.

Nerve fiber defects, also called Bejreens scotoma, occurred in 6; isolated scotoma was found in 12; and enlarged blind spots occurred in 8, often with scattered scotomata. Constricted fields were associated with cadmium exposure in two patients, and in one patient each with epoxy, chlordane, chlorine, formaldehyde, ammonia, methyl bromide, dripolene, carbon monoxide, and hypoxia. Chlorine-exposed patients had the highest prevalence of visual field defects, but other observations of these defects are fragmentary. Observation of abnormalities in nearly 70% of chemically exposed patients tested promotes visual fields to one of the most sensitive tests, joining reaction times and balance. Other patient groups should be assessed to extend these tentative observations. The possibility that these defects are spurious or were the result of malingering seems unlikely because of the high association rates with other CNS abnormalities, as well as worsening on interval retesting and the plausibility of the defects (i.e., absence of central scotomata and demonstration of the blind spots).

Although the visual field defects appear to be retinal, the pattern of damage from methyl alcohol, a well-studied poison, should caution us that occipital cortical lesions occur from poisons and may not be differentiated from retinal ones for some time. Also, these lesions may occur together.

Tests Correlated with Visual Fields

Visual fields defects had a small age coefficient by regression analysis ($p < 0.02$), which explained only 8% of the variance, and coefficients for educational level and

TABLE 4.9 Correlations of visual field with other abnormalities tests, showing significance and proportion of the variance explained (r^2)

	p value	r^2
Age	0.02	8
Education Level	0.903	2
Profile of Mood States	0.29	1.7
Culture Fair A	0.004	12
Color Discrimination	0.954	
Block Design	0.021	9
Digit Symbol	0.0001	28
Vocabulary	0.243	2.4
Contrast Sensitivity		
a	0.05	9
b	0.013	14
c	0.001	22
d	0.0001	27
e	0.006	17
Similarities	0.049	6.6
Visual Design Recall	0.0001	20

for POMS score were insignificant (Table 4.9). Contrast sensitivity measured by recognition of the direction of increasingly more closely spaced grids, a to e, of decreasing contrast, was correlated with visual field performance. The most significant relationship was with line d; line e (the faintest lines) had less significance than line d and explained less variance. A plausible array of diminishing relationships was found through lines c and b to a. Retinal rods must function for both contrast sensitivity and visual fields. Color discrimination, a cone function, was not related to impairment. Visual design reproduction, Culture Fair A, and block design, which depend on visual cortex and association areas, had significant correlations with visual field defects. Contrast sensitivity testing in these patients was less sensitive than visual fields and thus is expendable. Color discrimination stands by itself.

Defects in visual fields and delayed BRL R-1 were associated in patients with widespread brain damage despite their pathways being independent.

Hearing Tested by Audiometry

Loss of hearing acuity in the right ear was significantly correlated ($p < 0.0001$) with loss in the left, but the coefficient explained only 48% of the variance (Table 4.10). The right to left correlation was less than that for blink or visual fields. Hearing loss coefficients for visual field defects ($p < 0.002$ right and $p < 0.003$ left) explained almost 25% of the variance for both eyes, and hearing loss coefficients explained 20% of the variance in Culture Fair A ($p < 0.002$). The hearing loss coefficient for balance as sway speed with eyes open explained only 10% of the variance, and there was no correlation of hearing loss with sway speed with eyes closed. Hearing loss had no significant coefficients for reaction times, BRL R-1, finger writing errors, verbal recall, or vocabulary.

TABLE 4.10 Correlations of hearing loss with other tests, significance (p) and proportion of the variance explained (r^2)

	p Value	$r^2 \times 100$
Hearing Right to Left	.0001	48
Visual Fields Left	.002	25
Visual Fields Right	.003	24
Culture Fair A	.002	20
Sway Speed min Eyes Open	.030	10
Sway Speed min Eyes Closed	.172	0
Finger Writing Errors Total	.253	0
Vocabulary	.309	0
Blink Supraorbital Tap Left	.365	0
Choice Reaction Time	.408	0
Stories Recall	.587	0
Blink Supraorbital Tap Right	.648	0
Simple Reaction Time	.979	0

Number Writing Errors

Fingertip number writing is unique in the battery, as only it measures parietal lobe function (Table 4.11). Regression analysis showed that errors in finger writing had positive coefficients with balance with eyes open and with eyes closed and with both SRT and CRT, but not with age, blink reflex latency visual fields, hearing acuity, or POMS score, which are less intelligence-dependent. In contrast, educational level and the entire cognitive and embedded memory domains had significant coefficients (with negative signs) and relatively large variances explained, and perceptual motor speed tests, as well as reaction time and balance, had positive coefficients. The variance explained by the coefficients of cognition tests, perceptual motor speed tests, and embedded memory tests showed that avoiding errors in finger writing was a function of intelligence.

Frequency of Symptoms

These patients' most common abnormality was an elevated POMS score, which was greater than three times expected in 86% of patients and was accompanied by more than twofold elevations of symptom frequency in 91% of patients. These measures are subjective and confirm dis-ease as a "patient defined status of ill health"; so they would not be expected to help measure its functional impact. Interactions of POMS scores with the performance tests were complex in the regression analyses, which suggested that mood or emotions are strongly affected by chemicals (1). Psychological tests and POMS scores are subjective and might be deliberately manipulated by bright and insightful patients, particularly if they are test-wise, but evidence of this malingering style was not seen. Malingering should have been detected by inappropriate recall of the Rey 15-form test (2), failure to duplicate efforts in the several trials of reaction time, or balance testing. The worsening of performance during repeated trials in a few subjects was probably due to fatigue.

The median number of daily symptoms was 11 (of 35) in 135 adults. POMS scores

TABLE 4.11 Fingertip number writing errors compared by regression analysis with other tests

	Significance p	Percentage of Variance Explained ($r^2 \times 100$)	Number of Subjects n
Age	0.494	0	
Education Level	−0.003	6.6	132
Physiological Tests			
Sway Eyes Open min	0.030	4	
Eyes Closed min	0.004	7	
Simple Reaction Time	0.026	4.4	113
Choice Reaction Time	0.0001	11	133
Blink Supraorbital Right	0.294	0	72
Left	0.614	0	71
Visual Fields Right	0.373	1	66
Left	0.111	1	66
Hearing Right	0.111	5.6	46
Left	0.253	3.0	46
Cognition			
Culture Fair A	−0.0001	15.6	129
Digit Symbol	−0.0001	21.6	107
Block Score	−0.0001	18.0	127
Vocabulary	−0.008	9	75
Perceptual Motor Speed			
Pegboard	0.0001	20	
Trails A	0.0001	24	
Trails B	0.001	8	
Embedded Memory			
Information	−0.007	7	99
Picture Completion	−0.0001	17.5	108
Similarities	−0.000	17.7	106
Profile of Mood States	0.266	1	
Recall Stories	−0.013	4.7	132

and symptom frequency scores were highly correlated ($r = .617$, $p < 0.01$). Eight subjects had more than 14 symptoms per day. Symptoms usually had begun abruptly after a single episode of chemical exposure, but in subjects exposed to formaldehyde, benzene, or vinyl chloride for long periods they accrued gradually over months or years. A correlation matrix was developed for the symptom frequencies inventory in 255 adults after assigning each of 35 symptoms to one of eight groups: (1) chest, (2) irritation (of mucous membranes), (3) nausea (gastrointestinal), (4) balance, (5) mood disorders, (6) sleep disturbances, (7) memory impairment, and (8) limbic system (libido, etc.). Comparison frequencies for these groups showed that they moved together, and were one-dimensional in chemically exposed subjects and in unexposed subjects. Thus from this analysis it appears that the 35-question symptom inventory defines a category of disordered function that is affected by chemicals, in which the logical subdivisions are coordinated so that they move together in response, not separately. Thus rather than a single symptom or a group being a specific indicator, it appears that high frequency in one group indicates the frequency of symptoms in all groups. This effectively eliminates the entertaining idea of specificity of symptoms. Furthermore, it suggests that a minimal symptom inventory would measure what the 35 symptoms measure with high predictivity.

TABLE 4.12 Clinical criteria identified as "major" by at least 50% of physician practitioner respondents who had evaluated more than 200 affected individuals (upper quartile) +CE or less than 8 affected individuals (lower quartile) −CE

	Percent Responding			
	Less than 8		More than 200	
Criterion	+CE (n = 21)	−CE (n = 20)	+CE (n = 27)	−CE (n = 10)
Symptoms Reproducible	80	79	96	100
Condition Chronic	67	65	73	78
Responses at Low Exposure Levels	59	56	79	89
Symptoms Resolve When Incitants Removed	53	56	50	53
Reaction to Multiple Unrelated Substances	63	61	75	75
No Accepted Test Correlated	63	60	67	86
More Than One System Involved	25	21	54	56
Response Disturbs Patient	33	29	48	70
Neuropsychiatric Symptoms	31	27	40	50
Odor Sensitivity Altered	19	13	50	50

+CE includes respondents identifying themselves as clinical ecologists.

−CE excludes respondents identifying themselves as clinical ecologists.

Relationship to Multiple Chemical Sensitivity (MCS)

Thirty-four patients (26%) of the initial 135 adults complained specifically of multiple symptoms triggered consistently by "low levels" of many chemicals, including formaldehyde, gasoline, solvents, a paint, perfume, and usually cigarette smoke, and met the symptom-based criteria for multiple chemical sensitivity (MSC; Table 4.12) (8, 9, 10). All of these patients with multiple chemical sensitivity (MCS) had chemical encephalopathy (brain damage), but 74% of patients with chemical encephalopathy did not have MCS. The question that remains is the extent of overlap: what proportion of MCS groups seen by others (8, 9) have chemical encephalopathy? After nearly a decade of these investigations, sensitive performance testing has not been applied to groups of MCS patients as was used for these 255 clinic patients. Subjects exposed to indoor air should be compared as a separate inquiry, again to assess the overlap, as should patients with depression unexplained by life crises, those exposed to organophosphate pesticides, and those chronically reactive to irritant-toxic gases (chlorine, hydrogen sulfide, hydrogen chloride, formaldehyde, ammonia, etc.). Comparisons of the degree of overlap, using Venn diagrams or similar graphic methods, should help diagnosticians to understand the extent of cerebral toxicity, in contrast to dismissing these patients as having ill-defined psychiatric illnesses (10, 11).

Profile of Mood States Scores

The elevated profile of mood states (POMS) score, mean 82 (Table 4.13), indicated that distress was usually associated with impairment; the range was −22 to +174. A score of below 30, which is considered normal in a non-chemically exposed population,

TABLE 4.13 Coefficients of POMS score and other test scores with significance (p) and proportion of the variance (r^2)

	p	r^2(%)
Age	0.165	1.5
Education Level	−0.003	6.5
Cognitive		
Culture Fair A	−0.071*	2.5
Block Design	−0.0001	9.4
Digit Symbol	−0.026*	4.6
Vocabulary	0.834	0
Perceptual Motor Speed		
Pegboard	+0.008*	5
Trail Making B	0.909	0
Trail Making A	0.155	1
Finger Writing Errors (both hands)	0.266	0
Recall of Stories	0.186	1
Embedded Memory		
Information	−0.019*	15
Picture Completion	−0.0001	14
Similarities	0.113	2

* = Becomes insignificant with educational level in model.

was seen in 22 patients; the remainder were abnormal, with scores of 50 or greater in 103. The POMS score was without predictive capacity for physiological functions: balance, reaction time, vision, and hearing; no coefficients for independent variables were significant. In contrast, the POMS score was negatively correlated with educational level ($p < 0.003$) (Table 4.13) and had similar predictive value, significant coefficients, for cognitive measures of Culture Fair A, block design, and digit symbol, as well as for embedded memory, as information and picture completion.

OBJECTIVE 4: UNDERSTANDING THE CENTRAL NERVOUS SYSTEM

Is a delayed blink reflex R-1 an injury or simply a physiological indicator of toxicity? Reversibility is the key. To answer this question and several related ones concerning other test abnormalities, further follow-up of tested patients and carefully designed longitudinal studies of exposed groups are needed. For example, measurements of BRL R-1 baselines in hazardous material (HAZMAT) workers before they have any chemical exposure, and repeated measurements periodically during their (career-long) exposures, would determine whether protection strategies, including education, actually protect HAZMAT workers.

Brain's Distress Signals

It is useful to consider symptoms as the brain's "distress" signals (1) that correlate with functional deterioration, shown by repeated testing across time, after the effects of a chemical injury increase enough in severity to cause clinical impairment. When

TABLE 4.14 Seizures in 18 of 255 patients

		Exposure	Age	Type of Seizure
1	JD	Formaldehyde	48	Grand mal
2	RD	Formaldehyde	54	Temporal lobe
3	RH	Formaldehyde	11	Temporal lobe*
4	BR	Chlorine	54	Temporal lobe
5	LL	Chlorine	26	Temporal lobe
6	BG	Chlorine	54	Temporal lobe
7	JT	Hydrochloric acid	24	Temporal lobe
8	CO	Organophosphates	40	Temporal lobe
9	JY	Trichloroethylene	22	Temporal lobe
10	TH	Epoxy systems	33	Myoclonic
11	JA	Mixed (well head)	31	Grand mal
12	SB	Sodium azide	30	Temporal lobe
13	SC	Styrene monomer	35	Temporal lobe
14	DH	Chlordane	42	Temporal lobe
15	MM	Trichloroethylene	35	Temporal lobe, grand mal
16	JM	Hydrogen sulfide	14	Temporal lobe
17	DC	Ethylene dichloride	47	Temporal lobe
18	DH	Trimethyl benzene	34	Temporal lobe

* Also called partial motor seizures.

increased speed of sway with eyes closed exceeds 3 cm/sec, patients frequently notice clumsiness in the dark as at night. With even greater sway speeds, patients notice difficulty in walking straight even on a level surface, such as down a long hall; and as the sway speed further increases, they are unable to stand with their feet together, or to walk except with a broad-based gait (12).

Seizures as Signals of Chemical Damage

Seizures occurred in 7% of these patients, an unexpected finding (18/255) (Table 4.14). Seizures are regarded as extreme signs of CNS dysfunction (13). The onset of nearly half of these seizures came within a year or two after acute exposure to chlorine or after protracted exposures to formaldehyde. Seizures also followed exposures to sodium azide, styrene monomer, ethylene dichloride, trichloroethylene, epoxy, organophosphates, and leakage of chemical waste during injection into an exhausted oil well using a "Christmas tree." Major motor, grand mal, seizures occurred in three patients. One of them was a 48-year-old laboratory assistant in biology who had 15 years of exposure to formaldehyde and developed characteristic tonic-clonic (grand mal) seizures interspersed with staring episodes, often triggered by an olfactory aura, consistent with a diagnosis of temporal lobe epilepsy. The second was a 31-year-old waste injector from west Texas, and the third was a trichloroethylene-exposed individual. Myoclonic seizures appeared in a 33-year-old woman exposed to epoxy resin systems used in making prosthetic limbs, and thus to diethyl and 4,4-dimethyl aniline, after a second breakdown in her laboratory's ventilation system repeated an overwhelming exposure that had required her to obtain emergency room care for shortness of breath (i.e., pulmonary edema). Fifteen patients had temporal lobe (complex partial) seizures, which are thought to originate in the brain's limbic system (13, 14). In three patients chlorine was the associated chemical; formaldehyde was the major chemical in three; other exposures included sodium azide from a defective automobile air bag in a 26-year-old woman and severe organophosphate pesticide (chlorpyrifos) exposure in one man, a 40-year-old spray applicator. Seizures explain repeated auto accidents in two patients, including one who found himself and his car 40 feet down a ravine in New Hampshire. Subsequently, this patient's seizures occurred weekly with an olfactory aura, staring, and post-episode disorientation. Several patients with temporal lobe seizures had tried anticonvulsants, usually carbamazepine or ethosuximide, without relief.

Limbic Connections and Correlations

These patients' seizures probably arise in the limbic system (14). Its components, the amygdala, cingulate gyrus, and hippocampus, relay messages for ''fight or flight'' in response to noxious stimuli, including smells, and they control emotion, recall, and recent memory (14). In experimental animals, electrical or chemical limbic kindling causes seizures (14), which are signs of a hyperexcited, not depressed, brain. The most plausible explanation for the temporal lobe seizures that developed post-exposure in the 15 patients (6%) is chemically induced limbic kindling (15).

Results of Retesting across Intervals

Scores should improve with retesting for the tests responsive to familiarity and learning (4, 5, 16). The subconscious or involuntary tests would not be affected. Losses from aging have been estimated (see Chapter 3), but these patients' rates of deterioration suggest continuing toxic effects of chemicals (Table 4.15). Of the 22 subjects who were retested between 1 month and 6 years, 8 had improved on some tests. Four of these improved after leaving indoor environments (sick buildings), and two improved

TABLE 4.15 Patients reexamined: exposure and interval from first to second test

		Exposure	Interval in Months
1	TH	Epoxy	17, 11, 5, 11, 4, 26
2	RM	Hazardous materials	3, 23, 14
3	JH	Trichloroethylene	4, 5 (sauna)
4	BB	Indoor insulation	2 (sauna)
5	JC	Copying (NH_4SCN)	22
6	MS	Mobile home	57
7	RS	Mobile home	57
8	JW	Welding	1
9	CR	Chemical waste	47
10	NH	Cadmium	3, 7, 6
11	JL	Cadmium	3, 7, 6
12	DJ	HCHO	18
13	MF	HCHO	5, 5
14	BG	Chlorine	7, 7
15	JT	Hydrochloric acid	4
16	SF	*n*-Heptane, triphene	13
17	SB	Hydrogen sulfide	10
18	JS	Photography (NH_4SCN)	37
19	RK	Epoxy	47
20	PD	Chlorine (from sodium hypochlorite phosphoric acid)	4, 5 (sauna)
21	KM	Fire, vinyl chloride	24
22	MP	Phenol (intramuscular injection)	20

across 3 1/2 years and 6 years after initially getting worse. Of three who tried detoxification by exercise and sauna-induced sweating (9, 17), two improved and one got worse, an equivocal result. In contrast, functions deteriorated across intervals of 4 to 47 months in 14 patients. Of patients who got worse, ten had single chemical exposure, three to chlorine, two to formaldehyde, two to cadmium, and one each to hydrogen sulfide, *n*-heptane, and vinyl chloride. Two patients were exposed to epoxy systems and two to photographic chemicals containing ammonium thiocyanate, all in different incidents. More patient follow-up studies are needed to extend these provocative but inconclusive observations.

Interpretations of Brain Damage

Brain functions that seem “conceptually discrete” do not localize anatomically. The generalizations are that brains function slowly and imperfectly after major damage by chemicals (1, 12, 18, 19), and that multiple deficits were usually present. In order of frequency, deficits were found in reaction time, balance, recognition of fingertip numbers, block design (construction), recall of newly “learned” information, and dexterity coupled with attention and decision making, as in placing pegs and making trails. In these patients, slow and inaccurate function correlated with the highest symptom frequencies, suggesting that brain damage was severe and widespread. For example, balance with eyes closed, perhaps the most complex function, was more abnormal when finger writing errors, a parietal lobe function, were increased (2). In the chemically exposed subjects, when balance with the eyes open was the dependent variable, educational level and Culture Fair scores had significant coefficients, but these relationships were absent in unexposed subjects. Such associations suggest that cerebral dysfunction contributes to cerebellar dysfunction, as suggested earlier (19). Gross elevations of POMS scores and of complaint frequencies were strongly associated with overall neurobehavioral impairment. Thus, the affective or “emotion-driven” brain and the “psychomotor performance” brain were similarly susceptible to chemical damage.

Irritated eyes, conjunctiva, throat, and lower respiratory passages were attributed to direct effects of chemicals on these moist membranes. Reduced sense of smell is probably due to exquisite sensitivity of the olfactory bulbs to chemicals (6, 14). The role of immunological mechanisms is still unclear (20). Many patients had only *single brief exposures* to neurotoxic chemicals, followed by progressive impairment, suggesting neurodegenerative changes (18).

Predictions

Impaired neurobehavioral performance is probable when complaint and POMS scores are elevated by four times or more. To detect occupational or environmental neurotoxicity (6, 16, 21, 22) the use of sway speed, simple and two-choice visual reaction time, visual fields, Culture Fair, and vocabulary may be sufficient.

Generalizations

Uncertainty is greater as to which chemicals cause generalized brain damage when patients have been exposed to chemical mixtures rather than to a single chemical. Some of the “well-known mixtures of chemicals,” such as gasoline, diesel exhaust, chlorinated solvents, and epoxy resin systems, have one or two most plausible neurotoxic components and are becoming explicable by such probability ranking. This approach is the only reasonable one for ''contaminated'' chemicals and for chemical wastes, which are ill-defined mixtures. Problems of attribution multiply because of the probable creation of ''new'' chemicals by errors or breakdowns in chemical processing plants, the ''irreducibility of by-products,'' and the mixing of wastes. Chemical interactions and mixtures are inevitable in the ''real world.'' Thus, although ''hydrogen sulfide exposure'' is a convenient term, the exposure often includes other reduced sulfur gases; and ''formaldehyde vapor'' frequently contains formic acid, methanol, and traces of phenol. Perhaps the most poorly understood of the complex mixtures is ''indoor air.''

Mosaics to Fingerprints—A Giant Step

Distinct fingerprint effects of a chemical on brain function, that is, sentinel profiles, were not seen in these studies, and seem, from our current perspective, an unreasonable hope. The testable spectrum of brain functions is limited (12, 13, 23). Even delay of BRL R-1 was not specific for trichloroethylene (or even chlorinated solvents) as has been suggested (7). Delayed BRL R-1 was associated with inhalational exposures to chlorine, hydrochloric acid, chlordane, trimethoxysilane and tetrachlorosilane, ammonium thiocyanate (with other photographic chemicals), formaldehyde–phenol, monobutyl ether with butyl cellosolve, and hazardous material fires, and with the intramuscular injection of phenol in glycerin. More follow-up data are needed for us to judge the permanence of delayed BRL R-1.

Uncertainties and Contrasts

Many more chemicals disorder central nervous system functions than investigators were aware of a decade ago (13, 24). Their effects on the brain are generalized, resembling metabolic, degenerative, nutritional, or demyelinating diseases. A single toxic chemical may produce multiple syndromes. Although a quarter of these patients noted symptomatic exacerbation by other chemicals, suggesting multiple chemical sensitivity, and although removal of the offending agent often diminished symptoms, it brought slight or *no functional improvement.* No linear dose–response relationships have been suggested.

It is well accepted that each human subject is unique; thus people vary from being extremely sensitive to low doses of therapeutic drugs to being refractory even to high ones (3), even apart from their immune reactions. These drugs are simply chemicals used to treat diseases; so the wide spectrum of response to drugs applies also to human populations exposed to chemicals.

The chemically exposed populations differ remarkably from the groups of workers traditionally studied for the toxic effects of chemicals. The workers have been selected for fitness and have survived attrition of the more susceptible ones, leaving the resistant workers in the exposure tests. Thus, selection factors make these groups homogeneous compared to environmentally exposed subjects. Also, it is often overlooked that in congested industrial parks air movements and on-site spills expose workers, as bystanders, to manufacturing, transport, use, and disposal of many chemicals from adjoining industries. ''Chemically susceptible workers'' usually leave the workforce without a trace. Only occasionally do worker-bystanders, adversely affected by several chemicals, become multiply chemically sensitive (8–11, 20) before they leave their employment.

CONCLUSIONS

Many chemicals cause neurobehavioral impairment. However, impairment from single exposures to so-called irritant gases was unexpected. The damage was usually permanent, it worsened at rates faster than aging, and reversibility was rare. Brief acute exposures to "pure" chemicals were most informative. Insidious exposures to hydrogen sulfide, formaldehyde, organophosphates, chlordane, gasoline, PCBs, and diesel exhaust were slowly cumulative in their effects, but a brief "overdose" often initiated a clinical disorder and precipitated recognition of problems.

Improvement, that is, partial or complete return of function, depended on adaptation, relearning, and coping. Progressive deterioration of function usually continues for months or years after an acute chemical exposure. Use of the brain—in fact, its relentless stimulation—may modify this pattern. Recognition of slowing or loss of function or improvement depends upon sensitive tests that often involve the timing of phenomena.

With respect to sensitivity of the tests, balance was the most consistently abnormal function after chemical exposure, followed by simple and choice reaction times and blink reflex latency, which are physiological measures least influenced by educational attainment as a measure of innate ability. Adjusting for the effects of aging with prediction equations (see Chapter 3) aids interpretation.

Loss of visual receptive response, mapped by testing visual fields, may be the most common chemically induced brain defect, as it occurred in 80% of the 38 patients tested as a trial of efficacy. Hearing, the last test added to the battery, also shows promise. Blink reflex latency, another late addition, was prolonged to the abnormal range in 62% of the patients tested and was associated with many different chemicals.

In Chapters 5 through 14, studies of ten populations sharing exposure from "chemical accidents or incidents" or chronic exposure from sites of chemical waste help us to begin answering difficult questions concerning population-wide vs. individual sensitivity (i.e., how are effects distributed throughout the population?) and provide lessons concerning differential diagnosis (i.e., other explanations, including confounding factors and bias, are discussed). These considerations lead to limited generalizations about prognosis and therapy. Theories of chemical brain injury are considered as a prelude to a consideration of the crucial question: how can we prevent chemical brain damage? Hopefully much diagnosis and attribution can be reduced to clinical aphorisms, as outlined by Levine (25) more than half a century ago:

> . . . how is he to disentangle the complicated differential diagnosis without putting the patient to great expense? This type of clinical teaching has been neglected, for there are simple methods that can be used in what might be called the *destructive differential diagnosis,* which the older or more experienced physicians have learned and which they are really practicing, consciously or unconsciously. A physician finds that a patient has a palpable spleen and fever. Among the various conditions to be considered is subacute bacterial endocarditis. He learned in his hospital training that a positive blood culture would establish the diagnosis, but that a negative one does not eliminate it. He has not been taught, however, that if there are no murmurs whatever, he can with fair assurance dismiss the diagnosis of subacute bacterial endocarditis. This finding he can obtain in one minute and with no expense to the patient. This merely illustrates one example, of which there are many, where simple methods enable one to rule out possible diagnoses.

References

1. Kilburn KH: Evidence that the human nervous system is most sensitive to environmental toxins. *Environ Carcinog Rev* 1990–91;C8(2):327–337.

2. Lezak MD: *Neuropsychological Assessment.* New York: Oxford University Press, 1995.
3. Klaassen CD: Principles of toxicology. In: *The Pharmacological Basis of Therapeutics* (7th ed.), AG Gilman et al. (eds.). New York: Macmillan Co. 1985, pp. 1592–1604.
4. Kilburn KH and Warshaw RH: Neurobehavioral effects of formaldehyde and solvents on histology technicians: repeated testing across time. *Environ Res* 1992;58:134–146.
5. Ryan CM, Morrow LA, Bromet EJ, and Parkinson DK: Assessment of neuropsychological dysfunction in the work place: normative data from the Pittsburgh occupational exposures test battery. *J Clin Exper Neuropsych* 1987;9:665–679.
6. Ryan CM, Morrow LA, and Hodgson M: Cacosmia and neurobehavioral dysfunction associated with occupational exposure to mixtures of organic solvents. *Am J Psychiatry* 1988;145: 1552–1445.
7. Feldman RG, Chirico-Post J, and Proctor SP: Blink reflex latency after exposure to trichloroethylene in well water. *Arch Environ Health* 1988;43:143–148.
8. Cullen MR: The worker with multiple chemical sensitivities: an overview. *Occup Med* 1987; 2:655–661.
9. Ashford NA and Miller CS: *Chemical Exposures.* New York: Van Nostrand Reinhold, 1991.
10. Black DW, Rathe A, and Goldstein RB: Environmental illness: a controlled study of 26 subjects with "20th Century disease." *JAMA* 1990;264:3166–3170.
11. Simon GE, Katon WJ, and Sparks PJ: Allergic to life: psychological factors in environmental illness. *Am J Psychiatry* 1990;147:901–906.
12. Kilburn KH and Warshaw RH: Neurotoxic effects from residential exposure to chemicals from an oil reprocessing and Superfund site. *Neurotox Teratol* 1995;17:89–102.
13. Shaumburg HH and Spencer PS: *Experimental and Clinical Neurotoxicology.* Baltimore, MD: Williams & Wilkins, 1980.
14. Ordy JM, Brizzee KR, and Johnson HA: *Cellular Alterations in Visual Pathways and the Limbic System: Implications for Vision and Short-Term Memory in Aging and Human Visual Function.* New York: Allan R. Liss, 1982.
15. Post RM, Rubinow DR, and Ballenger JC: Conditioning, sensitization and kindling: implications for the course of affective illness. In: *Neurology of Mood Disorders,* RM Post and JC Ballenger (eds.). Baltimore, MD: Williams & Wilkins, 1984.
16. Williamson AH: The development of a neurobehavioral test battery for use in hazard evaluation in occupational settings. *Neurotox Teratol* 1990;12:509–514.
17. Kilburn KH, Warshaw RH, and Shields MG: Neurobehavioral dysfunction in firemen exposed to polychlorinated biphenyls (PCBs): possible improvement after detoxification. *Arch Environ Health* 1989;44:345–350.
18. Calne DB: Neurotoxins and degeneration in the central nervous system. *Neurotoxicology* 1991;12:335–340.
19. Schmahmann JD: An emerging concept: the cerebellar contribution to higher function. *Arch Neurol* 1991;48:1178–1187.
20. Levin AS and Byers VS: Environmental illness: a disorder of immune regulation. *Occup Med* 1987;2:669–681.
21. Savage EP, Keef TJ, Mounce LM, Heaton RK, Lewis JA, and Bucar PJ: Chronic neurological sequelae of acute organophosphate pesticide poisoning. *Arch Environ Health* 1988;43:38–45.
22. Anger WK: Worksite behavioral research; results, sensitive methods, test batteries and the transition from laboratory data to human health. *Neurotoxicology* 1990;11:629–720.
23. Fitzhugh LC, Fitzhugh KB, and Reitan RM: Sensorimotor deficits of brain-damaged subjects in relation to intellectual level. *Percept Motor Skills* 1962;15:603–608.
24. Schaumburg HH and Spencer PS: Recognizing neurotoxic disease. *Neurology* 1987;37: 276–278.
25. Levine SA: *Clinical Heart Disease* (3rd ed.). Philadelphia, PA: W. B. Saunders Co., 1945.

5

Hydrogen Sulfide Exposure from Refineries in Cities

Death by asphyxiation from hydrogen sulfide (H_2S) has been recognized for over 200 years (1). Christison described fatalities from working in sewers and with animal excreta in 1845 (2). Hydrogen sulfide poisons metallo-enzymes, particularly cytochrome oxidase, and paralyzes the human respiratory center (3). It also causes hyperpnea by stimulating the carotid body, similarly to cyanide (1). In fatal poisoning the cerebral cortices, basal nuclei, lentiform body, and putamen showed greenish discoloration (4). Computerized tomography has demonstrated abnormal low density of the basal ganglia and surrounding white matter in chronic H_2S poisoning (5), and after fatal exposure (6), but clinical neurological examinations have been normal after ''recovery'' (3, 7). Thirteen subjects died, and unconsciousness was reported in 75% of 221 subjects made ill by H_2S exposure in Alberta, Canada from 1969 to 1973 (8). Nearly all of them had headaches, altered behavior, confusion, and vertigo. Agitation or somnolence were noted in 28%, nausea and/or vomiting in 22%, and disequilibrium in 17%. The completeness of recovery, that is, whether the survivors had long-term impairment, is unknown because neurological testing was not done.

Persistent neurobehavioral impairment after H_2S induced unconsciousness has been described recently. Six workers rendered unconscious by H_2S and mercaptans from sewage, manure, decaying fish in fishing boats, a tannery, and an oil drilling platform had neurobehavioral testing after two to six years (9). Five men had abnormal balance, impaired dexterity (slowed placement of pegs in a pegboard) and slow trail making B performance, poor verbal and visual recall on Wechsler's memory scale, and reduced scores on block design, digit symbol, similarities, picture completion, and vocabulary from the Wechsler Adult Intelligence Scale (WAIS) (10). The sixth ex-worker was demented and bedfast. After three men had been overcome by H_2S, they had similar impairment and abnormal auditory evoked potentials (P-300 latency) (11).

Several case reports had added clues about the effects of H_2S, which are briefly reviewed. Thirty-nine months after an offshore oil worker was overcome by H_2S (12), he showed profound impairment of balance, slow simple and choice reaction times, impaired verbal and visual recall, prolonged trail making A and B, and reduced Culture Fair, block design, and digit symbol scores. His profile of mood states (POMS) score was greatly elevated with a low vigor score. A 20-month-old child was exposed for a year to 0.6 ppm H_2S downwind from a burning tip gas ignition point for a colliery. The H_2S levels exceeded the World Health Organization community standards of 0.003 to 0.01 ppm. Computerized tomography (5) showed subacute necrotizing encephalopathy in the basal ganglia and white matter. He had improved ten weeks after exposure ceased, but his final status was not described. A 45-year-old man showed similar bilateral symmetrical lucent lesions in the lentiform nucleus and basal ganglia on computerized tomography after unconsciousness due to H_2S (6). Acute coma due to H_2S has also been followed by periventricular leukomalacia (6).

Hydrogen sulfide and reduced sulfur gases from oil refineries in Canada (13) and from paper making in Finland (14) produced symptoms and impaired pulmonary function in residents downwind, but no neurological or psychological testing was done. Low level environmental exposure to H_2S has been ignored because mortality does not rise (15), or it is thought to trigger only mass psychogenic illness or "crowd disease" (16, 17). Before dismissing these gases as only nuisances, it would be prudent to examine exposed populations. The adverse CNS findings in 11 patients exposed to H_2S strongly supported the idea of permanent impairment from H_2S. The complaints of 9 workers triggered an epidemiological investigation of workers from a desulfurization unit of a California coastal oil refinery. Workers had shortness of breath, wheezing, eye and nose irritation and cough, skin rashes, depression, and headache and showed small airway obstruction on spirometry. Downwind neighbors of the refinery also had many symptoms, and 22 of them were studied with 13 former workers. Our hypothesis was that these symptoms were accompanied by impaired performance. Neurobehavioral impairment from chronic low-dose H_2S exposure has not been reported.

This chapter describes and analyzes patients and populations exposed to H_2S, which add strength to the hypothesis that H_2S causes chronic brain damage as shown by neurobehavioral dysfunction. As described in the following pages, there were several sources for these subjects. First were the H_2S-exposed patients seen in consultation from 1987 to 1995. The second group was from a pilot study in 1996 of 68 subjects who were exposed downwind from a Los Angeles area oil refinery explosion and gas leak in 1992. The third group included workers and downwind neighbors of an oil refinery near San Luis Obispo. The fourth group consisted of people in two communities with oil refineries who were studied as "unexposed" subjects for other chemical exposure groups but showed impairment most plausibly associated with being neighbors of oil refineries. The fifth and last group came from a study for balance and reaction time in Los Angeles oil refinery workers during their evaluation for asbestos exposure.

THE 16 PATIENTS

The 16 patients had been referred for evaluation of the effects of H_2S exposure (Table 5.1). They comprised nearly 10 percent of 160 consecutively examined chemically exposed patients. Five worked in oil fields, crude oil refining, and products shipping areas in Louisiana. Four were exposed downwind from oil fields in Kentucky and Texas, two were barge men hauling asphalt, two worked in a chemical plant downwind, one worked in sewage treatment, one was exposed to H_2S generated in a tank truck, and one was a dishwasher in a chemical process laboratory. Comparison and analysis was made to an unexposed group studied as the match for a chemical exposure group.

TABLE 5.1 Demographic and exposure data, H_2S exposure

Yr	Age	Sex	Ed Lev	Occupation	State	Exposure: Conditions	Exposure: Duration	Smoke	Major Symptoms
90	27	M	12	Oil field laborer	LA	Tank top oil depot	5–10 min	Never	Cognitive symptoms
91	62	M	0	Truck deliveries	LA	Next-door to H_2S release from well flameout	1 hr	Ex	Syncope
93	22	M	12	Tank cleaner	NV	Sodium hyposulfite and acid	2 hrs	Ex	Excess fatigue
93	21	M	13	Bargeman Miss. R.	LA	Pumping asphalt from oil refinery into barge	11/2 hrs	Ex	Headache
93	37	M	12	Bargeman Miss. R.	LA	Pumping asphalt from oil refinery into barge	5–6 hrs	Never	Pain in chest and back
94	62	M	18	Insurance business	KY	Downwind of crude oil pumping, with and without flare burning	2 yrs	Ex	Chest tightness
94	57	F	8	Farmer, homemaker	KY	Downwind of crude oil pumping, with and without flare burning	2 yrs	Never	Memory loss, asthma
92	42	M	16	Minister	TX	Downwind of refinery	12 yrs	Never	Memory loss
94	52	M	12	Water treatment worker	NV	Generated in sewage and ‘‘gray water’’ treatment	11 yrs	Ex 29 yrs	Extreme fatigue
94	35	F	12	Chemical plant process control 11 yrs	LA	Escape of H_2S and methyl mercapoproprionate into control room	1 day	Never	Unconsciousness
94	39	F	14	Chemical plant process control 10 yrs	LA	Loading area of plant as above	1 day	Never	Odor–headache
95	27	M	14	Contractor refinery	TX	Dug out pipeline leak	10 min	Never	Unconsciousness, recall memory loss
95	39	M	0	Contractor refinery	TX	Dug out pipeline leak	10 min	Ex	Unconsciousness, swelling legs and body
95	61	M	0	Contractor refinery	TX	Dug out pipeline leak	10 min	Ex	Unconsciousness, dizziness, fatigue
95	68	M	12	Contractor refinery	TX	Dug out pipeline leak	10 min	Ex	Unconsciousness, productive cough
95	63	F	9	Process laboratory	MO	Laboratory exposure	13 yrs	Never	Dizziness

The exposure, which rendered the first patient semiconscious, was monitored by his H_2S meter, which read to full scale at 10,000 parts per million (ppm). All the others smelled "rotten eggs" (H_2S); so their exposures are estimated to have been between 1 and 10 parts per million (ppm), that is, beneath the threshold for olfactory fatigue. However, exposure of the two barge men who were pumping asphalt from an oil refinery was probably 25 to 50 ppm, as they had headache and chest and back pain, and could not smell H_2S after an hour or more of exposure. One patient was delivering chicken feed for one to two hours downwind from H_2S released after the flame on an oil well vent pipe flared out. Exposure of another man, a tank cleaner, was to H_2S generated from sodium hyposulfite and acid within a tanker truck. A married couple, who lived downwind from wells pumping crude oil in Kentucky, associated the H_2S odor with an unlit vent flare and with memory loss and difficulty in concentrating. With the flame they noted a sharp pungent odor, and they had chest pain and tightness with asthma. Hydrogen sulfide escaped during the no-flame periods, and sulfur dioxide was released when the flare was lit. The sixth was a minister exposed to H_2S in Odessa, Texas, in his church and rectory immediately downwind from two H_2S-emitting oil refineries. When the wind shifted during church services, he had noted that numerous members of his congregation became nauseated and rushed outside to vomit. Chronic exposure to sewer gas in an aeration field for 20 years affected the sewerage treatment worker.

Exposed subjects ranged in age from 21 to 68 years with a mean of 44.7 years and had educational levels ranging from 0 to 18 years with a mean of 10.0 years, which was significantly below the unexposed subjects' mean because of three men without formal education (Table 5.1). Durations of H_2S exposures ranged from a few minutes in patients 1 and 13 through 16, who were most impaired, to 12 years in the minister. At the time of exposure 8 patients had never smoked and 8 were ex-smokers. Clinical physical and neurological examinations were essentially as expected for this age range of patients except for poor recall and diminished vibration sense. Data were analyzed by prevalence of abnormality and by comparison of means to the Arizona unexposed subjects. The prevalences of abnormality, as defined by test scores 1.5 standard deviations (±) from those of unexposed subjects (Chapter 3), were described for the 16 patients. In a second analysis, mean values of the 16 exposed patients were compared to unexposed subjects' means. Memory loss, excessive fatigue, and dizziness were the most common and most frequent symptoms, followed by difficulty in concentrating and chest pain and tightness (Table 5.2). Other symptoms included headache and memory loss, disorientation, nausea, decreased libido, and loss of strength. The woman with cough and asthma had also been exposed to sulfur dioxide intermittently when the flare above the upwind collection tank was burning.

Neurobehavioral testing showed that balance was impaired in 75% of subjects with eyes closed, as mean sway speed of the group was 2.95 cm/s compared to 1.18 cm/s in unexposed ($p < .0001$), and it was impaired in 56% of patients with eyes open, with mean 1.28 cm/s vs. 0.82 cm/s in unexposed ($p < .0001$) (see Tables 5.3 and 5.4). Choice reaction time was also prolonged in 63% of patients and the mean of the group was prolonged ($p < .0001$), whereas 44% had prolonged simple reaction time and the mean differences was significant ($p < .001$). Blink reflex latency (R-1) was lengthened in 75% of patients, but there were three with faster than average responses; so the mean was not different from the unexposed. Color discrimination was abnormal in 70% and visual fields were abnormal in 50% of those examined. Vibration sense was reduced in 82% of subjects tested.

Fingertip writing errors were the most common abnormality of psychological tests,

TABLE 5.2 Major complaints with frequencies greater than weekly, in H_2S-exposed patients

Symptom	Prevalence
Memory loss	11
Excessive fatigue	9
Dizziness	9
Headache	8
Decreased libido	8
Difficulty concentrating	5
Chest pain/tightness	5
Disorientation	5
Loss of strength	5
Nausea	4
Shortness of breath	4
Somnolence	2
Asthma	2
Cough	2
Sleep disturbed/dreams	2
Depression, severe	2
Blurred vision	2
Diarrhea	1
Syncope	1
Palpitations	1
Loss of appetite	1
Tinnitus	1
Body swelling and pain	1

and these errors were elevated in 75% with a significant difference in means ($p < .003$). Sixty-three percent had prolonged trail making B with a significant difference from unexposed; so the perceptual motor domain was impaired ($p < .0001$). Culture Fair and block design scores were each reduced in 69%, and means were significantly different from those of unexposed. Vocabulary score was diminished in 58%, and the means were significantly different. Immediate verbal recall was impaired in 63% and visual reproduction was impaired in 44%; neither difference was significant. Tests of long-term memory showed minimal impairment.

POMS score was elevated in 63% of patients, and the mean was significantly elevated (Table 5.3). Frequencies of 35 symptoms were elevated significantly above unexposed subjects' levels, as highlighted by the prevalence list of Table 5.2. Extensive questionnaires for medical and neurological diseases and for home and occupational chemical exposures did not show any pattern or combinations of confounding medical, neurological, or psychiatric diagnoses or exposure to other neurotoxins. All of these symptoms were rare, except that depression after H_2S exposures was frequent and needed treatment. These patients' symptoms are different from patterns identified for post-traumatic-stress syndrome, minimal head injury, or chronic fatigue syndrome.

A DISASTROUS INCIDENT IN TORRANCE, CALIFORNIA

On October 10, 1992, at 9:45 P.M. residents of the Los Angeles harbor area and north were shaken by two explosions at the TRM1 refinery hydrocracker, which registered

TABLE 5.3 Neurobehavioral performance of H_2S-exposed patients compared to unexposed means

	Unexposed		Exposed			Abnormal	
	Mean	Sd	Mean	Sd	p Value	Total	% Abnormal
Age yrs	42.4	15.4	44.7	16.7	NS		
Ed Level yrs	13.2	2.1	10.0	5.4	.004		
Balance cm/sec							
Eyes Open	0.82	0.21	1.28	0.47	.0001	9/16	56
Closed	1.18	0.41	2.95	1.54	.0001	12/16	75
Simple Reaction Time ms	285	64	422	192	.001	7/16	44
Choice Reaction Time ms	528	85	691	182	.0001	10/16	63
Blink Reflex Latency							
Supraorbital Tap ms							
Right	14.5	1.9	14.7	2.0	NS	9/12	38
Left	15.1	1.8	14.7	2.3	NS		75
Color Vision							70
Visual Fields						7/14	50
Vibration						9/11	82
Culture Fair sc	29.7	7.5	22.3	8.8	.001	11/16	69
Block Design sc	31.3	9.7	20.9	11.6	.0001	11/16	69
Digit Symbol sc	58.7	11.7	38.5	17.6	.001	9/16	56
Pegboard s	71.0	18.1	89.8	32.7	NS	6/16	38
Trails A sc	31.0	8.8	58.6	47.1	NS	5/16	31
Trails B sc	71.0	25.7	147.3	103.8	.0001	10/16	63
Fingertip Writing errors	3.9	1.9	10.8	8.7	.003	12/16	75
Recall							
Verbal, Immediate	23.3	4.2	15.6	10.0	NS	10/16	63
Visual, Immediate	35.4	3.9	24.6	8.5	NS	7/16	44
Vocabulary	24.2	9.2	12.3	5.7	.001	7/12	58
Information	17.9	5.6	14.6	7.0	NS	5/16	31
Picture Completion	14.4	3.0	13.3	4.5	NS	5/16	31
Similarities	19.8	4.6	16.5	6.1	NS	4/16	25
POMS Score	19.1	32.8	83.2	36.5	.0001	10/16	63
Symptom Freq. sc	0.7	0.6	4.8	2.5	.001	10/16	63
Depression			23.9			9/15	60

ms = milliseconds NS = normal
s = seconds (I/D) = immediate/30 min. delay)
sc = score

3.0 on the Richter scale (see Figure 5.1). Broken windows and blown-down walls caused hundreds of injuries, which were only a portent of the damage to lungs, skin (including hair loss), and brains that followed 6 to 8 days of sour gas leaks—hydrogen sulfide and related sulfur-containing gases—from this petroleum refinery. In high concentrations these gases kill, but at lower levels they damage exposed persons' brains to disturb and disorder balance, vision, memory recall, and ability to concentrate. Ammonia, chlorine, gasoline, phenols, and other refinery gases were also released. Exposure caused profound depression in many people, as well as asthma and progressively severe airway obstructive disease. Many persons were hospitalized for traumatic injuries, including those to the head, and for respiratory distress and insufficiency. OSHA cited Texaco for 28 serious violations and levied civil penalties of $147,500 (citation of May 21, 1993). Fries Avenue Elementary School and Wilmington Junior High School

TABLE 5.4 Neurobehavioral performance of H_2S-exposed patients

	1	2	3	4	5	6	7	8	9	10	11	12	13	14	15	16
Age/Ed Level yrs	27/12	39/0	68/12	61/0	27/14	62/0	21/13	27/12	37/12	39/14	35/12	62/18	57/8	52/12	42/16	63/9
Balance cm/sec																
Eyes Open	1.57*	0.49	1.18*	2.17*	1.73*	1.55*	0.84	1.19*	1.11	1.39*	0.76	1.26	1.01	0.76	1.91*	1.62
Eyes Closed	6.39*	1.40	3.36*	3.94*	2.83*	4.00*	1.12	1.80*	2.11*	5.73*	2.39*	1.26	2.35	1.37	2.73*	4.38
Simple Reaction Time ms	560*	575*	320*	249*	375*	550*	226	293*	423*	990*	421*	318	333	287	227	603*
Choice Reaction Time ms	676*	871*	699*	675*	600*	990*	467	558*	768*	1081*	549	615*	715*	500	416	875*
Blink Reflex Latency ms																
Right	18†	14.1	13.5	NR	12.6	18*	12.5	17*	16*	14.6	15.3*	13.5	13	15.4*	14	13.7
Left	18*	13.0	13.3	14.8*	11.8	20*	12.5	17*	16*	14.9	17*	13.5	13.6	13	14	
Color Vision sc	—	Ab	Ab	Ab	N	—	Ab	N	Ab*	Ab*	Ab*	—	Ab	Ab	—	Ab
Visual Fields	—	Ab	Ab	Ab	Ab	—	N	N	Ab	Ab	Ab(c)	Ab	Ab	N	—	Ab
Vibration	—	Ab	Ab	Ab	Ab	—	N	N	—	Ab	Ab	—	Ab	Ab	—	Ab
Culture Fair sc	20*	12*	19*	5*	24	18*	30	28	29	17*	34	21*	20*	24	41	14*
Block Design sc	25	2*	22	11*	22	13*	6*	45	28	10	29	16*	22*	21	41	21*
Digit Symbol sc	42	8*	36	14*	57	15*	49*	74	55	21*	42	41*	34*	40	52	36*
Pegboard sc	65	191*	99	88	67	112*	76	56	67	109*	76	92*	64	88*	61	136*
Trails A sc	43*	132*	91	129*	31	68	32	18	33	180*	23	38	37	37	21	54
Trails B sc	94*	—	238*	221*	50	335*	74	49	118*	180(e)*	55	111*	127*	94*	67	144*
Fingertip Writing errors	33*	16*	11*	7	2	19*	10*	5	0	16*	11*	15*	0	0	12*	16*
Recall immed/del																
Verbal	9*	0*	6*	7*	12	15/8*	33	22/1*	33	15/0*	14/14*	9*	18/12*	15/13*	33/13*	9*
Visual	15*	10*	24*	14*	16*	19/0*	34	35/32	36	30/0*	33/33	31	28/26	20/17	30/26	18*
Vocabulary sc	—	5	7*	2*	10*	—	15	—	16	13*	12*	20	10*	20	—	17
Information sc	21	3	15	9*	5*	6*	15	15	15	12*	17	24	12	23	26	16
Picture Completion sc	17	3	12	6*	15	10*	47	15	14	15	18	15	11*	15	20	10*
Similarities sc	16	0	18	6*	15	5*	23	19	19	23	22	21	13*	20	25	19
POMS sc	91*	137*	69*	96*	82	57	62*	48	155*	87	89	57	101*	34	31	138*
Depression	13	36*	20*	32*	24*	19*	12	17	54*	17	23*	18*	34*	6	2	40*
Symptom Freq. score	4.7*	9.9*	6.5*	5.4*	7.5*	—	3.1	2.1	3.4*	7.3*	3.7*	3.2	1.8	3.9*	1.9	7.9*

Ab = abnormal
N = normal
— = not measured
cm/s = centimeters per second
ms = milliseconds
sc = score
* = $p < .05$

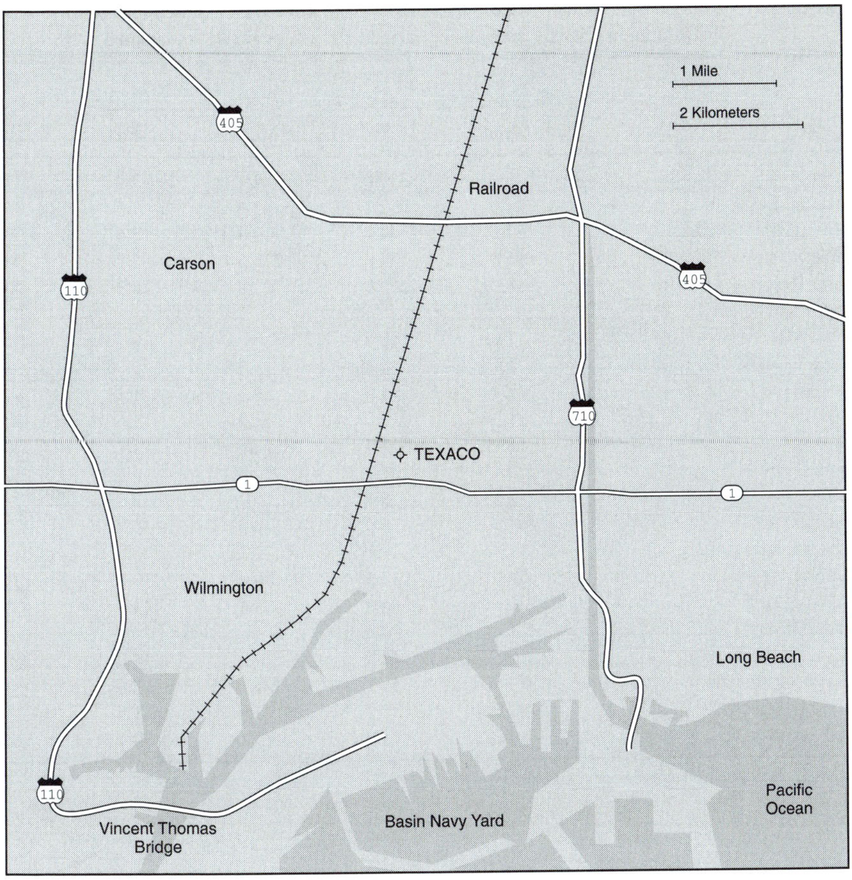

FIGURE 5.1. Wilmington, California, harbor area.

were primary and secondary evacuation sites, followed by Harbor College. The civil penalties were later raised to $231,000 (State $83,500; OSHA $147,500).

Subjects were divided on the basis of an examining physician's clinical judgment into four groups of ascending severity. Of the 68 pilot subjects, 25% were in Group 1, 21% in Group 2, 32% in Group 3, and 21% in Group 4. They included 24 African Americans and 20 Latino adults. Thirteen of the 20 children were Latino. Ethnically discrete comparisons were made to 20 African-American reference subjects from Oklahoma City and to 36 Latino unexposed subjects from Houston.

The ages of exposed African-Americans and unexposed were not different (Table 5.5, Figure 5.2). The figures were scaled by dividing the expected maximum for each test by 1,000 to create a scale factor. Because for some tests, for example, Culture Fair

TABLE 5.5a Comparison of unexposed African-American adults, 24 exposed at Torrance and 21 at Oklahoma City by analysis of variance; *p* values <0.05 underlined

	Exposed		Unexposed		
Variable	Mean	Sd	Mean	Sd	*p* value
Age yrs	46.9	17.0	42.4	7.4	.273
Education Level yrs	11.0	2.2	13.3	2.3	.001
Profile of Mood States	62.9	44.4	−0.4	15.6	.0001
Simple Reaction Time ms	491.0	274.0	278.5	53.2	.002
Choice Reaction Time ms	688.0	159.0	503.4	78.3	.0001
Sway–Balance cm/sec					
Eyes Open	1.06	0.73	0.75	0.20	.074
Eyes Closed	1.79	1.29	1.23	0.36	.057
Color Vision Lanthony Hue	13.4	1.5	12.1	1.1	.002
Blink Reflex R-1 ms Right	11.7	1.5	13.3	1.6	.005*
Left	11.1	1.4	13.4	1.7	.0005*
Culture Fair A	20.1	7.3	22.3	6.6	.300
Vocabulary	2.5	5.1	14.1	7.4	.0001
Digit Symbol	42.7	16.9			
Pegboard dominant sec	79.4	11.9	72.7	10.8	.056
Trail Making A	53.0	32.5	36.0	10.3	.027
Trail Making B	120.6	46.9	95.4	41.7	.066
Finger Writing	11.8	3.3			
FVC % of predicted	70.5	12.8	90.7	14.0	.0001
FEV_1 % of predicted	70.4	13.7	90.0	12.8	.0001
F_{25} % of predicted	80.0	35.2	97.6	21.5	.057
F_{75} % of predicted	80.0	38.0	95.1	30.1	.158

* Exposed are normal; unexposed are abnormal.

and vocabulary, higher scores were better, the exposed score was subtracted from the unexposed. In other tests, such as balance and reaction time, lower scores were better; thus unexposed were subtracted from exposed. In both cases the result was multiplied by the scale factor. Statistically significant differences ($p < 0.05$) were shown by hatched bars and insignificant results by clear bars. Educational level was two years lower in exposed subjects than in unexposed (significantly different), but this difference had no effect on physiological tests, nor would it decrease the substantial difference for vocabulary to change the interpretation. Reaction times, both simple and choice, and color discrimination were different in exposed vs. unexposed. Balance sway speed was nearly statistically significantly faster (more) abnormal and highly variable in exposed subjects. Perceptual motor speed tests, pegboard, trail making A and B and fingertip number writing, were worse and approached statistical significance in exposed subjects. Unexposed subjects had not been tested with recall or memory tests, or for visual fields. Compared to other unexposed groups, many of the visual fields were highly abnormal in exposed subjects, usually for both eyes, and nearly 50% showed arcuate scotomata or concentric field losses. Vital capacity and forced expiratory volume in 1 second, FEV_1, were 20% below the predicted and thus greatly different in exposed subjects, and midflow differences approached significance at $p < 0.057$. Blink reflex latency R-1 was abnormal in Oklahoma City subjects, presumably because of TCE, and was normal in the Torrance subjects, who were unexposed to chlorinated solvents.

The exposed Latino adults were well matched to Houston unexposed for age and

TABLE 5.5b Tests of exposed Torrance subjects

	Exposed		Unexposed*	
	Mean	Sd	Mean	Sd
Information	11.4	3.5		
Picture Completion	10.6	3.2		
Similarities	12.2	7.7		
Stories Immediate	17.3	3.5		
Delayed	13.5	3.1		
Visual Design Recall	21.6	7 7		
Visual Field Right	323	148		
Left	336	132		
Smell	3.3	0.9		

* No comparison data

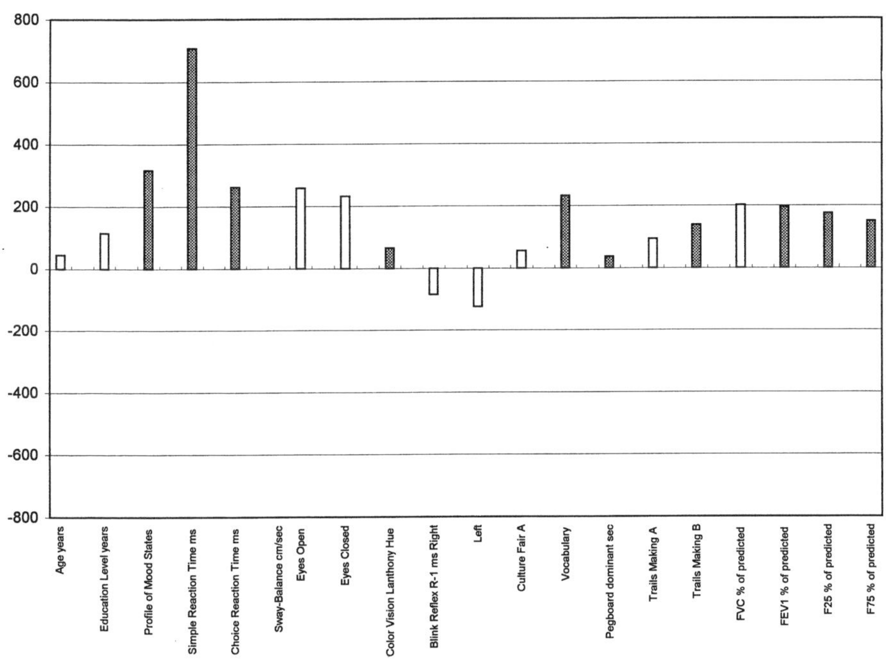

FIGURE 5.2. Comparison of African-American adults, 24 exposed to H_2S and 21 unexposed (Oklahoma City) subjects by ANOVA. Hatched bars are statistically significant. Scores for exposed (E) and unexposed (U) groups were divided by predicted values and the results expressed as a ratio E/U $\times$ 100.

TABLE 5.6 Comparison of Latino adults, 20 exposed at Torrance and 103 unexposed in Houston, by analysis of variance; *p* values <0.05 underlined

	Exposed		Unexposed		
	Mean	Sd	Mean	Sd	*p* Value
Age years	37.4	12.5	33.7	10.9	.176
Education Level years	10.1	2.7	11.0	2.8	.149
Simple Reaction Time min	403	149	323	106	.005
Choice Reaction Time min	569	131	537	112	.255
Sway–Balance Eyes Open	0.86	0.24	0.77	0.17	.059
Closed	1.40	0.56	1.15	0.35	.01
Blink Reflex R-1 ms Right	11.5	2.1	14.9*	2.3	.0001
Left	11.1	0.9	14.7*	2.3	.0001
Grip Strength Right	35.4	10.9	40.8	13.1	.01
Left	31.0	12.1	38.4	12.1	.0005
Visual Fields Right	447	96			
Left	424	99			
Color score	13.6	1.3	11.7	1.3	.0001
Contrast Sensitivity					
Smell	3.4	0.6			
Cognitive Function Domain					
Culture Fair A	20.9	8.3	25.1	7.8	.029
Digit Symbol	46.1	17.0	51.5	14.6	.05
Vocabulary	12.2	4.8	16.9	7.0	.005
Perceptual Motor Speed					
Pegboard	72.8	11.0	73.6	32.7	.908
Trail Making A	40.7	12.7	42.5	21.0	.713
Trail Making B	104.6	40.8	96.3	43.2	.430
Recall Domain					
Story Immediate	8.7	4.1	18.8	7.2	.0001
Story Delayed	6.8	4.8	15.6	7.4	.0001
Visual Design Recall	24.2	7.5	27.2	8.1	.122
Finger Writing Errors	7.8	3.8	5.06	6.6	.084
Long-Term Memory Domain					
Picture Completion	11.2	4.3	12.5	4.0	.183
Similarities	13.9	6.5	16.5	6.4	.103
Information	9.2	4.6	12.6	6.0	.02
Profile of Mood States	53	41	29.7	40.3	.02
Pulmonary Function Tests					
FVC % of pred	90.7	14.0	101.2	12.1	.0008
FEV_1 % of pred	90.0	12.8	96.9	12.4	.025
FEF_{25-75} % of pred	97.6	21.5	98.0	25.7	.956
FEF_{75-85} % of pred	95.1	30.1	87.5	43.4	.455

* Abnormal "control" values

education (Table 5.6, Figures 5.3a, b). The exposed had slower simple reaction times, and choice reaction times, balance sway speed was significantly faster in the exposed with eyes closed and almost significant with eyes open. Blink reflex latency R-1 was faster (normal) in exposed vs. abnormal in Houston subjects, which is a seeming paradox. Grip strength and color vision were abnormal in the exposed. Cognitive functions, Culture Fair, digit symbol, and vocabulary were much lower in the exposed. Similarly, verbal recall, immediate and delayed, was much lower in exposed, but the long-term memory tests were not different, a finding consistent with the equivalent ability in the

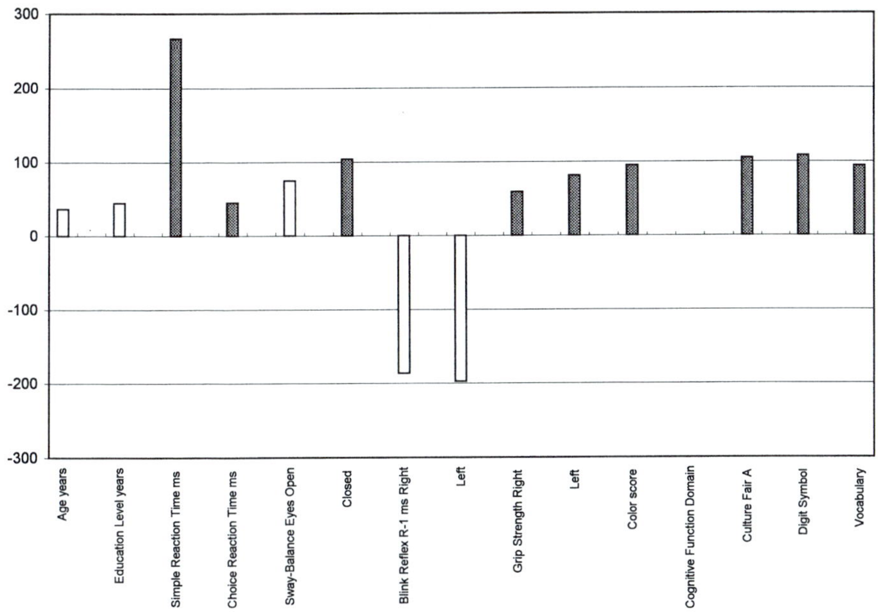

FIGURE 5.3a. Comparison of Latino adults, 20 exposed to H_2S (Torrance) and 103 unexposed (Houston) by ANOVA. Hatched bars are statistically significant.

groups before exposure. Perceptual motor speed tests were not different, but those values of the unexposed subjects were higher (more abnormal) than expected. In Latinos the vital capacity and FEV_1 were abnormal, although not low as in the African Americans, corrected for ethnic difference.

The 20 exposed children were mainly Latino and matched well for age and educational level to Houston children (Table 5.7, Figures 5.4a, b). Exposed children showed abnormal balance with eyes open but not eyes closed and more abnormal color vision. Reaction times were not increased in the exposed, and blink reflex latency R-1 was normal. Digit symbol score was lower in the exposed, perceptual motor speed was equivocal because of exceptionally high and probably abnormal trail making B scores in the unexposed, and recall was not different. Exposed children's vital capacities were lower, as were values for terminal flow (FEF_{75-85}).

Symptom frequency scores in adults compared to our standard unexposed group were elevated except for decreased alcohol tolerance (Table 5.8, Figures 5.5a, b). These frequencies of complaints elevations were consistent with the results of neurobehavioral tests.

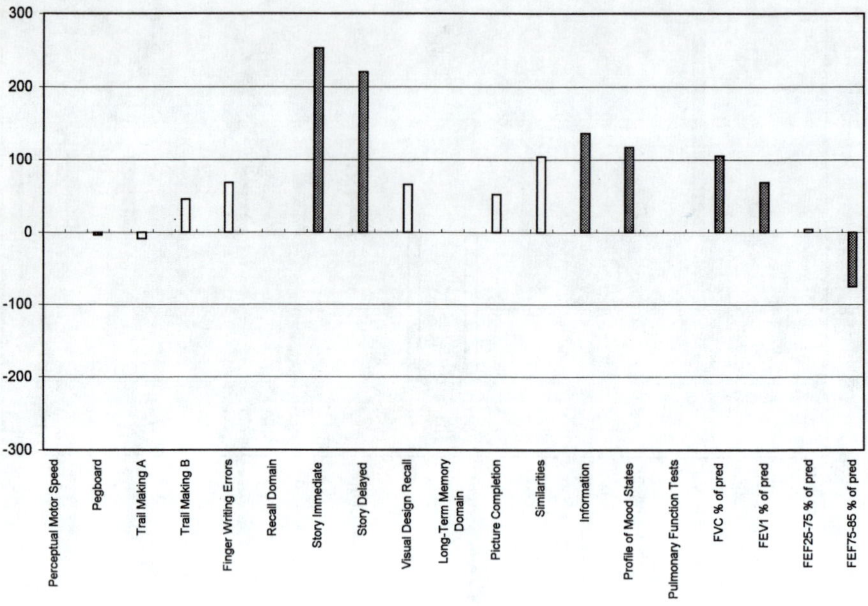

FIGURE 5.3b. Comparison of Latino adults, 20 exposed to H_2S (Torrance) and 103 unexposed (Houston) by ANOVA. Hatched bars are statistically significant.

No correlations were found between the clinical categories of ascending injury graded from 1 least to 4 greatest and any of these test results. The caveat is that when they were divided by ethnicity and the children were considered separately, the groups were small. As we also looked at the distributions of ethnicity and age within the groups and found no notable imbalances, we based this conclusion on the entire sample of 68 subjects.

THE UNOCAL REFINERY EXPOSURE

Unocal refinery workers and downwind neighbors had symptoms of asthma, depression, and dermatitis. We tested 13 former workers from the refinery and 22 downwind neighbors in Nipoma, California, before and after they filed suit against the refinery. When the 13 ex-workers were studied, the small airways obstruction, dermatitis, and depression had cleared.

Ten male ex-workers, mean age 38 years, who had worked in the desulfurization unit of the refinery for 1.5 to 3 years, and eight male and nine female neighbors of the

TABLE 5.7 20 exposed children vs. 44 Houston Latino children, means and standard deviations

	Unexposed		Exposed		
	Mean	Sd	Mean	Sd	*p* Value
Age yrs	10.9	3.0	12.5	3.0	.057
Education Level yrs	4.9	2.9	6.2	2.8	.118
Physiological Domain					
Simple Reaction Time ms	390	175	459	170	.137
Choice Reaction Time ms	613	192	650	173	.437
Sway-Balance cm/sec					
Eyes Open	1.12	0.42	0.87	0.30	.023
Eyes Closed	1.58	0.51	1.44	0.63	.338
Blink Reflex R-1 ms					
Right	14.6	1.7	11.0*	1.5	.0001*
Left	14.8	2.0	10.5*	1.1	.0001*
Color Vision (Lanthony Hue)	12.1		13.3		.017
Visual Fields Automated Perimetry					
Right			451		
Left			450		
Smell			3.4		
Cognitive Domain					
Culture Fair A score	22.9	8.0	23.4	7.1	.823
Digit Symbol	47.1	17.1	35.8	13.4	.007
Vocabulary	8.6	3.8	11.7	4.5	.224
Profile of Mood States	35.9	34.4	43.9	34.4	.388
Verbal Recall (Stories)					
Story 1 Immediate	7.7	4.4	8.6	4.1	.462
Story 2 Delayed	6.2	4.9	5.9	4.2	.819
Visual Recall			26.9	6.8	
Remote Memory					
Information	5.9	4.7	6.3	3.7	.711
Picture Completion	9.3	5.1	11.4	4.1	.114
Similarities	10.5	7.1	11.2	6.3	.724
Perceptual Motor Speed					
Pegboard	89.2	31.4	77.1	10.9	.10
Trail Making A	64.5	35.9	42.9	19.8	.015*
Trail Making B	124.6	46.6	95.9	47.7	.029*
Fingertip Number Writing	13.5	9.2	10.5	8.3	.223
Profile of Mood States Sc	35.0	37.0	53.0	41.4	
Pulmonary Function Tests					
FVC	87.4	21.4	74.8	14.2	.02
FEV_1	72.8	15.4	71.4	17.4	.743
FEF_{25-75}	60.3	23.5	71.3	29.0	.116
FEF_{75-85}	52.8	33.7	69.9	27.7	.053

* Exposed had better scores.

ms = millisecond

cm = centimeter

sec = second

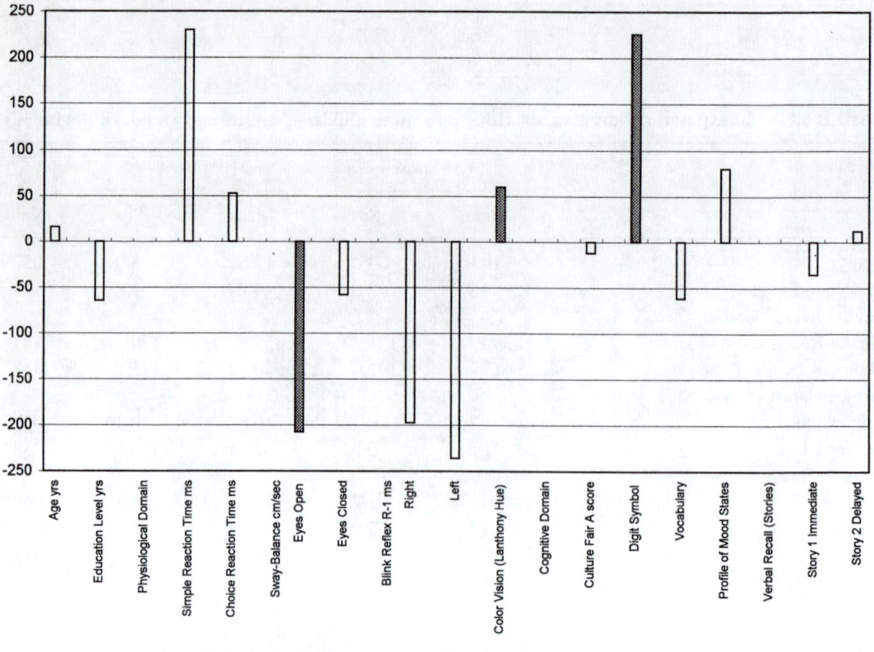

FIGURE 5.4a. Comparison of Latino children, 20 exposed to H_2S (Torrance) and 44 unexposed (Houston) by ANOVA. Hatched bars are statistically significant.

refinery, mean age 38.5 years, were studied in January 1989 and restudied in June 1991. In June we studied three additional ex-workers from oil refinery desulfurization and five additional neighbors (total 35 ex-workers and neighbors), and 32 unexposed (17 men and 15 women). The ex-workers had been pipe fitters, painters, laborers, and process handlers in the vanadium pentoxide (V_2O_5) desulfurization unit after its installation in 1986. None had ever been overcome by H_2S. Twelve workers studied had left the refinery by October 1988; one left in July 1989. One worker was lost to follow-up in 1991. These ex-workers and neighbors were plaintiffs in a class action lawsuit. Reference subjects were chosen from friends and relatives of the exposed subjects who had not worked at the refinery or resided in the downwind zone and were close matches for age, sex, and educational level.

Exposure Conditions and Air Monitoring Data

Residents lived within 1,200 meters east–northeast and at a lower elevation than the refinery and were within 2,400 meters of the sulfur plant and coking units (Figure 5.6).

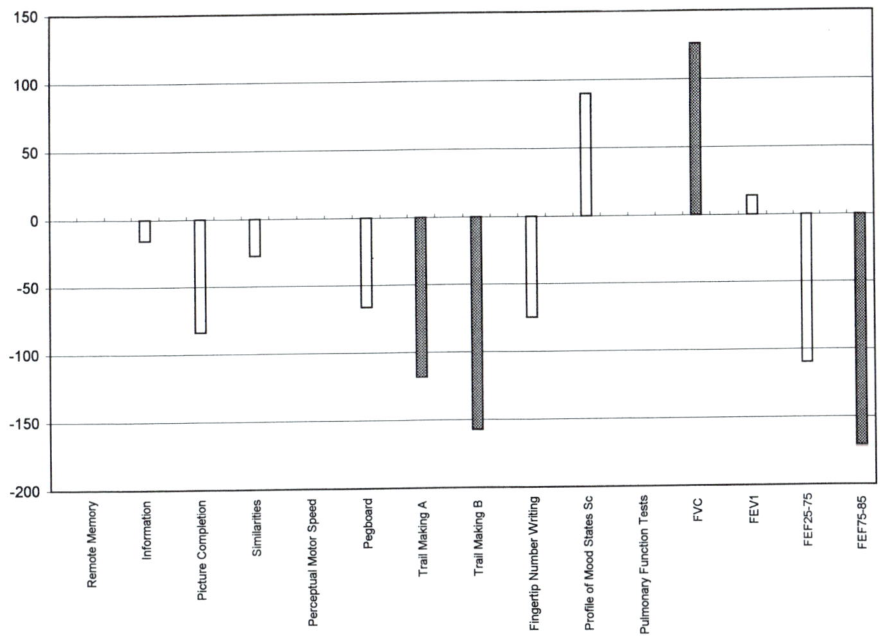

FIGURE 5.4b. Comparison of Latino children, 20 exposed to H_2S (Torrance) and 44 unexposed (Houston) by ANOVA. Hatched bars are statistically significant.

Almost daily coastal air inversions held the refinery's odorous stack gases close to the ground. These reduced sulfur gases are heavier than air. Air monitoring at street level on Calle Bendita near the center of the subjects' homes for one week in July 1990 showed H_2S at 10 parts per billion (ppb) with periodic peaks of 100 ppb, as well as dimethylsulfide 4 ppb, mercaptans 2 ppb, ethane 500 ppb, and propane 500 ppb. Also vanadium, as V_2O_5, and thiodiglycolic acid were detected by air and soil monitoring. Reduced sulfur gases outside the desulfurization unit between April 1987 and January 1991 showed 24-hour averages for mercaptans from 0.1 to 21.1 parts per million (ppm), hydrogen sulfide from 0.0 to 8.8 ppm, carbon oxide sulfide (COS) from 2.6 to 52.1 ppm, and total reduced sulfur from 6.1 to 70.7 ppm. Workers' exposures within this unit were not measured. The refinery's 24-hour emissions averaged 0 to 8.8 ppm for H_2S and 1.13 to 70.7 ppm for total reduced sulfur gases from 1987 to 1991. The regional air pollution monitoring station, located east of the refinery and south of the subjects' homes (Figure 5.6), often had the nation's highest ambient air SO_2 levels.

The mean test scores were pooled for the 35 ex-workers and neighbors and for men and women, as their ages, educational levels, and test scores showed only small

TABLE 5.8 Comparison of symptom frequencies in Torrance exposed subjects and the Wickenburg unexposed group (scale 1–11)

	Exposed	Unexposed
Skin itching	4.5	3.3
Deformed fingernails	2.3	1.6
Chest tightness	3.3	2.2
Palpitations	2.8	2.2
Pain or burning chest	3.4	2.1
Shortness of breath	4.0	2.5
Dry cough	4.5	2.6
Cough with mucus	4.3	2.8
Cough with blood in mucus	1.9	1.2
Dry mouth	4.7	3.2
Throat irritation	4.2	2.6
Eye irritation	6.0	2.8
Decreased sense of smell	3.6	2.1
Headache	6.1	4.4
Nausea	3.9	2.4
Dizziness	4.1	2.4
Lightheadedness	4.1	2.5
Unusual exhilaration	2.5	1.5
Loss of balance	3.3	2.0
Loss of consciousness	1.9	1.2
Extreme fatigue	5.1	3.4
Somnolence	3.8	2.6
Insomnia	4.4	2.9
Wake frequently	4.4	2.9
Sleep only a few hours	4.2	2.9
Irritability	5.4	3.4
Lack of concentration	5.7	3.2
Recent memory loss	5.1	3.1
Long-term memory loss	4.1	2.2
Mood swings	4.3	2.5
Loss of libido	3.6	3.1
Decreased alcohol tolerance	2.0	2.4
Indigestion	3.6	3.2
Loss of appetite	3.5	2.6
Stomach swollen	3.3	2.9

differences which were not statistically significant (Table 5.9 and 5.10, Figures 5.7a–c). Values of the entire exposed group were compared to unexposed in the first probability column, *p,* and scores of the 22 neighbors alone were compared in the p^* column.

Neurophysiological Domain

The simple reaction time of the exposed group was significantly longer than that of the unexposed, and the choice reaction time of the exposed subjects was also slower, by 71 ms ($p < 0.003$). Sway speed with eyes open was significantly faster in exposed subjects than unexposed, and with eyes closed the difference was also significant ($p < 0.04$). Color discrimination (Lanthony 15 hue test; 18) was significantly reduced in exposed compared to unexposed. In exposed subjects blink reflex latency (R-1) was

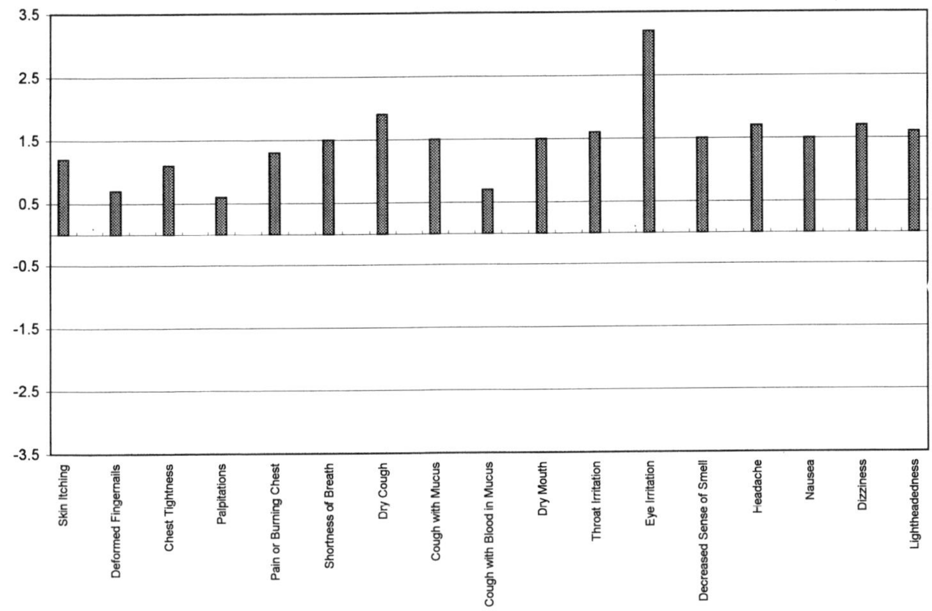

FIGURE 5.5a. Comparisons of symptom frequencies for H_2S-exposed adults (Torrance) and controls (Wickenburg), frequency scale 1–11. Hatched bars are statistically significant.

nearly identical on the right and the left, and neither result was significantly different from that for the unexposed. Thus exposed subjects, workers, and neighbors were significantly impaired compared to unexposed for three of four neurophysiological functions.

Neuropsychological Domain

Peg placement with the dominant hand was not significantly longer in exposed subjects than in unexposed, but trail making A and B times were significantly different between the exposed and unexposed groups when 22 exposed residents, excluding the ex-workers, were compared to unexposed. Differences between the groups for recall were equivocal. Thus the exposed group's verbal recall for story 1, immediate and delayed, was not significantly different from that of the unexposed, while the exposed group's immediate recall of story 2 was significantly less (Table 5.10, Figure 5.7b). Recall of

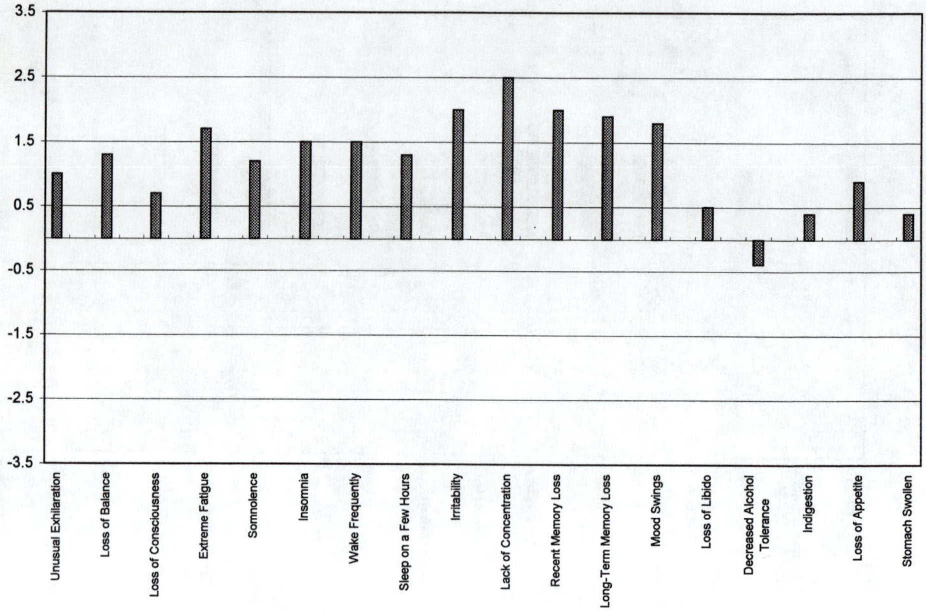

FIGURE 5.5b. Comparisons of symptom frequencies for H_2S-exposed adults (Torrance) and controls (Wickenburg), frequency scale 1–11. Hatched bars are statistically significant.

drawings and recall of numbers were not different for exposed compared to unexposed, but exposed residents scored significantly lower on immediate and delayed recall of drawings. The exposed group's scores for overlearned memory were not different from those of the unexposed group. Scores for Culture Fair, block design, and embedded figures were not significantly different in exposed and unexposed groups. Errors in recognition of numbers written on the fingertips were not different for the groups. Thus, although digit symbol scores were significantly lower, this domain appeared unaffected by exposure.

Affective Domain

The POMS score for the exposed group mean was seven times that of the unexposed (Table 5.11, Figure 5.8), whose scores equaled published normal values (19). Anger, confusion, depression, tension–anxiety, and fatigue scores were significantly elevated

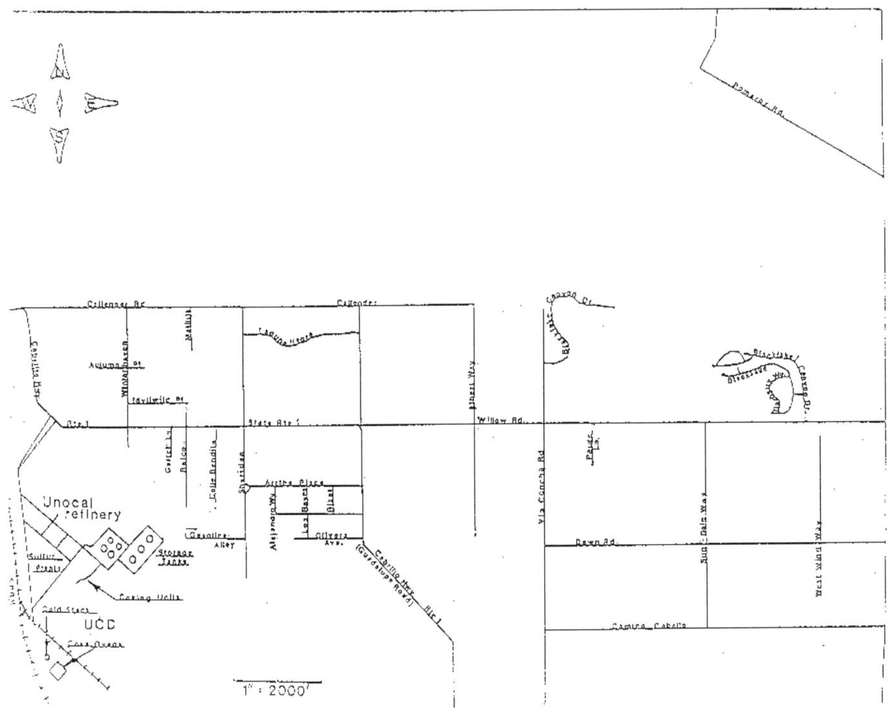

FIGURE 5.6. Unocal facility and vicinity.

TABLE 5.9 Neurophysiological functions in exposed and unexposed subjects (means and standard deviations with *p* values by t-test)

	35 Exp mean s.dev.	32 Ref mean s.dev.	*p*	*p**
Age yrs	39.7 ± 12.0	38.9 ± 12.5	NS	NS
Educ Level yrs	11.3 ± 2.2	12.2 ± 2.4	NS	NS
Reaction Time				
Simple ms	336 ± 145	268 ± 50	0.01	0.01
Choice ms	593 ± 106	522 ± 89	0.004	0.004
Sway Speed cm/s				
Eyes Open	0.92 ± 0.28	0.79 ± 0.19	0.037	0.000
Eyes Closed	1.47 ± 0.81	1.15 ± 0.31	0.04	0.000
Color Vision (Lanthony Hue Test)				
errors	12.1 ± 5.4	11.4 ± 4.3	0.005	0.000
Blink				
Glabellar Tap R-1				
Right ms	13.9 ± 1.7	13.8 ± 1.8	NS	NS
Left ms	14.1 ± 1.9	13.5 ± 2.0	NS	NS

* In 22 residents compared to unexposed.

ms = millisecond, cm/s centimeters per second

NS = not significant

TABLE 5.10 Comparison of immediate and 30-minute delayed recall, overlearned memory, and cognitive and psychomotor functions for exposed and unexposed subjects (means and standard deviations with *p* values by t-test)

		35 Exposed mean s. dev.	32 Unexposed mean s. dev.	*p*	*p**
Perceptual Motor					
Trail Making A		35.4 ± 15.4	28.8 ± 8.0	.033	.012
Trail Making B		87.8 ± 29.8	71.4 ± 35.8	.04	.01
Pegboard Dom. Hand		74.8 ± 21.3	69.7 ± 10.3	NS	NS (.09)
Recall					
Story 1	Immediate	9.6 ± 3.7	10.8 ± 3.8	NS	NS
	Delayed	7.9 ± 5.6	8.3 ± 4.0	NS	NS
Story 2	Immediate	9.4 ± 3.9	11.8 ± 4.3	.023	.0285
	Delayed	8.6 ± 4.7	9.9 ± 4.2	NS	NS
Visual	Immediate	29.6 ± 6.7	31.4 ± 4.6	NS	.016
	Delayed	23.2 ± 8.9	26.5 ± 7.0	NS	.021
Digit	Forward	6.4 ± 1.7	6.5 ± 1.4	NS	NS
	Backward	4.3 ± 1.3	4.7 ± 1.3	NS	NS
Overlearned Memory					
Information		16.8 ± 5.7	18.9 ± 6.2	NS	NS
Similarities		19.6 ± 5.0	20.1 ± 5.8	NS	NS
Picture Complet.		15.4 ± 2.3	14.7 ± 3.2	NS	NS
Cognitive					
Culture Fair		28.6 ± 6.5	30.7 ± 6.9	NS	NS (.08)
Block Design		30.8 ± 9.2	30.5 ± 11.5	NS	NS
Digit Symbol		50.6 ± 13.3	57.4 ± 13.7	.04	.03
Digit Symbol Recall		5.4 ± 2.4	5.7 ± 2.3	NS	NS
Embedded Figures		31.7 ± 4.1	32.2 ± 4.6	NS	NS
Fingertip Number Writing					
Errors Right		2.8 ± 2.9	3.0 ± 3.4	NS	NS
Errors Left		2.2 ± 2.8	2.4 ± 3.2	NS	NS

* 22 residents compared to unexposed

in exposed residents and in former workers, who were nearly identical. POMS score had significant coefficients in linear regression models for many symptom frequencies. However, POMS scores as independent variables, whether separately or together with age, sex, and educational level, had *no significant coefficients with the abnormal test scores,* including CRT, sway speed, color recognition, and trail making A and B.

Symptoms

Frequencies of 31 of 33 symptoms were significantly higher for exposed subjects than unexposed (Table 5.12, Figures 5.9a, b) when compared by t-test. Only a rare complaint, loss of consciousness, and loss of appetite were not significantly different. Respiratory and mucous membrane irritation were 10 to 30 times as frequent in exposed compared to unexposed, as were neurological symptoms, sleep disturbances, and general symptoms including headache. Skin complaints were three to six times higher in exposed subjects compared to unexposed.

Confounding Factors

The most frequent possible confounding factor was surgical anesthesia, which had been experienced by 50% of exposed subjects. Some of their test results were different from

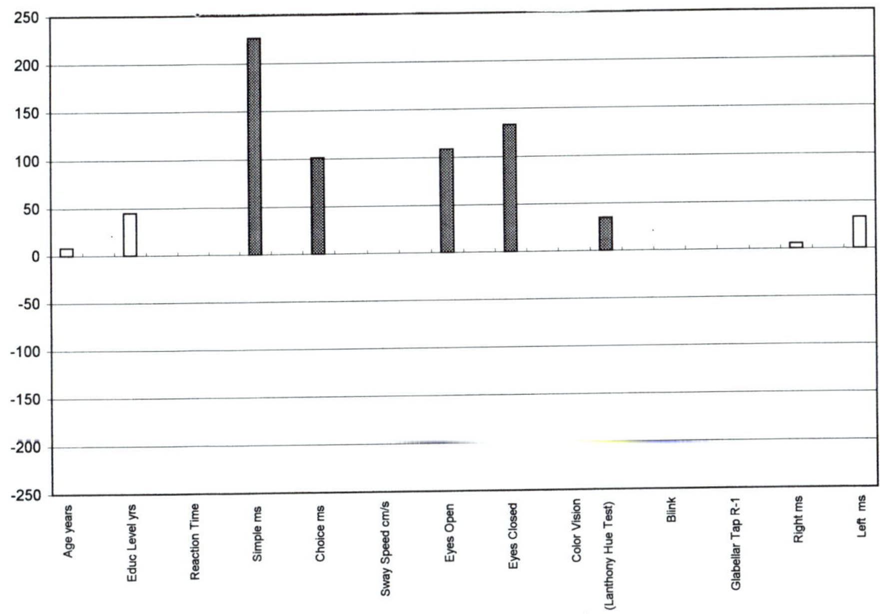

FIGURE 5.7a. Comparisons of 35 H_2S-exposed (Nipoma) and 32 unexposed (San Luis Obispo). Hatched bars are statistically significant.

those of subjects who had not received anesthesia. However, minutes of anesthesia as an independent variable had no significant coefficients in linear regression models for any neurophysiological test score. All of the ex-workers had been exposed to solvents; one was a painter. Half of them had used vibrating tools. Nine of the exposed residents had confounding factors, three used solvents at home, two used vibrating tools, one had received anesthesia numerous times, one had seizures and was on medication, and two had pesticide and herbicide exposures from their nursery. Excluding these nine subjects from analysis for each test category, in turn, did not change the outcomes significantly; so all subjects were retained. Alcohol use was not a confounding factor, as no subject had an elevated alveolar (air) alcohol on the day of testing, and only one neighbor and three ex-workers reported that they had ever been inebriated from alcohol.

Bias

As testers did not know the exposure status of the subjects, bias from this source is unlikely. Scores from testing the exposed group before and after they became clients

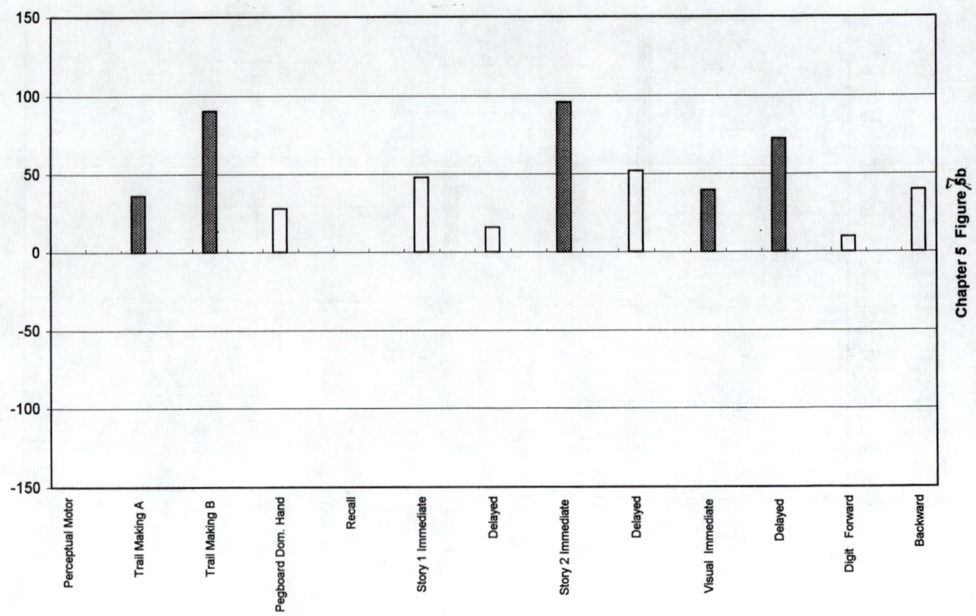

FIGURE 5.7b. Comparisons of 35 H_2S-exposed (Nipoma) and 32 unexposed (San Luis Obispo). Hatched bars are statistically significant.

did not vary, showing that becoming clients was not a bias. Groupwide bias in selection of a comparison subject is possible but unlikely, as subjects did not have insight into how to select better performers on the tests.

Repeat Testing

After 30 months, 21 residents and 9 workers showed statistically insignificant variation across the interval without a trend of improvement (see Chapter 16, Table 16.5.)

CASPER AND HOUSTON SUBJECTS

Casper, Wyoming Exposed and Unexposed Subjects

In 1991 approximately 100 residents of the Brookhurst section of northwest Casper, Wyoming brought suit against six chemical companies for causing adverse health effects

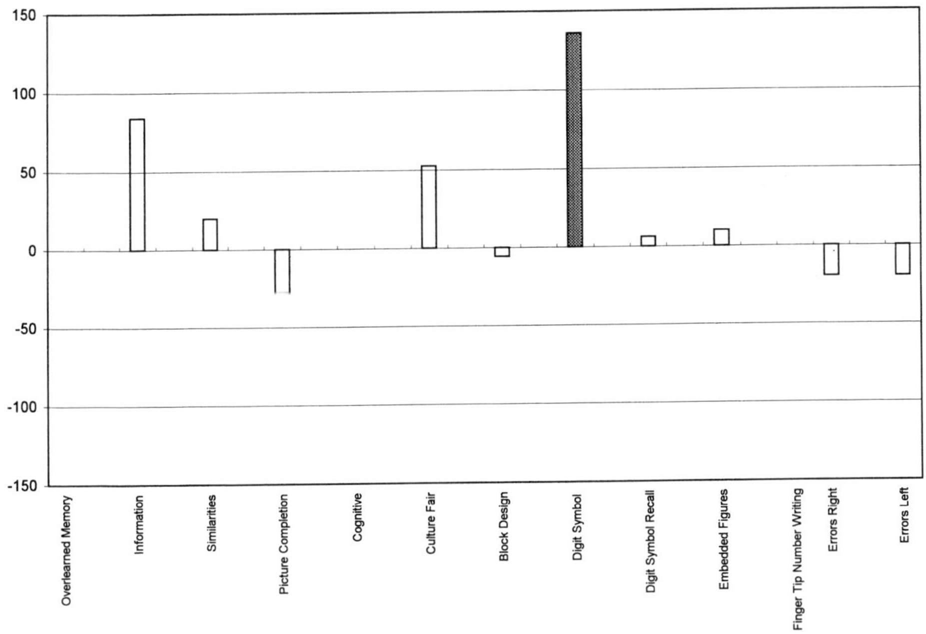

FIGURE 5.7c. Comparisons of 35 H_2S-exposed (Nipoma) and 32 unexposed (San Luis Obispo). Hatched bars are statistically significant.

TABLE 5.11 Profile of mood states, total score and components

	35 Exposed mean s.dev.	32 Unexposed mean s.dev.	p^*
Total	70.9 ± 40.7	10.3 ± 20.0	.0001
Anger	16.8 ± 11.3	5.6 ± 5.7	.0001
Depression	18.8 ± 11.7	5.1 ± 6.4	.0001
Tension	18.3 ± 7.3	7.8 ± 4.0	.0001
Confusion	13.3 ± 5.7	4.9 ± 2.8	.0001
Fatigue	15.5 ± 7.3	5.3 ± 3.7	.0001
Vigor	11.8 ± 7.0	18.5 ± 4.4	.0001

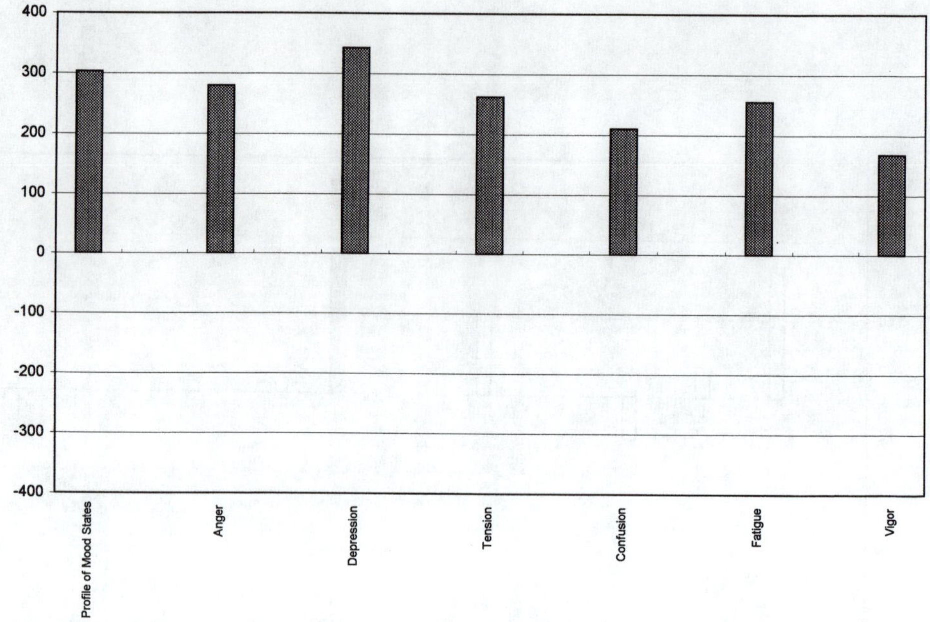

FIGURE 5.8. Comparisons of profile of mood states, H_2S-exposed and unexposed. Hatched bars are statistically significant.

and decreasing property values. They had lived in the subdivision for over ten years and contended that the plume of odorous fumes, together with surface and subsurface drainage of solvent-smelling chemicals, contaminated their yards and wells and was responsible for their numerous health complaints, cancers, and birth defects. Casper is a city of 51,000 located on the Platt River in central Wyoming. It is in an oil-producing area, and a refinery is located near the center of town. Six chemical companies were part of a corridor between Brookhurst and the city.

Eighty-four exposed individuals, whose ages ranged from 10 to 77 years, with a mean age of 38 and an educational level of 11 years, were compared with 50 unexposed subjects from the city of Casper with an average age of 50 years, range 14 to 82 years, and an educational level of 12.8 years. Although the strategy was for an exposed individual to nominate and contact a comparison person, this approach did not yield enough unexposed subjects; so we appealed to local organizations, including the Elks Lodge and the local hospital and medical center, to augment the comparison group.

TABLE 5.12 Frequencies of 33 respiratory, neurological, general, and skin complaints in exposed and unexposed subjects in 1991

	Exposed (35)	Unexposed (32)	
	mean Sd	mean Sd	*p*
Respiratory			
Chest tightness	91.7 ± 78.0	8.6 ± 18.9	.0000
Palpitations	68.5 ± 70.8	19.9 ± 54.6	.0022
Chest pain	69.7 ± 76.6	2.8 ± 8.9	.0000
Dry cough	82.4 ± 79.3	6.4 ± 18.3	.0000
Cough with blood	28.4 ± 51.4	1.0 ± 6.0	.0030
Dry mouth, nose, throat	97.1 ± 82.2	3.7 ± 9.9	.0000
Throat irritation	105.7 ± 78.0	11.1 ± 24.0	.0000
Eye irritation	125.1 ± 79.4	6.0 ± 21.6	.0000
Reduced smell	78.4 ± 80.7	7.7 ± 24.6	.0000
Neurological			
Dizziness	80.7 ± 75.5	4.2 ± 12.0	.0000
Lightheadness	93.6 ± 74.5	10.3 ± 17.7	.0000
Loss of balance	66.9 ± 66.8	5.4 ± 17.4	.0000
Loss of consciousness	2.5 ± 9.2	0	—
Lack of concentration	138.2 ± 86.1	8.3 ± 16.1	.0000
Recent memory loss	137.5 ± 90.7	8.3 ± 21.5	.0000
Long-term memory loss	84.4 ± 90.2	4.7 ± 13.4	.0000
Mood unstable	137.3 ± 93.3	2.4 ± 8.6	.0000
Irritability	131.3 ± 92.4	22.4 ± 36.7	.0000
Exhilaration	32.6 ± 60.3	1.9 ± 8.1	.0000
Sleep			
Somnolence	89.3 ± 101.4	1.4 ± 8.4	.0000
Insomnia			
Can't fall asleep	101.3 ± 88.5	17.0 ± 45.9	.0000
Wake frequently	126.9 ± 91.9	16.4 ± 46.9	.0000
Sleep few hours	121.4 ± 94.1	21.6 ± 57.4	.0000
General			
Headache	145.5 ± 76.6	31.3 ± 47.1	.0000
Nausea	90.5 ± 74.4	8.4 ± 17.7	.0000
Libido decreased	79.8 ± 89.2	17.6 ± 45.9	.0000
Excess fatigue	136.9 ± 88.2	18.1 ± 37.4	.0000
Alcohol tolerance decreased	32.3 ± 76.7	4.3 ± 21.8	.044
Indigestion	94.9 ± 105.7	9.2 ± 21.5	.0000
Loss of appetite	48.2 ± 76.4	20.6 ± 52.8	.086
Skin			
Itching	72.7 ± 81.8	19.0 ± 55.4	.002
Dryness	93.2 ± 93.1	16.2 ± 46.8	.0001
Redness	76.4 ± 72.9	21.4 ± 55.5	.0008

This effort resulted in a somewhat older and better-educated unexposed group than the exposed individuals. Age would reduce the difference between the exposed and unexposed, but in some tests this effect would be offset by the greater educational level in the unexposed.

The methods used for evaluating neurophysiological and neuropsychological performance are those outlined in Chapter 3. In brief we tested the simple and two-choice visual reaction time, color vision using the Lanthony desaturated hue test, balance as sway speed with eyes open and with eyes closed, blink reflex, and latency of R-1

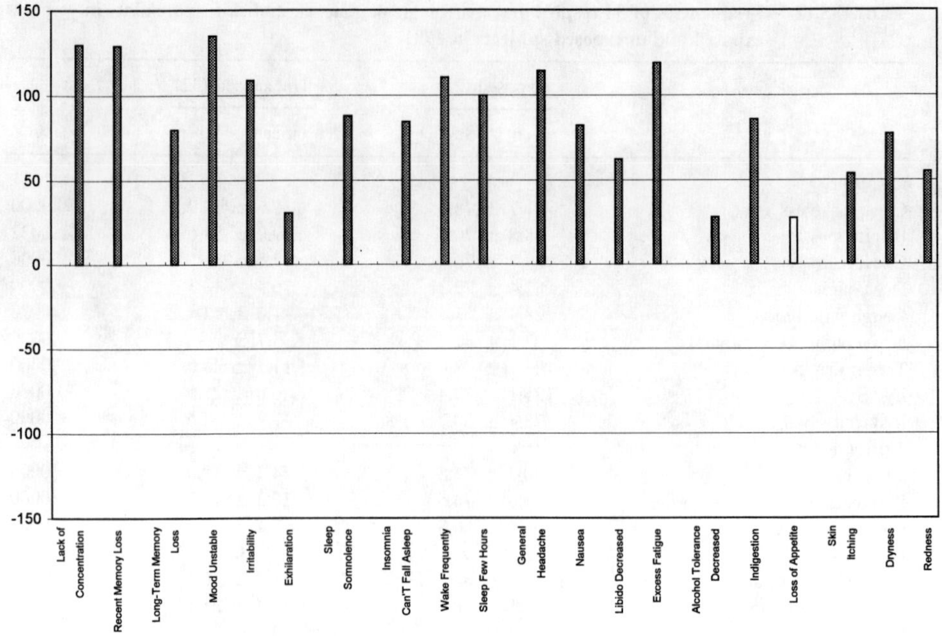

FIGURE 5.9a. Comparisons of symptom frequencies for 35 H_2S-exposed (Nipoma) and 32 unexposed (San Luis Obispo). Hatched bars are statistically significant.

stimulated by glabellar tap. Cognitive tests included Culture Fair 2A, a nonverbal and nonarithmetic design-solving test of constructional and cognitive performance, block design, and digit symbol from the WAIS. Perceptual motor speed was tested with a pegboard using slotted pegs, trail making A and B, and fingertip number writing errors from the Halstead-Reitan battery. Recall was tested with story 1 and story 2, visual reproduction, and digits forward and backward from the Wechsler memory scale. Embedded memory was evaluated with information, picture completion, and similarities from the WAIS.

Compared to the 50 Casper reference people, the exposed group had almost identical values for reaction time and for blink although fewer of the exposed had a delayed BRL R-1 on glabellar tap and considerably fewer responded to supraorbital tap stimulation (see Table 5.13, Figures 5.10a–d). Although sway speed appeared faster in the exposed group, particularly with eyes closed, this difference was not statistically significant. Similarly, the cognitive functions, although favoring the performance of the com-

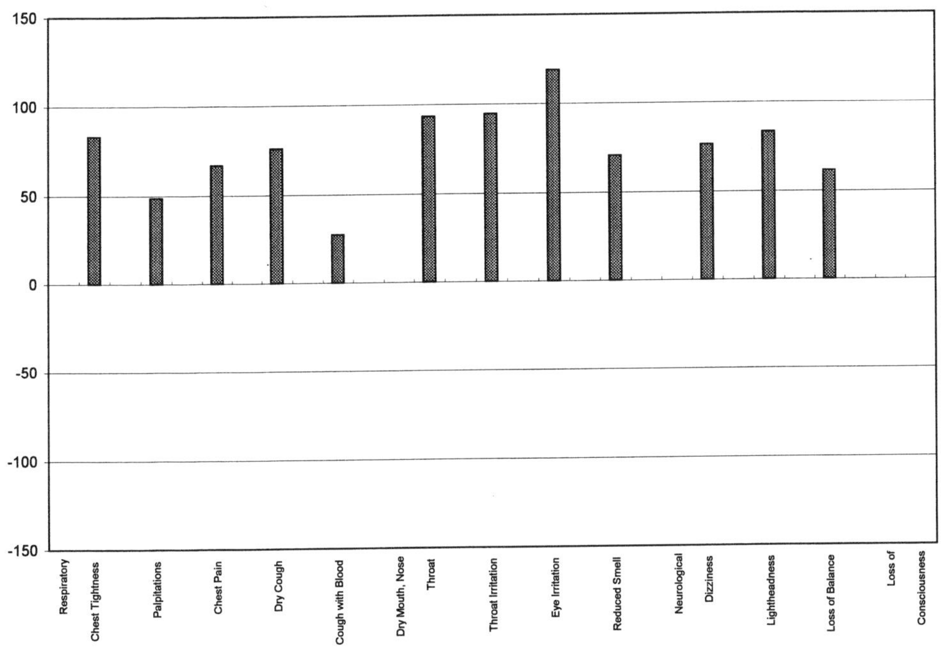

FIGURE 5.9b. Comparisons of symptom frequencies for 35 H_2S-exposed (Nipoma) and 32 unexposed (San Luis Obispo). Hatched bars are statistically significant.

parison group most times, actually showed a reversal, with more impairment for perceptual motor functions, pegboard, and trails A and trails B in unexposed controls, although these differences between the groups were not statistically significant. For recall functions the comparison group did slightly better, again without statistical significance, and this was also seen to be true for the embedded memory functions.

However, when the overall function was compared with the national predicted group based on Louisiana and California unexposed groups, there was a statistically significant slowing of choice reaction time in the exposed, and, most outstandingly, differences—both with eyes open and with eyes closed—for sway speed as a measure of balance (Figures 5.10c, d). Trail making B took longer in both exposed and unexposed Casper groups than in the national unexposed, whereas trail making A was prolonged in the comparison group only.

The interpretation of these differences, namely, that both the exposed and the comparison group had abnormalities of sway speed, choice reaction time, and trails B,

TABLE 5.13 Casper exposed compared to local unexposed and national unexposed, showing the intermediate scores for Casper unexposed

	Comparison (50)		Exposed (84)		National (66)		
	Mean	Sd	Mean	Sd	Mean	Sd	*p*
Age/years	50.4	20.1	38.1	17.5	38.0	12.8	
Ed Level	12.8	2.4	11.0	3.1	12.5	2.1	
POMS Score	18.1	27.9	56.6	51.5	16.0	28.4	
Physiological							
Simple Reaction Time	280	59.7	288	74	281	85	
Choice Reac. Time 1	542	107	553	115	519	88	
2	533	85	551	107	514	81	
3	539	94	559	94	524	88	.0067*
Color Score	12.1	7.06	12.3	6.6			
Blink Glabellar R ms	15.0	1.8 (92)	14.6	1.9 (67)			
L ms	15.5	1.8 (78)	15.4	1.9 (53)			
Supraorbital R ms	14.5	1.7 (94)	14.6	1.7 (39)			
L ms	14.4	1.9 (98)	14.2	1.6 (40)			
Sway Speed cm/sec							
Eyes Open	0.94	0.22	0.99	0.30	0.87	0.22	.0014*
Eyes Closed	1.40	0.41*	1.52	0.58	1.31	0.66	.01*
Cognitive							
Culture Fair A	27.6	7.9	29.3	7.3	30.6	6.1	
Block Design Score	28.7	10.6	31.0	9.2	31.0	10.3	
Digit Symbol	54.4	16.0	51.2	15.3	56.8	14.9	
Perceptual Motor							
Finger Writing Right	2.6	2.7	2.9	3.4	2.5	3.2	
Left	2.3	2.7	2.4	3.1	2.1	2.7	
Pegboard	82.7	25.8*	72.9	19.7	68.9	4.5	
Trails A	39.8	17.3*	34.6	13.0	33.8	14.1	
B	83.8	49.7*	79.2	45.1*	74.9	44.3	
Recall							
Story 1	11.7	4.4	10.6	4.2	10.5	3.8	
Story 2	11.4	4.5	9.8	4.4	9.7	4.1	
Visual Recall	11.7	4.3*	10.5	3.2	10.1	3.1	
Digits Forward	6.7	1.3	6.6	1.3	6.8	1.5	
Backward	4.5	1.1	4.4	1.4	4.7	1.2	
Embedded Memory							
Information	18.4	6.0	16.7	5.8	16.9	5.3	
Picture Completion	14.2	3.3	14.6	3.4	15.3	3.1	
Similarities	19.4	4.8	20.8	6.5	20.2	5.3	

* $p = <.05$

r = range

suggested a citywide exposure. There was a large oil refinery practically at the crossroads of the main east–west and north–south streets of Casper, which refined high sulfur crude from the basin fields in the Casper vicinity. There was gas flaring, with a perceptible odor of hydrogen sulfide. This observation suggested that the generalized effects observed were from the oil refinery exposure, which extended into the comparison group.

Certainly other interpretations should be considered, including the possibility that we are simply observing oddities due to the age deterioration factor and the physiologi-

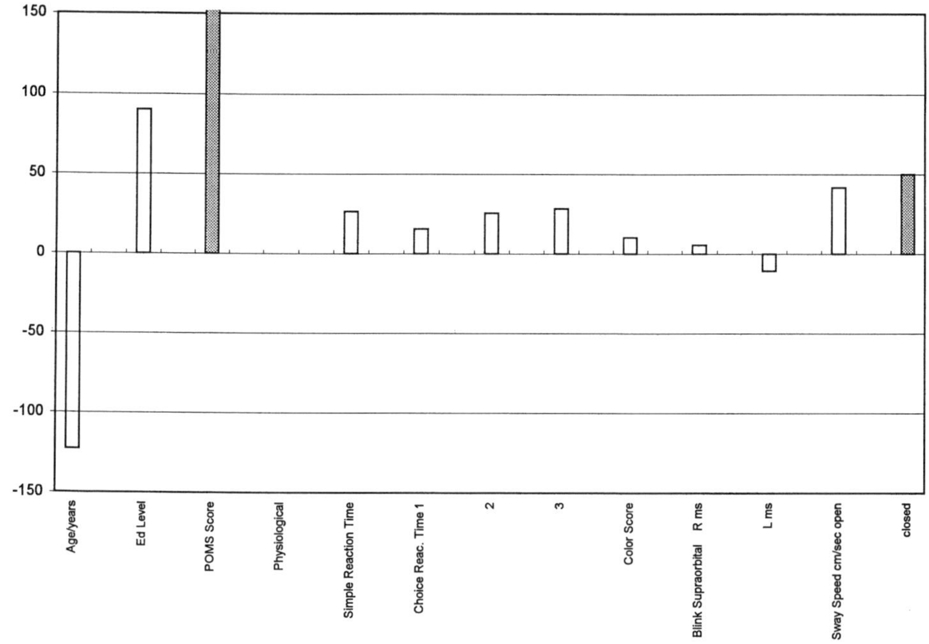

FIGURE 5.10a. Comparison of 80 exposed (Brookhurst) and 50 unexposed (Casper).

cal and perceptual motor responses. We reasoned that if further experience with the physiological tests shows that their sensitivity can be relied upon, then when they individually show differences of this magnitude, confounding exposure should be sought or some other factor that could explain the differences. Such differences do not seem to be methodological or site-specific, as we now have similar reference values from five different states in the United States.

The POMS score was more than three times as high in the exposed as the unexposed (56 compared to 18), and increased by component scores for anger, confusion, and depression. Objective tests showed a "Casper effect," which overlay both groups and did not distinguish them. Symptom frequencies and profile of mood states score (self-appraisal) were different, which may reflect concern or a sense of injury. This finding would tend to support, at least in a small way, the differences in objective tests compared to the national group.

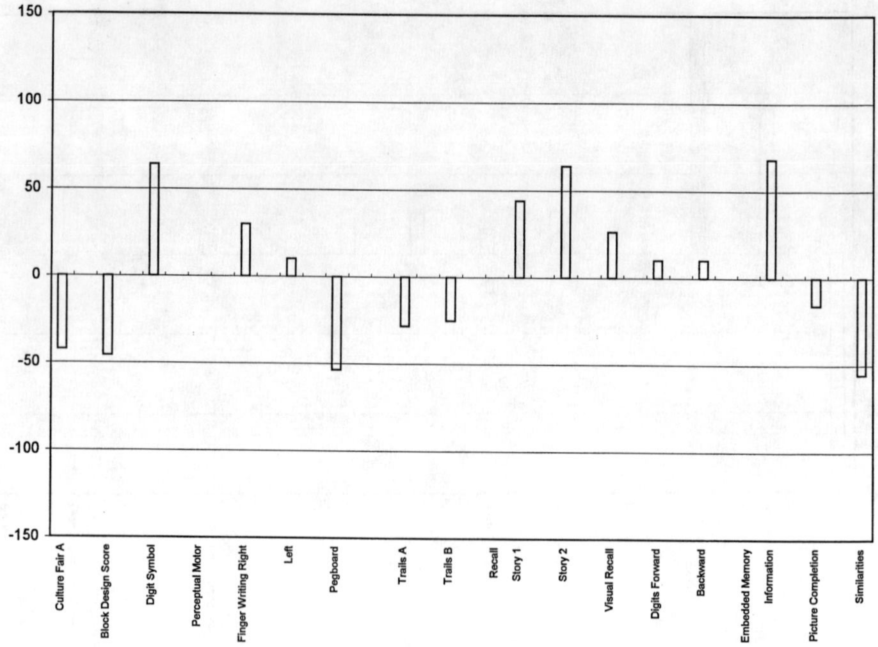

FIGURE 5.10b. Comparison of 80 exposed (Brookhurst) and 50 unexposed (Casper).

Houston Petroleum Refineries—Circumstantial Exposure

The Houston–Wickenburg comparison suggests abnormality for the Houston unexposed, who differ from Wickenburg unexposed for blink, recall, reaction time, vocabulary, and perhaps trails A and B. These differences are despite their being 10 years younger than thc Wickcnburg group with slightly higher POMS scores. Are Houston unexposed TCE-exposed? Blink abnormalities suggest that they are chemically affected, with chlorinated solvents as the prime possibility.

Consideration of children showed again a significant lengthening of blink reflex latency R-1 of 1.4 to 2.0 ms in all three ethnic groups (Caucasians, African-Americans, and Latinos), an increased sway speed, an impaired reaction time of 70 to 94 ms, and a general impairment of cognition (CFA, vocabulary, and digit symbol), recall, and long-term memory, despite a near match for age (Wickenburg 11.5 years, Caucasians 12 years, and Latino 11.4 years). Thus either living near the oil refinery–chemical region or being economically impoverished, unable to escape, was associated with impaired function scores.

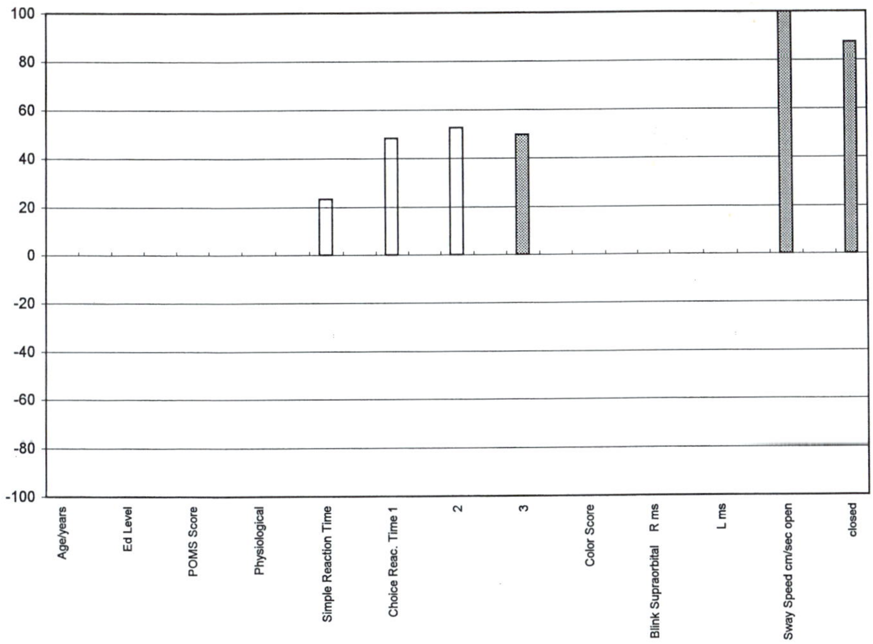

FIGURE 5.10c. Comparison of 80 exposed (Brookhurst) and national predicted groups.

Obviously, these differences could be reflecting ability, but that is unlikely for blink and balance. Thus, it is hypothesized that maladaptive performance has resulted from living near refineries and a major chemical manufacturing center where H_2S is the principal chemical exposure.

BALANCE FUNCTION AND REACTION TIMES IN REFINERY WORKERS EXPOSED TO H_2S

Balance function as sway speed and two-choice visual reaction time were measured in 38 refinery workers recruited from a group of 75 being examined for asbestos-related disease. The mean age was 42.7 ± 11.4 years, with a range from 22 to 63 years. Methods were the standard ones just described. Balance with eyes closed was abnormal, with sway speed 1.48 ± 78 cm/sec compared to 1.17 ± .32 cm/sec ($p < .0043$) in 68 unexposed subjects of mean age 37.6 years. Age means were not significantly different ($p < .06$). Sway speed with eyes open was also abnormal at 1.06 ± .44

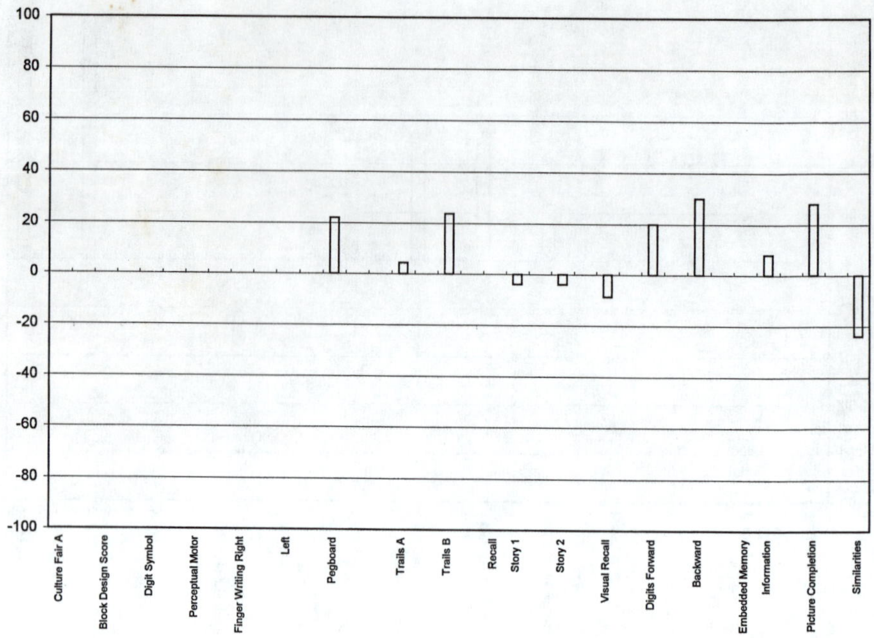

FIGURE 5.10d. Comparison of 80 exposed (Brookhurst) and national predicted groups.

cm/sec as compared to 0.81 ± .20 cm/sec ($p < .0001$) in unexposed subjects. Six subjects had sway speed with eyes closed greater than 2.0 cm/sec and should be considered to be an abnormal subgroup. One of these men has tinnitus, and another was in a spill of hydrogen chloride or hydrogen fluoride and had suffered lung damage. Otherwise, their other exposures and past medical disorders were not pertinent to balance abnormality. Choice reaction time was 537 ± 71 msec compared to 513 ± 79 msec, a difference that was not significant. Based on the previous study of ex-workers and downwind neighbors of a refinery processing Santa Barbara, California, channel crude oil rich in reduced sulfur gases, who had abnormal sway speed and abnormal choice reaction time at 593 ± 106 msec, the new data support the suggestion of toxic effects from these gases. Other exposures to hydrocarbons, sulfur oxides, hydrogen chloride, and fluoride included known neurotoxins. Stack emissions include manganese, chromium, mercury, lead, and vanadium, which are neurotoxic; so careful characterization of tank and stack emissions by environmental sampling is needed to establish which associations are causal. Of the metals, manganese and mercury should be accorded the highest index of suspicion because in occupational concentrations, as in mining and refining, they produce adverse effects on balance. Nevertheless, with our present insight into levels of exposure, mechanisms of action, and similarity to clinical poisoning, hydrogen sulfide is the most likely toxicant.

DISCUSSION

The 16 patients provide a scouting examination of the spectrum of H_2S effects. These ranged from serious neurobehavioral impairment, including balance and reaction time impairment from near fatal exposures, to insidious function loss from long-term exposure doses around refinery operations, gas flares, asphalt loading, and, most important, simple proximity to refineries. Skepticism about this novel interpretation seemingly was abolished by the observations of severe impairment, including visual field loss, in subjects around and downwind of the Torrance refinery explosion. Less intense impairment characterized the population exposed downwind and at work to the desulfurization plant oil refinery at San Luis Obispo. Probably refineries cannot be made safe for nearby residents or even those some miles away.

The downwind effect plus observations from other studies of chemical effects at Casper and Houston and in refinery workers has strengthened the social implications of these findings. In light of the adverse effects at Torrance and Nipoma, brain damage is implied at Casper and Houston, as populations unexposed to chemical manufacturing in Casper and to chlordane in Houston showed patterns of impairment consistent with the effects of reduced sulfur gases.

The most common neurophysiological impairment was for balance, followed by blink. In the neuropsychological testing, choice reaction time, fingertip number writing, and verbal recall were most commonly impaired, followed by trail making and Culture Fair. Thus, integrative functions with multiple inputs were impaired by H_2S exposure. Statistical certainty is a difficult problem in analyzing small groups of patients. Two available methods were used. One is to consider H_2S exposure as the definer of the group despite many differences in patients' exposure and previous status, so as to compare their average scores to those of an unexposed group. The other method is to use the 95% confidence limits of expected performance and determine prevalence of abnormality for each test score. The first analysis showed decreased performance for balance, reaction time, and cognitive and perceptual motor skills. The second, based on counting the prevalence, although more crude, showed that the same functions were impaired.

There are three conclusions. The first is that sensitive testing in subjects who were not made unconscious by H_2S or whose exposure was even lower showed protracted impairment when the subjects were tested at intervals from months to years after exposure. The second conclusion is that exposures causing impairment occurred in environmental situations, downwind as well as in the workplace, and the third is that the exposure did not have to be sublethal to cause permanent ill effects. A few hours of occupational H_2S exposure without unconsciousness or respiratory distress impaired neurobehavioral function, an effect that appeared to be permanent. Although alternative explanations may be possible in each individual, the composite experience suggests that well-planned epidemiological studies with sensitive methods should be performed on subjects environmentally exposed as well as on those occupationally exposed.

Occupational and downwind residential exposures to a California coastal refinery processing high sulfur crude oil and emitting reduced sulfur gases, rich in H_2S, were associated with abnormal objective physiological tests: slower simple and choice reaction times, excessive speed of sway with eyes open and with eyes closed, and reduced color discrimination. Thus the automatic (subconscious) parts of the neuroaxis except for blink showed impairment. The impaired performance was accompanied by reduced perceptual motor speed and perhaps recall. Impairment was less severe than in subjects who had recovered from H_2S-induced unconsciousness (9, 11, 12). Most of the psychometric differences were small and not significant, which implied that these tests were less sensitive than the physiological ones, or that the subjects studied had less damage to the cerebral cortex than did our groups. There was a sevenfold greater affective disturbance as shown by mood states and an excessive frequency of 31 of 33 symptoms.

The objective and subjective abnormalities followed activation of a petroleum desulfurization unit in the nearby refinery. Reduced sulfur gases exemplified by H_2S are the most plausible explanation of the neurotoxic effects, but mercury, manganese, and vanadium pentoxide, as potent inhibitors of signal transduction pathways conveyed in airborne dust, may have contributed. It is unclear whether the desulfurization plant had a specific causal role in the health disorders above that of the refinery. Clearly it added more irritative complaints, which made the burden of being downwind ''unbearable'' to the subjects. Because ex-workers had greater proximity to the source, one might have expected them to be more severely affected than the downwind neighbors. Because they were not, workers may have recovered somewhat in the interval of nearly a year between leaving work and being tested. Alternately they may have had better initial performance than the neighbors but lost more, so as to average with them. Finally, it is possible that intermittent exposure, for 40 hours per week for 3 or 4 years, at the refinery was not equivalent to neighbors exposed at presumably lower doses for up to 168 hours per week for 10 to 15 years. Exploration of the dose–response relationships needs more subjects and continuous monitoring of concentrations of reduced sulfur gases and other neurotoxins. Ex-workers had minimal changes during the 1989 to 1991 interval although their balance improved slightly, whereas the residents, all of whom continued to be exposed, remained impaired.

Alternate Explanations

Clients in environmental chemical lawsuits have been viewed as seeking personal gain and thus as unreliable and undeserving as ''whiplash'' or ''back strain'' plaintiffs. In checking the group scores for possible evidences of bias from poor performance, poor attention, or early termination of effort was not observed. Being party to a lawsuit could have motivated them to raise their symptom frequencies and conceivably could even influence scores on psychological tests, but this seems unlikely because a majority of exposed subjects would have to do this in a consistent pattern without rehearsal, and they were all naive concerning these tests. Furthermore, scores were nearly identical on retesting after two years, which also argues against this explanation (see Chapter 16, Table 16.5). Balance by sway speed, choice reaction time, and blink reflex are multiple-trial tests in which the subjects' scores improve and become stable. If the exposed were test-wise subjects, poor performance would be anticipated in all tests in the battery, not just in the most sensitive ones. Moreover, the pattern of abnormality was similar to but less severe than that in workers overcome by H_2S (9, 11, 12).

Inappropriate Comparison Group

If comparison subjects were ''supranormals'' they could bias interpretation of average results wrongly, causing investigators to consider them abnormal. However, comparison of the mean scores of these 32 reference subjects to those of three reference groups showed virtual identity in the neurophysiological and neuropsychological domains (20–22). Thus the choice of the comparison group seems appropriate.

Somatization disorder or chronic post-traumatic stress (DSM III, 1980) triggered by odors and health fears might elevate POMS scores and symptom frequencies, but this seems unlikely in these subjects because POMS scores had no significant coefficients in linear regression models for any abnormal physiological or psychological test score. It is more probable that the exposed subjects' elevated POMS scores and excess frequency of symptoms were neuropsychological consequences of chemicals acting on the brain. Moreover, stress does not impair balance and choice reaction time, but improves them (23).

Attribution of Effects

The desulfurization workers' complaints that initiated the study, mainly dermatitis, depression, and asthma, gradually disappeared when they were away from the refinery. Asthma and dermatitis but not depression were attributed to sulfur dioxide (SO_2) and vanadium pentoxide. In contrast, the neighbors' symptoms did not improve as they continued exposure downwind of reduced sulfur gases. Workers and neighbors developed airway and skin irritation shortly after the installation of a vanadium pentoxide desulfurization unit. However, H_2S and carbon oxide sulfide (COS) were measured in the residential area for 5 years, and this refinery had processed ''sour'' crude oil, with reduced sulfur gases, for nearly 40 years. Hydrogen sulfide, COS, and mercaptans are heavier than air, collect in low places such as sewers and holds of ships from decomposition of sulfur compounds under hypoxic conditions (7, 9, 14), and have caused deaths (8, 9).

Mechanisms

Reduced sulfur gases cause death quickly by respiratory paralysis at exposures above 500 ppm of H_2S. Levels between 100 and 500 ppm irritate the eyes and respiratory tract, and unconsciousness and death have been reported from prolonged breathing of 50 ppm. Fortunately, the odor threshold is 25 ppb. The mechanism of brain damage from low doses of H_2S is unclear, but soluble sulfides may interfere with cellular utilization of oxygen by combining with iron in the cytochrome oxidase respiratory enzyme in mitochondria (3). Primates exposed to 500 ppm of H_2S for 22 minutes showed cerebral cortical necrosis, reduction in Purkinje cells of the cerebellar cortex, and focal gliosis. Repeated exposures of mice to H_2S reduced brain RNA and inhibited cytochrome oxidase activity (3).

CONCLUSIONS

It would be prudent to assess the neurobehavioral performance of workers before their employment in oil fields and refineries (23) and periodically thereafter. By coupling the results with careful measurements of reduced sulfur gases and ''trace'' components, dose–response relationships would emerge. Meanwhile refineries with H_2S desulfurization should be viewed with caution.

References

1. Smith RP and Gosselin E: Hydrogen sulfide poisoning. *J Occup Med* 1979;21:93–96.
2. Christison R: A Treatise on Poisons in Relation to Medical Jurisprudence, Physiology and the Practice of Physic (4th ed.). Edinburgh: Adam and Charles Black, 1845, pp. 805–810.
3. Beauchamp RO, Jr., Bus JS, Popp JA, Boreiko CJ, and Andjelkovich DA: A critical review of the literature on hydrogen sulfide toxicity. *CRC Crit Rev Toxicol* 1984;13:25–97.
4. Adelson L and Sunshine I: Fatal hydrogen sulfide intoxication. *Arch Path* 1966;81:375–380.
5. Gaitonde UB, Sellar RJ, and O'Hare AE: Long term exposure to hydrogen sulphide producing subacute encephalopathy in a child. *Brit Med J* 1987;294:614.
6. Matsuo F and Cummins JW: Neurological sequelae of massive hydrogen sulfide inhalation. *Arch Neurol* 1979;36:451–452.
7. Goldsmith JR: The 20-minute disaster: hydrogen sulfide spill at Poza Rica. In: *Environmental Epidemiology,* JR Goldsmith (ed.), Boca Raton, FL: CRC Press, 1987.
8. Burnett WW, King EG, Grac M, and Hall WF: Hydrogen sulfide poisoning: review of 5 years experience. *Canadian Med Assoc J* 1977;117:1277–1280.
9. Tvedt B, Skyberg K, Aaserud O, Hobbesland A, and Mathiesen T: Brain damage caused by hydrogen sulfide: a follow-up study of 6 patients. *Am J Indust Med* 1991;20:91–101.
10. Wechsler D: *Adult Intelligence Scale Manual* (revised). New York: The Psychological Corporation, 1971.
11. Wasch HH, Estrin WJ, Yip P, et al.: Prolongation of the P-300 latency associated with hydrogen sulfide exposure. *Arch Neurol* 1989;46:902–904.
12. Kilburn KH: Profound neurobehavioral deficit in an oil field worker exposed to hydrogen sulfide. *Am J Med Sci* 1993;306:301–305.
13. Dales RE, Spitzer WO, Suissa S, Schechter MT, Tousignant P, and Steimetz N: Respiratory health of a population living downwind from natural gas refineries. *Am Rev Respir Dis* 1989; 139:595–600.
14. Jaakkola JJK, Marttila O, Vilkka V, Silakoski I, and Haahtela T: The South-Karelia air pollution study: the quantitative effect of malodorous sulfur compounds on daily symptoms: a longitudinal study. *Am Rev Respir Dis* 1990;141:A75.
15. Spitzer WO, Dales RE, Schechter MT, et al.: Chronic exposure to sour gas emissions: meeting a community concern with epidemiologic evidence. *Can Med Assoc J* 1989;141: 685–691.
16. Modan B, Swartz TA, Tirosh M, et al.: The Arjenyattah epidemic, a mass phenomenon: spread and triggering factors. *Lancet* 1983;2:1472–1474.
17. Landrigan PJ and Miller B: The Arjenyattah epidemic. Home interview data and toxicological aspects. *Lancet* 1983;2:1474–1476.
18. Lanthony P: The desaturated panel D-15. *Doc Ophthalmol* 1978;46:185–189.
19. McNair DM, Lorr M, and Droppleman LF: *Profile of Mood States.* San Diego, CA: Educational and Industrial Testing Service, 1971/1981.
20. Kilburn KH, Warshaw RH, and Shields MG: Neurobehavioral dysfunction in firemen exposed to polychlorinated biphenyls (PCBs): possible improvement after detoxification. *Arch Environ Health* 1989;44:345–350.
21. Kilburn KH and Warshaw RH: Neurobehavioral effects of formaldehyde and solvents on histology technicians: repeated testing across time. *Environ Res* 1992;58:134–146.
22. Kilburn KH and Warshaw RH: Neurotoxic effects from residential exposure to chemicals from an oil reprocessing facility and Superfund site. *Neurotox Teratol* 1995;17:89–102.
23. Gamberale F and Kjellberg A: Behavioral performance assessment as a biological control of occupational exposure to neurotoxic substances in neurobehavioral methods in occupational health. *Adv Biosci* 1983;46:137–144.

6

Chlorine and Cresylate from a Train Derailment

Derailment and puncture of a tank car carrying chlorine and one carrying "spent" potassium cresylate created a noxious aerosol over Alberton, Montana, and 4 km to the southwest, which began at 4 15 A.M. on April 11, 1996 (see Figure 6.1). Within minutes some of the 500 residents awoke and evacuated the area, traveling 54 km to Missoula. Others moved out because of pungent and acrid fumes that lasted for up to 3 days. Burning of the eyes, nose, and throat and of the skin were frequent. Chest tightness and trouble in breathing were nearly universal. Four passersby on the interstate highway were hospitalized in intensive care for pulmonary edema, and a dozen others were treated in hospital with various severities of respiratory decompensation. Recurrence and/or persistence of voice changes, skin burning, and respiratory symptoms were coupled with difficulty in recalling and concentrating, trouble sleeping, headaches, and other complaints, which led to neurobehavioral investigation 7 weeks after the spill. Many residents remained displaced because of recurrence of chest tightness, headaches, nausea, and memory disorders within minutes after they returned home. An odor described frequently as being "like pesticide sprays" persisted at the derailment site and in Alberton for two months or more. The 500 subjects in a 4.8 km radius near the spill (the hot zone) were invited for testing, and 97 were examined on June 1 and 2, 1996.

TESTING OF SUBJECTS

Fifty-five exposed subjects had symptom questionnaires and profile of mood states measured in mid-May 1996. Ninety-seven subjects were tested, 81 adults (ages 18 to 63 years) and 16 children (17 years and under) on June 1 and 2, 1996, in Missoula. Sixteen adults were tested subsequently and 97 were analyzed. All were residents of Alberton or adjoining areas, including Lothrop and Petty Creek. The exposure duration averaged 117 minutes with a range from 0 minutes to 3 days in adults. In children the average was 54 minutes and the range 2 to 240 minutes. Subjects were almost equally divided between nonclients and clients of three law firms.

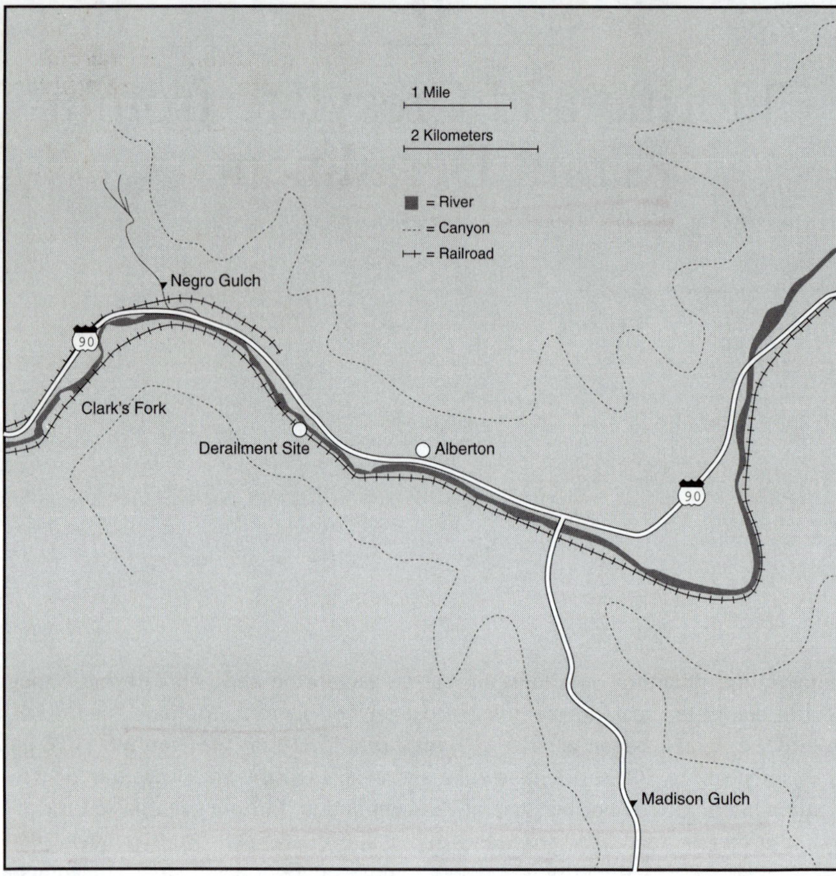

FIGURE 6.1. Alberton, Montana in the canyon of the Clark's Fork River.

culture Fair ≡ intelligence test.

The methods of measurement were those used in previous studies of the effects of chemicals on the central and peripheral nervous systems and the respiratory system. Included were mapping of visual fields, color discrimination, hearing, balance, blink (reflex latency R-1), simple and choice reaction time, and grip strength. Neurobehavioral tests included Culture Fair (an intelligence test), vocabulary, digit symbol, peg placement in a grooved (Lafayette) pegboard, trail making A and B, fingertip number writing errors, and verbal recall (stories 1 and 2) from the Wechsler memory scale. A profile of mood states (POMS) was self-administered, which assayed tension, depression, anger, fatigue, vigor, and confusion. The frequency of each of 35 symptoms covering general health, respiration, and nervous system was scaled from absent to daily (11). Comparisons were made to a national group of 202 adults and 145 children

TABLE 6.1 Alberton chlorine-exposed adult subjects compared to national control subjects

	Exposed 97		Unexposed 202		
	Mean	Sd	Mean	Sd	*p* value
Age yrs	38.4	9.9	44.1	20.6	.017*
Education Level yrs	13.4	2.4	12.9	2.3	.126
Simple Reaction Time ms	281	142	290	65	.909
Choice Reaction Time ms	511	126	503	86	.539
Balance Sway Speed cm/sec					
Eyes Open	0.81	0.29	0.77	0.19	.185
Eyes Closed	1.38	0.61	1.23	0.40	.015*
Blink Reflex Latency R-1 ms	13.6	2.1	12.7	2.0	.004*
Right					
Left	13.4	2.1	12.4	2.1	.005*
Color Score	12.2	1.4	11.8	1.6	.088 b
Visual Fields Right	1352	215	1419	233	.174
Left	1343	211	1431	205	.067
Pegs	67.2	10.1	76.1	23.6	.001 R
Trails A	31.3	11.2	33.9	12.6	.107
Trails B	68.4	27.5	77.5	32.8	.029 R
Culture Fair	30.9	5.6	27.7	7.4	.0005R
Digit Symbol	53.7	16.0	56.0	13.5	.217
Vocabulary	24.4	9.4	23.3	8.8	.342
Information	17.9	6.1	17.9	5.6	.980
Picture Completion	14.9	3.2	15.0	2.7	.657
Similarities	20.7	5.3	20.2	4.9	.471
Fingertip Writing Right	3.3	3.5	1.9	2.0	.0001*
Left	2.9	3.6	1.3	1.8	.0001*
Stories Immediate	19.9	8.2	21.9	8.2	.172
Delayed	16.2	8.3	17.9	8.5	.322
POMS Score	80.2	43.7	21.0	31.6	.0001*
Grip Strength					
Women Right	34.4	8.3	30.2	7.5	.005 R
Left	31.4	7.6	28.1	6.8	.014 R
Men Right	54.1	11.8	50.6	10.4	.082
Left	51.5	10.5	48.8	10.9	.179
	Children, 16				
	Exposed 16		Unexposed 14.5		
Blink Reflex Latency					
R-1 ms Right	14.1	2.7	11.2	1.5	.0001*
Left	13.2	2.2	11.3	1.7	.0002*
Story 1	8.3	4.4	10.4	4.6	.089 b
POMS	55.9	43.2	26.0	31.6	.0009*
	All Exposed, 97				

Vision: 48/90 abnormal visual fields.

Pulmonary Function Test: 46% (45) were abnormal; 38% showed a greater than 5% improvement in FEV_1 after a bronchodilator.

* = Statistically significant
b = Bordering statistical significance
R = Statistically significantly better than unexposed
Lt = Compared to Tennessee unexposed

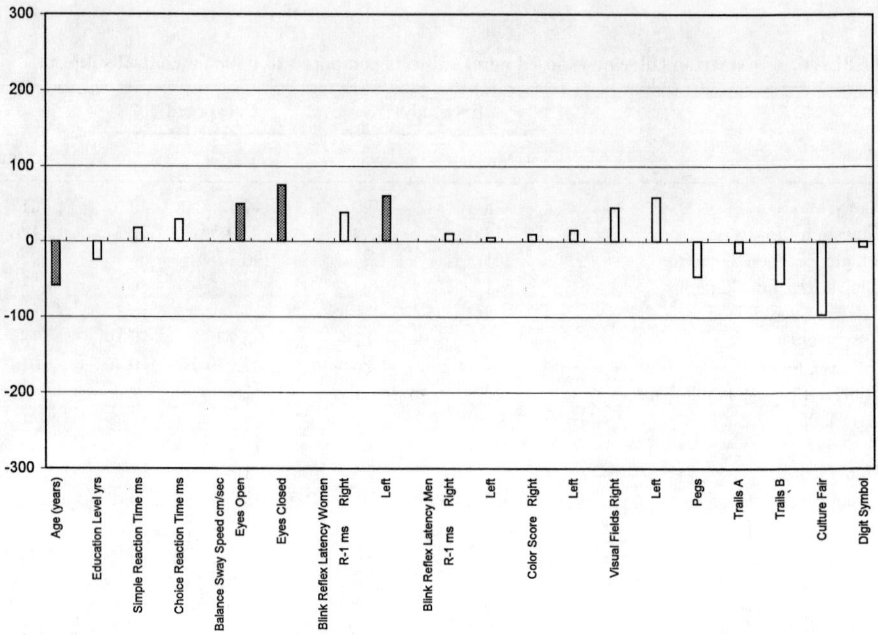

FIGURE 6.2a. Comparison of 97 chlorine-exposed adults and 202 unexposed adults by ANOVA. Hatched bars are statistically significant.

unexposed to chemicals. Abnormality was defined as a statistically significant difference in mean (average) values for the exposed group compared to the unexposed.

In adults, abnormalities included balance with the eyes closed, blink reflex latency left, finger writing errors, and POMS score, which was four times the score of the unexposed group (Table 6.1, Figures 6.2a, b). In addition, visual fields were abnormal in 48 of 90 tested subjects (in addition 9 children had abnormal visual fields) (Table 6.1). Pulmonary function was abnormal by conventional criteria (<80% of predicted) in 45, and FEV_1 improved more than 5% after administration of a bronchodilator aerosol in 37 members of the entire group, meaning that 70% of exposed subjects had bronchoconstriction. Production of phlegm, shortness of breath, and wheezing were all significantly more prevalent in exposed than in unexposed subjects.

The 16 Alberton children had abnormal blink reflex latency, abnormal POMS, and borderline abnormal verbal recall (Table 6.1). Also, they shared in the visual field and pulmonary function abnormalities. Nonclients and clients showed no significant differences in any test. Thus, none of 20 tests was abnormal, below the expectation

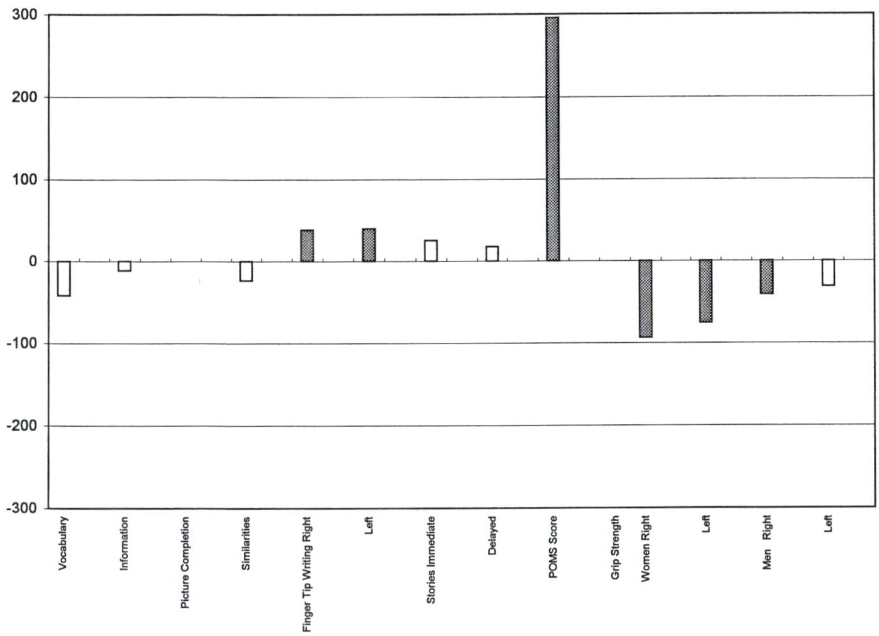

FIGURE 6.2b. Comparison of 97 chlorine-exposed adults and 202 unexposed adults by ANOVA. Hatched bars are statistically significant.

of 5% abnormal, by chance alone. Twenty subjects had five or more impaired tests abnormalities, and ten additional subjects had four abnormalities each.

The frequencies of 35 symptoms were higher (statistically significantly) in the chlorine-exposed Alberton subjects compared to the Arizona unexposed group (Table 6.2, Figures 6.3a, b). The symptom frequencies of the 55 prestudied Alberton residents and the 51 appraised at the time of testing were not significantly different for rheumatic and lupus erythematosus symptoms, respiratory complaints, or psychiatric disorders. Only 2 of 35 symptoms, palpitation and deformed fingernails, were significantly more frequent in the prestudied group. In summary, those people studied initially by questionnaire and POMS and those who had complete testing had similar questionnaire responses. The POMS scores of 92.4 vs. 74.6 and tension and anger were significantly higher in the prestudied subjects, but both groups were highly abnormal—the unexposed value was 30. Occupational exposures to chemicals that are neurotoxic did not differ between exposed subjects and unexposed.

Neurobehavioral and pulmonary impairments were found in chlorine-exposed Alberton, residents tested 7 weeks after the spill by comparison to national unexposed sub-

TABLE 6.2 Symptom frequencies, Alberton, Montana

	Exposed	Unexposed	*p*
Skin itching	4.9	3.2	.0001
Fingernail changes	2.8	1.9	.008
Chest tightness	5.0	2.2	.0001
Palpitations	4.1	2.1	.0001
Burning in chest	4.3	2.0	.0001
Shortness of breath	5.4	2.5	.0001
Dry cough	5.0	2.6	.0001
Cough with mucus	5.0	3.0	.0001
Cough with blood	1.9	1.2	.0003
Dry mouth	5.9	3.2	.0001
Throat irritation	5.9	2.8	.0001
Eye irritation	5.8	2.8	.0001
Decreased smell	3.9	2.1	.0001
Headache	6.1	4.1	.0001
Nausea	4.6	2.4	.0001
Dizziness	3.9	2.1	.0001
Lightheadedness	4.5	2.5	.0001
Exhilaration	1.7	1.7	.876
Loss of balance	3.3	2.2	.0003
Loss of consciousness	1.2	1.3	.849
Extreme fatigue	5.9	3.2	.0001
Somnolence	4.7	2.5	.0001
Insomnia			
Cannot fall asleep	4.4	3.0	.0005
Wake frequently	4.7	2.8	.0001
Sleep few hours	4.5	2.9	.0003
Irritability	5.8	3.5	.0001
Loss of concentration	5.7	3.5	.0001
Recent memory loss	5.6	3.5	.0001
Long-term memory loss	3.7	2.5	.0008
Mood swings	4.3	2.6	.0001
Loss of libido	5.1	3.2	.0001
Decreased alcohol tolerance	3.3	2.5	.076
Indigestion	4.9	3.2	.0001
Loss of appetite	4.0	2.6	.0001
Swollen stomach	3.5	2.7	.03

* Statistically significant.

jects. The impairments were in the tests that generally are affected earliest by chemicals and were similar to those observed earlier in chlorine-exposed subjects (1, 2). These impairments were not explained by existing medical disorders, by occupational or other prior chemical exposures, or by subjects' being participants in the lawsuit; they are attributed, more probably than not, to the airborne products of the derailment, particularly to chlorine but also to creosotic acid and chlorinated by-products of potassium cresylate reacting with chlorine.

These data are consistent with the conclusions from seven previous patients studied many months after exposure to chlorine (1), namely, that neurobehavioral impairment is associated with chronic respiratory symptoms and impairment. The new finding is a latent period of only 7 weeks from exposure to recognition of impairment. This implies that impairments developed rapidly and were monitored by the patients' symp-

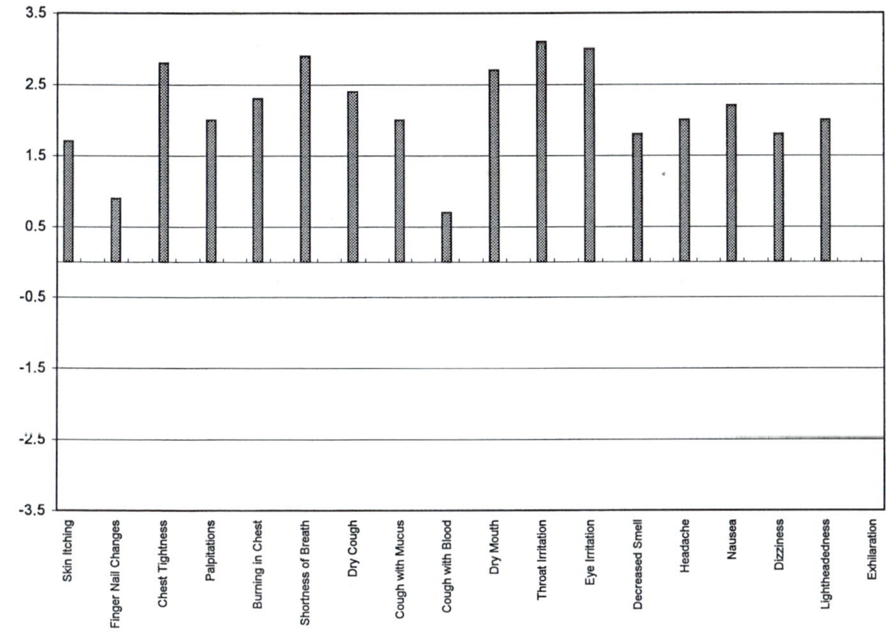

FIGURE 6.3a. Comparison of symptom frequencies in 97 chlorine-exposed adults and 202 unexposed adults by ANOVA. Hatched bars are statistically significant.

toms, which developed acutely, and suggests a continuing process. Although chlorine and creosate doses, levels of exposure, and their precise durations are forever unavailable, no other associations could be made. These 97 subjects had significant impairment of neurobehavioral function compared to regional and to national reference groups. They shared exposure to the chlorine–creosote mixture created by the derailment. No other common factors of exposure or disease were found as possible causes (confounders), including chemical exposures. Personal factors and medical illnesses were ruled out by careful histories. Associations of impairment and exposure were clear by comparisons to regional and to national unexposed. Balance and simple and choice reaction time, which are especially sensitive and reliable for detecting brain injury (3–5), were abnormal. Impairment of cognitive function, as reflected in Culture Fair, a broad intelligence test that is not language-dependent, and in trail making B, the most discriminatory of the perceptual motor speed tests, was not detected at this point. Verbal recall was not impaired. Thus, overall these subjects who were exposed briefly to chlorine and perhaps other chlorinated chemicals have chronic neurobehavioral impairment, particularly of unconscious and automatic functions of the nervous system. Additionally, they

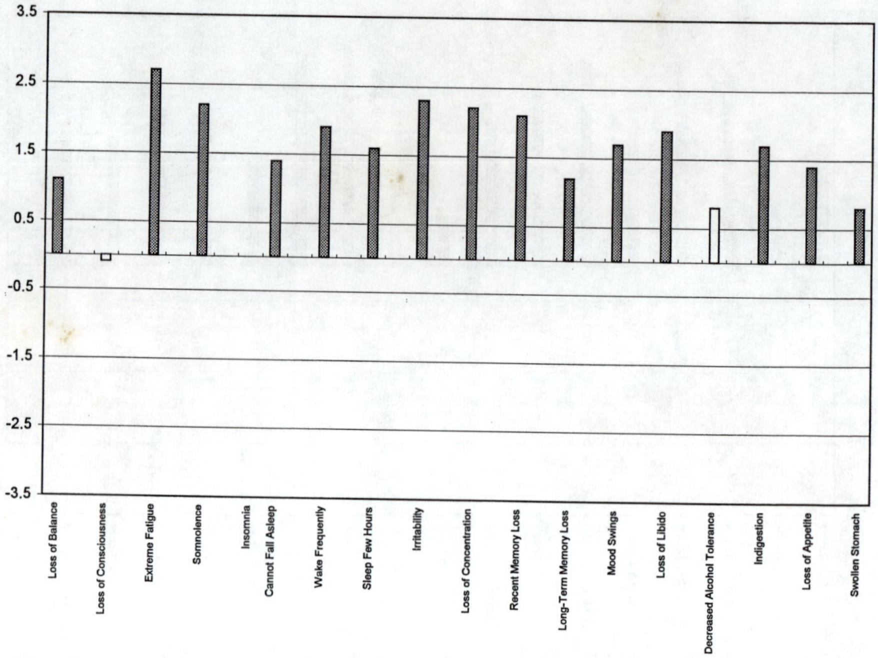

FIGURE 6.3b. Comparison of symptom frequencies in 97 chlorine-exposed adults and 202 unexposed adults by ANOVA. Hatched bars are statistically significant.

had reduced expiratory flow rates, indicating bronchoconstriction, and increased respiratory tract symptoms.

Their findings resemble those of six patients exposed at home to a 43-ton chlorine gas release in Henderson, Nevada, in whom balance, simple and choice reaction time, recall for verbal and visual information, and vocabulary were impaired (1). In another incident, 13 women were exposed to chlorine given off by disinfectant bleach in Benton, Arkansas (2).

One of our subjects (1) was an engineer installing a water treatment system who was sprayed in the face with chlorine and continued to inhale some gas for 3 days in March 1993. When he was tested 18 months later (September 1994), his deficits included prolonged reaction time, impaired balance, loss of grip strength, impaired hearing, severely constricted visual fields, decreased vibration sense, hearing loss, and cognitive, perceptual motor speed, and recall impairment. Retesting 30 months after exposure showed constricted visual fields and additional impairment of reaction time, balance, grip strength, verbal recall, and perceptual motor speed.

DISCUSSION

Analyzing the test results by comparison of means was convenient and suggested many significant differences, but it should be regarded with some caution until regional unexposed have been studied.

In the light of these findings, why were chlorine's effects on the central nervous system not recognized previously? There are several plausible explanations: (1) the nervous system effects were not looked for or ever considered; (2) those effects were manifested late, after pulmonary effects; (3) because findings were not clinically obvious they were not tested; and (4) the test methods used were not sensitive enough to detect impairment (5). Follow-up for chlorine exposure has usually been done by pulmonary function tests and respiratory questionnaires. Recent studies from Canada showed chronic airways obstruction and symptoms of asthma and chronic bronchitis, notably phlegm production (6, 7), similar to effects in the men and women described in this paper; but they paid no attention to neurobehavioral function.

What mechanism might explain immediate and delayed central nervous system effects of chlorine? Chlorine produces chlorine dioxide and reacts with organic chemicals to make chloramines and other organic chlorine products (8). Chlorine absorption from the lungs into circulating blood transports chlorine or chlorinated by-products to the brain where they may be offloaded into astrocytes and neurons. Interval observations of the effects of chlorine exposure in the engineer, described above, showed functional worsening, which may relate to continuing dying-back of neurons or enhanced toxic stimulation of astrocytes as aging and chemical damage are superimposed (9). Reports of chlorine-induced cerebral lesions include localization by pathologic (10) and imaging (9) methods.

The most disturbing outcome reported was that in which 3 of 20 patients, seen previously within 2 years of chlorine exposure, developed temporal lobe seizures (11). The seizures were characterized by brief periods of staring and disorientation without loss of motor control and without frothing at the mouth, incontinence, or tonic or clonic movements, but were followed by ''postictal confusion and depression.'' As seizures represent an ''ultimate dysfunction'' (12) of the central nervous system and occurred months after exposure, they may be complications of a healing process such as astrocytic scars. An alternative hypothesis is kindling of the limbic system to cause temporal lobe seizures after inhalation of other chemicals (12–15). Seizures have been associated with many chemicals that are used as pharmaceuticals, including penicillin, cyclosporin, and chloramphenicol, narcotics, analgesics, and prednisone (12, 13), and with environmental chemicals, including organochlorines (14), chlordane, deldrin, heptachlor, and endosulfur, which kindle seizures experimentally (15).

Our conclusions, which are based on observations of yet another ''unnatural experiment,'' are tentative. There are plans to compare these subjects to regional unexposed subjects and to restudy them after a year's interval to measure rates of deterioration. Other investigators should be stimulated to test chlorine-exposed individuals to chronicle the evolution of the central nervous system impairment at intervals. Nevertheless, chlorine exposure should be avoided to prevent serious central nervous system impairment. The concordance of findings in this incident-exposed group reinforces those in subjects who lived near an industrial chlorine release (11) and those in a consumer chlorine bleach incident. These observations should stimulate critical reevaluation of the cavalier attitude often taken toward gaseous chlorine stored under pressure—based on ''it seems safe'' when highly diluted in water. Noxious chlorine concentrations that are irritating to people are reached in public swimming pools, sewage treatment plants, cleaning of floors in hospitals and nursing homes, and sterilization of dishes and utensils. Railway transport of compressed chlorine gas produced the massive release at Alberton, which was similar to one that occurred in Nevada from a stationary site (1).

Future Needs

The next logical step is to examine an unexposed group of Montana unexposed subjects so that these comparisons can be verified. Also, follow-up studies should be conducted one year after the derailment (as planned for the spring of 1997 when this was written).

References

1. Kilburn KH: Evidence that inhaled chlorine is neurotoxic and causes airways obstruction. *Intl J Occup Med Toxicol* 1995;4:267–270.
2. Kilburn KH: Chronic neural and pulmonary effects from inhaled chlorine: 4.5 years after exposure. *J Occup Environ Med* 1997 in press.
3. Kilburn KH and Warshaw RH: Effects on neurobehavioral performance of chronic exposure to chemically contaminated well water. *Intl Toxicol Indust Health* 1993;39:391–404.
4. Kilburn KH and Warshaw RH: Neurobehavioral effects of formaldehyde and solvents on histology technicians: repeated testing across time. *Environ Res* 1992;58:134–146.
5. Kilburn KH, Warshaw RH, and Shields MG: Neurobehavioral dysfunction in firemen exposed to polychlorinated biphenyls (PCBs): possible improvement after detoxification. *Arch Environ Health* 1989;44:345–350.
6. Courteau JP, Cushman R, Bouchard F, Quevillon M, Chartrand A, and Bherer L: Survey of construction workers repeatedly exposed to chlorine over a three to six month period in a pulpmill. I. Exposure and symptomatology. *Occup Environ Med* 1994;51:219–224.
7. Bherer L, Cushman R, Courteau JP, Quevillon M, Cote G, Bourbeau J, et al.: Survey of construction workers repeatedly exposed to chlorine over a three to six month period in a pulpmill. II. Follow up of affected workers by questionnaire, spirometry, and assessment of bronchial responsiveness 18 to 24 months after exposure ended. *Occup Environ Med* 1994; 51:225–228.
8. Okun DA: Water quality management. In: *Maxy-Roseneau-Last, Public Health & Preventive Medicine.* JM Last and RB Wallace (eds.). Norwalk, CT: Appleton and Lang, 1992, Chap. 35.
9. Levy JM, Hessel SJ, Nykamp PW, Stegman CJ, Crowe JK, Spiegel RM, Horsley WW, and Cook GC: Detection of the cerebral lesions of chlorine intoxication by magnetic resonance imaging. *Magnet Reson Imaging* 1986;4:51–52.
10. Adelson L and Kaufman J: Fatal chlorine poisoning: report of two cases with clinicopathologic correlation. *Am J Clin Path* 1971;56:430–442.
11. Streit W and Kincaid-Colton CA: The brain's immune system. *Scientif Am* 1995;Nov.:54–61.
12. Engel J, Jr.: *Seizures and Epilepsy.* Philadelphia, PA: F. A. Davis Co., 1989.
13. Bear DM: Temporal lobe epilepsy—a syndrome of sensory–limbic hyperconnection. *Cortex* 1979;15:357–384.
14. Messing RO, Closson RG, and Simon RP: Drug-induced seizures: a 10 year experience. *Neurology* 1984;34:1582–1586.
15. Gilbert ME: A characterization of chemical kindling with the pesticide endosulfan. *Neurotox Teratol* 1992;14:151–158.

7

Adverse Effects from Hydrogen Chloride

The escape of large quantities of hydrochloric acid caused much annoyance and destruction of vegetation in the neighborhood and the local land owners sought redress in the courts. The problem was solved in 1830 by William Gossage, who knocked the floor out of a derelict stone windmill near his factory, filled the interior with brushwood and passed the waste gas upward against a descending stream of water which effectively washed out the acid.

—D. Hunter (1)

The widespread use of hydrochloric acid (HCl) and other acids led to the Alkali Act in Great Britain to register acid production and to regulate releases to protect the public. Erosion of the teeth of workers by HCl fumes, which was quite different from caries, was an early adverse effect of the chemical; and HCl damage to airways and the lung leading to aspiration necrosis and pneumonia was well known early in the twentieth century. Recognition of this damage paralleled in time the discovery that HCl is a principal digestive agent in the stomach. Asthma and pulmonary edema from acid inhalation have been described repeatedly in the nineteenth (1) and twentieth centuries (2, 3).

In 1993, mischance, legally an accident, provided our investigators the opportunity to study associations between an environmental exposure to HCl fumes and adverse health effects. A leaking container (Baker-Hughes) truck spread over 800 liters (200 gallons) of HCl onto the ground and into the air adjoining a mobile home park in Louisiana. The investigating officer and several residents became acutely ill with burning and tearing eyes and throats, headache, chest pain, shortness of breath, and flu-like complaints. Persistence and worsening of these symptoms led to a study of all of the available exposed subjects 20 months later.

Forty-five exposed adult subjects and a cohort comparison group of 56 adults had neurobehavioral testing, including balance, reaction time, blink reflex latency, and spirometry. They also completed health questionnaires and a profile of mood states (POMS).

These adults (exposed and unexposed) did not differ in mean age, but the exposed had completed 1.2 fewer years of school (educational attainment, $p < 0.002$). Data were analyzed by comparing means by analysis of variance and by covariance analysis. The exposed differed significantly from unexposed for balance tested with eyes open and eyes closed, simple and two-choice visual reaction, digit symbol, and placing pegs in a pegboard (in women only). Scores on POMS and all six components were also significantly different. Balance sway speeds greater than the mean value for unexposed subjects were associated with proximity to the HCl leak, as were reduced midflow rates (FEF_{25-75} and FEV_1). The most exposed subject, the proband of the study, had further functional deterioration 5 months after initial testing.

THE RELEASE

The release of HCl occurred on Saturday afternoon August 14, 1993, when, in a flatbed truck loaded with four individual plastic tanks containing 1,000 liters of HCl, the driver noticed that each tank was leaking. He drove by two sides of a mobile home court and parked within a few dozen yards of several homes and south and east of most of the court. Fumes were noted to be ascending from the last tank on the truck, which was leaking and collapsing and had annealed the tractor to the trailer.

The subsequent study's proband was the sheriff's officer who investigated the truck loaded with HCl that was leaking and had pulled off the road next to the mobile home park. He began warning the people in the court soon after the truck stopped, without knowing its contents. He called for a Hazardous Materials (HAZMAT) team and for ambulances, as he found that several of the people were having trouble breathing. He continued to contact people in the court, warning them to leave, and he returned repeatedly to the spill. Another officer and ambulance attendants accompanied him after a short time and assisted in the evacuation. Within a year he developed serious impairment of his gait and balance, a sharp decrease in memory, weakness of his left side, headaches, and loss of the ability to concentrate. Similar memory loss, headaches, and respiratory illnesses in another law officer and people downwind of this release led to the investigation described below.

TESTING OF SUBJECTS

The ages of both groups of adults, exposed and unexposed, were 35 years with no difference; but their educational levels, 10.6 years in the exposed group and 11.8 years in the unexposed group, were different (see Table 7.1, Figures 7.1a, b). Men's and women's heights, weights, and grip strengths by gender did not differ between groups. The 45 exposed adults (21 women and 24 men) were compared to 41 women and 15 men in the unexposed group.

Simple and choice reaction times were significantly delayed in the exposed group compared to unexposed with p values $<.0001$. Balance measured as sway speed eyes open and eyes closed was significantly more rapid in the exposed. Blink reflex latency was exactly the same in the two groups (Table 7.1). There was no difference in color discrimination. Analysis by comparison of means showed significant differences for digit symbol in the cognitive function domain but not for Culture Fair A or vocabulary.

TABLE 7.1 Demographic data and neurobehavioral function score for exposed and unexposed groups of adults

	Exposed		Unexposed		
	45		56		
	Mean	Sd	Mean	Sd	*p* Value
Age yrs	34.6	13.4	34.9	11.3	0.9
Educational Level yrs	10.6	2.4	11.8	1.3	0.002*
Simple Reaction Time ms	389	174	280	59	0.0001*
Choice Reaction Time ms	619	193	479	66	0.0001*
Balance (minimum)					
Eyes Open cm/s	0.81	0.66	0.66	0.12	0.022*
Eyes Closed cm/s	1.65	1.12	1.10	0.27	0.004*
Blink Supraorbital ms					
Right	13.4	2.3	12.9	2.2	0.318
Left	13.2	2.0	12.8	2.4	0.462
Blink Glabellar Tap ms					
Right	14.1	2.0	14.0	1.6	0.826
Left	14.2	2.1	14.2	2.1	0.976
Color Score	12.1	2.4	11.6	2.0	0.250
Cognitive Function					
Culture Fair A score	25.6	8.2	27.2	7.2	0.304
Vocabulary score	15.7	7.7	16.7	7.3	0.487
Digit Symbol score	46.3	15.3	61.3	13.9	0.0001*
Perceptual Motor Speed					
Pegboard s	76.9	21.9	70.4	20.5	0.132
Trail Making A s	46.5	25.2	37.9	23.1	0.078
Trail Making B s	90.8	44.4	67.7	24.0	0.001*
Fingertip Writing Errors					
Right	4.7	4.5	3.3	3.4	0.09
Left	4.0	4.2	2.5	2.9	0.04*
Recall					
Story 1	9.5	3.8	9.6	4.0	0.869
Story 2	9.4	4.2	9.3	4.0	0.934
Visual Design	31.1	6.4	31.6	6.5	0.733
Digits Forward	6.4	1.4	7.1	1.4	0.018*
Digits Backward	4.3	1.2	4.5	1.4	0.437
Long-Term Memory					
Information	12.5	5.0	13.8	4.9	0.191
Picture Completion	12.7	4.0	13.0	2.9	0.670
Similarities	16.1	5.4	17.6	4.6	0.146
POMS Score	70.5	44.4	28.5	29.7	0.0001*
Tension	18.8	7.4	11.2	5.8	0.0001*
Depression	18.6	15.7	9.9	9.6	0.0001*
Anger	15.3	10.2	9.2	7.4	0.0009*
Vigor	10.6	6.6	17.4	5.7	0.0001*
Extreme Fatigue	16.1	7.3	8.3	5.3	0.0001*
Confusion	12.2	5.4	7.3	4.4	0.0001*

* = $p < 0.05$

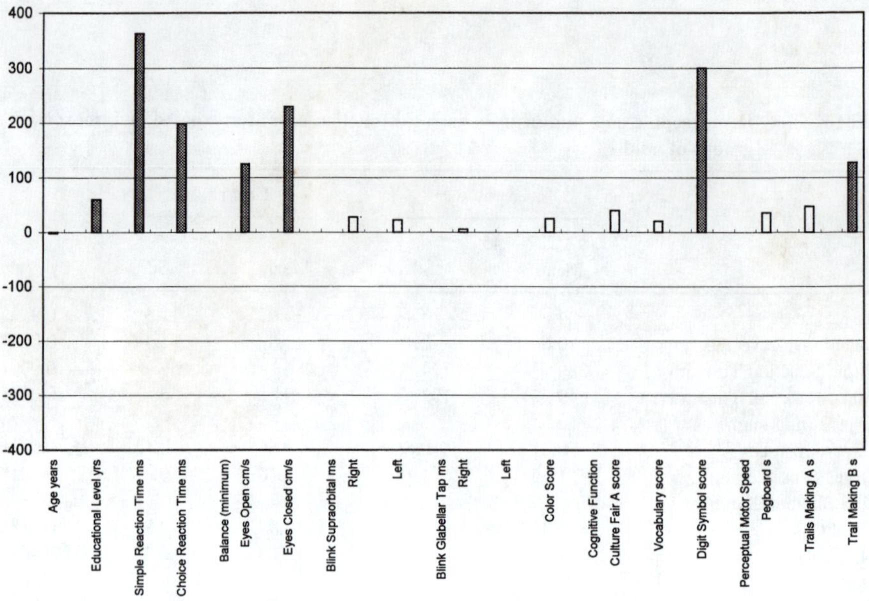

FIGURE 7.1a. Comparison of 45 hydrogen chloride–exposed adults and 56 unexposed adults by ANOVA. Hatched bars are statistically significant.

In the perceptual motor speed domain, trail making B and finger writing errors on the left were significantly different, but pegboard and trail making A were not different. The only difference in the recall and long-term memory domains was a difference in recall of digits forward, suggesting that memory and recall were not affected by this exposure. The affective scores (POMS scores) were significantly different with a 70.5 mean in exposed compared to 28.5 in unexposed. The POMS components of tension, depression, anger, fatigue, and confusion were all significantly elevated, and vigor was significantly decreased in the exposed compared to unexposed subjects.

Because the exposed women were more likely than the men to have been home during the hours of the initial exposure, the women were analyzed separately by comparison of means with unexposed women (Table 7.2, Figures 7.2a, b). This comparison confirmed the differences shown for the entire cohort (men and women) and added differences for Culture Fair to that for digit symbol in the cognitive domain, added a difference for trails A in the perceptual motor domain, and in the recall domain added visual recall measured the Rey 15 form test. The 14 children between 8 and 17 also showed significant differences for choice reaction time ($p < 0.01$) and for balance

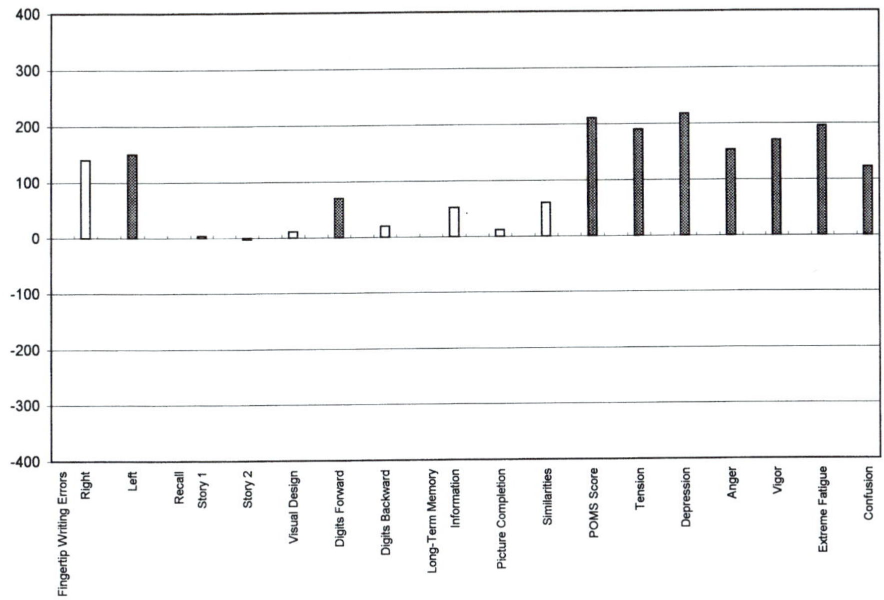

FIGURE 7.1b. Comparison of 45 hydrogen chloride–exposed adults and 56 unexposed adults by ANOVA. Hatched bars are statistically significant.

with eyes closed ($p < 0.007$) from the 29 unexposed children (not shown in the tables). Others showed trends toward deficits that were not significant.

Further examination of these data by covariance analysis, to reconcile effects due to age and other factors, showed that the adjusted differences for both the ln of simple and choice reaction time, which were the modeling transformations with the best linearity, were significantly different ($p < .0001$) (Table 7.3). The differences for ln of sway speed eyes opened and eyes closed were significantly different ($p < .02$ and $p < .004$). The difference for digit symbol was also significant, as was that for the inverse of pegboard (in men only) ($p < .007$).

The symptom frequency scores for 33 of 35 respiratory, neurobehavioral, general, and vegetative function symptoms were all significantly greater in the exposed group (Table 7.4, Figures 7.3a, b). Only two rare symptoms, loss of consciousness and decreased alcohol tolerance, were not different. These subjects' histories of infrequent alcohol consumption were confirmed by there being no elevated alveolar alcohol levels. The ARA lupus erythematosus questionnaire showed differences of significance for

TABLE 7.2 Age, education, and neurobehavioral scores compared in exposed and unexposed women

		Exposed		Unexposed		
		21		41		
		Mean	Sd	Mean	Sd	*p* Value
Age yrs		37.1	12.9	34.0	10.5	0.3
Educational Level yrs		10.9	1.7	11.9	1.2	0.01
Reaction Time ms						
Simple		392	127	290	60	0.0001
Choice		627	173	519	76	0.001
Balance as Sway Speed cms						
Eyes Open		0.96	0.63	0.73	0.15	0.027
Eyes Closed		1.69	0.77	1.28	0.34	0.005
Blink Reflex Latency ms						
Glabellar	Right	13.9	1.6	13.9	2.2	0.95
	Left	14.0	2.6	13.9	2.0	0.352
Supraorbital	Right	12.5	2.3	12.6	2.1	0.115
	Left	12.1	1.8	12.4	2.4	0.036
Cognitive Functions						
Culture Fair sc		23.8	8.6	27.9	6.2	0.034
Vocabulary sc		16.0	6.9	17.9	7.7	0.364
Digit Symbol sc		50.5	17.1	64.1	12.8	0.001
Perceptual Motor Speed						
Pegboard sec		71.4	15.3	68.8	15.6	0.526
Trails A sec		46.4	22.0	34.2	9.1	0.003
Trails B sec		88.7	45.3	63.8	20.7	0.004
Long-Term Memory						
Information sc		11.3	4.3	13.1	5.1	0.165
Picture Completion sc		12.3	3.1	13.0	2.7	0.373
Similarities sc		15.8	5.3	17.9	4.8	0.120
Recall						
Story 1 sc		10.7	3.6	10.4	3.4	0.824
Story 2 sc		9.7	4.7	9.8	4.3	0.925
Visual Recall sc		29.1	6.1	32.1	5.8	0.064
Rey 15 Form Test sc		11.8	3.3	13.9	1.8	0.002

yrs = years cms = centimeters
ms = milliseconds sc = score

cold and numb fingers, excessive sun rash, painful breathing, and hair loss, but not for anemia, protein in the urine, seizures, rash on the cheeks, or mouth ulcers.

Respiratory symptoms were much more common in the exposed group, including production of phlegm, shortness of breath while walking and when climbing stairs, and shortness of breath with wheezing. The spirometric measurements showed that vital capacity was decreased in both groups, exposed and unexposed, as was FEV_1, to 87% and 84% of predicted (Table 7.5). The midflows FEF_{27-75} were 77% in exposed and 75% in unexposed, and the terminal flows (FEF_{75-85}) were similar, at 76% and 74%. Thus, objective evidence of difference in pulmonary function was not seen, but both groups were significantly below the baseline unexposed population (4). However, the exposed children's pulmonary functions were reduced significantly compared to the unexposed (Table 7.6).

The examination for confounding by exposure to a variety of chemicals and occupations, pesticides, solvents, and other industrial operations showed that more exposed

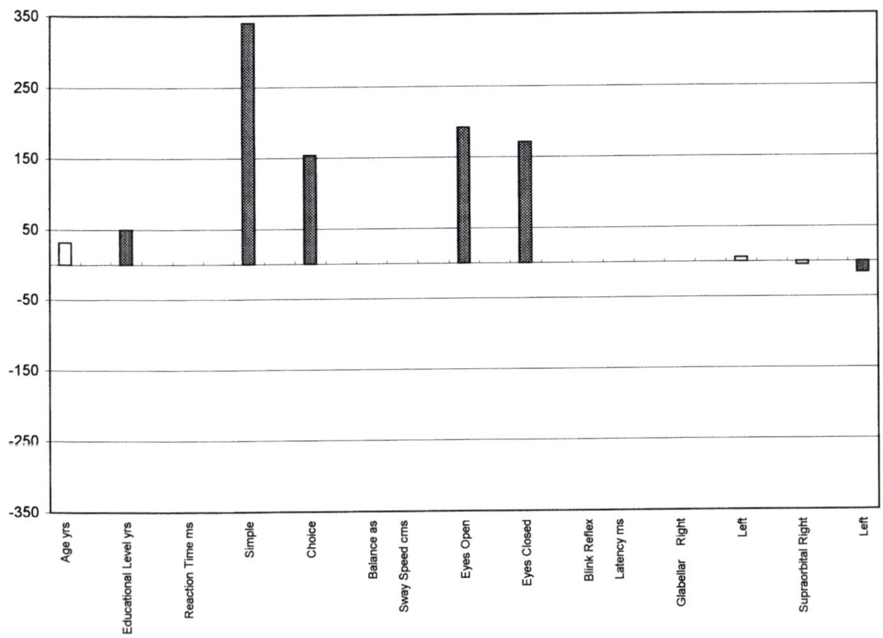

FIGURE 7.2a. Comparison of 21 hydrogen chloride–exposed women and 41 unexposed women by ANOVA. Hatched bars are statistically significant.

subjects than unexposed had worked in chemical refining and been exposed to solvents and to spray painting. However, analysis of these factors in regression equations, which included age and other significant coefficients, showed that they did not contribute to the variation in the tests. Similarly, exposures to general anesthesia, periods of unconsciousness, head injury, automobile accidents, and medical and neurological diseases did not explain the differences. However, the exposed people had significantly more depression, recognized by self-appraisal, than did the unexposed group.

Examination of the effect on balance with eyes open showed greater impairment in the exposed people closest to the site of the HCl spill. Most of these near individuals also had trends at a 10% <0.1 level of significance for simple and choice reaction time impairment.

DISCUSSION

An environmental exposure to hydrochloric acid was followed by impairment of reaction time and of body balance, together with diminished scores on digit symbol and

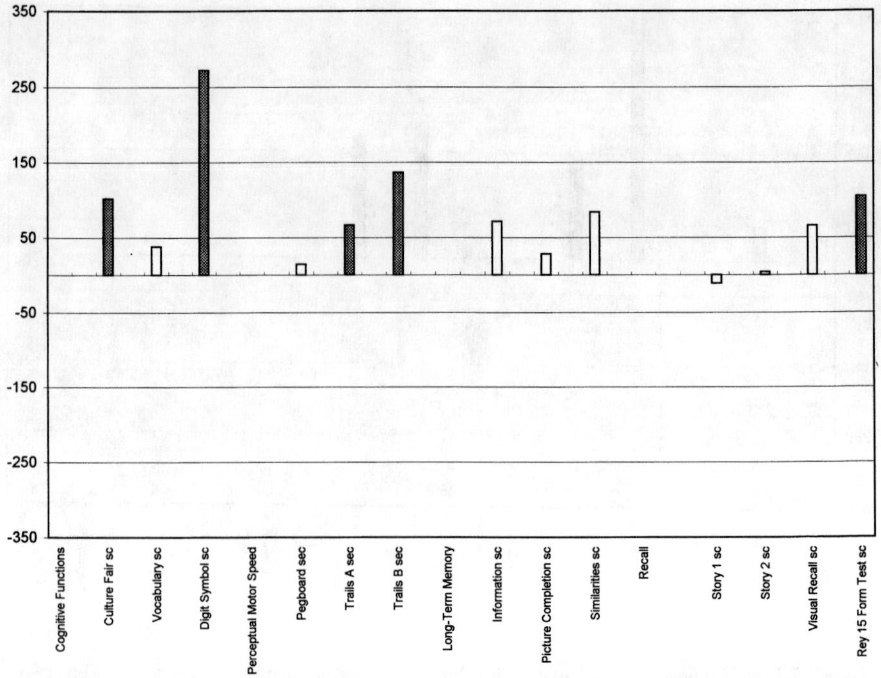

FIGURE 7.2b. Comparison of 21 hydrogen chloride–exposed women and 41 unexposed women by ANOVA. Hatched bars are statistically significant.

TABLE 7.3 Analysis of covariance, which adjusted all for significant factors: age, educational level, gender for digit symbol and pegboard and height for balance (Sway)

	Adjusted Difference	*p* Value
ln SRT ms	0.273	0.0001
ln CRT ms	0.195	0.0001
Sway Eyes Open min cm/sec	0.121	0.02
Sway eyes Closed min cm/sec	0.197	0.004
$\sqrt{}$Digit Symbol sc	0.676	0.001
1/Pegboard (in men) sc	−0.0021	0.007

ms = milliseconds sec = seconds
min = minimum sc = score
cm = centimeters

TABLE 7.4 Symptom frequencies, means and standard deviations, for exposed and unexposed groups compared by analysis of variance

	Exposed		Unexposed		
	Mean	Sd	Mean	Sd	*p* Value
Skin itch	5.9	3.4	3.3	2.7	0.0001
Deformed nails	2.9	3.1	1.4	1.4	0.0026
Chest tightness	5.1	3.3	2.1	1.8	0.0001
Palpitations	4.8	3.2	1.9	1.6	0.0001
Burning chest	4.9	3.3	1.7	1.7	0.0001
Shortness of breath	6.4	3.6	2.5	2.0	0.0001
Dry cough	4.6	2.6	2.8	2.1	0.0004
Cough with mucus	5.8	3.1	3.1	2.4	0.0001
Cough with blood	2.4	2.5	1.1	0.3	0.0001
Dry mouth	5.6	2.7	2.5	1.9	0.0001
Throat irritation	5.0	2.5	2.6	1.6	0.0001
Eye irritation	4.9	3.4	2.3	1.7	0.0001
Decreased sense of smell	4.6	4.0	2.2	2.4	0.0003
Headache	8.2	2.6	4.5	2.5	0.0001
Nausea	5.1	3.0	2.5	2.0	0.0001
Dizziness	5.7	3.2	2.4	2.1	0.0001
Lightheadness	5.2	2.9	2.3	1.9	0.0001
Unusual exhilaration	1.8	2.0	1.5	1.5	0.0001
Abnormal balance	4.8	3.3	2.0	1.8	0.0001
Loss of consciousness	1.5	1.3	1.2	0.7	0.09
Extreme fatigue	7.8	3.7	3.5	2.6	0.0001
Somnolence	5.6	3.7	1.8	1.6	0.0001
Insomnia	4.6	3.8	2.6	2.2	0.0018
Wake frequently	5.3	3.8	2.6	2.5	0.0001
Sleep only few hours	4.8	3.9	2.8	2.6	0.003
Irritability	7.2	3.3	3.8	2.5	0.0001
Impaired concentration	6.4	3.4	3.1	2.3	0.0001
Recent memory loss	6.4	3.6	2.6	2.3	0.0001
Long-term memory loss	5.0	3.5	2.0	2.0	0.0001
Mood swing	5.4	3.9	2.4	2.0	0.0001
Decreased libido	4.2	3.1	2.3	2.4	0.0011
Decreased alcohol tolerance	3.5	3.0	3.1	2.3	0.424
Indigestion	6.2	3.8	2.6	1.7	0.0001
Loss of appetite	4.0	2.7	2.3	1.9	0.0005
Swollen stomach	5.1	3.2	2.6	1.9	0.0001

trail making B and on peg placement (by men only). Women showed additional abnormalities, including lower scores on Culture Fair and trail making A as well as B, and on Wechsler's visual recall and the Rey 15 form recall test. In addition, frequencies of 35 symptoms were much higher in the exposed individuals of both genders and suggested chronic effects from the exposure. Pulmonary functions of adults were reduced below national baselines but did not distinguish exposed from the local unexposed population, whose performance was also comparatively low. However, exposed children's pulmonary functions were definitely reduced; so they may be affected primarily by this exposure, with the effects not obscured by accumulation of other damage.

This is not the first report of impaired neurobehavioral performance in subjects who were exposed environmentally to hydrochloric acid, but it appears to be the first time that neurobehavioral examinations and testing have been done. Thus, we open a new area of concern about this strong mineral acid. Its history in toxicology, on the other hand, is well known, its escape to the environment during production having led to the Alkali Act in Great Britain after the LeBlanc process for making sodium carbonate gave rise to large quantities of HCl in the 1830s in England (1). There was concern during World War I about the acute affects of chlorine, as it was used as a war gas; but many concluded that phosgene, a frequent HCl contaminant, was largely the reason for the pulmonary edema it produced. However, there also have been concerns that chlorine is hydrated to hypochlorous acid, and that this strong mineral acid is responsible for respiratory irritation, eye irritation, and also erosion of the teeth. All these effects have been attributed to HCl (1). Alternately, the oxygen ion (O^-) produced in this process gives Cl_2 its sterilizing properties.

This exposed population's balance and reaction time functions showed evidence of a proximity effect, seen previously for pulmonary responses (2, 3). As is typical for such incidents, air measurements of HCl were not made, which would have been essential for dose–effect calculations. Nevertheless, the mobile home court occupants' descriptions of the position of the yellow-green cloud mapped for investigators the locations of

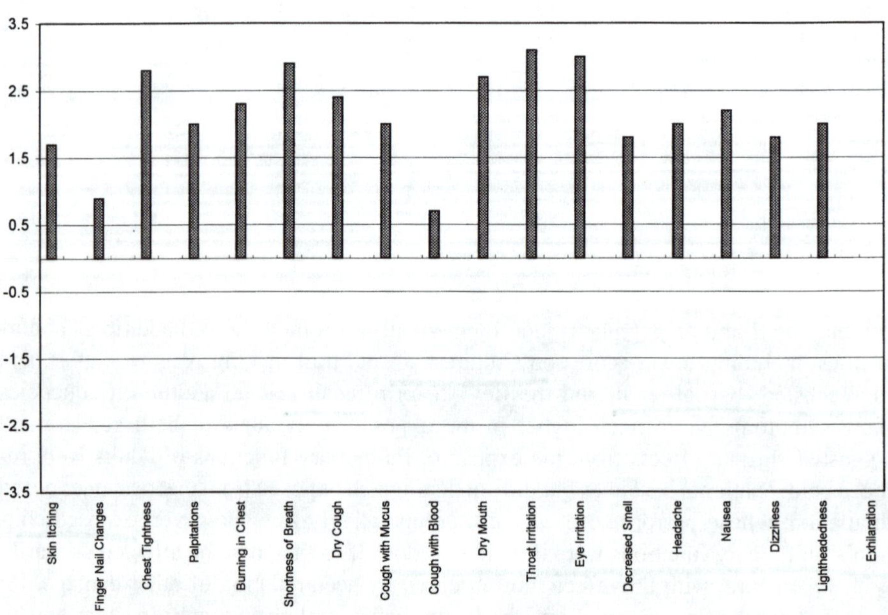

FIGURE 7.3a. Comparison of symptom frequencies of 45 hydrogen chloride–exposed adults and 56 unexposed adults by ANOVA. Hatched bars are statistically significant.

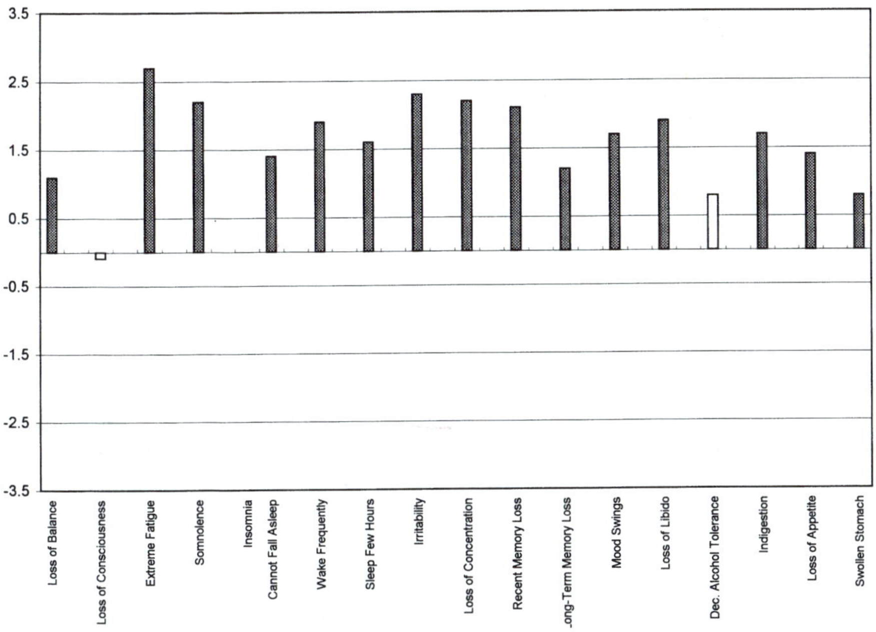

FIGURE 7.3b. Comparison of symptom frequencies of 45 hydrogen chloride–exposed adults and 56 unexposed adults by ANOVA. Hatched bars are statistically significant.

those subjects with the greatest abnormalities of balance, reaction time, and pulmonary midflow. In contrast, blink reflex latency R-1, a sensitive trigeminal-nerve-dependent response that is highly sensitive to chlorinated solvents, showed no effect. Perhaps the most provocative finding was that the magnitudes of impairment of balance were related to distance and direction from the HCl source.

The similarity chemically of HCl to chlorine provides a plausible hypothetical mech-

TABLE 7.5 Prevalence of respiratory symptoms and pulmonary function tests as percentage of predicted in men and women of exposed and unexposed groups

	Exposed		Unexposed		
	Mean	Sd	Mean	Sd	*p* Value
FVC	94.6	15.3	92.6	14.8	NS
FEV_1	87.3	15.0	83.9	14.9	NS
FEF_{25-75}	77.2	25.0	75.2	30.4	NS
FEF_{75-85}	76.1	40.9	73.5	35.7	NS

TABLE 7.6 Pulmonary function measurements adjusted for gender, age, and height for exposed and unexposed children

	Exposed 14		Unexposed 29		
	Mean	Sd	Mean	Sd	p Value
FVC	70.1	12.9	78.7	14.3	.066
FEV_1	61.2	11.4	71.6	15.9	.036

anism for its toxicity, as chlorine has been recently shown to have detrimental central nervous system effects (5) (see also Chapter 6). Although, just as for chlorine, most reported effects of HCl have been on the airways and the respiratory system, the nervous system was impaired for blink, balance, hearing, reaction time, and vision. Exposed subjects also complained of impaired verbal recall although testing did not show it.

In predicting the future course of these subjects, two observations are relevant. One is that the functions of the proband for this study, the sheriff's officer, deteriorated between two examinations, 6 months apart. His course suggests a slow dying-back of axons or some other chronic progressive toxic effect that resembles that seen in accumulative disorders rather than recovery, which has been assumed for single acute exposures to asphyxiant gases. The second is that similar progressive deterioration was observed after chlorine exposure (Chapter 6) (5), and is important after exposures to formaldehyde (Chapter 4) and hydrogen sulfide (Chapter 5) as well (6, 7). A possible mechanism involves the combination of chlorine with available circulating compounds, particularly carbon fragments, to make chlorinated derivatives such as chloramines and chloroform (8, 9). Such a hypothesis would postulate impairment of the neuroaxis involving the blink pathways (5). It may be that only a fraction of these individuals were exposed to the extent of those studied after exposure to chlorine, and that blink had not yet slowed significantly. Follow-up studies are needed.

Hydrogen chloride is a common industrial product, frequently transported on the highways; so opportunities abound for such exposures. Regulations and posting are mandatory so that the propensity for damage is clearly known by those persons at the sites at the time of spills and does not depend upon subsequent, often flawed, recognition and notification.

The proximity effect in this population's balance function suggests that the central nervous effects must include the pathways—vestibular, cerebellar, and visual—that interact with the afferent information for balance. Similar effects were seen on reaction time although no effects were seen on blink, a response highly sensitive to chlorinated solvents. Finally, as noted earlier, the magnitudes of impairments of balance, just as for pulmonary effects, were related to the distance from the site of the leak of HCl.

In summary, chronic neurobehavioral dysfunction and airways obstruction occurred after environmental HCl exposure, adding these effects to those on the lungs, cornea, and teeth reported previously in workers. Widespread use of HCl makes a repetition of this incident probable; so safer methods of transporting HCl are clearly indicated.

References

1. Hunter D: *Diseases of Occupations* (4th ed.). Boston: Little, Brown and Co., 1969.
2. Promisloff RA, Lenchner GS, and Cichelli AV: Reactive airway dysfunction syndrome in three police officers following a roadside chemical spill. *Chest* 1990;98:928–929.

3. Rosenau JM. *Preventive Medicine and Hygiene.* New York: Appleton and Co., 1913.
4. Miller A, Thornton JC, Warshaw R, Bernstein J, Selikoff IJ, and Teirstein AS: Mean and instantaneous expiratory flows, FVC and FEV_1: prediction equations from a probability sample of Michigan, a large industrial state. *Bull Eur Physiopathol Respir* 1986;22:589–597.
5. Kilburn KH: Evidence that inhaled chlorine is neurotoxic and causes airways obstruction. *Intl J Occup Med* 1995;4:267–272.
6. Kilburn KH: Neurobehavioral impairment and seizures from formaldehyde. *Arch Environ Health* 1994;49:37–43.
7. Kilburn KH: Case report: profound neurobehavioral deficits in an oil field worker overcome by hydrogen sulfide. *Am J Med Sci* 1993;306:301–305.
8. Kern DG: Outbreak of the reactive airway dysfunction syndrome after a spill of glacial acetic acid. *Am Rev Respir Dis* 1991;144:1058–1064.
9. Okun DA: Water quality management. In: *Maxy-Roseneau-Last Public Health & Preventive Medicine,* JM Last and RB Wallace (eds.). Norwalk, CT: Appleton and Lang, 1992, pp. 619–648.

8

Effects of Airborne Arsenic at Bryan/College Station, Texas

We evaluated the effects of arsenic and possible other chemical exposures from an arsenic trioxide–arsenic acid plant on residents of Bryan, Texas. We asked for volunteers from 156 plaintiffs in a class action suit certified to include 20,000 to 30,000 people exposed to arsenic by living within the concentration isopleths of exposure to 5 nanograms of arsenic trioxide per cubic meter (ng/m^3) of air defined by the United States District Court for the Southern District of Texas, Houston division (Figure 8.1). At this Atochem plant arsenic trioxide was produced for use as a defoliant for cotton, and was converted to arsenic acid (pentavalent form) for treating wood used in playground equipment. Other chemicals of potential concern packaged there included parathion, methylparathion, diazinon, and manganese ethylene bisdithiocarbamate and zinc dimethyl dithiocarbamate.

The plant's arsenic water plume caused the Texas Water Commission to cite Atochem in 1992 for solid waste and water pollution by arsenic. Water contaminated with arsenic was used in the plant's cooling tower. The spread of arsenic in air was modeled and mapped by Dr. Colin Baynes with isopleths representing from 100 to 5 ng/m^3 arsenic trioxide (Figure 8.1). Dust taken from 64 attics of homes in the vicinity of Atochem had median levels of arsenic of 16 $\mu g/g$, with levels ranging from 1 to 813 $\mu g/g$. Within the 20 ng/m^3 isopleth attic dust levels were >90 $\mu g/g$, and even in the 10 ng/m^3 isopleth levels were above 10 $\mu g/g$. A further water remediation plan was designed to react arsenic with ferric sulfate and sodium hydroxide and evaporate the residue. Organophosphates and carbamates were not found in attic dust samples.

The hypothesis was that arsenic impaired central nervous system function. These patients' symptoms suggested such impairment, and a review of the literature did not show any reason to reject it. Thus, our objective was to determine whether a sample of the Bryan/College Station subjects named as class representatives in the lawsuit and of nonparticipants from the same areas had neurological and psychological impairment. At the site, for several decades arsenic trioxide had been converted to arsenic acid to treat wood used to make playground equipment.

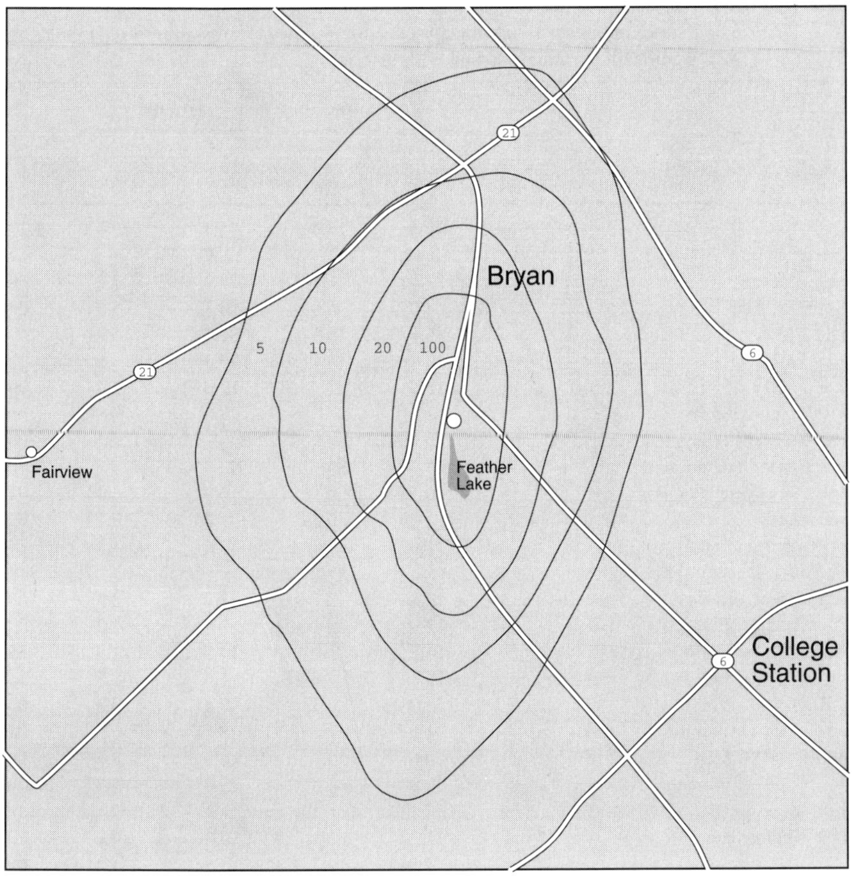

FIGURE 8.1. Bryan/College Station, Texas. Atochem plant indicated by open circle. Isopleths from center for 100, 20, 10, and 5 ng/m^3 arsenic trioxide.

TESTING OF SUBJECTS

Methods

The 78 subjects, aged 17 to 70 years, were all of the participants from a recruitment canvas of 156 who accepted an invitation to be examined, representing over 400 residents who surrounded the Atochem site at 702 Dodge Street in Bryan. Included were 31 subjects who had joined a class action lawsuit in 1991. Recruitment was aimed at those who had lived in the area 5 to 25 years, and they matched in income, sex, and educational level the demographics of the entire residential area. We recruited 156 subjects who lived from 0.3 to 9 km from the chemical plant and examined 78 subjects (31 clients and 47 volunteers). Most of the clients lived within 1.0 km of the site.

A matched cohort design was used with 39 women and 39 men in the exposed group between the ages of 17 and 70 years, compared to 68 women and 49 men as regional unexposed. The southwestern unexposed used as controls were from Wickenburg, Arizona, and were recruited to match the exposed group in sex, age, and years of educational attainment (highest school grade attained). There was no evidence of chemical

TABLE 8.1 Neurophysiological measurements, scores on tests, neuropsychological and profile of mood states in exposed and unexposed subjects, mean and standard deviation (Sd), with significant *p* values marked with asterisk

		Unexposed		Exposed		
		117		78		
n		Mean	Sd	Mean	Sd	*p*
Age yrs		42.4	15.4	45.3	16.0	.208
Women/Men		68/49		39/39		
Height Men		177.0	6.4	172.9	7.2	.006*
Women		164.0	6.6	160.5	5.8	.009*
Weight Men		86.6	15.5	84.7	15.9	.570*
Women		69.9	15.4	75.5	18.3	.100
Educational Level yrs		13.2	2.1	12.0	3.4	.004*
Neurophysiological Tests						
Simple Reaction Time ms		285	64	341	124	.000*
Choice Reaction Time ms		528	85	593	177	.001*
Balance Sway Speed cm/sec	Eyes Open	0.78	0.18	0.92	0.47	.029*
	Eyes Closed	1.26	0.39	1.43	0.72	.029*
Color Score Lanthony		11.6	1.4	11.6	1.1	.746
Blink Reflex Latency ms						
Supraorbital Right		12.8	2.1	13.8	2.3	.007*
Left		12.9	2.1	13.7	2.2	.027*
Glabellar Right		14.5	1.9	14.7	1.9	.557
Left		15.1	1.8	15.5	2.3	.316
Grip Right kg Men		52.0	10.5	47.5	9.3	.038*
Women		31.6	7.2	28.1	6.2	.015*
Grip Left kg Men		50.6	10.7	44.9	8.7	.008*
Women		29.9	6.3	25.8	5.3	.001*
Recall (Wechsler)						
Story 1 Immediate		12.2	3.9	9.8	4.1	.0005*
Delayed		9.5	4.3	7.7	4.4	.005*
Story 2 Immediate		11.1	4.2	9.9	4.2	.05*
Delayed		9.4	4.3	7.9	4.9	.029*
Picture Recall		35.4	3.9	30.6	7.5	.0005*
Cognitive Function						
Culture Fair A		29.7	7.5	25.0	9.0	.0005*
Vocabulary		24.2	9.2	18.2	11.7	.0005*
Digit Symbol		58.7	11.7	51.5	16.3	.0005*
Perceptual Motor Speed						
Pegboard Dominant		71.3	18.1	79.1	21.3	.007*
Trail Making A		31.0	8.8	42.3	23.3	.0005*
Trail Making B		71.0	27.0	88.7	39.4	.0005*
Long-Term or "Crystallized" Memory						
Information		18.5	5.6	16.7	6.4	.043*
Picture Completion		15.2	3.0	14.2	4.1	.099
Similarities		20.8	4.6	18.6	6.6	.005*
POMS Score		19.1	32.8	48.0	37.7	.0005*
Tension		8.6	6.0	14.2	7.4	.0005*
Depression		7.8	9.1	14.1	11.7	.0005*
Anger		8.2	7.8	12.3	9.1	.001*
Vigor		18.6	6.4	13.4	5.8	.0005*
Fatigue		7.7	6.4	11.6	6.6	.0005*
Confusion		5.4	4.4	9.2	5.4	.0005*

contamination of air or of water in Wickenburg, where subjects were picked at random from voter registration rolls and were contacted by telephone to ascertain whether they met the matching criteria and were willing to be tested. Testees were reimbursed for their time and mileage. During the testing, examiners were blinded as to subjects' legal category and exposure status, expressed as distance of their residence from the Atochem site in Bryan. However, the Wickenburg unexposed subjects' status was known to the testers. Also, unexposed comparisons for peripheral nervous system symptoms were our 18 testers. All subjects gave their informed consent, and the protocol was approved by the Human Studies Research Committee of the University of Southern California School of Medicine. Subjects were evaluated by using a neurobehavioral battery consisting of balance, reaction time, blink, and others, together with neuropsychological tests as adopted in the patient group and previous epidemiological studies (Chapters 3 and 4). Comparisons were made to the Wickenburg unexposed group (Chapter 11).

Results

The 39 women and 39 men tested had a mean age of 45 years and ranged from 19 to 78 years. Their educational level was 12 years. Thus, they were almost 3 years older,

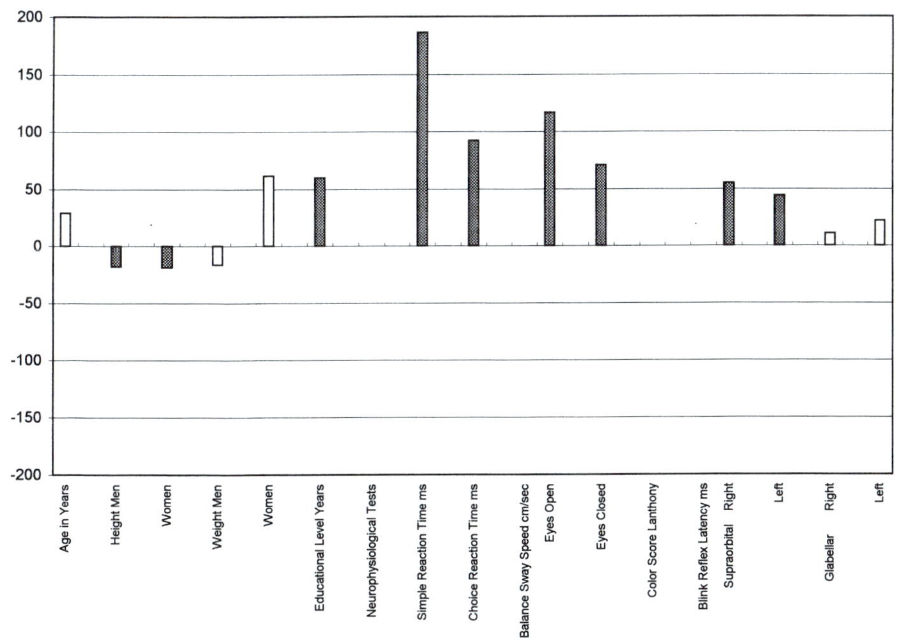

FIGURE 8.2a. Comparisons of 78 arsenic-exposed adults and 117 unexposed adults by ANOVA. Hatched bars are statistically significant.

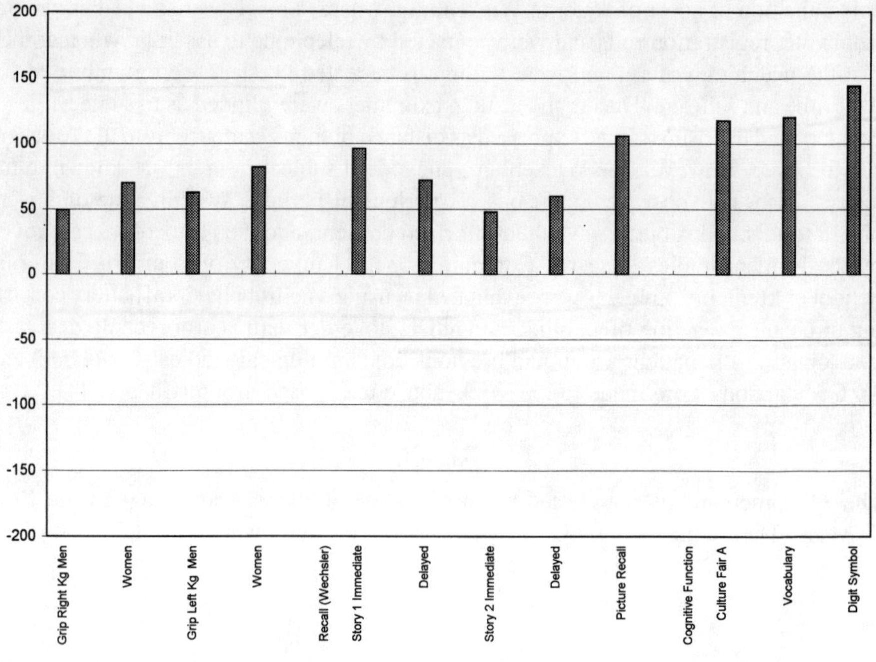

FIGURE 8.2b. Comparisons of 78 arsenic-exposed adults and 117 unexposed adults by ANOVA. Hatched bars are statistically significant.

an insignificant difference, and 1.2 years less educated than the unexposed group, a difference that was significant (Table 8.1, Figures 8.2a–c). The 31 clients and the 47 nonclients had no differences for age, educational level, or physiological and psychological test results; so their results were pooled.

Neurophysiological Testing

Performances of simple and two-choice visual reaction time both were significantly slower in the exposed subjects, with correspondingly greater standard deviations. Balance measured as sway speed was significantly faster (abnormal) with eyes open and with eyes closed in the exposed. Color discrimination scores were virtually identical and normal in both groups. Exposed subjects' blink reflex latency R-1 was significantly slower by a full millisecond (ms) on the right and 0.8 ms on the left, and both were statistically significant. Response to glabellar tap showed no significant difference, but the number of nonresponders was higher in the exposed group. Finally, grip strength in both men and women was lower in the exposed group, by an average of 6 kg in

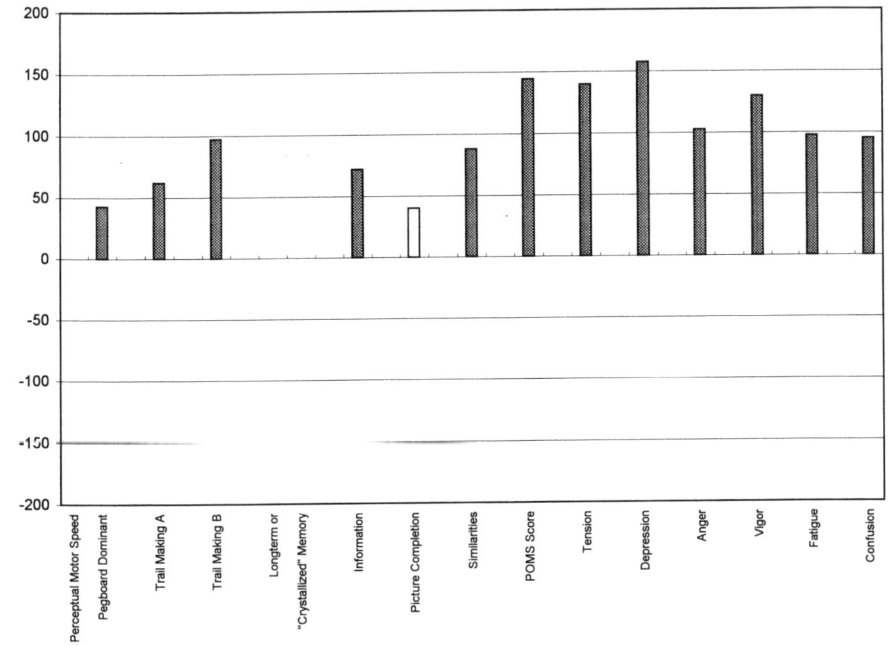

FIGURE 8.2c. Comparisons of 78 arsenic-exposed adults and 117 unexposed adults by ANOVA. Hatched bars are statistically significant.

men and 3 kg in women. Thus the physiological tests separated the exposed from the unexposed group.

Neuropsychological Testing

Less verbal information, in the Wechsler story 1 and story 2, was recalled in the exposed than in the unexposed group, both immediately and after a 30-minute delay. Similarly, visual or picture recall was lower for immediate recall (delayed was not tested). In the cognitive domain, exposed subjects had lower Culture Fair scores, vocabulary scores, and digit symbol scores than the unexposed, which were all statistically significant. For perceptual motor speed, the exposed had lower scores and larger standard deviations for putting slotted pegs in the pegboard with the dominant hand, trail making A, and trail making B; so this was clearly a positive domain. Three long-term or crystallized memory tests from the WAIS-R (1) showed small but significant differences for information and for similarities but no difference for picture completion, for a positive domain. The POMS score was significantly higher in exposed compared to unexposed subjects as were the component scores, except vigor, which was lower.

When 31 clients who were all in the inner area of the arsenic plume with estimated air concentrations above 20 ng/m^3 were compared with the 47 class members, there were no significant differences although the choice reaction time difference was borderline significant. No gradients of effect were found in subjects living from 0.32 to 5.6 km from Atochem.

Peripheral Neuritis

Nine symptoms for peripheral effects, emphasizing the feet and the legs, showed a striking difference between the 75 subjects who completed this questionnaire and 18 unexposed (Table 8.2). Pain in the hands and numbness and tingling of the legs and feet were most common, currently and in the past. Tender feet and weakness of the fingers were also frequent, and more than a quarter of the exposed subjects had been unable to stand. Skin peeling had occurred in 31%. Only tender calves and excessive sweating were not significantly different from unexposed.

Symptom Frequencies

The frequencies of 32 of 35 symptoms, including eye and throat irritation, chest complaints, and neurologic, sleep, and vegetative complaints, were significantly higher in

TABLE 8.2 Peripheral neuritis in 75 exposed subjects and 18 unexposed compared by analysis of variance (ANOVA)

	Number	Now	Past	In Both	Ever %	*p*
Feet tender or painful						
Exposed	42	13	14	6	44	
Unexposed	17	0	0	1	6	0.017*
"Pins and needles" in toes and feet						
Exposed	47	9	14	5	37	
Unexposed	17	0	0	1	6	0.038*
Numbness and tingling of legs and feet						
Exposed	43	16	11	5	43	
Unexposed	16	1	0	1	11	0.047*
Pains in hands						
Exposed	41	17	10	7	45	
Unexposed	17	0	1	0	6	0.008*
Tender calves						
Exposed	52	11	8	4	31	
Unexposed	17	0	0	1	6	0.121
Weakness of fingers						
Exposed	42	13	11	9	44	
Unexposed	18	0	0	0	0	0.002*
Periods when unable to stand						
Exposed	54	10	7	4	28	
Unexposed	18	0	0	0	0	0.023*
Skin peeling						
Exposed	52	7	13	3	31	
Unexposed	18	0	0	0	0	0.012*
Excessive sweating						
Exposed	49	12	8	6	35	
Unexposed	16	1	0	1	11	0.113

exposed than in unexposed groups (Table 8.3, Figures 8.3a, b). Most frequent were skin complaints, irritability, lack of concentration, recent memory loss, and extreme fatigue. Only the differences in headache, decreased alcohol tolerance, and loss of appetite were not significant.

Respiratory Symptoms

Chronic bronchitis, by MRC (Medical Research Council) criteria (2), was significantly more common in the exposed group, and shortness of breath with wheezing was more than twice as frequent (Table 8.4). There was a fivefold increase in shortness of breath while walking, a doubling in shortness of breath while climbing stairs, and a threefold increase in wheezing.

TABLE 8.3 Frequencies of complaints on an 11-step scale, with insignificant differences underlined

	Exposed (78)	Unexposed (117)	*p*
Skin itching	5.4	3.3	.0000
Fingernail changes	2.4	1.6	.005
Chest tightness	3.1	2.2	.0008
Palpitations	3.4	2.2	.0003
Burning in chest	3.1	2.1	.0019
Shortness of breath	4.0	2.5	.0000
Dry cough	3.7	2.6	.0003
Cough with mucus	4.3	2.8	.0000
Cough with blood	1.8	1.2	.0000
Dry mouth	4.3	3.2	.003
Throat irritation	3.7	2.6	.0009
Eye irritation	4.3	2.8	.0000
Reduced sense of smell	3.6	2.1	.0001
Headache	4.8	4.4	<u>.3208</u>
Nausea	3.3	2.4	.0044
Dizziness	3.7	2.4	.0000
Lightheadedness	3.9	2.5	.0000
Unusual exhilaration	2.0	1.5	.03
Balance disturbance	3.3	2.0	.0000
Loss of consciousness	1.8	1.2	.0007
Extreme fatigue	4.9	3.4	.0009
Somnolence	3.9	2.6	.0015
Insomnia	4.4	2.9	.0001
Wake frequently	4.7	2.9	.0000
Wake every few hours	4.8	2.9	.0000
Irritability	5.2	3.4	.0000
Lack of concentration	5.1	3.2	.0000
Recent memory loss	5.1	3.1	.0000
Long-term memory loss	4.2	2.2	.0000
Mood instability	4.5	2.5	.0000
Decreased libido	4.4	3.1	.0025
Decreased alcohol tolerance	3.2	2.4	<u>.0702</u>
Indigestion	4.7	3.2	.0003
Loss of appetite	3.0	2.6	<u>.2472</u>
Stomach bloats/swells	3.8	2.9	.0231

<u>Underlined</u> = Probabilities are not significant.

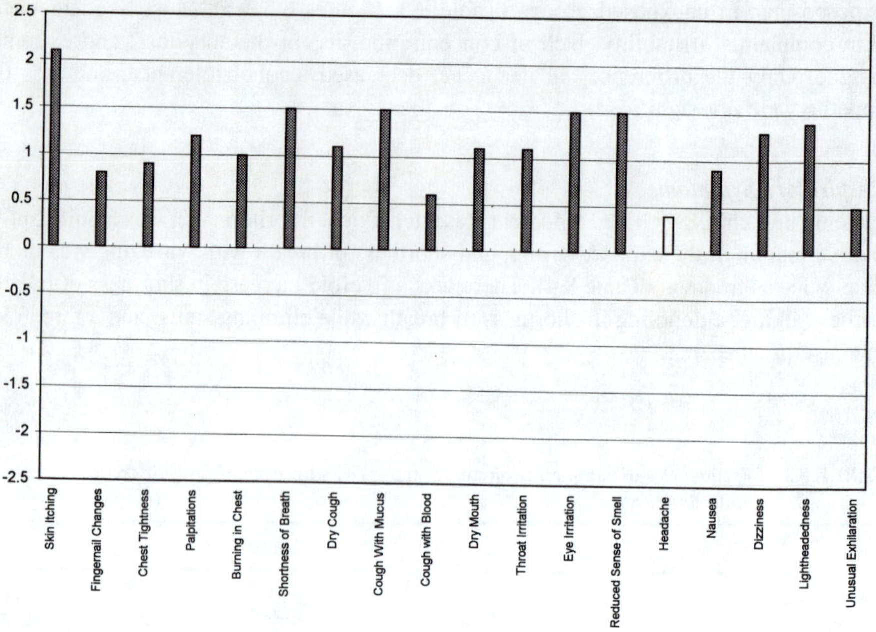

FIGURE 8.3a. Comparisons of symptom frequencies in 78 arsenic-exposed adults and 117 unexposed adults by ANOVA. Hatched bars are statistically significant.

Pulmonary Functions

The exposed group had a significantly lower forced vital capacity (FVC), but there were no significant reductions in FEV_1 and flows although the FEV_{75-85} difference bordered on significant (Table 8.5).

The medical disease questionnaire showed that significantly more exposed subjects had a history of cancer, but further data were unavailable. There were no differences between exposed and unexposed for childhood diseases, heart disease, neurological and psychiatric illness, and use or overdose of drugs and alcohol. More unexposed than exposed had received general anesthesia.

ARA Questionnaire

The frequency of four rheumatic complaints suggestive of lupus erythematosus was significantly higher for the exposed group, including numb and white fingers, mouth sores, protein in the urine, and hair loss (Table 8.6). Other elevated symptoms were not statistically significantly different, and the serum antinuclear antibodies, antithyroid, and antirheumatoid antibodies were not elevated.

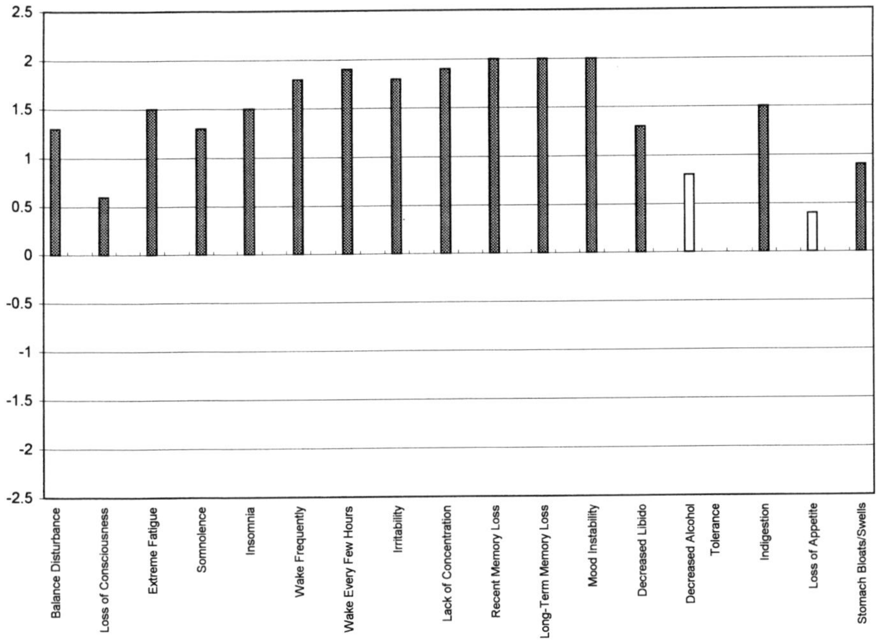

FIGURE 8.3b. Comparisons of symptom frequencies in 78 arsenic-exposed adults and 117 unexposed adults by ANOVA. Hatched bars are statistically significant.

TABLE 8.4 Respiratory symptoms

Numbers	Exposed (78)	Unexposed (117)	*p*
Phlegm	30.8	12.8	.002
Chronic bronchitis by criteria of MRC	44.9	26.8	.001
Shortness of breath			
At rest	16.7	5.1	.008
Walking	33.3	6.0	.000
Climbing stairs	61.5	33.1	.000
Wheezing	34.6	11.1	.000
Shortness of breath with wheezing	33.3	7.1	.000
Normal breathing between attacks	77.1	41.1	.000

TABLE 8.5 Comparison of pulmonary function tests in 78 exposed workers and 115 unexposed subjects presented as percentage of predicted values (based on Michigan populations of Miller et al. 1986)[32]

	All Subjects				
	Exposed		Unexposed		
	(n = 78)		(n = 115)		
	Mean	Sd	Mean	Sd	p
FVC % pred	95.7	16.2	100.8	11.9	.012
FEV_1 % pred	92.2	18.0	94.2	13.1	.372
FEF_{25-75} % pred	92.2	31.9	92.2	30.3	.997
FEF_{75-85} % pred	95.2	44.0	82.6	51.1	.077

Confounding from Occupational Exposures

Comparison of the frequency of exposure to 22 occupations and work sites known to have neurotoxic chemical exposures showed only small differences for exposed subjects, who had more chemical or pharmaceutical industry employment, whereas more unexposed had been employed in electronics manufacturing.

DISCUSSION

Arsenic-exposed subjects were significantly impaired compared to unexposed for all six domains: neurophysiological tests, recall both immediate and delayed, cognitive function, perceptual motor speed, long-term or crystallized memory, and POMS score. This environmental arsenic exposure had lasted 50 years or more for some people. The obvious attribution is to arsenic, but several factors should be considered before we accept this choice. First, the delayed blink reflex latency for R-1 has been associated in the past almost exclusively with chlorinated solvents. Such trigeminal nerve effects have not previously been associated with arsenic and so are problematic until confirmed. The outright attribution of these effects to arsenic is tempting, but there are only a few papers reporting central nervous system (CNS) effects of arsenic (3–5) in addition to patient reports of delirium and convulsions (6, 7). Only a few environmentally exposed people have been tested for neurobehavioral effects of arsenic (8, 9). Peripheral neuritis symptoms (6, 10, 11) were found in these exposed subjects, but they also had distur-

TABLE 8.6 Prevalences of American Rheumatism Association criteria for lupus erythematosus

	Exposed (78)	Unexposed (117)	p
Rheumatism	25.6	17.9	.198
Numb fingers	43.6	27.4	.019*
Mouth sores	16.7	6.8	.030*
Anemia	23.1	19.7	.568
Rash on cheeks	9.0	3.4	.101
Sun rash	14.1	9.4	.312
Painful breathing	15.4	12.8	.614
Protein in urine	10.3	2.5	.022*
Hair loss	24.4	5.1	.000*
Seizures	3.4	2.6	.614

bances of sleep, weakness, and cognitive and memory impairment. Such symptoms are regarded as uncommon in industrial practice (12). The neurobehavioral impairments seen at Bryan are tentatively attributed to arsenic and constitute a first epidemiological confirmation of reports attributing delirium (8) and permanent (9, 13, 14) or reversible encephalopathy (7) to arsenic.

That observation obviously leads to the next question: were these subjects affected by exposure to neurotoxic chemicals besides arsenic? Organophosphates and carbamates must be considered because they were sometimes handled and packaged at the site. Their chronic toxicity is generally attributed to stimulation of a neurotoxic esterase in the brain rather than inhibition of acetylcholine esterase. Organophosphates and carbamates generally cause chronic and protracted neurobehavioral dysfunction only after field workers are ''knocked down'' (15) although insidious poisoning has occurred (16). Neurobehavioral impairment 9 km from the Atochem site makes this mechanism unlikely because of intermittent contact with small and probably insufficient quantities of these chemicals. Our tests could not distinguish between these substances' effects on the brain and those of arsenic.

It appears highly likely that the central nervous system effects of arsenic have been overlooked—that investigators have traditionally focused on the peripheral nervous manifestations, the gastrointestinal tract and the skin. Workers have rarely been tested with methods that would show central nervous system effects. An exception is that hearing loss was found in boys exposed to environmental arsenic (17).

What would resolve this dilemma? Arsenic residues have been measured in soil, water, and attic dust. Preliminary sampling of attic dust in homes at varying distances from the site showed a 100-fold gradient of arsenic levels but no residues of carbamates or organophosphates. After extending the isopleth map model and calculating doses received by the tested subjects, investigators should test more distant subjects. Air levels of 10 to 100 ng/m^3 of arsenic produce a human daily dose of 144 to 1440 μg, a range that equals or surpasses the doses that in Taiwan were associated with increases in cancer (18). Although this class action has a potential size of 20,000 to 30,000 people, it may need enlarging, as the population of Bryan and College Station is nearly 100,000. In this regard, a cluster of neural tube defects occurred near Atochem. Also, cancer rates were excessive among the exposed group, and this lead needs following. We found excessive respiratory complaints and only marginal functional evidence of respiratory impairment, but that function may be clearly reduced in a larger population.

The question of how arsenic damages or injures the brain apparently has not been asked previously—so right there we have a license to speculate. Starting with the facts, arsenic is a well-known cause of Raynaud's phenomenon and other vasospastic responses (19) leading to peripheral neuropathy, black foot, and ischemic gangrene of the extremities (20). Therefore, a vascular or a microvascular disorder seems a prime possibility. This idea ignores the seeming differences in blood vessel reactivity in the brain vs. peripherally but plays into the hands of ''microvascular dementia,'' a major alternate diagnosis to Alzheimer's disease (21, 22). These disorders are separated by major findings on brain imaging. Further exploration along these lines, novel as it may seem, should be tempered by the realization that astrocytes and mediators also are competing for roles in brain disruption by arsenic (23, 24).

Arsenic is a general protoplasmic poison and carcinogen with a long history as such (25). For example, arsenic contamination of sugar used in making beer caused 70 deaths among 6,000 people in northern England in 1903 (26). In 1928 in France, 40,000 people were poisoned when wine and bread were contaminated with arsenic. In the 1950s in Georgia, North Carolina, and South Carolina, moonshiners fermented mash-distilled alcohol in auto radiators soldered with lead and decanted it into arsenic pesticide bottles, causing arsenic, lead, and alcohol poisoning (6, 7). Arsenic combined with hydrogen, arsine gas, is a particularly severe poison. When arsine leaked in the hold of a container ship, the 17-man crew had serious gastrointestinal, constitutional, and neurological symptoms plus severe hemolytic anemia and renal toxicity (27).

Arsenic adversely affects energy metabolism, in part, by replacing phosphate (11). Some of the effects of arsenic on the brain resemble vitamin B_1 deficiency (28). Patients receiving large doses of arsenic during intravenous therapy for syphilis developed nausea, vomiting, and diarrhea, followed by tachycardia, hypotension, vasomotor collapse, and death. Chronic poisoning is characterized first by weakness, malaise, anorexia, and vomiting; second by irritation of the mucous membranes, hyperkeratosis and darkening of the skin, striae of the nails, and pitting edema; and third by numbness and burning of the hands and the feet, signs of overt peripheral neuropathy.

Chronic arsenic poisoning is manifested by mental slowing, somnolence, headache, poor memory, irrational speech, and toxic delirium (3, 14). Optic neuritis has occurred in arsenical treatment of syphilis and in combined alcohol, lead, and arsenic poisoning (6, 7). Peripheral neuropathy is thought to be more common than are neurological symptoms such as memory loss (4). Polyneuropathy is symmetrical with sensory and motor involvement, causing tingling, numbness, and pins and needles, usually extending from distal to proximal sites. Nerve biopsies, in both poisoned human patients and experimental animals, show degeneration of axons with bulkiness and loss of the normal structures (3). Arsenic smelter workers with peripheral neuropathy had slowed conduction of the ulnar motor nerve and the peroneal and sural nerves, compared to exposed workers without neuropathy, whereas control (aluminum smelter) workers had normal conduction (5). Thus nerve conduction abnormalities are not early signs of neurological impairment.

Concern about arsenic as a carcinogen was restimulated in Taiwan, where, particularly in malnourished subjects, excessive risks of liver, lung, bladder, and kidney cancer were associated with 170 to 800 micrograms of arsenic per liter (μg/l) of water (18). Risks for cancer from arsenic in the United States have been estimated at 13 excess deaths per thousand persons from drinking 1 liter of water (29). Water supplies of at least 350,000 people in the United States have arsenic levels above 50 μg/l (the EPA standard), and another 2.5 million have levels between 25 and 50 μg/l. Average mortality rates from lung cancer among white males and females in the United States from 1950 to 1969 were significantly increased in counties with copper, lead, or zinc smelting and refining, with probable arsenic effluents, but not in counties where other nonferrous ores were processed (30). In addition, an increased risk for vascular disease has been defined (31), including coronary and peripheral arterial insufficiency.

References

1. Wechsler D: *Adult Intelligence Scale Manual* (revised). New York: Psychological Corporation, 1971.
2. Ferris BG, Jr.: Epidemiology standardization project. *Am Rev Respir Dis* 1978;118:7–54.
3. Schaumburg HH, Spencer PS, and Thomas PK: *Disorders of Peripheral Nerves.* Philadelphia, PA: F. A. Davis Co., 1983.
4. Bleecker ML and Bolla-Wilson K: Occupational inorganic arsenic exposure unmasking a memory disorder. In: *Neurobehavioural Methods in Occupational and Environmental Health.* Copenhagen: WHO, 1985.
5. Feldman RG, Niles CA, Kelly-Hayes M, Sax DS, Dixon WJ, Thompson DJ, and Landau E: Peripheral neuropathy in arsenic smelter workers. *Neurology* 1979;29:939–944.
6. Heyman A, Pfeiffer JB, Willett RW, and Taylor HM: Peripheral neuropathy caused by arsenical intoxication. *NEJM* 1956;254:401–409.

7. Jenkins RB: Inorganic arsenic and the nervous system. *Brain* 1966;89:479–498.
8. Franzblau A and Lilis R: Acute arsenic intoxication from environmental arsenic exposure. *Arch Environ Health* 1989;44:385–390.
9. Bolla-Wilson K and Bleecker ML: Neuropsychological impairment following inorganic arsenic exposure. *J Occup Med* 1987;29:500–503.
10. DeWolf FA and Edelbroek PM: Neurotoxicity of arsenic and its compounds. In: *Handbook of Clinical Neurology 20: Intoxications of the Nervous System,* Part 1, FA deWolff (ed.). Amsterdam: Elsevier Science BV, 1994.
11. Massey EW: Arsenic neuropathy. *Neurology* 1981;31:1057–1058.
12. *Proctor and Hughes: Chemical Hazards of the Workplace* (3rd ed.), GJ Hathaway, NH Proctor, JP Hughes, and ML Fischman (eds.). New York: Van Nostrand Reinhold, 1991, pp. 92–95.
13. Freeman JW and Couch JR: Prolonged encephalopathy with arsenic poisoning. *Neurology* 1978;28:853–855.
14. Beckett WS, Moore JL, Keogh JP, and Bleecker ML: Acute encephalopathy due to occupational exposure to arsenic. *Brit J Indust Med* 1986;43:66–67.
15. Savage EP, Keefe TJ, Mounce LM, Heaton RK, Lewis JA, and Buren PJ: Chronic neuropsychological sequelae of acute organophosphate pesticide poisoning. *Arch Environ Health* 1988;43:38–45.
16. Lotti M: The pathogenesis of organophosphate polyneuropathy. *Crit Rev Toxicol* 1992;22: 465–487.
17. Bencko V and Symon K: Test of environmental exposure to arsenic and hearing changes in exposed children. *Environ Health Perspect* 1977;19:95–101.
18. Wu MM, Kuo TL, Hwang YJ, and Chen CJ: Dose–response relationships between arsenic well water and mortality from cancer. *Am J Epidem* 1989;130:1123–1132.
19. Lagerkvist B, Linderholm H, and Nordberg GF: Vasospastic tendency and Raynaud's phenomenon in smelter workers exposed to arsenic. *Environ Res* 1986;39:465–474.
20. Ch'i I-C and Blackwell RQ: A controlled retrospective study of blackfoot disease, an endemic peripheral gangrene disease in Taiwan. *Am J Epidem* 1968;88:7–24.
21. Roth M: The association of clinical and neurological findings and its bearing on the classification and aetiology of Alzheimer's disease. *Brit Med Bull* 1986;42:42–50.
22. Larson EB, Kukull WA, and Katzman RL: Cognitive impairment: dementia and Alzheimer's disease. *Annu Rev Publ Health* 1992;13:431–449.
23. Jacobs BL: Serotonin, motor activity and depression-related disorders. *Am Scientist* 1994; 82:456–463.
24. Streit WJ and Kincaid-Colton CA: The brain's immune system. *Scientif Am* 1995;Nov.: 54–61.
25. Windebank AJ, McCall JT, and Dyck PJ: Metal neuropathy. In: *Peripheral Neuropathy,* Vol. II, PJ Dyck, PK Thomas, EH Lambert, and R Bunge (eds.). Philadelphia, PA: W. B. Saunders Co., 1984.
26. Reynolds ES: An account of the epidemic outbreak of arsenical poisoning occurring in beer drinkers in the north of England and the midland countries in 1900. *Lancet* 1901;1:166–170.
27. Fowler BA and Weissberg JB: Arsine poisoning. *NEJM* 1974;291:1171–1174.
28. Sexton GB and Gowdey CW: Relation between thiamine and arsenical toxicity. *Arch Dermatol Syph* 1963;56:634–647.
29. Smith AH, Hopenhayn-Rich C, Bates MN, Goeden HM, Hertz-Picciotto I, Duggan HM, Wood R, Kosnett MJ, and Smith MT: Cancer risks from arsenic in drinking water. *Environ Health Perspect* 1992;97:259–267.
30. Blot WJ and Fraumeni JF: Arsenical air pollution and lung cancer. *Lancet* 1975;II:142–144.
31. Engel RT and Smith AH: Arsenic in drinking water and mortality from vascular disease: an ecologic analysis in 30 U.S. counties. *Arch Environ Health* 1994;49:418–427.
32. Miller, A, Thornton JC, and Warshaw RH: Mean and instantaneous expiratory flows FVC and FEV_1: prediction equations from a probability sample of Michigan, a large industrial state. *Bull Env Physiopathol Resp* 1986;22:589–597.

9

Neurobehavioral Effects of Residential Chlordane

Chlordane was introduced in 1948 and used extensively as a termiticide until 1975, when its use was interdicted by the Environmental Protection Agency. For some uses it was banned in 1988 because of human neurotoxicity. Unfortunately, on-hand stocks remained in circulation, and the chemical was probably illegally imported from Mexico. Chlordane accumulates in fatty tissues and has been classified as a probable human carcinogen.

In April of 1987 the outside of an apartment complex in Houston, Texas had all wooden surfaces sprayed for termites with chlordane in unknown concentration. Later, in 1987 and 1988, chlorpyrifos (Dursban) and chlordane were combined, and many of these wooden surfaces were resprayed with the mixture. The apartment units were tested for chlordane residue in 1990 and 1991, and 85% of 81 wipe samples from wood surfaces were found to have 0.5 μg/929 cm^2 or more chlordane. Indoor concentrations were as high as 13.6 μg/929 cm^2 on wipe samples, and 24 of the 294 apartments from which air samples were obtained had levels above 0.5 μg/m^3 for 8-hour samples. Eight current occupants of the apartments had blood or fat chlordane content measured, and all samples were elevated.

Over 250 people were exposed to chlordane in the 1987 spraying. Our investigators measured neurobehavioral function and administered a questionnaire for symptom frequency, mood status, confounding factors and medical, rheumatic, and respiratory disorders to 216 of these adults available for study in 1994. Measurements included simple and choice reaction time, balance, blink reflex latency, color vision, and cognitive, perceptual motor, memory, and recall functions. The analysis included 104 exposed and 137 unexposed adult subjects tested in English and 112 exposed and 36 unexposed adult subjects tested in Spanish. Age, educational level, weight, height, and sex ratios were similar for the exposed and unexposed groups. Results of tests of long-term memory functions, which usually are spared by chemical injury, were not different in the groups. This was consistent with their having had similar levels of psychological function before exposure. There were no biases identified, and confounding factors were generally balanced in the groups. Chlordane appeared to be associated with protracted impairment of physiological and psychological functions of the central nervous system, which is an important target of chlorinated cyclodiene insecticides. Human exposure to chlordane should be prohibited and guarded against.

TESTING OF SUBJECTS

In June of 1994, 216 adult occupants or former residents of the apartments were tested with our standard neurobehavioral battery and a series of questionnaires. Exposed subjects and (invited) unexposed groups (both English-speaking and Spanish-speaking adults, as well as children, most of whom were tested in English) were compared for their neurobehavioral function, pulmonary function, symptoms, and factors that might confound or bias the results.

Methods

A matched cohort design was used with 77 women and 60 men in the English-speaking exposed group between the ages of 17 and 70 years, compared to 58 women and 46 men in the local English-speaking unexposed group. The groups tested in Spanish included 22 women and 14 men as unexposed subjects and 56 women and 56 men who were exposed. The unexposed were local subjects who had been recruited by the exposed subjects to match them, and those recruited by our staff to match the exposed group for sex, age, and years of educational level (highest school grade completed). As the results did not differ by the method of recruiting, these unexposed groups were combined. There was no evidence of chemical contamination of either exposed or unexposed subjects from their jobs. However, all subjects shared air and water in southeast Houston near the ship channel, probably contaminated from numerous oil refineries and chemical companies. Potential unexposed subjects were contacted to ascertain if they met the matching criteria and their willingness to be tested. They were reimbursed for their time and for mileage. Examiners were blinded as to subjects' category and exposure status. All subjects gave informed consent, and the protocol was university-approved. Standardized methods as described in Chapter 3 and 4 were used.

Results

The 216 exposed subjects tested, 55% women and 45% men, had an average age of 32.5 years and an average educational attainment of 10.3 years. The 173 unexposed subjects had the same ratio of women and men, an average age of 34.0 years and an educational level of 11.5 years. Analysis of covariance was relied upon because of the 2-year differences in educational level and in age, which favored the performance of the unexposed group, and a large difference in numbers of the Spanish-speaking exposed individuals (112) vs. the unexposed group (36). Although these differences were smaller in the adults tested in English, analysis of covariance was used for uniformity. Effects were compared in language-specific groups but not along traditional surname lines. It was a preferred-language separation.

The English-speaking exposed subjects had a mean age of 32.9 years and an educational level average of 11.5 years, which were similar to the average age of 32.2 and educational level of 12.0 in the 137 unexposed; and 56% of both groups were women.

TABLE 9.1 Neurophysiological and neuropsychological scores and profile of mood states in exposed and unexposed subjects tested in English compared by analysis of variance (ANOVA) and covariance analysis (CA)

	Unexposed (137)		Exposed (104)		ANOVA	CA
n	Mean	Sd	Mean	Sd	*p*	*p*
Age yrs	32.2	11.3	32.9	11.4	0.6629	
Educational Level yrs	12.0	2.4	11.5	2.1	0.0892+	
Women/Men	77/60		58/46			
Height cm Men	173.8	7.0	173.4	8.4	0.8033	
Women	160.7	7.0	160.1	7.6	0.6660	
Weight kg Men	87.4	21.2	87.7	17.5	0.9431	
Women	70.9	19.7	73.8	22.1	0.4295	
Grip Right kg Men	49.8	8.7	49.8	8.7	0.9990	.060
Women	33.1	8.2	30.7	6.3	0.0836	.060
Grip Left kg Men	47.8	7.6	46.8	9.9	0.5652	.495
Women	30.7	8.0	28.1	5.7	0.0400*	.039*
Neurophysiological Tests						
ln Simple Reaction Time ms	309	92	414	235	0.0001*	.0005*
ln Choice Reaction Time ms	564	122	639	226	0.0006*	.0005*
ln Balance Sway Speed cm/sec Eyes Open	0.82	0.20	0.95	0.35	0.0008*	.002*
Eyes Closed	1.26	0.35	1.48	0.60	0.0005*	.0005*
Color Score Lanthony[4]	11.6	1.3	11.9	1.5	0.0956	.239
Blink Reflex Latency Tap ms						
Supraorbital Tap Right	14.5	2.4	13.5	2.3	0.0038*	.005**
Left	14.3	2.5	13.2	2.3	0.0015*	.002**
Glabellar Tap Right	15.8	2.0	15.6	1.8	0.3715	.244
Left	15.6	2.0	15.1	2.1	0.1061	.056
Recall (Wechsler)						
Story 1 Immediate	10.5	4.2	8.7	3.7	0.0010*	.008*+
Delayed	8.3	4.5	6.7	3.7	0.0038*	.007*+
Story 2 Immediate	9.4	4.0	8.2	3.9	0.0324*	
Delayed	8.3	4.2	6.6	4.1	0.0028*	
Visual Recall	29.5	7.7	29.6	6.9	0.9666++	
Digit Span Forward	6.8	1.5	6.7	1.7	0.5963	
Backward	4.4	1.4	4.3	1.5	0.4405	
Cognitive Function						
Culture Fair A score	28.1	7.7	25.4	8.1	0.0079*	.023*
Vocabulary score	18.5	8.3	16.0	7.7	0.0254*	.129
Digit Symbol score	57.5	15.0	48.5	15.0	0.00005*	.0005*
Perceptual Motor Speed						
1/Pegboard Dominant score	72.4	27.6	76.1	20.5	0.2597	.015w* .188m
ln Trail Making A score	37.3	17.1	44.7	19.4	0.0027*	.005*
ln Trail Making B score	79.8	37.7	93.1	37.1	0.0092*	.0005*
Sensoro-interpretive						
Finger Writing Errors Right	2.4	3.4	2.9	3.5	0.3309	
Left	2.0	3.2	2.4	3.4	0.3707	
Long-Term or "Crystallized" Memory						
Information score[1,5]	14.6	6.1	13.1	5.9	0.0567	.141
Picture Completion score[2]	13.7	4.0	13.2	3.9	0.3627	.459
Similarities score[2]	17.7	6.1	16.6	5.9	0.1989	.515
POMS Score	32.3	38.8	72.2	43.6	0.0001*	
Tension	10.9	7.3	18.5	8.0	0.0001*	
Depression	11.9	11.8	20.7	14.3	0.0001*	
Anger	10.8	9.6	18.2	11.0	0.0001*	
Vigor	17.1	6.4	12.4	5.7	0.0001*	
Fatigue	8.1	6.3	14.2	7.3	0.0001*	
Confusion	7.7	5.4	12.9	6.0	0.0001*	

* Statistically significant. ++ No prediction model. w = women

\+ Stories combined. ** References more abnormal than exposed. m = men

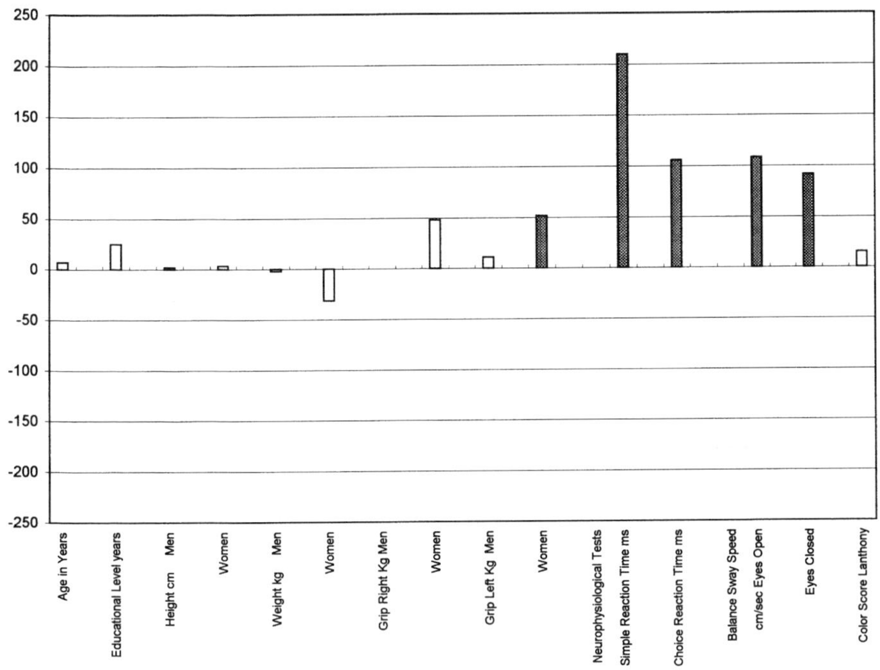

FIGURE 9.1a. Comparison of 104 chlordane-exposed English-speaking adults and 137 unexposed English-speaking adults by ANOVA. Hatched bars are statistically significant.

The exposed group's weights and heights were not statistically significantly different from the unexposed for men or women (Table 9.1, Figures 9.1a–c).

The following description is based on the relatively conservative and certain analysis of covariance, which adjusts for differences between the groups in age and other determinative factors; see *p* values in the far-right column of Tables 9.1 and 9.2. Simple reaction time was slowed to an average of 414 in the exposed compared to 309 ms in the unexposed, and the choice reaction times at 639 vs. 564 was similar, and both differences were statistically significant. Spanish-speaking tested groups showed similar significant differences (see Table 9.2, Figures 9.2a–c). For balance measured as sway speed with eyes open the difference of 0.95 cm/sec in the exposed vs. 0.82 cm/sec in the English-tested was significantly different, as was the difference of 1.48 vs. 1.26 for sway speed eyes closed. Significant differences in balance were also found in the Spanish-speaking tested. The color score on the Lanthony desaturated hue test was insignificantly higher in the exposed for both language groups. Blink reflex latency R-1 for English-speaking and Spanish-speaking tested (Tables 9.1 and 9.2) was faster in the exposed than in the unexposed when elicited by supraorbital taps (right and left),

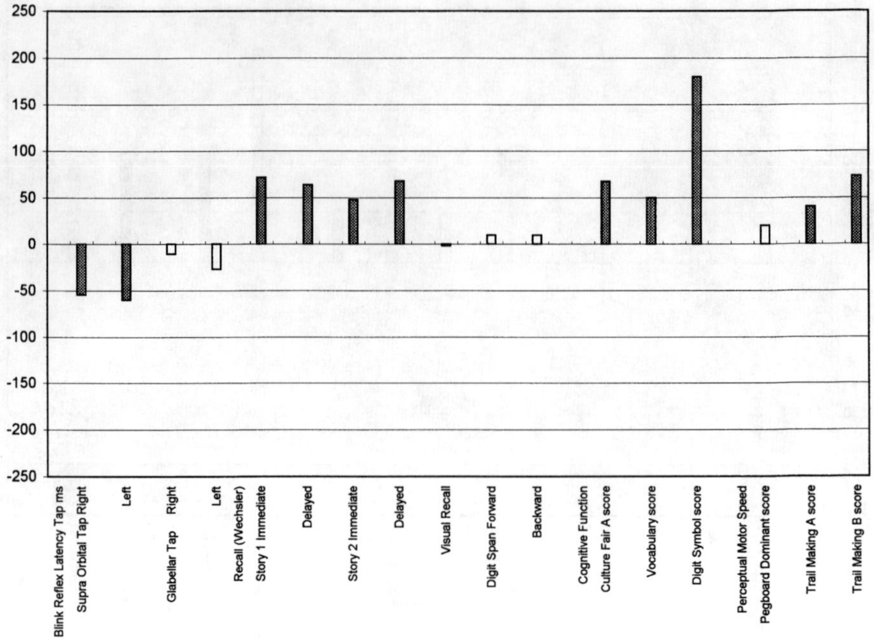

FIGURE 9.1b. Comparison of 104 chlordane-exposed English-speaking adults and 137 unexposed English-speaking adults by ANOVA. Hatched bars are statistically significant.

but not by glabellar taps and recorded from the right and the left. Grip strength was similarly not significantly different except in women tested in English (Table 9.1).

Immediate and delayed recall of the Wechsler stories were significantly less in the exposed English-speaking group vs. unexposed, but not for the Spanish-speaking one, but neither was significant using analysis of covariance. Visual recall and digit span forwards and backwards were not significantly different by covariance analysis. The cognitive functions domain in English-tested subjects showed a significant difference in means for Culture Fair A (at 25.4 in exposed vs. 28.1 in the reference group), as did digit symbol. Similar differences were significant in those tested in Spanish. Vocabulary averaged 16.0 in exposed and 18.5 in unexposed tested in English and approached statistical significance; in those tested in Spanish, the difference of 11.6 vs. 17.5 was statistically significant. The perceptual motor speed tests showed statistically significant differences in both language groups for trail making A and trail making B basic variance analysis; but the difference for grooved pegboard with the dominant hand was only statistically significant in women. In the long-term or crystallized memory domain (information, picture completion, and similarities) there were no significant differences

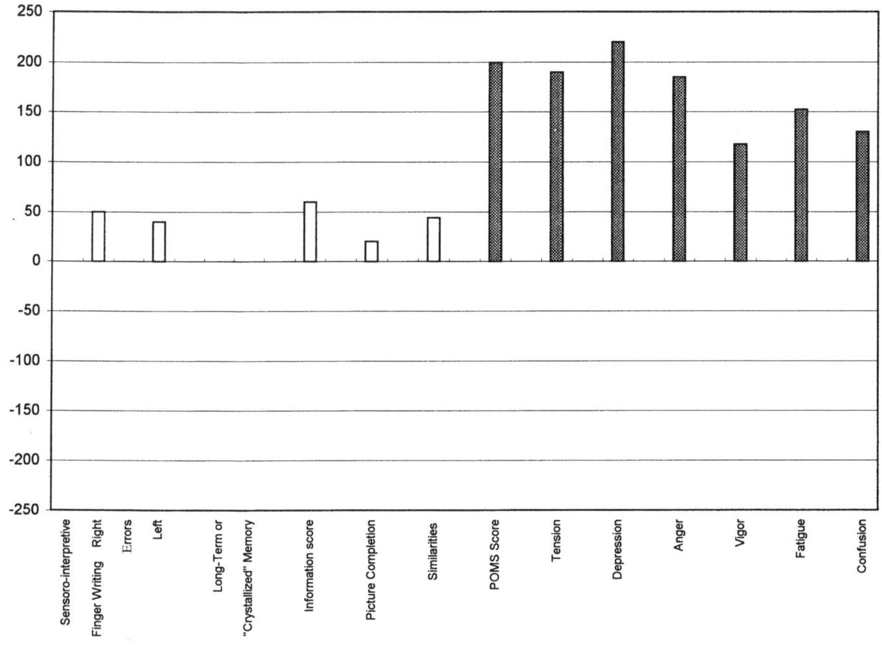

FIGURE 9.1c. Comparison of 104 chlordane-exposed English-speaking adults and 137 unexposed English-speaking adults by ANOVA. Hatched bars are statistically significant.

between exposed and unexposed groups tested in English, but the Spanish-speaking exposed subjects had unusually low scores for information and picture completion. If this difference were cultural, it should have included the reference group; so it is tentatively attributed to other chemical exposures. This assumption is consistent with both groups' being in the same population prior to exposure. Fingertip writing errors were not different between the groups in either language.

Affective status, as revealed by POMS score, showed a large and statistically significant difference, with averages of 72.2 for the English-tested exposed vs. 32.3 for the unexposed. For the Spanish-tested, the difference between exposed and reference subjects was similar although scores were lower in both groups. Significant differences were found in all six component factors, tension, depression, anger, fatigue, and confusion all being significantly higher and vigor significantly lower.

The children's test results were confined to English-tested because the Spanish-tested group had only 16 exposed and 7 unexposed, too few to analyze. There were no differences between the 59 exposed children tested in English and 76 unexposed (Table 9.3, Figures 9.3a, b) by covariance analyses. Thus, the key measurements of

TABLE 9.2 Neurophysiological and neuropsychological tests and profile of mood states scores of exposed and unexposed subjects tested in Spanish compared by analysis of variance (ANOVA) and covariance analysis (CA)

Variable			Unexposed (36)		Exposed (112)		ANOVA	CA
			Mean	Sd	Mean	Sd	*p*	*p*
Age yrs			39.9	10.8	32.0	9.0	.0005*	
Educational Level yrs			10.1	3.2	8.8	3.7	.0535	
Women/Men			22/14		56/56			
Height cm	Men		169.5	7.7	166.4	6.4	.1505	
	Women		156.4	35.1	155.9	6.0	.6859	
Weight kg	Men		83.0	14.0	76.5	10.5	.0572	
	Women		65.8	12.7	66.8	11.6	.7413	
Grip Right kg	Men		47.9	7.6	46.4	8.1	.5564	.303
	Women		29.8	5.6	28.5	5.1	.3288	.303
Grip Left kg	Men		46.4	6.2	44.3	9.4	.4419	.443
	Women		27.7	4.8	26.8	5.0	.4546	.087
Neurophysiological Tests								
ln Simple Reaction Time ms			334	99	456	220	.0016*	.0005*
ln Choice Reaction Time ms			609	111	694	146	.0018*	.0005*
ln Balance Sway Speed cm/sec		Eyes Open	0.81	0.20	0.96	0.32	.0102*	.015*
		Eyes Closed	1.17	0.32	1.40	0.48	.0076*	.004*
Color Score Lanthony[4]			11.7	1.0	12.1	1.5	.1174	.254
Blink Reflex Latency Tap ms								
Supraorbital Tap	Right		14.5	1.6	14.6	2.2	.8545	.915
	Left		14.1	1.8	14.1	2.1	.9928	.820
Glabellar Tap	Right		15.9	1.5	15.6	1.6	.2928	.401
	Left		15.5	1.3	15.3	1.9	.4609	.513
Recall (Wechsler)								
Story 1	Immediate		10.4	3.8	8.4	4.3	.0133*	.168⁺
	Delayed		8.5	3.5	6.4	4.6	.0149*	.097⁺
Story 2	Immediate		9.5	4.7	8.0	3.8	.0574	
	Delayed		8.0	4.4	6.4	3.9	.0529	
Visual Recall			27.3	7.8	25.0	8.7	.1624⁺⁺	
Digit Span	Forward		6.0	1.4	5.3	1.5	.0148*	
	Backward		4.0	1.4	3.5	1.3	.0612	
Cognitive Function								
Culture Fair A			21.2	6.7	17.7	9.5	.0418*	.018*
Vocabulary			17.5	8.3	11.6	7.4	.0001*	.0005*
Digit Symbol			46.9	12.2	38.3	16.4	.0046*	.0005*
Perceptual Motor Speed								
1/Pegboard Dominant			73.2	25.5	82.2	31.6	.1299	.008w* .151m
ln Trail Making A			47.7	21.4	69.7	40.0	.0021*	.0005*
ln Trail Making B			114.7	47.9	131.4	51.4	.0932	.056
Sensoro-Interpretive								
Finger Writing Errors	Right		2.8	3.4	3.5	3.7	.2878	
	Left		2.1	3.1	3.1	4.0	.1959	
Long-Term or "Crystallized" Memory								
Information[1,5]			12.5	6.5	8.3	5.3	.0002*	.015*
Picture Completion[2]			12.0	3.8	9.3	5.3	.0065*	.032*
Similarities[2]			16.7	6.7	14.0	7.1	.0532	.275
POMS Score			11.9	29.2	52.5	36.0	.0001*	
Tension			8.4	6.9	15.2	6.5	.0001*	
Depression			6.1	8.0	14.0	10.1	.0001*	
Anger			5.2	6.0	14.6	10.0	.0001*	
Vigor			16.9	5.4	12.8	6.1	.0005*	
Fatigue			4.1	4.4	11.1	6.0	.0001*	
Confusion			4.9	4.3	10.4	4.8	.0001*	

* Statistically significant ⁺⁺ No prediction model m = men

⁺ Stories combined w = women

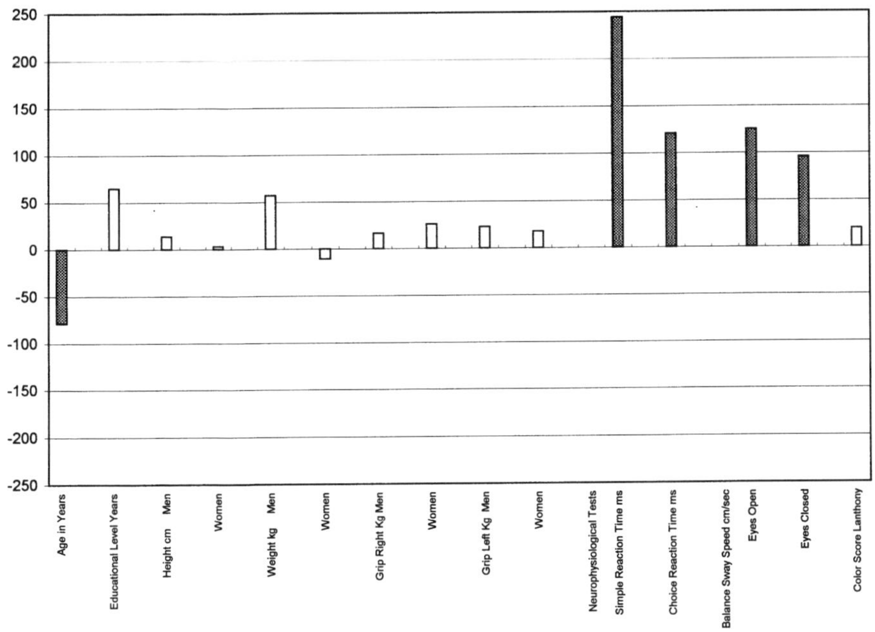

FIGURE 9.2a. Comparison of 104 chlordane-exposed Spanish-speaking adults and 137 unexposed Spanish-speaking adults by ANOVA. Hatched bars are statistically significant.

balance, reaction time, and color showed no differences. The generally delayed blink reflex latency R-1 found in adults was also seen in children, but they showed a greater degree of slowing, that is, worse impairment than adults showed. Blink reflex latency R-1 in another major unexposed population of children, that of Wickenburg, Arizona (see Chapter 11), was significantly faster than in these presumably ''unexposed'' Houston children. In fact, blink reflex latency R-1 has a linear relationship with age, gradually slowing from age 5 to 83 years (see Chapter 3). This paradoxical finding is unexplained but may be another clue to a pervasive ''southeast Houston effect,'' which is associated with proximity to oil refineries, chemical industries, and the ship channel from Galveston Bay to Houston.

The frequency of 35 symptoms in exposed subjects was uniformly greater, from skin complaints through complaints of the chest, throat, and eye to the central nervous system, including recall, memory, concentration, sleep disturbances, irritability, dizziness, and balance, as well as vegetative symptoms including indigestion, loss of libido, loss of appetite, and swollen stomach. All symptoms were statistically significantly more common in the exposed vs. the unexposed groups.

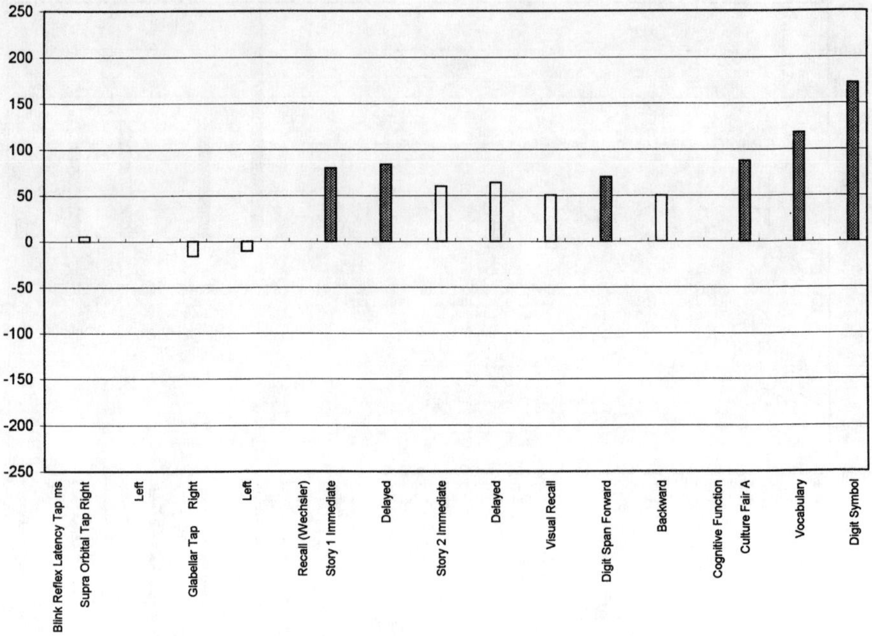

FIGURE 9.2b. Comparison of 104 chlordane-exposed Spanish-speaking adults and 137 unexposed Spanish-speaking adults by ANOVA. Hatched bars are statistically significant.

Respiratory symptoms were examined in this manner, and an allergy history, the production of phlegm, and chronic bronchitis by MRC criteria were statistically significantly more common in exposed subjects. Shortness of breath at rest, walking, and climbing stairs was also significantly different, as were wheezing and shortness of breath with wheezing. Curiously, asthma by history was not significantly different, despite being almost twice as common in the exposed group. The pulmonary function studies as percentage of predicted level averaged 97% for FVC, 91% for FEV_1, 91% for FEF_{25-75}, and 83% predicted for FEF_{75-85}, but there were no statistically significant differences between the groups.

Comparative prevalences of mumps, chicken pox, and measles were not different. There were no differences for diagnosed neurological or psychiatric disease. There had been more exposed subjects under general anesthesia but more head injuries in the unexposed group. Significantly more birth defects had occurred in the exposed group than the unexposed. Also, the exposed group had significant excesses of angina pectoris ($p < 0.0001$) and kidney disease ($p < 0.016$). However, histories of myocardial disease, lupus erythematosus, and cancer were not different for exposed and unexposed. Life-

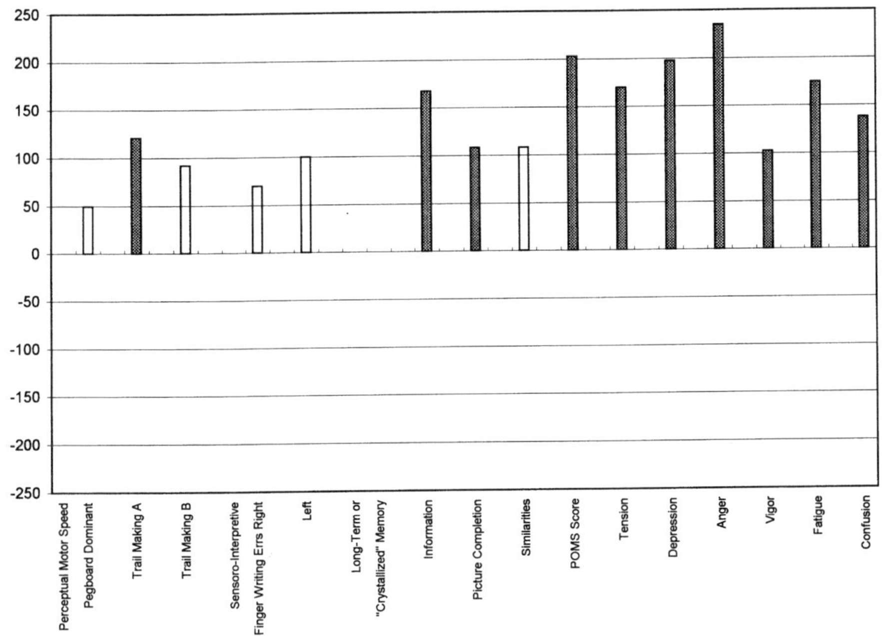

FIGURE 9.2c. Comparison of 104 Chlordane-exposed Spanish-speaking adults and 137 unexposed Spanish-speaking adults by ANOVA. Hatched bars are statistically significant.

style factors, drug overdoses and alcohol consumption on a weekly, monthly, or seldom basis, were not significantly different; however, significantly more of the exposed group had never used alcohol (at 44.9% vs. 28.4%), and more unexposed had had alcohol overdoses (4.2% vs. 0.6%). Both factors (use and overdosing) would tend to narrow the differences between exposed and unexposed subjects. There were no differences in illicit drug use or tranquilizer drug use, and only about 5% of both groups used illicit drugs currently.

The American Rheumatism Association criteria for lupus erythematosus showed that significantly more of the exposed group had numb and cold fingers, mouth sores, rash on cheeks, rash elicited by sunlight, painful breathing (pleuritic chest pain), and hair loss. In contrast, there were no differences for general rheumatic complaints of anemia, protein in urine, or seizures. Ten percent of the exposed group had five or more ARA symptoms vs. zero percent of the unexposed group. Occupational exposures to chemicals with possible confounding effects were more common in the unexposed than in the exposed group, particularly for dry cleaning, photo finishing, printing, and home pesticide exposure. In summary, there were no differences that would do other

TABLE 9.3 Children in Houston

	Unexposed		Exposed	
	76		59	
	Mean	Sd	Mean	Sd
Age yrs	11.6	3.0	11.6	3.1
Educational Level yrs	5.7	2.9	5.3	3.0
Simple Reaction Time ms	414	161	424	176
Choice Reaction Time ms	641	186	712	199
Sway cm/sec Eyes Open	1.23	0.54	1.31	0.53
Eyes Closed	1.70	0.60	1.74	0.72
Glabellar Tap Right	15.5	2.1	15.4	1.7
Left	15.3	2.1	15.3	2.1
Supraorbital Right	13.8	2.0	14.5	2.1
Left	14.0	2.3	13.8	2.0
Story 1 Immediate	8.1	4.2	7.4	4.6
Delayed	6.7	4.4	6.0	4.6
Story 2 Immediate	8.2	4.2	7.2	4.3
Delayed	7.1	4.3	5.2	4.2
Picture Completion	25.0	8.0	24.2	8.5
Vocabulary	9.5	5.4	8.1	6.1
Culture Fair A	25.0	7.6	24.4	8.9
Digit Symbol	40.0	15.6	38.5	16.8
Color score	141	44	145.4	34.7
POMS	40.0	35.1	46.6	34.2
Pegboard	82.3	26.1	80.5	21.3
Trails A	57.3	34.9	56.2	36.0
Trails B	113.4	46.5	108.3	46.5
Finger Writing Right	7.0	12.4	5.3	5.7
Left	6.6	12.6	5.0	5.6
Information	7.6	5.4	7.4	5.2
Picture Completion	10.6	4.7	11.4	4.1
Similarities	11.9	6.8	12.2	6.6

than to reduce the difference between the unexposed and exposed and favor the null hypothesis.

DISCUSSION

This first large-scale examination of subjects exposed in their homes to chlordane as compared to unexposed subjects showed significant differences in both the neurophysiologic and the psychological realms, including mood states. Accompanying these differences were large and significant differences in symptom frequency and in respiratory, rheumatic, and cardiovascular disease symptoms. The most notable changes were slowing of reaction time and increase in the balance dysfunction as revealed by sway speed, together with a general reduction in cognitive function, perceptual motor speed, and immediate and delayed verbal recall. This pattern is similar to that noted in 10 individual patients referred for environmental chlordane exposure (see Chapter 4).

Chlordane is a chlorinated cyclodiene insecticide known as a neuropoison. Many of its signs and symptoms of poisoning resemble those produced by DDT (1, 2). One striking difference is the ability of chlordane to induce convulsions, as well as the

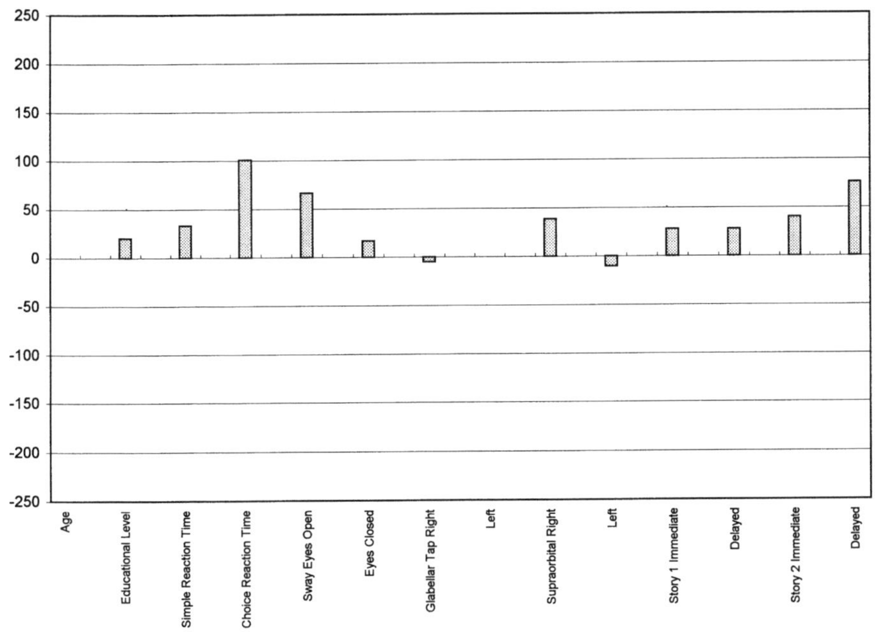

FIGURE 9.3a. Comparison of 59 children exposed to chlordane and 76 unexposed children by ANOVA. (All were tested in English.)

frequency of headache, nausea, vomiting, dizziness, and chronic jerking movements it produces. In this study the exposure appears to be from the air, the outgassing of chlordane from the wooden surfaces of apartments, and perhaps the soil. Analyses showed elevated chlordane levels in the blood as well as elevated levels on wipe samples and in the air of some of these apartments.

It is thought that the cyclodienes interact with the picrotoxin receptor in the nervous system, increasing the release of excitatory transmitters and interfering with the GABA neurotransmission system (1). The primary target appears to be those synapses that have the highest number of converging presynaptic elements so that the threshold for excitation is lowered, and there is an increase in the number and frequency of action potentials (1, 3). This is a kindling type of process that ''avalanches'' through the limbic system so that postsynaptic pathway responses are 10 to 100 times more intense than normal. In view of the likelihood that hyperresponsiveness occurs from an interference with inhibitory activity or from an increase of excitation (1, 4), it is strange that, aside from their symptoms, these subjects showed depression of function, particularly of basic responses such as balance and reaction time, trail making A and B, and Culture

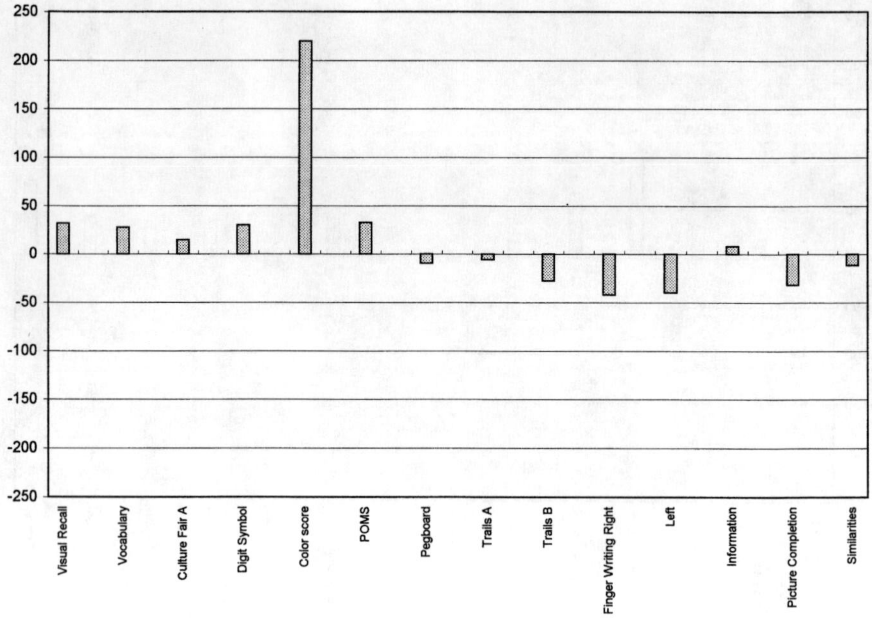

FIGURE 9.3b. Comparison of 59 children exposed to chlordane and 76 unexposed children by ANOVA. (All were tested in English.)

Fair, instead of showing excitation. They did show the psychological disorders that were previously associated with the exposure: anxiety, irritability, insomnia, and motor pathology.

It is tragic indeed that exposure is still occurring with these cyclodiene pesticides, which the National Research Council in 1982 (5) characterized as a hazard in any dose: "there is not a level of exposure of the cyclodiene termiticides below which there is no biological effect; therefore every effort should be made to minimize exposure." Also, in 1986 the EPA found that chlordane was the most frequently misused or misapplied of the termiticides (6). As of 1987, under an agreement with the EPA, Velsicol ceased to sell chlordane for consumer use in the United States although it still was licensed to export it. It is peculiar, therefore, that in 1988 the EPA allowed chlordane to be applied at 150 residences across the United States and decided that air monitoring would be done for two years to detect whether there were levels of chlordane in the air. The Houston experience presented here makes it regrettable that chlordane has been applied to at least 30 million homes in the United States. It accounted for 11% of calls about pesticides to poison control centers in Minnesota in 1991 (7).

References

1. Murphy SD: Toxic effects of pesticides. In: *Casarett and Doull's Toxicology* (3rd ed.), CD Klaassen, MO Amdur, and J Doull (eds.). New York: Macmillan Co., 1986.
2. Singer R: *Neurotoxicity Guidebook.* New York: Van Nostrand Reinhold, 1990.
3. Matsumura F and Tanaka K: The molecular basis of neurotoxicity actions of cyclodiene-type insecticides. In: *Cellular and Molecular Neurotoxicology.* New York: Raven Press, 1984.
4. Ecobichon D and Joy R: *Pesticides and Neurological Diseases* (2nd ed.). Boca Raton, FL: CRC Press, 1992.
5. National Research Council: *An Assessment of the Health Risks of Seven Pesticides Used for Termite Control.* Washington, D.C.: National Academy Press, 1982.
6. EPA: Restricted use classification of pesticides used for subterranean termite control and consumer advisory sheet distribution; criteria and procedures, August 21, 1986.
7. Olson DK, Sax L, Gunderson P, and Storis L: Pesticide poisoning surveillance through regional poison control centers. *Am J Public Health* 1991;81:750–753.

10

Visual and Neurobehavioral Impairment Associated with Polychlorinated Biphenyls (PCBs)

Residents of a small community surrounding a pumping station on a natural gas pipeline in Tennessee had noted cancers, skin rashes, tumors, irritability, and difficulty with recall and concentration that they associated with PCBs, which comprised 50% of the pydrol used as pumping fluid. We tested (together) and compared the neurobehavioral performance of 98 persons exposed to PCB-contaminated water and soil, intermixed with 58 unexposed people.

All subjects had visual, balance, blink, and reaction time measured and completed a neurobehavioral test battery, a profile of mood states (POMS), and extensive questionnaires for symptoms, chemical exposures, and medical history. The 98 exposed adults were three years older than 58 unexposed and had 2 years less schooling vs. unexposed. Compared to unexposed subjects, the exposed had significantly slower simple and choice reaction times; balance measured as sway speed was significantly faster with eyes closed and open. Color discrimination and contrast sensitivity scores were significantly different, and many exposed subjects had reduced visual fields with constriction or loss in four quadrants. Culture Fair, digit symbol, and vocabulary scores were significantly lower for the exposed, as was verbal recall. Perceptual motor speed was impaired, as peg placement in a pegboard and trail making A and B took longer; and embedded memory scores on information, picture completion, and similarities were lower. POMS scores were significantly elevated. In children the significant differences were elevated color scores on the right and elevated POMS scores, particularly confusion. No confounding factors or other attributable causes were found, and with this design tester bias was minimal. Residential exposure to PCBs since the mid-1950s was associated with severe visual defects and impairment of neurophysiologic and neuropsychologic function. These findings are explained by prolonged exposure to PCBs. Children's changes, which are less apparent than adults', now are attributed to proportionately more reserve, that is, larger populations of uncommitted neurons, in children.

THE EXPOSURE

Marr's Branch drains into the Buffalo River, a tributary of the Tennessee River. Natural gas pipeline pumping station #79 of the Tennessee Gas Pipeline Company (TGPC), owned by Tenneco, put the community of Lobelville, Tennessee on the map in 1951 (Figure 10.1). The reciprocating and turbine pumps that push the natural gas north across Tennessee from the pipeline's origin in the gas fields of Texas were lubricated with pydrol containing 50% polychlorinated biphenyls, PCBs. Pydrol was used as pump lubricant until the mid-1970s. One neighbor, a swine farmer, was reimbursed for the deaths of 18 hogs in 1966 near a watering hole on a drainage ditch from the pumping

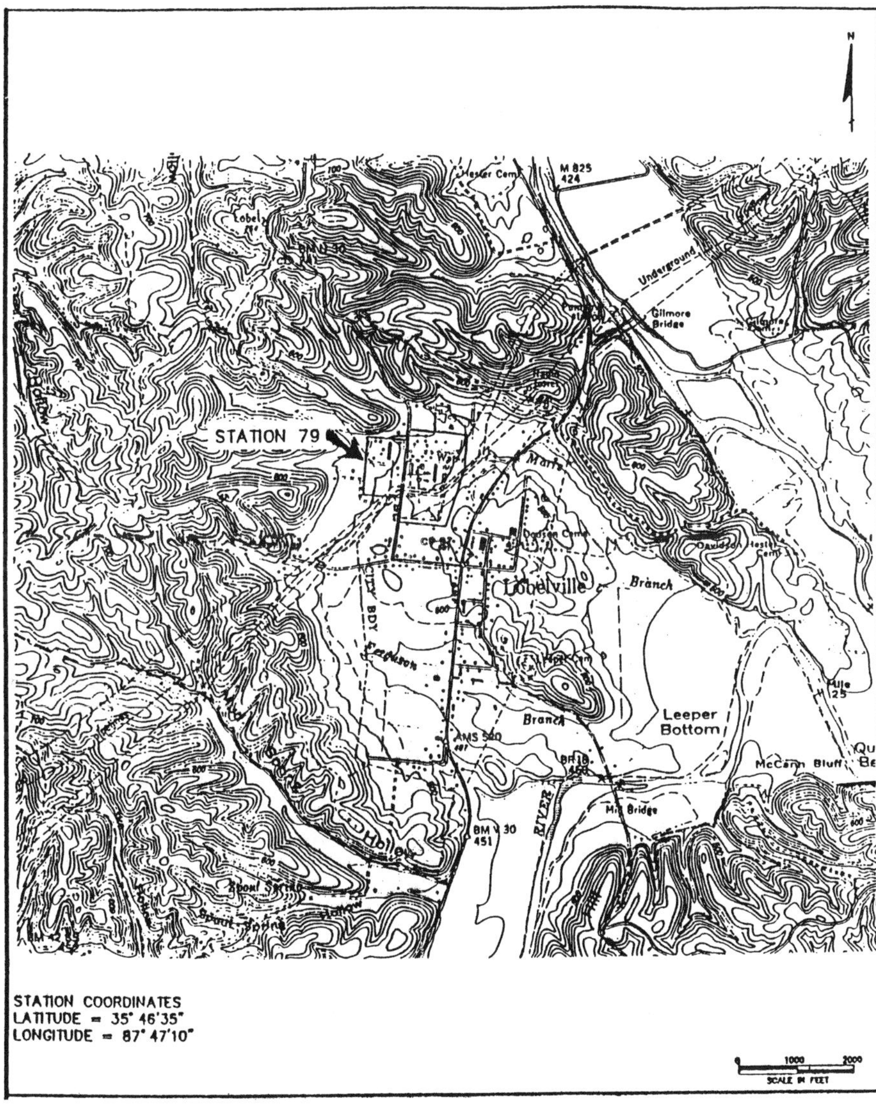

FIGURE 10.1. Lobelville, Tennessee and environs. *Source:* USGS topographic quadrangle, Lobelville, TN (1950, photo revised 1968).

plant. By 1990 one Marr's Branch neighbor had severely diminished recall memory, diminishing eyesight, rashes, tumors, and general ill health. School failures were noted among adolescents. Investigation showed that PCBs were in farmland, pumping station drainages, Marr's Branch, and the Buffalo River, and in the blood of retired TGPC workers and neighbors at or above 80 ppb. Neurobehavioral and pulmonary testing of two exposed neighbors in August 1994 showed impairment for balance, blink reaction time, vision, recall, and depression and high frequencies of 35 symptoms encompassing mucous membrane irritation, the respiratory tract, nausea, headache, and other general ill feeling, and sleep, thought, memory, and mood disorder symptoms. Following those findings, this pilot study compared 98 Lobelville exposed residents with 36 residents of Columbia–Springhill, Tennessee about 100 km to the east and outside of the Buffalo River drainage area, and 32 residents of Hurricane Mills 24 km to the north, beyond the Buffalo River and the pipeline.

TESTING OF SUBJECTS

Methods

Fifty-four women, 44 men, and 24 children in the exposed group were compared to 30 women, 28 men, and 10 children who were not exposed at the PCB site. The standard battery of tests was given as described in Chapter 3. Visual fields in the mode of threshold testing with a Biorad automated perimeter recording to a computer were mapped for the central 30° of right and left eyes of all adults and children over 8 years. Other tests were administered in the same manner as in previous groups (Chapters 5–9).

Results

Ages of adult exposed and unexposed subjects matched, but educational attainment was significantly greater in unexposed vs. exposed. The exposed subjects were impaired compared to unexposed for all tests in all domains (Table 10.1a, b, Figures 10.2a, b) except blink on the left (BRL R-1) and grip strength on the left in men. Even vocabulary and the embedded memory tests (information, picture completion, and similarities), which frequently are unaffected by chemical exposures, were impaired. Of most importance, balance (minimum value of three trials) was impaired, both with eyes open and with eyes closed. Similarly, simple and choice reaction times were greatly prolonged. Covariance analysis, a regression method that adjusts for differences in age and other factors such as educational level and height when necessary, was applied to further test the differences in mean values. This method also distinguishes between exposure differences that are fixed across the age range, so that exposed subjects plot parallel to unexposed from 17 to 80 years of age, with increased (i.e., divergent) cumulative exposure differences with age. As seen in Table 10.2, balance measured with eyes open in exposed was parallel to that of unexposed, whereas balance with eyes closed increased with age; and these equations explained 27.5% and 18.5% of the variance, respectively. Simple reaction time was parallel, but choice reaction time diverged, with r^2 of 16.3% and 25.6%, respectively. Supraorbital BRL R-1 right and left were parallel, with r^2 of 16.8% and 7.5%. Color discrimination (4th power) diverged with r^2 of 24.5%.

Culture Fair A, square root of digit symbol ($\sqrt{ds}$), and vocabulary all diverged, with r^2 of 43.4%, 52.2%, and 48.3%, respectively. Story recall immediate and delayed

TABLE 10.1a Comparison by analysis of variance with *p* values

	Exposed		Unexposed		
	98		58		
	Mean	Sd	Mean	Sd	*p*
Age yrs	39.5	14.7	34.3	13.5	.029
Educational Level yrs	10.9	1.9	12.9	2.3	.0001
Simple Reaction Time ms	409	202	278	71	.0001*
Choice Reaction Time ms	613	177	478	81	.0001*
Balance Sway Speed cm/sec					
Eyes Open	0.89	0.42	0.69	0.15	.001*
Eyes Closed	1.52	1.03	1.06	0.3	.001*
Blink Reflex Latency					
R-1 ms Right	11.8	1.50	11.0	1.6	.006*
Left	11.4	1.4	11.4	1.9	.918
Hearing Losses Both Ears	367	216	228	109	.002*
Color Score Right	13.1	2.0	11.6	1.2	.0001*
Left	13.0	2.1	11.5	1.3	.0001*
Contrast Sensitivity					
Right	24.9	10.3	30.7	6.4	.011*
Left	27.7	10.6	31.2	6.4	.006*
Visual Performance Right	1135	394	1386	251	.0001*
Left	1133	390	1378	274	.0001*
Culture Fair A	23.4	7.9	31.0	6.4	.0001*
Digit Symbol	46.5	15.6	61.8	12.7	.0001*
Vocabulary	12.9	6.3	21.0	8.2	.0001*
Grip Strength					
Women Right	28.7	6.6	33.5	6.4	.002*
Left	26.4	5.7	30.3	6.6	.005*
Men Right	49.9	9.2	55.0	8.5	.02*
Left	47.8	12.4	51.2	8.3	.201
Story 1 Immediate	7.0	3.7	11.5	4.1	.0001*
Delayed	5.0	3.7	9.7	4.5	.0001*
Story 2 Immediate	8.0	4.2	11.6	3.7	.0001*
Delayed	4.8	4.0	9.9	4.1	.0001*
Pegboard	75.1	21.4	64.6	10.1	.0006*
Trails A	43.1	24.1	30.5	12.1	.003*
Trails B	98.7	42.1	62.3	29.6	.0001*
Finger Writing Right	5.2	4.1	3.2	3.7	.003*
Left	4.4	4.1	3.1	3.7	.038*
Information	11.6	5.1	17.0	5.3	.0001*
Picture Completion	11.9	3.8	14.7	2.2	.0001*
Similarities	13.5	6.3	20.0	5.1	.0001*

* Statistically significant

TABLE 10.1b Profile of mood states scores and component scores, means, standard deviations, and significance (*p* values)

	Exposed 98		Unexposed 58		
	Mean	Sd	Mean	Sd	*p*
POMS Score	72.6	38.9	22.1	25.0	.0001*
Tension	18.5	7.3	8.9	4.6	.0001*
Depression	20.7	13.4	7.9	7.1	.0001*
Anger	15.9	10.4	7.7	6.5	.0001*
Vigor	11.6	6.2	17.0	6.2	.0001*
Fatigue	15.7	6.2	8.3	5.6	.0001*
Confusion	13.4	5.3	6.4	3.6	.0001*

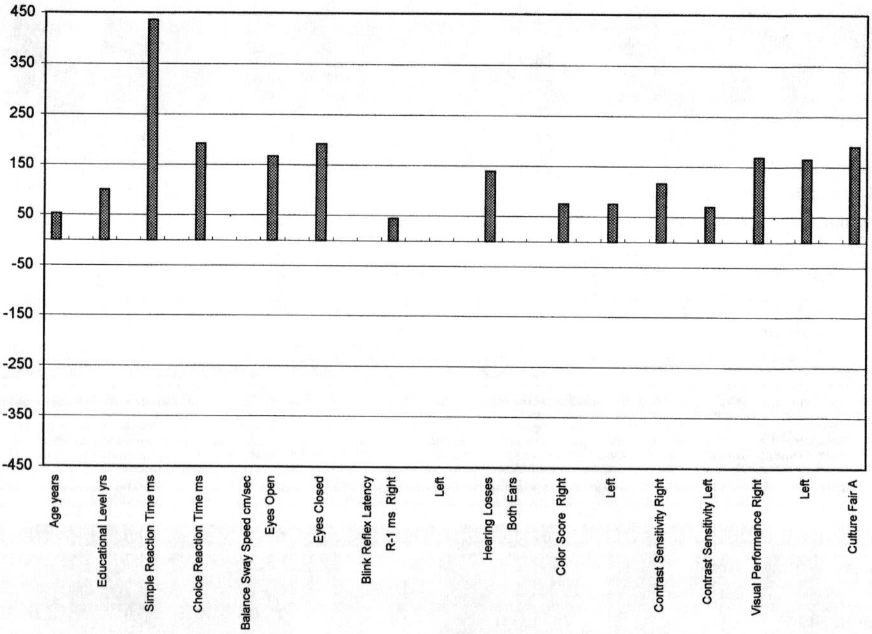

FIGURE 10.2a. Comparisons of 98 PCB-exposed adults and 58 unexposed adults by ANOVA. Hatched bars are statistically significant.

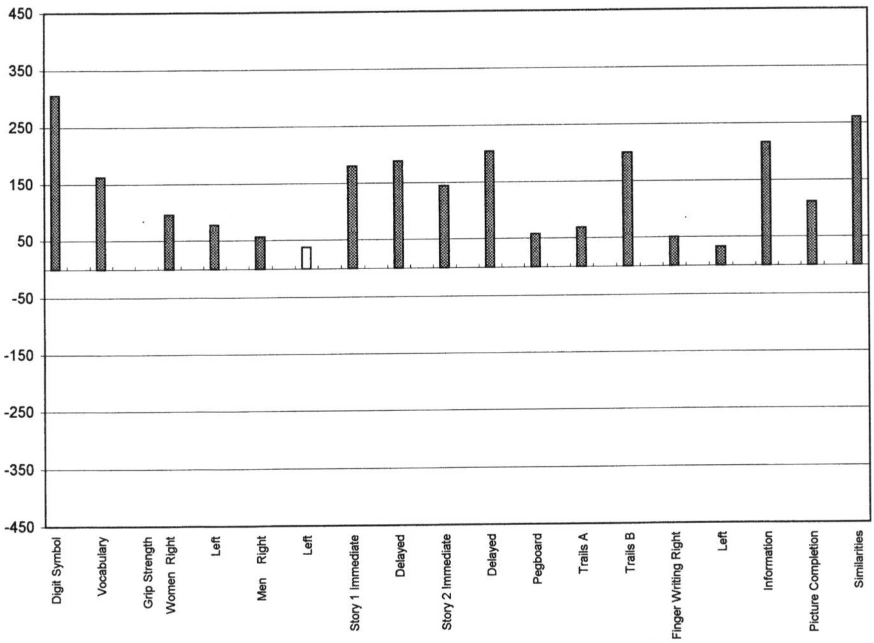

FIGURE 10.2b. Comparisons of 98 PCB-exposed adults and 58 unexposed adults by ANOVA. Hatched bars are statistically significant.

both diverged, with r^2 of 28.1% and 29.4%. Information[1.5] was flat, in that exposed and unexposed were not different; r^2 was 46.5%. Picture completion and similarities were both parallel, with r^2 of 26.7% and 24.8%. The inverse of peg placement was parallel in women with r^2 of 31.1% and in men with r^2 of 18.9%. The ln trail making A diverged with r^2 of 23.2%, and the ln trail making B was parallel with r^2 of 33.8%.

There were visual field abnormalities in 85% of adults; 19% had constricted fields, 13% had losses in four quadrants, 19% had losses in two or three quadrants, and 32% had minor (i.e., one quadrant) defects (scotomata) (Figure 10.3a). Only 26% of the Tennessee *unexposed* had abnormal visual fields; all defects were minor except one in a 75-year-old man (Figure 10.3b). Quantified visual performance in the six rings at equal distances outward from the focal spot corresponding to the macula confirmed these differences in prevalences.

The 35 symptom frequencies assessed on the 11-point scale were statistically significantly higher for exposed subjects (Table 10.3) with the single exception of decreased alcohol tolerance, which is of dubious value as most subjects report no drinking. Even common frequent complaints such as headache, lightheadedness, irritability, and mood

TABLE 10.2 Covariance analysis for 96 exposed adults in Lobelville, TN

	Coefficient	SE	*p* Value	Age Interpretation	r^2
ln Balance Eyes Open	−0.7897	0.313	.0001	Parallel	27.5
Eyes Closed	−2.297	0.904	.0001	Diverge	18.5
ln Simple Reaction Time	0.346	0.062	.001	Parallel	16.3
ln Choice Reaction Time	0.209	0.039	.001	Diverge	25.6
Supraorbital Right	1.287	0.269	.138	Parallel	16.8
Left	0.018	0.814	.921	Parallel	7.5
Clrm[4] (Color)	$2.25e^{-10}$	$2.06e^{-9}$	.0001	Diverge	24.5
Culture Fair A	16.159	8.363	.0001	Diverge	43.4
Digit Symbol score	0.049	1.154	.0001	Diverge	52.2
Vocabulary	10.546	7.691	.0002	Diverge	48.3
Stories Immediate	4.591	4.043	.0001	Diverge	28.1
Delayed	6.628	4.158	.0001	Diverge	29.4
Information[1.5]	6.413	32.636	.0001	Flat	46.5
Picture Completion[1.5]	143.132	99.334	.0002	Parallel	26.7
Similarities[2]	50.244	80.255	.0001	Parallel	24.8
1/peg Males	0.0044	0.0033	.037	Parallel	18.9
Females	0.012	0.006	.01	Parallel	31.1
ln Trails A	1.163	0.468	.0001	Diverge	23.2
ln Trails B	1.044	0.732	.0016	Parallel	33.8

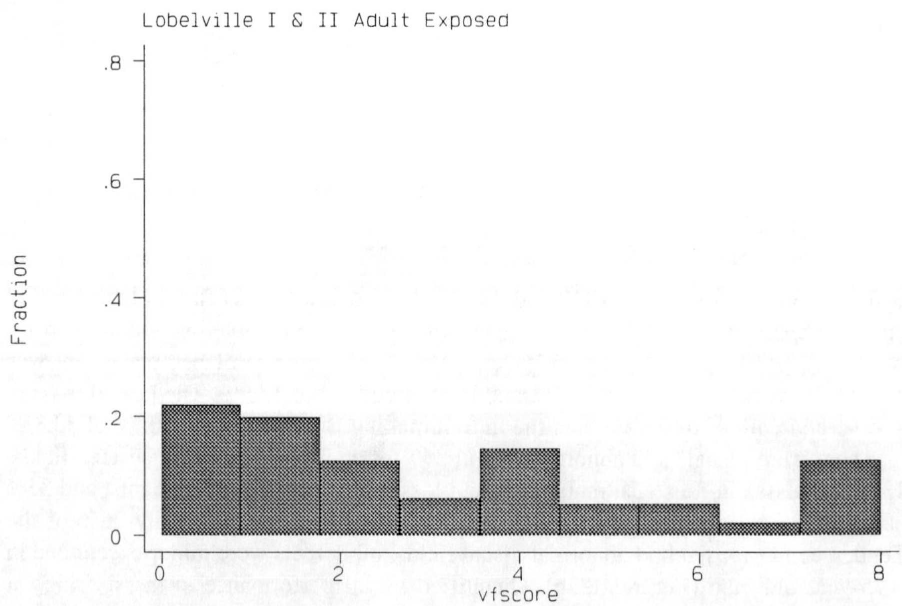

FIGURE 10.3a. Visual field score, adult exposed.

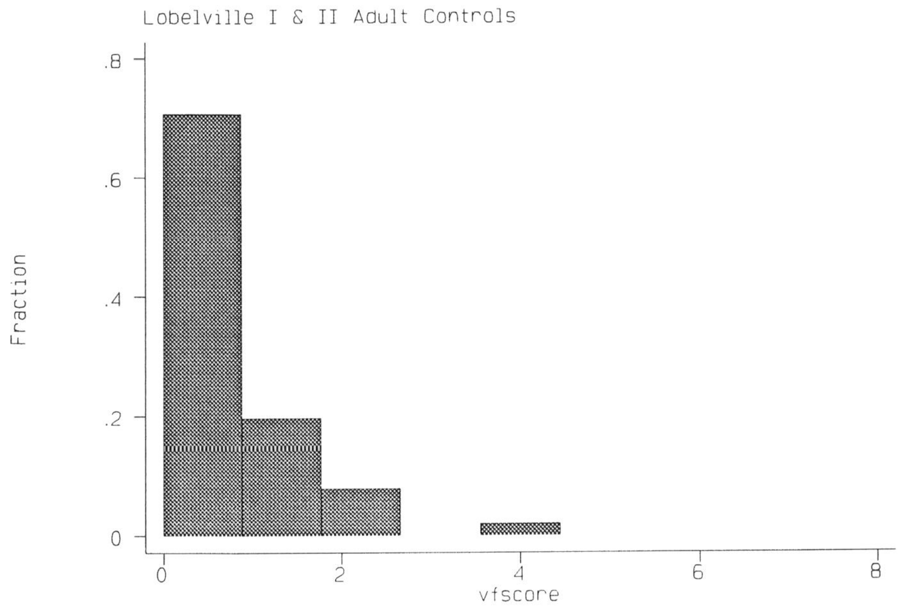

FIGURE 10.3b. Visual field score, adult controls.

swings were two to three times more frequent in exposed subjects. The malingerer symptoms were almost never found in both groups, below a frequency of 2. The exposed children had fewer, only nine, differences from unexposed and lower frequencies (Table 10.4). Seven of ten rheumatic and lupus erythematosus symptoms were significantly more frequent in the exposed group than the unexposed, and the differences were large (Table 10.5).

The respiratory questionnaire showed even greater differences in prevalence, with 62% of exposed producing phlegm vs. 12% unexposed, 80% short of breath on stairs vs. 31%, and 50% with wheezing vs. 8% (Table 10.6). When standard pulmonary functions were expressed as percentage of predicted, which adjusted for age, height, and sex, exposed subjects showed no significant differences from unexposed (Table 10.7).

The children studied at Lobelville (Figures 10.4a, b) were virtually identical to their Tennessee unexposed controls although younger and less educated by a year.

DISCUSSION

The severity of the impact of ''PCBs'' on brain function across the test battery exceeds the effects of chemicals on the brain in most of the patients of Chapter 4 and the other chemically exposed populations (Chapters 5–9, 11–14). It most resembles the effects of hydrogen sulfide exposure from the refinery explosion and fire (Chapter 5). As the PCB exposure began 40 years ago, the subjects tested were born of parents exposed before the children's conception and had been exposed for their entire lives. Thus, the unexpected low years of education may reflect inhibited or misdirected development of the brain. The lifetime duration of exposure makes poor brain development a possible explanation for the low educational achievement of these adults. Also the retina-optic

TABLE 10.3 Symptom frequencies in adults

	Exposed (98)		Unexposed (58)		
	Mean	Sd	Mean	Sd	*p*
Skin itching	6.9	3.3	3.2	2.5	.0001*
Fingernail changes	4.0	3.1	1.5	1.3	.0001*
Chest tightness	5.0	3.2	2.0	1.5	.001*
Palpitations	4.4	3.1	2.3	2.0	.0001*
Burning in chest	4.7	3.3	1.9	1.6	.0001*
Shortness of breath	5.6	3.3	3.1	2.0	.0001*
Dry cough	4.9	3.1	2.5	1.8	.0001*
Cough with mucus	5.2	3.2	2.6	1.9	.0001*
Cough with blood	1.8	1.7	1.1	.6	.002*
Dry mouth	6.0	3.1	3.1	2.5	.0001*
Throat irritation	4.7	3.1	2.8	1.9	.0001*
Eye irritation	5.6	3.2	2.4	2.1	.0001*
Reduced sense of smell	3.6	3.1	2.1	2.0	.0012*
Headache	6.8	3.2	4.1	2.4	.0001*
Nausea	4.6	3.0	2.5	1.7	.0001*
Dizziness	5.3	2.9	2.1	1.6	.0001*
Lightheadedness	5.7	3.2	5.8	4.7	.0001*
Exhilaration	2.6	2.6	1.8	1.5	.042*
Loss of balance	4.7	3.0	1.9	1.2	.0001*
Loss of consciousness	1.9	1.9	1.2	0.4	.002*
Extreme fatigue	7.4	3.2	3.1	2.3	.0001*
Somnolence	5.6	3.7	2.5	2.2	.0001*
Insomnia					
Cannot fall asleep	5.0	3.5	2.6	2.5	.0001*
Wake frequently	5.7	3.6	2.7	2.5	.0001*
Sleep few hours	4.9	3.4	2.6	2.5	.0001*
Irritability	7.4	3.0	3.7	2.4	.0001*
Loss of concentration	7.3	3.1	3.2	2.1	.0001*
Recent memory loss	7.2	3.4	3.2	2.6	.0001*
Remote memory loss	5.9	3.7	2.4	2.2	.0001*
Mood swings	6.5	3.5	2.4	2.1	.0001*
Loss of libido	5.8	3.7	3.8	3.3	.001*
Decreased alcohol tolerance	2.2	2.2	2.2	1.8	.993
Indigestion	6.3	3.3	2.8	2.2	.0001*
Loss of appetite	4.1	2.8	2.4	1.9	.0001*
Swollen stomach	4.8	3.5	2.8	2.5	.0003*
Tingling navel	1.6	1.3	1.2	.8	.026
Itching gums	1.7	1.5	1.2	.5	.006

* Statistically significant.

TABLE 10.4 Children's symptom frequencies

	Exposed		Unexposed		
	24		10		
	Mean	Sd	Mean	Sd	*p*
Skin itching	5.1	3.4	2.0	1.9	.011*
Fingernail changes	2.1	2.5	1.2	0.4	.259
Chest tightness	2.3	2.3	1.8	1.9	.549
Palpitations	1.8	1.5	1.1	0.3	.183
Burning in chest	1.8	1.7	1.6	1.3	.697
Shortness of breath	3.6	3.2	1.7	0.8	.094
Dry cough	3.3	2.2	2.5	1.4	.30
Cough with mucus	2.8	2.7	2.0	0.9	.408
Cough with blood	1.3	0.7	1.0	0.9	.296
Dry mouth	4.4	3.4	2.1	1.0	.043*
Throat irritation	3.9	2.4	1.8	1.0	.012*
Eye irritation	4.5	3.4	2.3	2.0	.067
Reduced sense of smell	1.8	1.1	1.7	1.6	.844
Headache	6.5	3.2	3.0	1.6	.003*
Nausea	4.0	3.2	1.8	1.6	.049*
Dizziness	4.1	3.1	1.6	1.0	.019*
Lightheadedness	3.5	3.0	1.2	0.4	.026*
Exhilaration	3.0	2.9	1.6	1.3	.149
Loss of balance	2.6	2.4	1.6	1.0	.199
Loss of consciousness	1.4	1.1	1.1	0.3	.445
Extreme fatigue	4.2	3.2	1.9	1.3	.040*
Somnolence	3.0	2.4	1.7	1.6	.111
Insomnia					
Cannot fall asleep	2.0	1.5	2.1	1.1	.913
Wake frequently	3.0	2.8	1.8	1.2	.197
Sleep few hours	2.1	1.7	1.3	0.5	.139
Irritability	4.2	2.9	2.5	2.7	.130
Loss of concentration	6.4	3.3	3.9	2.6	.043*
Recent memory loss	3.9	3.0	2.4	1.7	.145
Remote memory loss	3.4	3.0	1.6	0.8	.080
Mood swings	4.4	3.4	2.1	2.5	.066
Loss of libido	2.6	3.3	1.0	0.0	.169
Decreased alcohol tolerance	1.4	1.3	1.1	0.3	.510
Indigestion	2.4	2.0	2.7	3.3	.756
Loss of appetite	2.9	2.3	1.9	1.5	.227
Swollen stomach	1.8	1.7	1.5	1.3	.579
Tingling navel	1.5	1.6	1.0	0.0	.285
Itching gums	1.2	0.6	1.1	0.3	.588

* Statistically significant.

TABLE 10.5 Adults' percentage of rheumatism and disseminated lupus erythematosus questions answered yes (ARA criteria)

	Exposed (98)	Unexposed (58)	
	Mean	Mean	*p*
Immune	3.03	0	.183
Rheumatism	37.4	12.1	.0006*
Numb fingers	67.7	31.0	.0001*
Mouth sores	33.3	1.7	.0001*
Anemia	32.3	15.5	.021*
Rash on cheeks	11.1	0	.008*
Sun rash	29.3	12.1	.0130*
Pleuritic pain	41.4	3.4	.0001*
Protein in urine	11.1	12.1	.857
Hair loss	36.4	0.08	
Seizures	0	0	

* Statistically significant.

TABLE 10.6 Prevalences of respiratory symptoms in exposed and referent subjects compared by analysis of variance with significant *p* values*

Group:	Exposed	Referent	*p*
Phlegm (prevalence = p)	0.62	0.12	0.0001*
Chronic bronchitis by history score	2.1	1.4	0.049*
Shortness of breath			
At rest p	0.52	0.08	0.0001*
Walking p	0.66	0.04	0.0001*
Climbing stairs p	0.80	0.31	0.0001*
Wheezing p	0.50	0.08	0.0002*
Wheezing, short of breath p	0.36	0.12	0.234

* Statistically significant.

TABLE 10.7 Pulmonary function tests expressed as percentage of predicted

	Exposed		Referents		
	Mean	Sd	Mean	Sd	*p* Values
Adults					
FVC	97.0	11.8	93.1	12.8	0.196
FEV_1	91.4	16.4	89.2	14.5	0.574
FEF_{25-75}	96.9	36.6	101.5	36.1	0.612
FEF_{75-85}	80.0	43.0	77.9	35.2	0.83
FEF_1/FVC	76.9	8.9	78.4	5.7	0.442
Children					
FVC	86.8	14.5	87.3	14.7	0.945
FEV_1	79.7	20.0	75.9	17.1	0.648
FEF_{25-75}	79.5	39.6	66.5	26.7	0.392
FEF_{75-85}	86.8	70.7	58.9	38.1	0.282

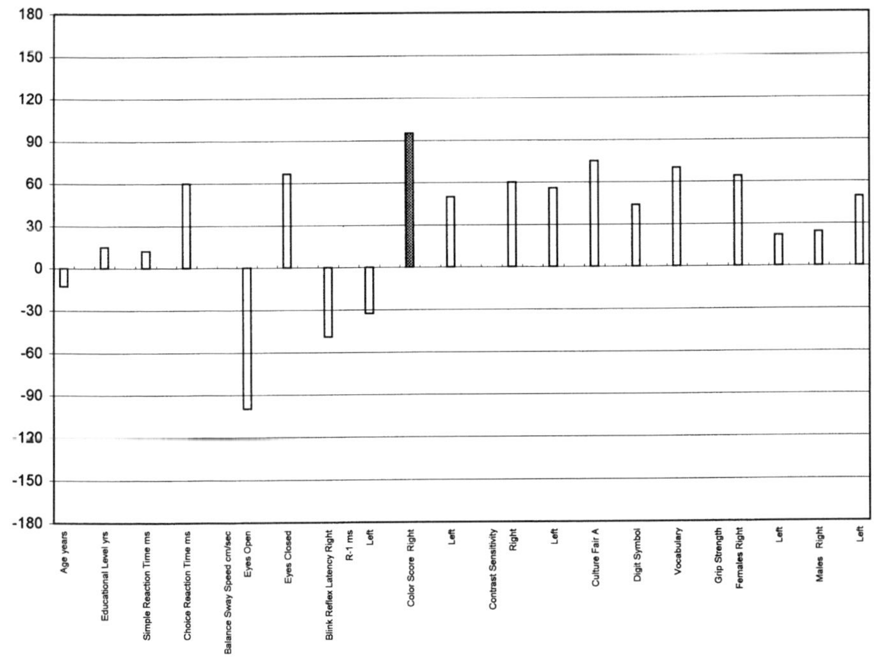

FIGURE 10.4a. Comparison of 24 PCB-exposed children and 10 unexposed children by ANOVA. Hatched bars are statistically significant.

cortex apparatus and the trigeminal-pons-facial nerve apparatus may behave discretely compared to the multi-brain center interactive functions governing balance, reaction, recall, and cognition.

The children's measurements resembled those from other exposed children groups in showing no measured effects from chemicals even when the matched adults, their parents, were impaired. One explanation, that children have uncommitted neurons in reserve that permit compensation for chemically damaged ones, should have proved advantageous for those in this population studied in early adulthood and thus seems contradicted. Another possibility is that these children had been less exposed than their parents, as PCB use at TGPC #79 pumping station reputedly ceased before they were conceived. Thus, we may have a chemically induced generational effect. The comparison of this Tennessee reference group to the aging composite, which is in effect a national unexposed "control" group (Chapter 11), also showed no difference. In fact, these Tennessee unexposed scores on some tests exceeded the national ones, slightly. Thus, the severity of impairment of the PCB-exposed subjects was unprecedented.

There have been two exceptions to the generalization that adverse effects were not

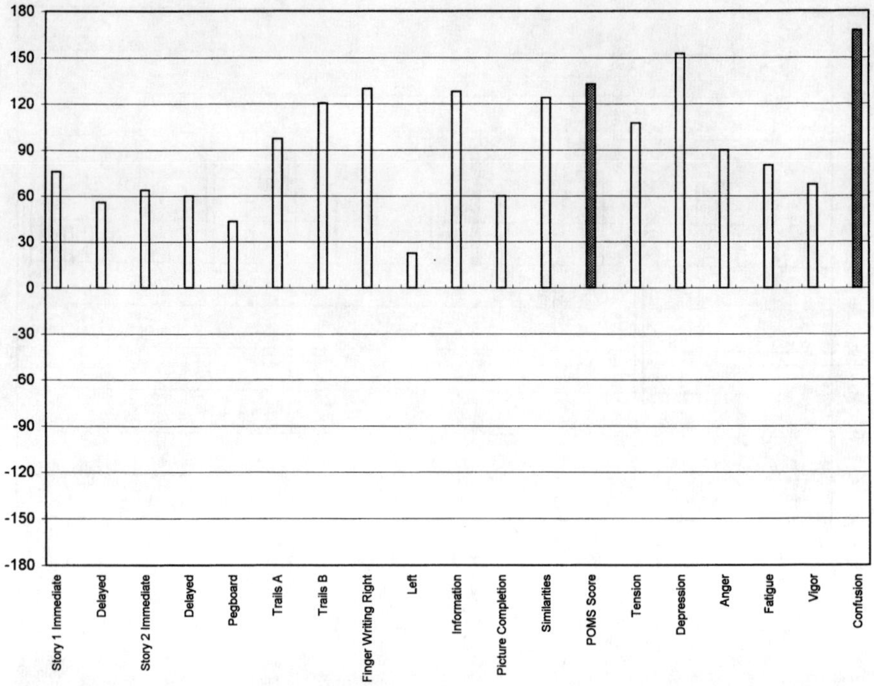

FIGURE 10.4b. Comparison of 24 PCB-exposed children and 10 unexposed children by ANOVA. Hatched bars are statistically significant.

shown in children. Exception one was that, in these Lobelville children, visual fields were abnormal, just as they were in the hydrogen sulfide–exposed Wilmington/Torrance group (see Chapter 5), whose major exposure was acute for a duration of hours and then intermittent to lesser quantities of the chemical for a month. The second exception occurred at Phoenix (see Chapter 11), where children not only had slowed blink (BRL R-1), as did their parents and other adults, but had slowing of perceptual motor performance. When Phoenix children's performance was analyzed by covariance, which simultaneously adjusted for age, education, and other factors, the exposed group showed a gradient of increased loss with age. There were so few children studied in exposed and unexposed for Lobelville that covariance analysis was not done.

Compared to the Muscle Shoals population (Chapter 11), which was also studied for the effects of PCBs (1), this Lobelville population yielded a much cleaner attribution. A probable explanation is that the Muscle Shoals population had been exposed to volatile organic chemicals and trichloroethylene in quantity, in addition to PCBs, via contaminated well water. In addition, the interpretation for the Muscle Shoals population was more difficult because simple and choice reaction time, balance measured as sway eyes open and eyes closed, and the blink reflex latencies for R-1 were *the* abnormalities, together with affective domain measured with POMS. Compared to the local unexposed, the Muscle Shoals exposed had no other abnormalities in the cognitive, recall memory, and perceptual motor domains. Another problem in interpreting this study was an urban–rural difference accompanied by an ethnic difference. Both the exposed and the unexposed populations at Muscle Shoals were African-American and had no overlap in their psychological performance described herein with the Caucasian unexposed populations from Wickenburg, Springfield, and San Luis Obispo that serve as our overall reference standard. Thus, we are faced with the probability that the Muscle Shoals population selection, which was not a conscious (human) one but was one of nature's (industry's) experiments, was an exclusive phenomenon and is not yet verifiable by comparison with other unexposed groups. Also, as mentioned earlier, exposure in Muscle Shoals was to multiple chemicals, which certainly provides an explanation for abnormal blink reflex latency R-1, which can be plausibly attributed to TCE. This is a striking difference vs. the Lobelville PCB-exposed population, who had no TCE exposure and in whom BRL R-1 was typical of unexposed subjects and thus probably normal.

PCBs cause "Yusho," which is a poisoning identified by acne-like lesions and, as the Japanese first described, constitutional symptoms, observed after an outbreak in 1968 in the Kyushu prefect (2). This poisoning was due to contamination of rice oil with Kanechlor, used in heat transfer. Also, in the Yusho experience analyses showed that patients who died had large quantities of polychlorinated dibenzofurans, 1,000 times higher than in the comparison population in Japan. Also, large quantities of polychlorinated quaterphenyls were found in these people, and they persisted like the PCBs although the dibenzofurans (DCDFs) tended to disappear. By the early 1980s, neuroexaminations showed sensory deficits in the exposed, but apparently little attention was paid to the patients' central nervous systems (2, 3). The Japanese subjects in the Yusho epidemic studied at Kyushu showed general fatigue, weight loss, anorexia, headache, numbness, hypostesia, and neuralgic limbs, considered comparable by Hariyama to DDT poisoning (4). It is interesting that he listed neurological diseases first and showed motor conduction velocities that were occasionally low in the sural nerve although the mean values were not actually different from those of the unexposed. An additional 2,000 PCB-exposed subjects were studied in Taiwan, and by 1984 (5) that 1978 epidemic was characterized. Affected subjects had pigmentation of the skin, cheese-like discharge from the eyes, and many neurological manifestations, which for the first time extended from headache to dizziness and muscle pain as well as neuralgia. Nerve conduction velocities were prolonged, most pronounced in the sural nerve, but the central nervous system was ignored again. Thus, these data unequivocally showed central nervous system effects of PCBs for the first time.

The pumping station's use of PCBs in pydrol may be a special case for thermal conversion of PCBs to PCDF and dibenzodioxins (PCDD), both with up to 1,000 times the neurotoxicity of PCBs (6). Although the Arochlor 1260, 1254, and 1248 used are produced with relatively low contents of PCDF and PCDD, the friction of pumping could cause temperatures to reach 270°C along pump cylinders and fittings and convert quantities of PCBs to PCDFs and PCDDs. Without question the literature for over a decade has emphasized the greater (compared to PCBs) neurotoxicity of PCDF and PCDD, building on the Yusho experience, particularly over a number of years of follow-up (7). The neurobehavioral disorder of these Lobelville subjects resembled at that seen in firefighters who fought a blaze in a medical school transformer room where PCB-containing transformers heated and exploded (8). Such incidents continue to occur, and surveillance over some years is needed for a complete evaluation (9).

References

1. Kilburn KH and Warshaw RH: Neurobehavioral testing of subjects exposed residentially to groundwater contaminated from an aluminum die-casting plant and local referents. *J Toxicol Environ Health* 1993;39:483–496.
2. Okumura M: Past and current medical states of Yusho patients. *Am J Indust Med* 1984;5: 13–18.
3. Kashimoto T, Tung TC, and Ohi G: Role of polychlorinated dibenzofuran in Yusho (PCB) poisoning. *Arch Environ Health* 1981;36:321–326.
4. Hirayama C: Clinical aspects of PCB poisoning. In: *Poisoning and Pollution,* K. Higuchi (ed.). New York: Academic Press, 1976.
5. Chia LG and Chu FL: Neurological studies on polychlorinated biphenyl (PCB)–poisoned patients. *Am J Indust Med* 1984;5:117–126.
6. Hutzinger O, Choudhry GG, Chittim BG, and Johnston LE: Formation of polychlorinated dibenzofurans and dioxins during combustion, electrical equipment fires and PCB incineration. *Environ Health Perspect* 1985;60:3–9.
7. Reggiani G and Bruppacher R: Symptoms, signs and findings in humans exposed to PCBs and their derivatives. *Environ Health Perspect* 1985;60:225–232.
8. Kilburn KH, Warahaw RH, and Shields MG: Neurobehavioral dysfunction in firemen exposed to polychlorinated biphenyls (PCBs): possible improvement after detoxification. *Arch Environ Health* 1989;44:345–350.
9. Schecter A: Medical surveillance of exposed persons after exposure to PCBs, chlorinated dibenzodioxins and dibenzofurans after PCB transformer or capacitor incidents. *Environ Health Perspect* 1985;60:333–338.

11

Exposures to Chemical Mixtures Rich in Trichloroethylene (TCE): Residential and Occupational

ABSORPTION AND TOXICOLOGY OF TCE

The lung absorbs TCE quickly, as it does other anesthetic gases, because of a blood–gas partition coefficient of 9.12 at 37°C and a high lipid solubility (olive oil to gas coefficient of 960 at 37°C) (1). TCE's partition to brain is rapid (1), supporting its historical use as an anesthetic (2). Cranial neuropathies and cardiac arrhythmias that followed its use in inhalational anesthesia led to its being abandoned for this purpose. Surface anesthesia and intoxication were noted after industrial TCE exposure (3). Chronic TCE exposure of 31 printers reduced impulse transmission (nerve conduction) in sural and trigeminal nerves (4). Slowing of blink reflex latency was seen in Woburn, Massachusetts TCE-exposed neighbors of a Superfund site (5). Widespread adverse central nervous system effects were first shown from exposure in Tucson, Arizona, including delayed blink reflex latency, slowing of reaction time, and speeding of the speed of sway (balance), which were combined with cognitive, recall, and perceptual motor impairment and impaired trail making A and B (6). Irreversibility of these changes is likely based on stable findings in a subgroup of subjects restudied after one year. Also, antinuclear antibodies (7) and cardiac birth defects (8) were found after TCE exposure.

Four groups of residents environmentally exposed to TCE in water and/or air were investigated by using the methods described in Chapters 3 and 4. Each group of exposed subjects was compared to suitable unexposed groups. For three of them (Phoenix, Tinker, and Muscle Shoals), comparison was to regional unexposed subjects recruited through tax rolls or from associates of the exposed. In Tucson, a composite unexposed group (Chapters 5 and 12) was used, whose scores were statistically indistinguishable from those of the unexposed group for Phoenix.

STUDY 1: THE NORTHEASTERN PHOENIX, ARIZONA COMMUNITY

The objective was to determine whether neighborhood exposure to chemicals emitted from two microchip manufacturing plants had produced adverse human effects. For over two decades, residents west and south of these Motorola plants noted unpleasant, pungent, or nauseating odors within and outside their homes, which were associated with headache, nausea, extreme fatigue, difficulty in concentrating, irritability, dizziness, and impaired recall. Odors came directly from the plants, from sewers, and from a canal that went northwest from the plant through the neighborhood. Analysis of air and of water from preexisting water wells and new test wells (9) showed many halogenated volatile organic chemicals (HVOCs). The most common neurotoxic chemicals were trichloroethylene (TCE), 1,1,1-trichloroethane, tetrachloroethylene, and vinyl chloride. In addition, there were other di- and trichloroethanes, several chlorinated benzenes, carbon tetrachloride, and several metals including arsenic (9).

Reasons for Inconclusive Past Studies

Past efforts to quantify risks for neurotoxicity, cancer, and birth defects from chemicals often have been inconclusive. Thus, tests for the neurotoxic effects of occupational exposures to chemicals rarely have been applied to chemically exposed neighborhood residents (10–15). Cancers, including leukemia, are reputed to be excessive based on neighborhood clusters (14, 15), as are birth defects (8, 11), but their small numbers have yielded only borderline statistical significance. The problem of assessing differences in infrequent events in small populations is irresolvable. Another approach has been to compare prevalences of symptoms or of diseases, which have only approached statistical significance. Thus, questionnaires for medical disorders and for complaints such as foul odors, headache, and fatigue have been used (10, 13), but they have been criticized for recall and other bias. So much concern and community pressure (12, 13) are generally needed to get to this stage that only rarely has objective testing followed (5, 6).

Development of This Study

Some participants in this study had sued Motorola. Others were studied because they had not become clients. The local unexposed group lived in Phoenix but away from this zone and from other known chemical exposures. Because the complaints of the pilot subjects suggested impairment of the central nervous system and the chemicals were known neurotoxins (13, 15, 16), neurophysiological and neuropsychological testing were done (6, 17).

This study developed a set of interrelated objectives that emerged in stepwise fashion as data accrued and were examined. The objective of the *first phase* was to determine whether neurobehavioral function of persons who had lived as neighbors to microchip manufacturing (exposure-zone subjects) differed from that of an unexposed reference group.

After neurobehavioral impairments were found in exposure-zone subjects (EZS), the *second phase* was to determine whether such impairment was generalized to Phoenix. Was it an ambient air pollution or another urban effect? What was found was that Phoenix subjects away from this site and other known sources of chemical contamination were nearly the same as regional unexposed and were distinct from the exposure-zone subjects.

The *third phase* addressed the issue of subjects' legal status as plaintiffs in a civil action. It was intended to answer the question of how nonplaintiffs did in the exposure-zone function. Were they more like plaintiffs or like reference subjects? This led to our mapping each EZ subject's location (thus distance) from Motorola plants. They were functionally like exposed clients. The defining variable was distance, as most of them were farther away and were somewhat less functionally impaired than the plaintiffs or clients. No other factors were found.

The *fourth phase* was to determine whether the duration of residence in the exposure-zone predicted impairment—although those subjects exposed after 1983 (exposed from 1983 to 1993) were less impaired than those exposed within the interval from 1957 to 1993.

The *fifth phase* extended the exposure-zone question of phase one to children. Children in the exposure zone were only minimally impaired compared to children from the reference group.

People Investigated

The cohort comparison design had 294 exposure zone (EZ) subjects compared to 156 regional unexposed and 67 Phoenix unexposed who lived away from the plume (Figure 11.1). The 58 nonclient EZS were neighbors of the 236 plaintiffs in lawsuits against Motorola. All were between the ages of 17 and 83 years and had lived in those areas for 5 to 25 years. The regional unexposed were from Wickenburg, Arizona and had been recruited from voter registration rolls to match Phoenix exposed subjects for sex, age, and years of educational attainment (highest school grade completed). There was neither current nor historical evidence of chemical contamination of air or water in Wickenburg. The 67 Phoenix reference subjects were recruited as associates of the EZ subjects who had never resided near the Motorola plants or on another known toxic chemical plume. Regional reference subjects were picked at random from voter registration rolls and contacted by telephone to ascertain if they met the matching criteria, were free of chemical exposure, and were willing to be tested. Nonclients and reference subjects were reimbursed for time and mileage. During the testing, examiners were blinded as to subjects' exposure status in Phoenix. However, the Wickenburg unexposed subjects' status was known to the testers. All subjects gave informed consent, and the protocol was approved by the Human Studies Research Committee of the University of Southern California School of Medicine.

Exposure Estimates

Exposure estimates were based on the known groundwater plume of halogenated volatile organic chemicals (HVOCs), TCE, trichloroethane (TCA), 1,1- and 1,2-dichloroethylene (1,1-DCE, 1,2-DCE), tetrachloroethylene (PCE), and vinyl chloride (VC). Their concentrations were measured during an Arizona Department of Environmental Quality sweep sampling in October to December 1992, which included quarterly or semiannual sampling programs for individual source facilities (9). If more than one value was available from a well during this quarter, the highest one was used in contour mapping of the alluvial plume, using 130 samples. Concentrations of TCE varied from less than 0.2 to >10,000 ppb, TCA from <0.2 to 260,000 ppb, 1,1-DCE from <0.2 to 6,900

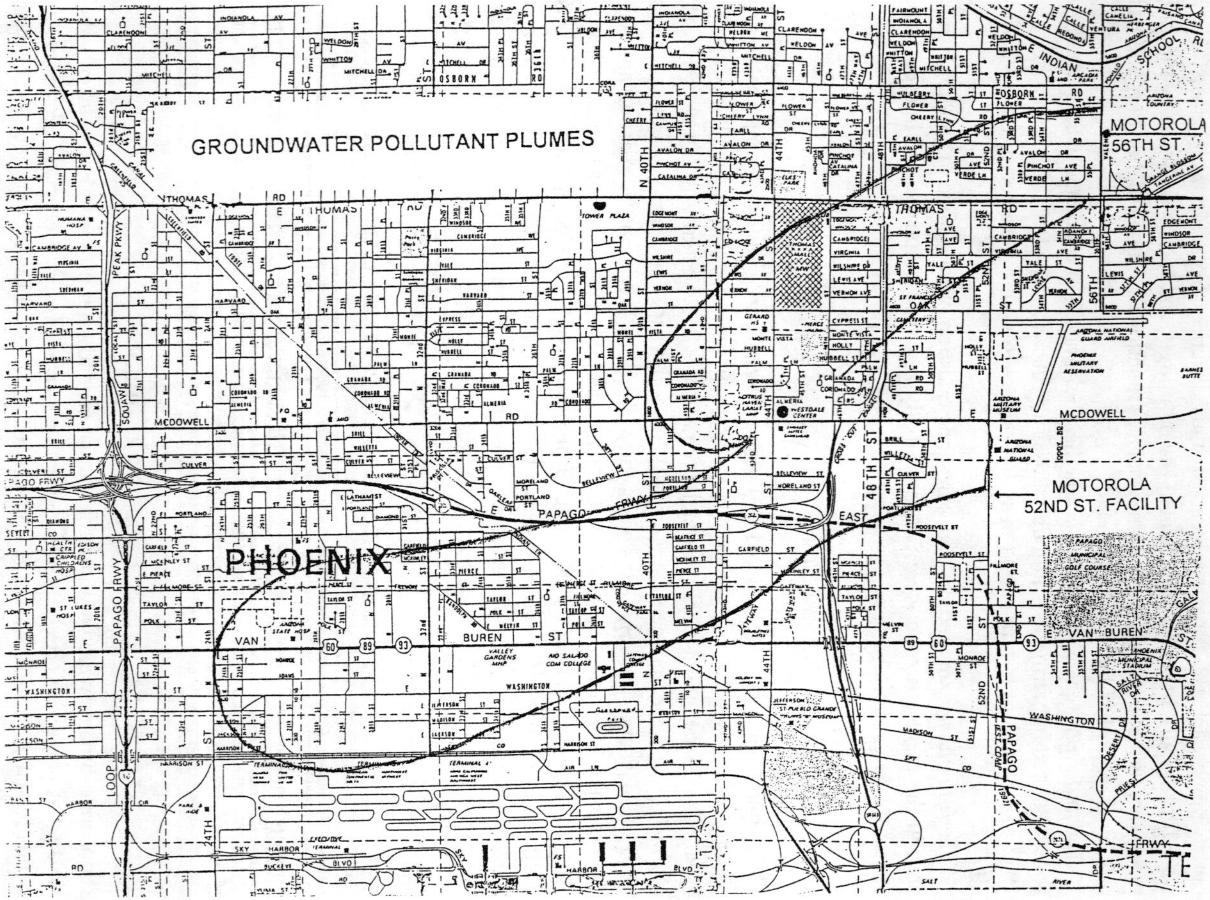

FIGURE 11.1. The extent of pollutant plumes in groundwater in October to December 1992 is shown related to the Motorola plants at 56th and 52nd Streets. Trichloroethylene concentrations are found in the alluvium (at all wells).

ppb, 1,2-DCE from <0.2 to 1,600 ppb, PCE from <0.2 to 23,000 ppb, and VC from <0.2 to 330 ppb. Because TCE and TCA are the best-known neurotoxins of these HVOCs and were the most widely distributed chemicals, their two groundwater plumes are shown (in Figure 11.1) spread in 64 km^2 and to 25,000 residents.

Magnitude of TCE Disposal

Motorola's first plant, which opened in 1949 at 52nd Street and McDowell on a 93-acre site, had by 1965 dumped over 135,000 liters of solvents per year into lagoons on the property. Other thousands of liters went into Phoenix sewers. The total TCE disposal on-site after 1955 was estimated at 4.5 million liters by the Arizona Department of Environmental Quality in 1991 (9). Water from a well on this Motorola property had a TCE level of 1.4% in 1982.

After 1982 Motorola discharged chemical wastes into the air at an estimated annual rate of 818,182 kg, by federal and state records. Thus, the atmospheric contamination zone included much of the same area as the groundwater plume.

A groundwater treatment plant opened at the Motorola 52nd Street plant in 1983, and it has had occasional releases such as one of vinyl chloride on May 10, 1993. Maximal levels of TCE in the plume in 1992 were found from Papago Heights between McDowell and Harrison, from 52nd Street west to 40th Street, and then angled south from Papago Street to Harrison and west to 32nd Street (Figure 11.1). Over 70% of tested subjects who resided on the plume came from this area, and about 20% were from west of the 56th Street Motorola plant.

A Critique of Methods

Methods of proven value for testing subjects for the effects of occupational exposures to chemicals have rarely been applied to investigate chemically exposed neighborhood residents (10, 13, 18). Often neighborhoods have had clusters of leukemia, cancer, and birth defects, but numbers have been small, yielding borderline or no statistical significance. Preliminary studies of the prevalences of symptoms or diseases do not show them clearly elevated although sometimes they have verged on statistical significance. This is a problem when infrequent events are assessed in small populations. Questionnaires for medical disorders and for complaints such as foul odors, headache, and fatigue have been used most (10, 11) but are subject to recall bias. Because many chemicals emitted from these sites are neurotoxins and the complaints of the pilot subjects suggested impairment of the central nervous system (15, 19), neurophysiological and neuropsychological testing were done (5, 6). Also questionnaires were given for lupus erythematosus (7, 20).

Description of Exposed Subjects

The 236 EZ women and men who were clients, mean age 51.8 years and educational level 12.2 years, were compared to 161 regional unexposed, mean age 50.7 years and educational level 13.2 years (see Tables 11.1a and 11.1b, Figures 11.2a,b). Also the 58 EZ nonclients were compared to exposed clients, and the 67 out-of-exposure Phoenix residents were compared to exposed clients (see below for results). The out-of-exposure group was significantly younger than the clients, and their educational levels were

TABLE 11.1a Neurophysiological and neuropsychological scores in 236 Phoenix exposed and 161 regional unexposed subjects, means and standard deviations (Sd) with p values, by analysis of covariance

		Unexposed		Exposed		
		161		236		
		Mean	Sd	Mean	Sd	p^c
Age yrs		50.7	20.0	51.8	17.6	.551
Educational Level yrs		13.2	2.4	12.2	2.7	.001
Simple Reaction Time ms		282	62	334	118	.0001
Choice Reaction Time ms		543	90	618	153	.0001
Balance Sway Speed						
Eyes Open cm/sec		0.83	0.20	0.87	0.49	.266
Eyes Closed cm/sec		1.34	0.46	1.59	0.77	.0003
Color Score		11.9	1.6	12.6	2.0	.003
Blink Reflex Latency ms						
Supraorbital Tap	Right	13.3	2.2	14.2	2.1	.0001
	Left	13.3	2.2	13.9	2.1	.008
Glabellar Tap	Right	14.9	2.2	15.4	2.0	.03
	Left	15.3	2.2	15.4	2.0	.8
Cognitive Function						
Culture Fair A sc		26.7	7.6	23.5	9.0	.0003
Vocabulary sc		24.4	8.9	19.3	9.6	.0001
Perceptual Motor Speed						
Pegboard Dominant s		82.0	28.9	90.0	32.4	.013
Trail Making A s		37.8	23.5	46.6	28.2	.001
Trail Making B s		82.2	35.3	101.8	44.7	.000
Recall (Wechsler) score						
Stories Immediate score		22.1	7.2	17.7	7.1	.001
Profile of Mood States						
POMS Score		18.9	31.8	50.4	39.3	.0001
Tension score		8.5	5.7	14.2	7.8	.0001
Depression score		7.9	9.2	14.2	11.9	.0001
Anger score		7.4	7.5	12.1	9.8	.0001
Vigor score		18.5	6.5	13.6	6.4	.0001
Fatigue score		7.6	6.4	12.8	7.0	.0001
Confusion score		5.9	4.5	10.6	5.4	.0001

* By t-test, no prediction equations. sc = score
ms = milliseconds p^c = significance by covariance analysis
s = seconds

significantly different from those of the clients; so these groups were compared by analysis of covariance.

Testing of Subjects

Neurophysiological Testing

The performances of simple and choice reaction time were significantly delayed for the exposed group as compared to unexposed (Table 11.1a). The EZ client group was abnormal for balance as shown by sway speed with eyes closed, but did not differ from unexposed with eyes open. Color discrimination was decreased significantly in the exposed subjects as well. The blink reflex latency (R-1) was prolonged on both sides

TABLE 11.1b Descriptive statistics for the adjusted difference between 236 Phoenix exposed and 161 regional unexposed adults

Variable		Mean Difference	Standard Error of the Difference	p Value
ln (so)		0.0190	0.0285	0.506
ln (sc)*		n/a	n/a	0.001
ln (srt)		0.1415	0.0273	0.001
ln (crt)		0.1131	0.0191	0.001
Glabellar Tap	Right	0.4685	0.2091	0.026
	Left	−0.0041	0.2072	0.984
Supraorbital Tap	Right	0.8475	0.2047	0.001
	Left	0.5196	0.2026	0.011
$1/(\text{clscr})^4$		−0.000000000848	0.000000000167	0.001
Culture Fair A		−2.3747	0.6038	0.001
Vocabulary		−4.1238	0.8397	0.001
1/pegd		−0.0011	0.0003	0.001
ln (tra)		0.1962	0.0359	0.001
ln (trb)		0.1677	0.0352	0.001

* There were interactions between group and covariates.

for the exposed when stimulated by supraorbital tap and was significantly different from that of the unexposed for the right side but not the left after a glabellar tap. Covariance analysis confirmed the significance of the differences for balance with the eyes closed, reaction time, and BRL-R-1 (Table 11.1b).

Neuropsychological Testing

Exposed subjects were significantly different from unexposed for cognitive and psychomotor functions and for verbal recall (Table 11.1a). The EZ client subjects' scores on Culture Fair 2A and vocabulary were also impaired compared to unexposed subjects, and scores on grooved pegboard (dominant hand) and trail making A and B were also significantly below those of the unexposed. Verbal recall (memory) function was significantly reduced. EZ client subjects' POMS scores were greatly increased and more than doubled those of the unexposed, and all six component scores were also significantly increased except for vigor, which was decreased. Covariance analysis confirmed the differences for Culture Fair, vocabulary pegboard, and trail making A and B (Table 11.1b).

Symptom Frequencies

Symptom frequencies were significantly higher in the EZ clients than in the reference subjects, with the frequencies for EZ nonclient subjects in between (see Table 11.2 and Figure 11.3a, b). Thus, significant differences were present in all categories, including mucous irritation, abnormal skin and nails, and respiratory, general (vegetative), sleep, and neurobehavioral symptoms, including mood and memory. Loss of recent memory, extreme fatigue, headache, inability to concentrate, and skin itching were more frequent in EZ client subjects as compared to unexposed subjects (Figure 11.3a).

ARA Criteria

Eight of 10 American Rheumatism Association criteria for lupus erythematosus were significantly more frequent in the EZ client subjects as compared to unexposed (Table

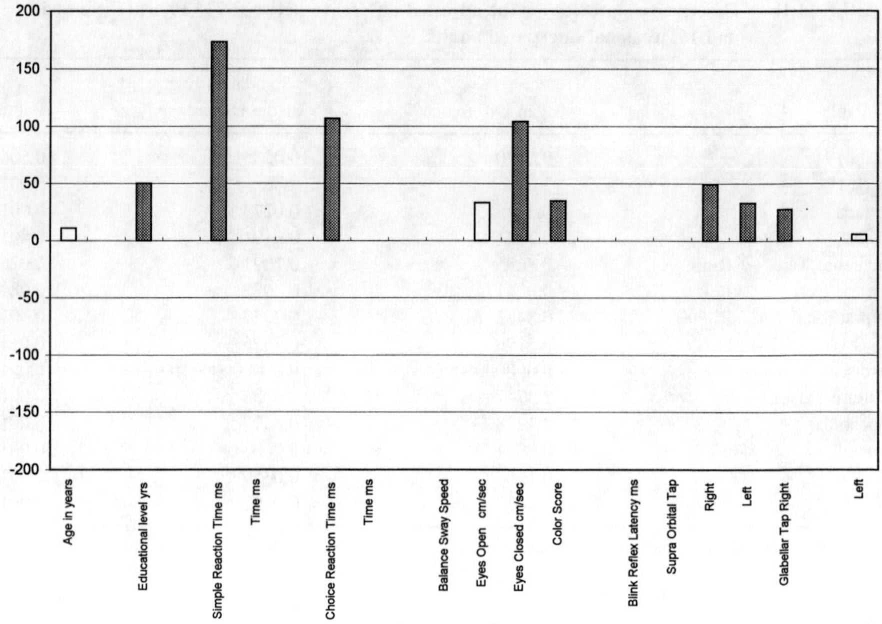

FIGURE 11.2a. Comparison of 236 exposed adults (Phoenix) and 161 unexposed adults by ANOVA. Hatched bars are statistically significant.

11.3). The exceptions were anemia and seizures. Antinuclear antibody titers (criterion 11) were not elevated compared to the unexposed group. Twelve percent of the Phoenix on-plume subjects had five or more rheumatic symptoms compared to only 4.3% of unexposed, and 25.8% of Phoenix subjects compared to 7.7% of unexposed had four or more symptoms, needed for a presumptive diagnosis of lupus. These differences were both significant ($p < .001$).

Pulmonary Status

All respiratory symptoms were significantly more prevalent in EZ client subjects than in unexposed. Pulmonary functions after adjusting for height, age, sex, and duration of cigarette smoking were significantly decreased, including mean FEV_1 and FVC, compared to unexposed referents (Table 11.4). The 67 out-of-exposure-zone Phoenix subjects (PU) and the 58 in-zone nonclients (NC) were not different from unexposed, but particularly the 67 differed from the in-zone exposed (C) for FVC, FEV_1, and FEV_{25-75}. The 58 EZ nonclients resembled the EZ clients, differing only for FVC.

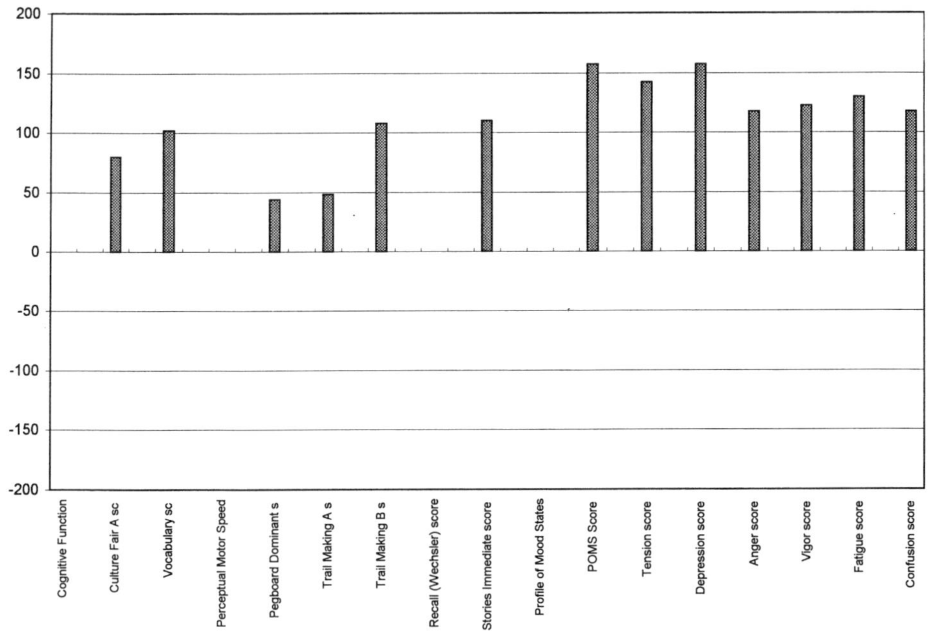

FIGURE 11.2b. Comparison of 236 exposed adults (Phoenix) and 161 unexposed adults by ANOVA. Hatched bars are statistically significant.

Confounding

Possible occupational confounding factors showed that a higher proportion of *unexposed* than EZ client subjects had seven occupational exposures. Exposed clients exceeded unexposed for no factor. The prevalences of childhood disease were similar in the groups, suggesting that they reported accurately. However, histories of cancer, angina pectoris, and stroke (possible results of exposure to solvents) were significantly more prevalent in the EZ clients than in unexposed subjects, and depression was more common in EZ clients. In contrast there were no significant differences in other psychiatric illnesses, neurologic illnesses, or cardiovascular diseases, including peripheral vascular disease.

Alveolar alcohol was below .01 μl/dl in all subjects. Because hospitalizations with general anesthesia were commonly reported, minutes of anesthesia was inserted as an independent variable with age and educational level in regression analysis of several tests, including reaction time, sway speed, and blink latency. None of the coefficients for minutes of anesthesia was significant.

TABLE 11.2 Symptom frequencies in unexposed Wickenburg and exposed Phoenix populations

	Unexposed		Exposed		
	117		236		
	Mean	Sd	Mean	Sd	*p*
Skin itch	3.27	2.87	5.16	3.31	.0000
Fingernail changes	1.62	1.73	2.73	2.87	.0001
Chest tightness	2.15	1.66	3.64	2.86	.0000
Palpitations	2.20	1.93	3.53	2.83	.0000
Burning chest	2.13	1.78	3.28	2.78	.0000
Shortness of breath	2.52	1.86	4.49	3.05	.0000
Dry cough	2.55	1.58	3.60	2.63	.0000
Cough with mucus	2.85	1.06	4.65	3.09	.0000
Cough with blood	1.16	0.47	1.61	1.54	.0023
Dry mouth	3.16	2.48	4.91	3.24	.0000
Throat irritation	2.64	1.84	4.29	2.88	.0000
Eye irritation	2.82	2.31	4.90	3.40	.0000
Reduced sense of smell	2.13	1.87	3.61	3.32	.0000
Headache	4.38	2.69	5.73	3.32	.0002
Nausea	2.43	1.79	3.46	2.76	.0003
Dizziness	2.35	1.83	4.01	2.98	.0000
Lightheaded	2.53	1.95	4.17	3.00	.0000
Unusual exhilaration	1.49	1.03	1.84	1.81	.0517
Balance	2.00	1.58	3.93	2.89	.0000
Loss of consciousness	1.18	0.54	1.57	1.57	.0094
Extreme fatigue	3.38	2.79	6.01	3.39	.0000
Somnolence	2.65	2.78	4.74	3.57	.0000
Insomnia	2.85	2.37	4.56	3.36	.0000
Wake frequently	2.87	2.41	4.90	3.34	.0000
Sleep only a few hours	2.90	2.73	4.61	3.46	.0000
Irritability	3.42	2.25	4.68	3.01	.0000
Concentration	3.18	2.44	5.57	3.31	.0000
Recent memory	3.14	2.37	6.24	3.44	.0000
Long-term memory	2.17	1.85	4.85	3.27	.0000
Instability of mood	2.49	2.36	4.00	3.17	.0000
Decreased libido	3.13	2.57	4.84	3.58	.0000
Decreased alcohol tolerance	2.43	2.68	3.57	3.56	.003
Indigestion	3.25	2.19	4.65	3.09	.0000
Loss of appetite	2.61	2.02	3.61	2.78	.0007
Stomach swells or bloats	2.94	2.29	4.08	3.28	.003

Comparisons with Nonclients

Neurobehavioral function measurements for 67 out-of-the-exposure-zone subjects, who were younger than the 161 unexposed subjects from outside Phoenix, differed little from EZ subjects' values for BRL-R-1 supraorbital, glabellar left, pegboard, and trails A but were better than measurements for EZ subjects in 10 other tests (Tables 11.5a and 11.5b, Figure 11.4). This finding is consistent with exposure zone chemical (TCE) effects and argues against a ''Phoenix effect.'' Analysis of covariance showed that differences for reaction times, Culture Fair, peg placement, and trails B remained significant. Only sway speed with the eyes open lost significance, and sway speed with eyes closed showed complex interactions with age, gender, height, and exposure.

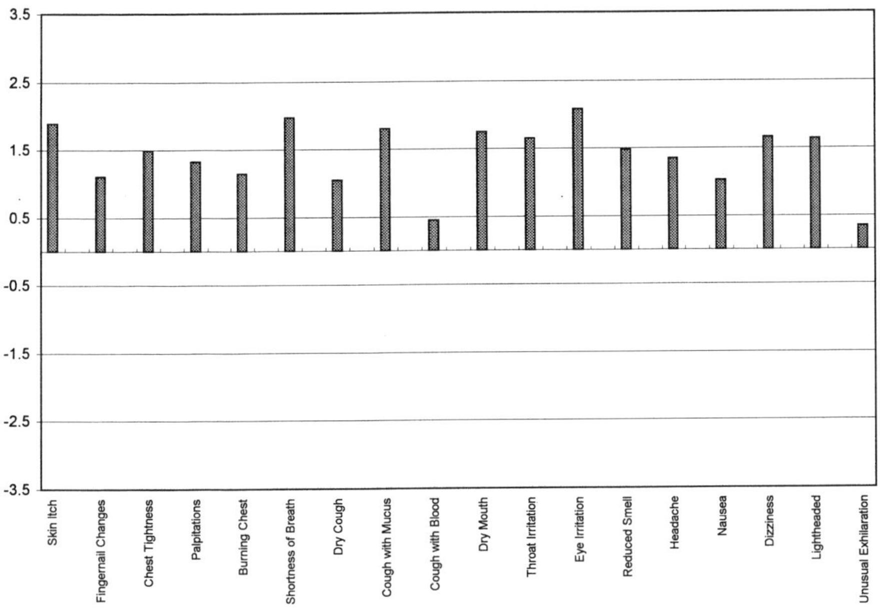

FIGURE 11.3a. Comparison of symptom frequencies in 236 exposed adults (Phoenix) and 117 unexposed adults by ANOVA. Hatched bars are statistically significant.

The 58 nonclient subjects in the exposure zone showed no significant differences from clients (Tables 11.6a and 11.6b, Figure 11.5) for supraorbital blink reflex latency, sway speed eyes open, reaction times, vocabulary, Culture Fair A, and POMS score, but differed significantly for sway speed eyes closed color score, and for the perceptual motor tests (pegboard and trail making A and B). These observations suggested that they were less impaired than the clients. When the exposed nonclients were compared to the unexposed subjects, they were significantly different when analyzed by covariance except for sway speed and the perceptual motor tests. Thus, the nonclients' functions were impaired by their being in the exposure zone, except for their sway speeds; so their balance was unusually stable, and their perceptual motor performance was midway between that of exposed clients and that of unexposed.

When these 58 nonclients were added to the 236 clients, and the 294 subjects were compared to the 159 unexposed, all of the differences between the groups remained statistically significant.

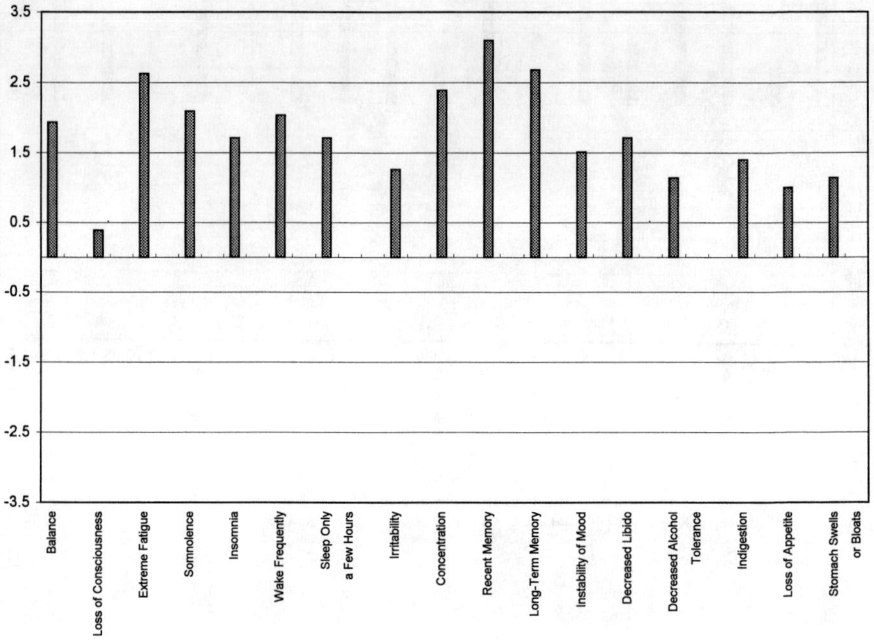

FIGURE 11.3b. Comparison of symptom frequencies in 236 exposed adults (Phoenix) and 117 unexposed adults by ANOVA. Hatched bars are statistically significant.

TABLE 11.3 American Rheumatism Association criteria for lupus erythematosus

	Unexposed (117)	Exposed (236)	
	Mean	Mean	*p*
Rheumatism	17.9	31.6	.006
Numb fingers	27.3	46.0	.001
Mouth sores	6.8	14.8	.032
Anemia	19.6	27.0	.132
Rash on cheeks	3.4	9.7	.036
Sun rash	9.4	21.5	.005
Painful breathing (pleurisy)	12.8	23.2	.021
Urinary protein	2.6	9.3	.020
Hair loss	5.1	20.3	.0002
Seizures	3.4	7.6	.126

TABLE 11.4 Pulmonary function tests in 294 Phoenix exposed (236 clients and 58 nonclients) and 67 Phoenix unexposed and 156 unexposed subjects*

Group:	Referent (ref) Wickenburg Unexposed		Phoenix Exposed Clients (PEC)		Phoenix Unexposed (PU)		Phoenix Exposed Nonclients (PEN)	
Number:	156		236		67		58	
	Mean	Sd	Mean	Sd	Mean	Sd	Mean	Sd
Comparison			(p vs. ref) PEC vs. ref		(p vs. ref) PU vs. ref	(p vs. exp) PU vs. PE	(p vs. ref) PEN vs. ref	(p vs. exp) PEN vs. PE
FVC %pred	100.5	14.9	95.0	15.4	101.9	16.0	103.0	16.6
			(.0005+)		(.5217)	(.0017+)	(.2775)	(.0005+)
FEV 1%pred	93.7	16.7	88.0	19.2	97.1	17.6	93.3	19.6
			(.0024+)		(.1833)	(.0007+)	(.8759)	(.0602)
FEF 25 75%pred	85.7	36.5	83.3	35.7	93.6	36.7	80.8	43.4
			(.787)		(.1344)	(.0376+)	(.4171)	(.6554)
FEF 75–85%pred	83.4	62.4	86.6	65.1	84.8	56.2	69.2	36.1
			(.639)		(.8764)	(.8355)	(.1028)	(.0505)
FEV_1/FVC	72.3	10.6	71.5	9.8	75.6	6.2	70.8	8.4
			(.4474)		(.0171+)	(.0012+)	(.3604)	(.6552)

* Three subjects could not do spirometry.

+ Significant difference compared to unexposed.

Subjects in the Exposure Zone since 1983

Client subjects who resided in the EZ only after 1983 (as defined in 1992) were almost 10 years (significantly) younger and had almost the same educational level as the unexposed (Table 11.7a, Figure 11.6a). These 80 subjects were 10 years younger and had nearly one year more education than those who began their EZ residence earlier. Blink reflex latency was significantly longer in the 156 subjects in group C, who were on the plume earlier and longer, and who had abnormal Culture Fair, vocabulary pegboard, and trail making B times (longer), as compared to the 80 subjects in group B, exposed only since 1983 (10 years or less) (see Table 11.7b). Thus the scores of those EZ client subjects exposed only after 1983 were between the no effect of unexposed subjects and the scores of the EZ group with longer exposure. They differed from the unexposed (Figure 11.6b) for being younger, for being closer to unexposed for simple and choice reaction time, and in balance as sway speed with eyes closed, vocabulary, and POMS score (Table 11.7c). Subjects who were in the EZ earlier and thus frequently longer (1955–93), group C, were different in every test from the unexposed group, group A, except for balance with eyes open.

Children in the EZ were significantly different from unexposed for blink (BRL R-1), for peg placement, trail making A, recall of stories, and POMS score (see below, Table 11.8, Figure 11.7). Thus, they were measured as less severely affected than adults.

The comparison of the EZ subjects' performance on neurophysiological and neuropsychological tests to regional unexposed showed many substantial and significant differences. These differences remained after adjustments for age and other factors by covariant analysis; and after adding in the nonclient group, they were consistent with diffuse central nervous system impairment. Such impairment was accompanied by a higher frequency of respiratory, irritative, and neurological symptoms. Their disordered

TABLE 11.5a Comparison of 67 non-exposure-zone nonclient adults and 236 exposure-zone subjects (Phoenix)

Status:	Off-Exposure (67)	Exposed (236)	
Number:	Mean/Sd	Mean/Sd	p^c
Age yrs	44.5/15.4	51.6/17.7	.002
Ed Level yrs	13.3/2.7	12.2/2.7	.005
Simple Reaction Time ms	289/60	334/118	.003
Choice Reaction Time ms	551/109	619/153	.001
Sway Balance			
Eyes Open	.75/.21	.87/.49	.048
Eyes Closed	1.21/.37	1.59/.76	.0001
Color Score	11.4/1.0	12.6/2.6	.0001
Blink Reflex Supraorbital Tap ms			
Right	14.0/2.2	14.2/2.1	.37
Left	13.9/2.1	13.9/2.1	.966
Blink Reflex Glabellar Tap ms			
Right	14.7/1.9	15.3/2.0	.046
Left	14.9/2.6	15.4/2.0	.133
Culture Fair A sc	29.4/7.0	23.6/9.0	.0001
Vocabulary sc	24.9/7.0	19.2/9.6	.0001
Pegboard s	86.3/36.3	87.9/29.9	.422
Trail Making A s	49.5/40.6	44.3/22.2	.503
Trail Making B s	86.0/43.9	101.8/44.7	.011
POMS Score	32.1/43.3	50.1/39.4	.0001

sc = score, s = seconds, ms = milliseconds

p^c = covariance analysis adjusting for age, educational level, gender, and weight as applicable.

The only significant difference between off plume nonclient adults and unexposed subjects was for blink reflex latency after supraorbital tap on right and left.

TABLE 11.5b Descriptive statistics for the adjusted difference between 236 clients and 67 nonexposed adults in Phoenix

Variable	Mean	Sd	*p* Value
Sway Eyes Open	0.0576	0.0437	0.189
Closed	0.2138	0.0526	0.001
Simple Reaction Time	0.113	0.039	0.004
Choice Reaction Time	0.074	0.0283	0.009
Glabellar Tap Right	0.4227	0.3065	0.169
Left	0.3249	0.336	0.335
Supraorbital Tap Right	−0.0632	0.2967	0.831
Left	−0.2551	0.2868	0.374
Color Score	−0.00000000121	0.000000000228	0.001
Pegboard	0.00002	0.00041	0.963
Trail Making A	−0.0707	0.0613	0.249
Trail Making B	0.0682	0.0552	0.218
Culture Fair A	−2.6611	0.8596	0.002
Vocabulary	−3.4014	1.1292	0.002
Profile of Mood States	24.9136	5.5844	0.001

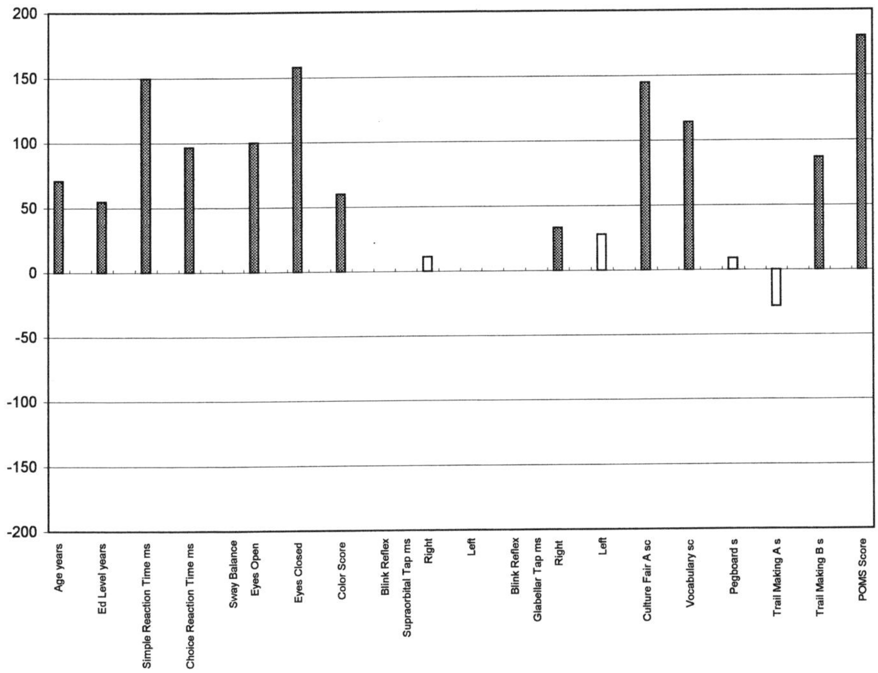

FIGURE 11.4. Comparison of 236 exposed adults (Phoenix) and 67 off-exposure nonclient adults. Hatched bars are statistically significant.

moods states, recall memory, and mental, emotional, and sleep functions suggested involvement of the limbic system of the brain (21). Rheumatic symptoms (20), cancer, angina, and stroke were also elevated significantly and were similar to the findings in a TCE-exposed population in Tucson, Arizona (7). EZ subjects had respiratory symptoms, particularly shortness of breath, associated with airway obstruction, as shown by pulmonary function testing.

Conclusions

The major conclusions of this study are:

1. There were adverse effects on neurobehavioral function of the EZ Phoenix subjects. Those most impaired were immediately west of the 52nd Street plant.
2. The exposure zone clients, who were, on average, nearer the 52nd Street plant than were nonclient subjects, were more impaired than nonclients. In fact, nonclient EZ subjects' performance was indistinguishable from that of equally distant client subjects.

TABLE 11.6a Comparison of 58 nonclient adults to 236 client adults in the exposure zone

	Nonclients		Clients		
Status:	58		236		
Number:	Mean	Sd	Mean	Sd	p^c
Age yrs	53.6	13.3	51.8	17.6	.459
Ed Level yrs	12.1	2.3	12.2	2.7	.799
Simple Reaction Time s	310	115	334	118	.162
Choice Reaction Time s	602	160	619	153	.457
Sway Balance					
Eyes Open	0.75	0.20	0.87	0.49	.072
Eyes Closed	1.22	0.39	1.59	0.76	.0004
Color sc	11.9	1.8	12.6	2.0	.017
Blink Reflex Supraorbital Tap ms					
Right	14.2	2.2	14.2	2.1	.808
Left	13.8	1.8	13.9	2.1	.717
Blink Reflex Glabellar Tap ms					
Right	15.2	2.2	15.3	2.0	.773
Left	14.5	2.4	15.4	2.0	.011
Culture Fair A sc	25.6	8.1	23.5	9.0	.104
Vocabulary sc	21.3	12.0	19.3	9.6	.165
Pegboard s	77.6	21.4	90.0	32.4	.006
Trail Making A s	38.7	14.5	46.6	28.2	.04
Trail Making B s	89.1	41.4	101.8	44.7	.049
POMS sc	34.4	43.0	50.1	39.4	.396

* Covariance analysis.

sc = score, s = seconds, ms = milliseconds

The only significant difference between the off plume nonclient adults and unexposed subjects was for blink reflex latency after supraorbital tap on right and left.

TABLE 11.6b Descriptive statistics for the adjusted difference between 236 clients and 58 nonclient adults in Phoenix

Variable		Mean	Sd	*p* Value
Sway Eyes Open		0.0954	0.0454	0.037
Eyes Closed		0.2312	0.0532	0.001
Simple Reaction Time		0.0672	0.0438	0.126
Choice Reaction Time		0.0339	0.305	0.268
Glabellar Tap	Right	0.2004	0.3250	0.538
	Left	1.0321	0.3381	0.003
Supraorbital	Right	0.1724	0.3183	0.589
	Left	n/a	n/a	0.0956
$1/(clscr)^4$		n/a	n/a	0.001
Pegboard		−0.0014	0.0004	0.001
Trails A		9.0287	3.5117	0.011
Trails B		0.1663	0.0523	0.002
Culture Fair		−2.4067	0.9324	0.010
Vocabulary		n/a	n/a	0.006
POMS		16.6143	5.8632	0.005

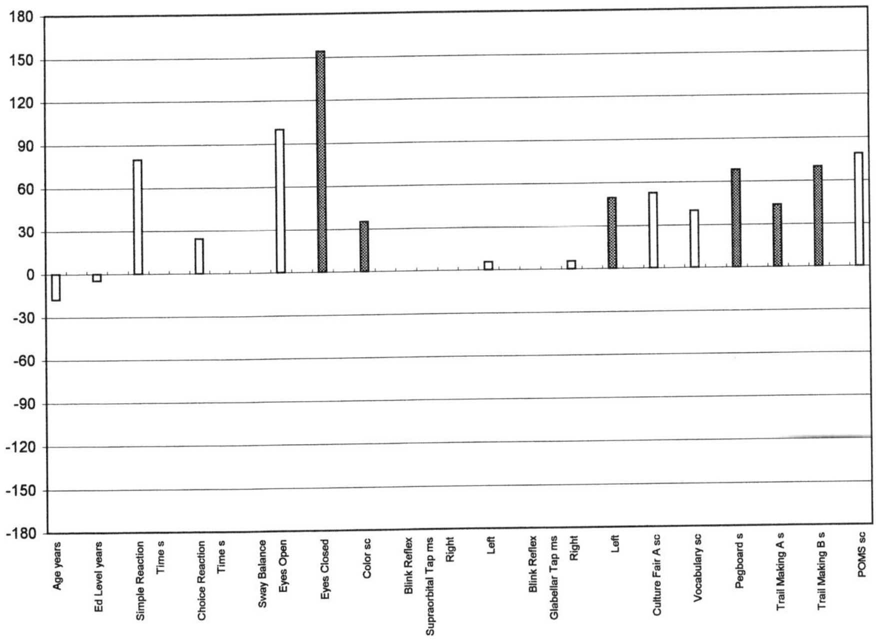

FIGURE 11.5. Comparison of 58 exposed nonclient adults and 236 exposed client adults by ANOVA. (Both Phoenix.) Hatched bars are statistically significant.

3. This EZ group also showed airways obstruction, which was most likely due to prolonged exposure to airborne chemicals in the EZ.
4. Subjects who lived in the EZ only after 1983 had intermediate impairment that was consistent with less exposure. However, as they were exposed for a shorter interval, a reduction in exposure doses since 1983 cannot be inferred.
5. Subjects who were nonclients and lived outside the plume resembled regional unexposed except for delayed blink reflex latency. This finding is consistent with widespread TCE exposure in northeast Phoenix.
6. Children were affected for the ''sentinal'' TCE function BRL R-1, for verbal recall, and for perceptual motor function and mood state. They are notable as the only children's group to show such differences, which may reflect duration of their exposure and/or loss or exhaustion of brain reserve (Table 11.8, Figure 11.7).

Minimal Confounding

The impairments shown in these exposed subjects were similar to those shown previously from environmental exposures to HVOCs, predominantly TCE, in Tucson, Ari-

TABLE 11.7a Comparison of subjects who were exposed, that is, lived on the plume only after 1983, with those who lived there in the 1955–93 period

	Unexposed		Exposed after 1983		Exposed before 1983		*p* Values	
	161 (A)		80 (B)		156 (C)			
Variable	Mean	Sd	Mean	Sd	Mean	Sd	C vs. B	B vs. A
Age yrs	50.7	20.0	45.6	15.0	55.0	18.1	0.0001	0.0451
Ed Level yrs	13.2	2.4	12.6	2.5	12.1	2.8	0.1453	0.0904
Simple Reaction Time	282	62	346	112	328	121	0.2906	0.0001
Choice Reaction Time	543	90	612	157	622	152	0.6531	0.0001
Sway Eyes Open cm/s	0.83	0.2	0.9	0.7	0.86	0.34	0.5067	0.2084
Closed	1.34	0.46	1.62	0.95	1.57	0.65	0.6874	0.0025
Glabellar Tap Right	14.8	2.1	15.0	2.1	15.5	2.0	0.0437	0.6903
Left	15.3	2.0	14.8	1.9	15.6	2.0	0.0055	0.0976
Supraorbital Tap Right	13.3	2.2	14.0	2.1	14.4	2.1	0.2397	0.0668
Left	13.3	2.2	13.5	2.2	14.1	1.9	0.0321	0.5201
Color	11.9	1.6	12.3	1.8	12.7	2.1	0.2331	0.0648
Culture Fair A	26.7	7.6	23.0	7.8	22.3	9.3	0.0023	0.5222
Vocabulary	24.4	8.9	21.7	9.3	18.0	9.5	0.0064	0.0315
Pegboard	82.0	28.9	83.3	26.2	93.4	34.7	0.0229	0.7473
Trail Making A	37.8	23.5	44.1	26.0	47.9	09.3	0.3313	0.0584
Trail Making B	82.2	35.3	90.9	41.2	107.4	45.6	0.007	0.0913
Profile of Mood States	19.1	31.4	59.3	44.9	45.8	35.3	0.0127	0.0001

TABLE 11.7b Descriptive statistics for the adjusted difference between adults exposed before 1983 and after 1983

Variable	Mean	Sd	*p* Value
Simple Reaction Time	−0.066	0.0418	0.116
Choice Reaction Time	−0.0258	0.0299	0.39
Sway Eyes Open	−0.0915	0.0463	0.049
Eyes Closed	n/a	n/a	0.0048
Glabellar Tap Right	0.3141	0.2882	0.277
Left	0.5614	0.2953	0.059
Supraorbital Tap Right	−0.0662	0.2837	0.816
Left	0.212	0.2728	0.438
Color	−0.000000000133	0.000000000229	0.562
Culture Fair A	−0.3086	0.882	0.727
Vocabulary	−2.2485	1.1593	0.054
Pegboard	0.00014	0.00039	0.712
Trail Making A	−0.0463	0.547	0.398
Trail Making B	0.0285	0.0506	0.573
Profile of Mood States	−13.361	8.3628	0.013

zona (6, 7). They are different from findings from residential exposure to a toluene-rich mixture of HVOCs (22). Although the value of total minutes of general anesthesia was higher in exposed subjects, it had no significant coefficients for any tests in regression models. In the present cohort, other chemical exposures, illness, occupational exposures, medications, and medical histories or misadventures that might explain these abnormalities were absent; so there is no plausible alternate hypothesis.

Litigation Bias

It has been claimed that being plaintiffs in litigation alters subjects' symptoms, behavior, and even test results. Most tests in the battery showed minimal difference between EZ plaintiffs and nonplaintiffs and thus no evidence for malingering (23). Balance and perceptual motor speed measures, which showed the only differences, may be equally well explained by distances of subjects from the Motorola site. Thus, the nonclients resembled clients more than unexposed subjects. Nonclients lived farther from the site, and adding the nonclients to the client exposure zone subjects did not abolish any test differences between exposed and unexposed. That EZ nonclients had better balance than would be predicted, which is unexplained. The possibility that nonclients might also be less sensitive to TCE could not be determined.

Exposures

It was impossible to measure the individual chemical exposures from 1955 to 1993 (12), but exposure status was inferred from residence in the EZ and was caused by chemicals spreading from these electronics manufacturing plants. Modeling, based on analysis of well water and soil borings for TCE and trichloroethane (9), defined a groundwater plume. However, exposure was not limited to these chemicals and probably had an airborne component, especially after 1983, when disposal into air replaced dumping of these chemicals on the soil. Residents within the exposure zone demonstrated effects consistent with these HVOCs that were not shown by 67 Phoenix subjects away from the exposure zone or in regional unexposed.

TABLE 11.7c Descriptive statistics for the adjusted difference between adults exposed after 1983 and unexposed

Variable		Mean	Sd	*p* Value
Simple Reaction Time		0.1851	0.0305	0.001
Choice Reaction Time		0.1259	0.0241	0.001
Sway	Eyes Open	0.073	0.0383	0.058
	Eyes Closed	n/a	n/a	0.001
Glabellar Tap	Right	0.3777	0.2802	0.179
	Left	−0.3099	0.2782	0.267
Supraorbital Tap	Right	0.9524	0.2615	0.001
	Left	0.4012	0.2814	0.155
Color score		−0.000000000739	0.000000000236	0.002
Culture Fair A		−2.4417	0.8052	0.003
Vocabulary		−2.4352	1.1348	0.033
Pegboard		−0.0012	0.0004	0.008
Trail Making A		0.2294	0.0442	0.001
Trail Making B		0.1495	0.0473	0.002
Profile of Mood States		40.1609	5.0113	0.001

Attribution

It seems logical to suggest that the neurotoxic effects observed in these neighborhood exposed subjects can be attributed to HVOCs, especially TCE. The extended blink reflex latency specifically suggests exposure to TCE from both occupational (16) and environmental exposures (5, 6). TCE and other chemicals are spreading from the electronics manufacturing plants through soil and water (including sewers) following disposal of TCE into ''dry wells'' at Motorola, which drain into the Salt River aquifer. Fugitive losses of TCE and other VOCs into the air from the same plant would contribute to residential exposure although the dose has not been modeled. Subjects within the exposure zone had airways obstruction, which, contrasted with normal spirometric values of 67 Phoenix residents away from the zone and the Wickenburg unexposed, suggest substantial effect.

Exposure Duration

Those subjects exposed after 1983 had test scores that were between those of the group with earlier and longer (1955–93) exposure and those of the unexposed or the off-zone Phoenix groups, but were more like those of persons exposed for the longer period than the unexposed. Thus, the tentative conclusions are: (1) exposure continued after 1983, despite ameliorative efforts; and (2) impairment may not yet be maximal in subjects exposed since 1983.

Environmental Epidemiology

Studies of this new type are difficult to relate to those conducted in the past for at least seven reasons: (1) Effects of nearly continuous residential exposure to low doses of solvents may substantially exceed those from intermittent, occupational exposure, just as animals continuously exposed (24) to *n*-hexane showed more neurobehavioral impairment and nerve destruction than was predicted from 8 hours per day of animal experiments (25). (2) Human functional impairment may require several years at these levels of exposure to be measurable. (3) The calculations of indoor air exposures over

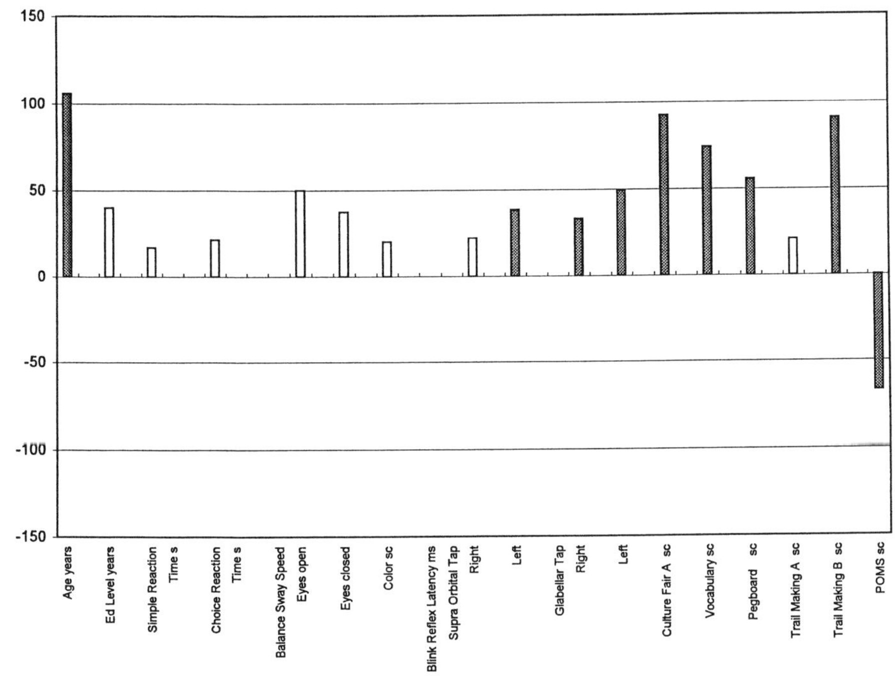

FIGURE 11.6a. Comparison of 80 adults exposed after 1983 and 156 adults exposed between 1955 and 1993 by ANOVA. (Both Phoenix.) Hatched bars are statistically significant.

years would present difficulties even if household or neighborhood doses had been measured intermittently. In addition, exposure levels over time are "moving targets" modified by factors due to instrument sensitivity (minimum level detected), which has improved greatly since 1955, and by rates of production or release, spills, and ecological factors such as wind direction and velocity, temperature, humidity, and soil permeation rates. (4) Absence of measurements and lack of models makes environmental chemical estimates much more difficult to reconstruct historically than are occupational exposures such as those to asbestos fibers (26) or to lead (27). (5) There are no biomarkers for long-term HVOC exposure. (6) More than a decade of examining human risk from environmental chemicals at manufacturing or dump sites shows that meaningful or even plausible associations between impaired human performance and presumed exposure doses are rare (10, 11, 14). Bridging this chasm probably requires a new paradigm. (7) Even the best exposure models are largely untried against sensitive adverse human health effects; so their predictive ability is unknown.

Lack of public health involvement with the human aspects of these exposures has been attributed to logistical and methodological problems (10, 11), but it also may be

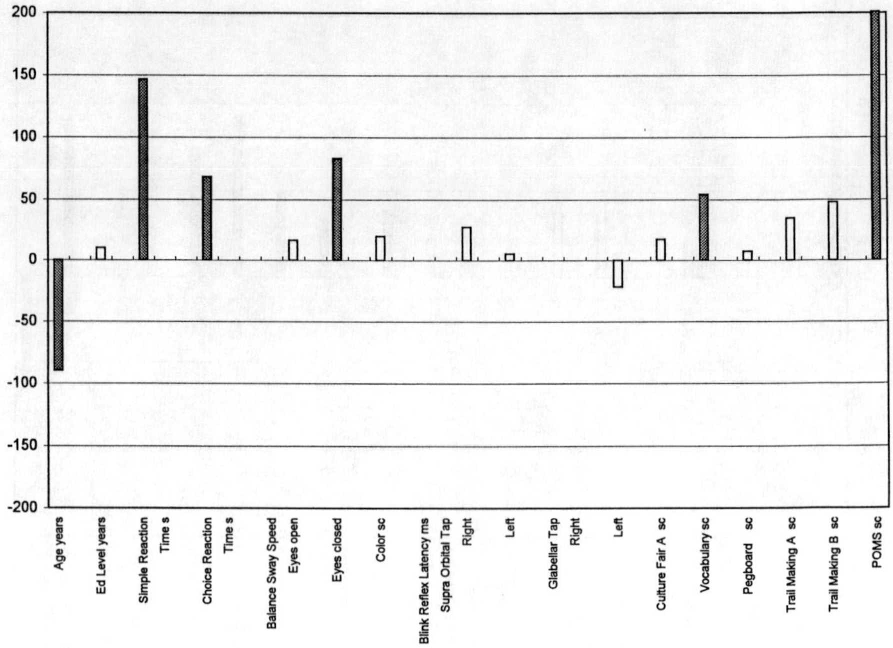

FIGURE 11.6b. Comparison of 80 adults exposed after 1983 and 161 unexposed by ANOVA. (Both Phoenix.) Hatched bars are statistically significant.

due to their novelty and uncertainty. Usually there are several questions (13, 28). Should the alleged complaints be taken seriously? Do they justify scientific study? What health disturbances should be measured? Intervals of years pass between exposure and investigation. Compared to occupational levels, environmental exposures are "low dose" but nearly continuous; so their cumulative effects may be greater than the effects of occupational exposure (11). Despite shifts in responsibility from public health to environmental agencies, adequate studies are rarely completed. Perhaps public agencies fear censure if they *do* identify adverse health effects from a longstanding problem that they should have addressed earlier (28). Also, litigation for property damage and personal injury has been argued as introducing bias (29). (In this instance, bias was unsubstantiated.) These issues create a reluctance for investigators to generate findings that have social or economic consequences. Finally, few methods, even those with proven worth in occupational health epidemiology, have been used in environmental epidemiology, perhaps because of lack of agreement about their sensitivity and the anticipated results.

TABLE 11.8 Comparison of neurophysiological and psychological function in exposed and unexposed children

	Unexposed		Exposed		
	144		50		
	Mean	Sd	Mean	Sd	*p*
Age	11.4	3.3	11.3	3.4	.858
Educational Level	6.0	3.0	5.2	3.2	.122
Simple Reaction	344	114	376	109	.093
Choice Reaction	576	145	610	149	.168
Sway Balance Eyes Open	0.89	0.23	0.91	0.24	.640
Eyes Closed	1.37	0.38	1.39	0.39	.810
Blink Reflex Latency R-1					
Supraorbital Tap Right	12.2	1.9	13.4	1.9	.0007
Left	12.4	2.0	13.2	1.6	.0093
Color score	12.1	1.9	12.5	2.1	.253
Vocabulary	11.2	7.0	9.7	5.7	.213
Culture Fair A	27.4	8.1	25.6	6.9	.174
Pegboard	77.2	16.6	88.1	30.9	.004
Trails A	40.9	20.1	58.2	40.8	.0004
Trails B	93.4	48.3	107.3	51.9	.113
Story Combined (1 and 2)	21.8	8.4	17.2	8.6	.002
POMS Score	26.0	31.6	47.2	41.3	.0005

STUDY 2: SOUTHWESTERN TUCSON, ARIZONA COMMUNITY

Groundwater contamination occurred in southwestern Tucson, Arizona from 1957 to 1981 or afterward, due to leaching of metal cleaning solvents from aircraft refitting operations into the aquifer of the Santa Cruz River (Figure 11.8). The principal solvent was trichloroethylene (TCE), but others included 1,1-dichloroethylene, 1,2-dichloroethylene, chloroform, benzene, xylene, 1,2-dichloroethane, and bis(2-ethyhexyl) phthalate. Hexavalent chromium was also found. Many other organic chemicals were detected once or twice over this interval. The solvents were used by companies located around Tucson Airport to degrease and clean metal parts in aircraft and missile production and refitting.

Tucson's water supply is entirely subsurface, and between 1952 and 1981 had received an estimated 2,000 gallons of TCE. Southwest Tucson, which is northwest of the airport, developed rapidly from the 1950s to 1981, and many wells tapped the Santa Cruz River aquifer. During this period water from many of these wells contained TCE above the EPA maximum contamination level of 5 ppb. TCE concentrations averaged >500 ppb for 28 of 30 years before 1981 and were from 25 to 100 ppb thereafter.

Each resident's domestic water contained TCE in concentrations from 6 ppb to over 500 ppb for 1 to 25 years (30). A combination of multisystem symptoms and what were perceived by residents to be excessive numbers of birth defects, particularly of the cardiovascular system (8), and excessive cancers of breast, brain, thyroid, and testis, as well as leukemias and lymphomas, triggered a class action lawsuit against the companies. Residents' frequent complaints were of impaired memory, inability to

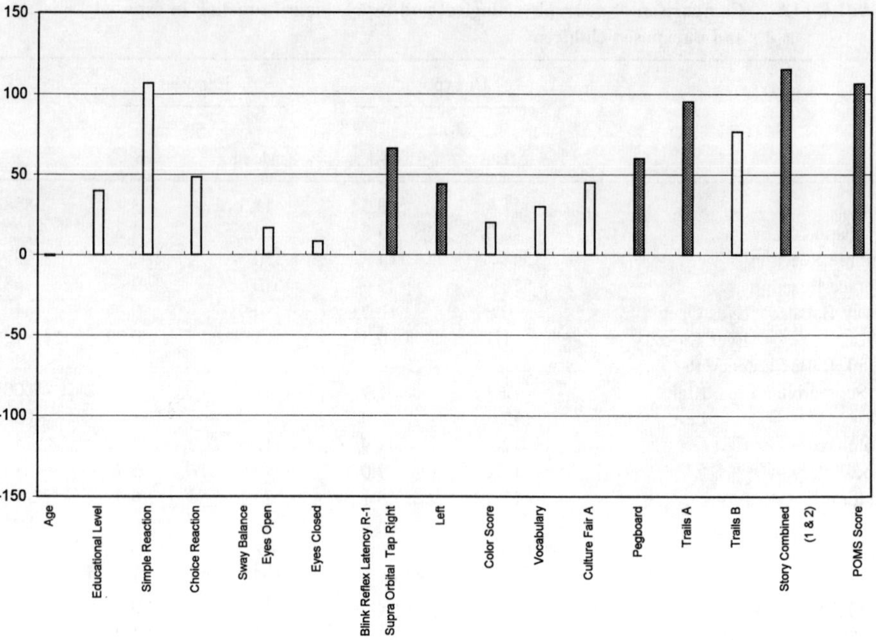

FIGURE 11.7. Comparisons of 50 exposed children (Phoenix) and 144 unexposed children. Hatched bars are statistically significant.

concentrate, dizziness, unsteady gait, disturbed sleep, irritability, and distress, which led to objective testing. Neurobehavioral test (NBT) scores of 170 residents of Southwest Tucson were compared with scores from a combined residential unexposed population (6), and the subjects were compared for blink reflex latency to histology technicians whose blink had been studied by identical methods in 1987 (17, 30), prior to the Arizona unexposed population study of 1993.

Exposed Population

From 1,250 clients, 544 test subjects were recruited into three groups. The clients represented slightly over 20% of residents within the zone of the contaminated water wells. Each member of the three groups had used water from contaminated wells for at least a year between 1957 and 1981, and was examined in 1986, 1987, or 1989. By 1991, testing having been completed in 1989, there were 1,250 clients. Some 196 "worst case" subjects had family members with cancers or birth defects or many health complaints. A

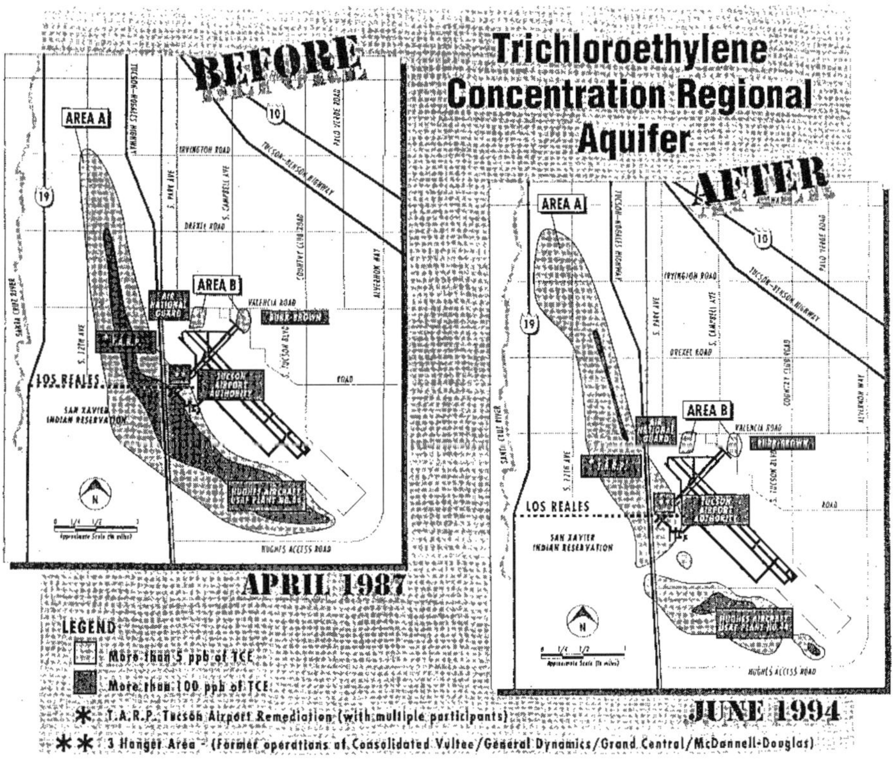

FIGURE 11.8. Tucson Airport area, showing aquifer TCE contamination.

second group of 178 were from families without cancers or birth defects. A third group of 170 subjects included some parents of children with birth defects and subjects with lupus erythematosus and rheumatic disorders. Test scores for the three groups had virtually identical mean values. The third group had more extensive testing, including blink reflex and speed of sway; so they are reported on in detail. All subjects spoke fluent English and were tested in English. Approximately one-third had Spanish surnames.

Unexposed Subjects

Three groups of subjects, who had been studied by identical methods (22, 31–33) for comparison to three chemically exposed populations, served as unexposed subjects in the physiological and psychological tests. Only for blink reflex latency R-1, Tucson exposed subjects were compared to a national volunteer sample of histology technicians who had been minimally exposed at work to formaldehyde and to solvents, mainly toluene and xylene (31). The 68 residential unexposed came from two groups, the first of which contained 21 women and 15 men, mean age 38.9 years + 12.5 years standard deviation (sd) and educational level 12.4 years ± 2.4 years sd, who were the matched unexposed group for men and women exposed residentially to waste oil recovery (22). The second group included 14 women and 18 men mean, age 37.4 years ± 12.7 years sd and educational level 12.7 years ± 1.7 years sd, who were the matched unexposed for ex-workers and residents exposed to gases from a oil refinery (33). The first unexposed group was picked at random from voter registration rolls and matched for age, sex, and educational attainment to the waste oil exposed subjects. The second unexposed group was composed of close friends but not neighbors of the ex-refinery workers and nearby residents exposed downwind, and matched the exposed group for age, sex, and educational attainment. Despite their living in Louisiana and California and differing in their manner of recruitment, there were no statistically significant differences for these subjects in their age, sex, educational attainment, or the outcome variables, their mean neurobehavioral tests scores; thus the two unexposed groups were combined for comparison to the Tucson TCE exposed subjects. All comparisons except blink used this combined national group. Originally another ''unexposed'' group of 165 subjects from Phoenix, Arizona, who matched the Tucson exposed group for age, sex, and educational level, were compared. However, their neurobehavioral test scores were practically identical to those of the exposed subjects and statistically significantly below those of other published reference groups (22, 31–33) as well as the Wickenburg, Arizona unexposed subjects described earlier in this chapter. Further investigation showed that members of the original ''unexposed'' group had themselves been exposed to TCE and other solvents and to chemicals in air, surface drainage, and well water in Phoenix.

Environmental Measurements

Because TCE was invariably present and at higher concentrations than other chemicals (30), it was the marker chemical to model the well water contaminants. TCE concentrations in the wells had been measured from 1957 to 1981 by the city of Tucson, by the Arizona Department of Health Services Bureau of Water Quality Control, by the U.S. Geological Survey, and by the U.S. Environmental Protection Agency. From these measurements, average annual, peak year, and (life maximum) TCE exposures were calculated. By multiplying each individual's years of residence (exposure duration) by average annual TCE concentration, the lifetime (cumulative) TCE exposures were calculated for 170 tested subjects (30). Estimates were based on measurements at the nearest well to a residence, as modified by distribution factors such as pressure, pipe diameters, and reservoir capacity. These data were aggregated from wells serving a series of residential addresses. The TCE plume area for each year and concentration models served to confirm or reject TCE exposures, based on well head samples, that is, to reject outlier values when average and maximal exposure were calculated (30). To compare predictive capacity for neurobehavioral test scores, the four TCE exposure parameters (duration of exposure and lifetime average, life maximum, and cumulative exposure) for each subject were entered as independent variables, along with age, sex, and educational level in the regression equations. None of the coefficients was significant for any neurobehavioral test.

Group Comparisons

Although the exposed group was 4.2 years older than the combined unexposed, this difference was not statistically significant (Table 11.9, Figure 11.9). Moreover, their age distributions were similar, with young adult peaks 6 years below the means. Small test-score differences between men and women were not significant and disappeared when scores were adjusted for age; so the sexes were combined. Increasing age diminished and more educational attainment increased some test scores. Family income, sex,

TABLE 11.9 Tucson age, educational attainment, balance function (sway), simple and two-choice visual reaction time, finger writing errors, and profile of moods states in exposed and combined unexposed populations compared by Students "t" for unequal groups

		Exposed 170 M Sd	Combined Unexposed 68 M Sd	p
Age yrs		42.2 ± 13.9	38.0 ± 12.8	.2
Range		16 to 78	14 to 82	
Ed Level yrs		10.8 ± 3.1	12.5 ± 2.1	.0001
Range		2 to 18	5 to 19	
Sway Speed cm/sec	Eyes Open	1.13 ± 0.39	0.82 ± 0.22	.0001
	Eyes Closed	1.41 ± 0.52	1.24 ± 0.66	.05
Reaction Time				
Simple msec		348 ± 96	281 ± 55	.0001
Choice 1 msec		619 ± 159	519 ± 88	.0001
Choice 2 msec		608 ± 131	514 ± 81	.0001
Choice 3 msec		606 ± 135	513 ± 79	.0001
Choice RT as % Predicted*		118 ± 22	102 ± 15	.0001
Finger Writing Errors	Right	2.6 ± 3.2	2.5 ± 3.2	.73
	Left	2.2 ± 2.8	2.1 ± 2.7	.86
POMS score		45.5 ± 43.4	16.0 ± 28.4	.0001
Tension		13.7 ± 8.7	8.6 ± 4.1	.0001
Depression		13.9 ± 12.9	6.7 ± 6.3	.0001
Anger		12.8 ± 11.1	7.8 ± 5.7	.0001
Vigor		14.4 ± 5.8	16.7 ± 5.0	.0001
Fatigue		10.6 ± 7.1	7.2 ± 3.8	.31
Confusion		9.0 ± 6.4	5.7 ± 2.9	.0001

* Regression equation: Choice reaction time = 1.858 age + 433, r = .061.

and POMS score had no significant influence on any test score. As part of the test differences may be due to the exposed group's being 4 years older than and having 1.7 years less education than that of the unexposed group, unexposed scores were adjusted for educational level and age with appropriate coefficients before comparison. Coefficients for age and educational attainment level were not significant in blink or eye closure; so adjustments were not needed for those measurements. Differences in ages and educational attainment simply did not account for the exposed group's poorer performance on neurobehavioral tests.

Mean speeds of sway were greater with eyes open ($p < 0.0001$) and with eyes closed ($p < 0.05$) in the exposed group compared to the combined unexposed (Table 11.9, Figure 11.9). The exposed group mean simple reaction time was 67 milliseconds (msec) longer than that of the unexposed group ($p < 0.0001$). Choice reaction time of the exposed subjects was 93 msec longer in the third trial ($p < 0.0001$) than that of the unexposed, was longer in all trials, and remained longer after age adjustment.

Eye closure latency was greater for both eyes in the exposed and significantly different ($p < 0.0014$) on the right compared to the HT unexposed group (Table 11.10, Figure 11.10). Times to reach peak closure speed were longer in exposed than unexposed for both eyes, and differences were statistically significant. Onsets of closure times were not different. Blink reflex latency on the right was also greater than left R-1, by about 1 msec, in exposed and in unexposed groups. The prevalences of failure of left and

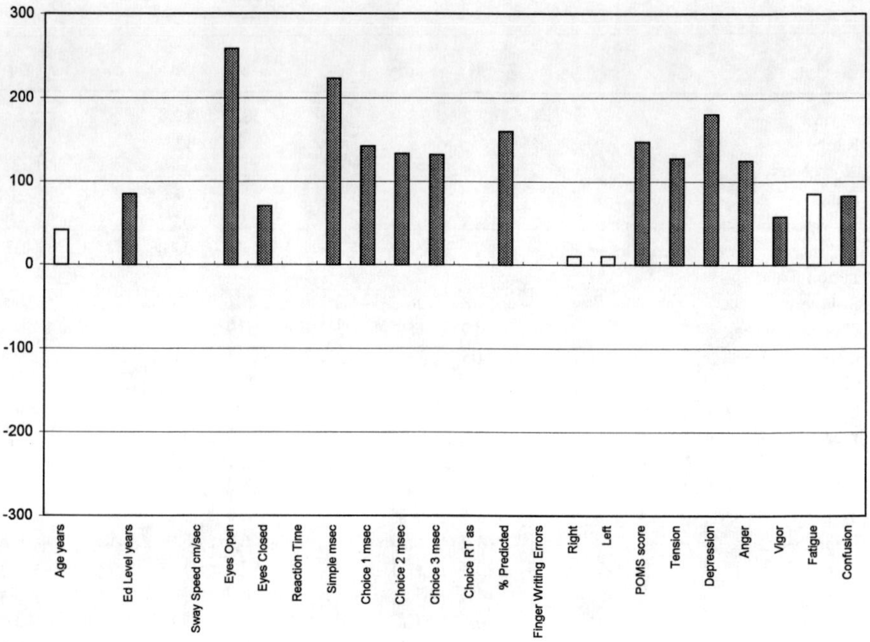

FIGURE 11.9. Comparison of 170 exposed adults (Tucson) and 68 unexposed adults by ANOVA. Hatched bars are statistically significant.

TABLE 11.10 Eye closure and blink reflex in 160 Tucson men and women compared to 113 unexposed men and women*

	Exposed	HT-1 Unexposed	
	160	113	*p*
Eye Closure			
Latency R msec	46.4 + 8.0	49.4 + 7.2	.0014
L	54.1 + 8.0	55.9 + 7.2	.09
Peak R	85.6 + 10.2	60.5 + 7.3	.0001
L	89.5 + 15.4	68.4 + 9.6	.0001
Blink Reflex	m sd	m sd	
right R-1 msec	10.9 + 2.6	10.2 + 1.6	.008
left R-1 msec	11.7 + 2.4**	11.2 + 2.0†	.0754
diff msec	0.8 + 2.0	1.0 + 1.7	

* Blink testing was incomplete in both groups.

** $p < 0.005$ and † $p < 0.001$ compared to right.

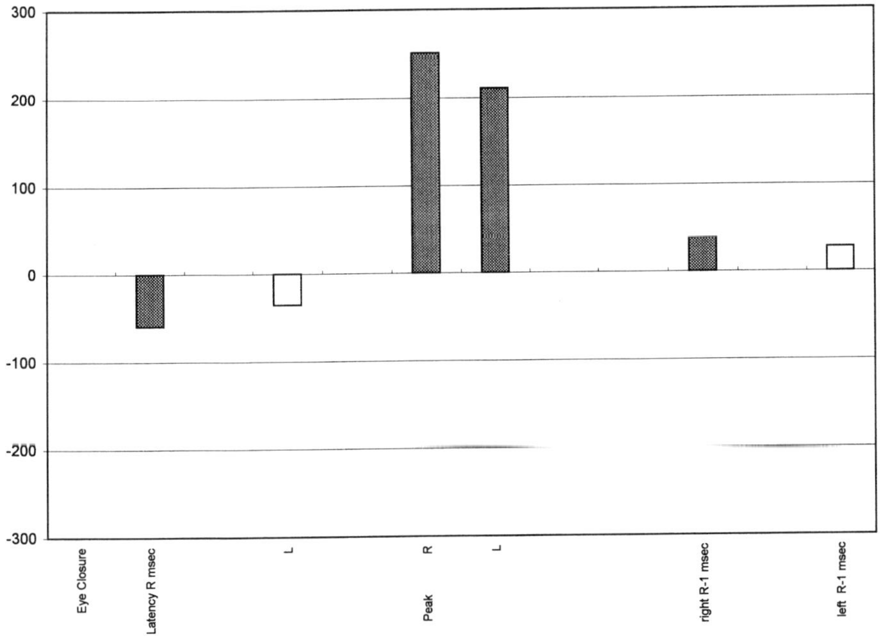

FIGURE 11.10. Eye closure and blink reflex in 160 exposed adults (Tucson) and 113 unexposed adults by ANOVA. Hatched bars are statistically significant.

right R-1 were similar. Thus, the differences between exposed and unexposed groups were reliable, but the mean values were low compared to those published (6, 16).

Profile of mood states score was statistically significantly higher in the exposed population than in the unexposed, as were the component scores except for fatigue. Thus exposed subjects had lower intelligence scores and more mood disorders. Mood status as ascertained by POMS score or individual mood scores had no significant effects on neurobehavioral test scores as ascertained by regression models, which were adjusted because they had coefficients for age and educational levels.

Performance by the exposed group on verbal recall and visual reproduction of the Wechsler Memory Scale was significantly below that of the combined unexposed except for story 1 (Table 11.11, Figure 11.11). The mean scores on Culture Fair 2A, digit symbol, and block design were statistically significantly lower in the exposed group than in the unexposed. They were correlated (positively) with educational attainment and (negatively) with age. Peg placement took 7.5 seconds longer (mean) in the exposed,

TABLE 11.11 Memory, perceptual, and cognitive functions of 170 Tucson men and women compared to 68 combined unexposed

	Exposed	Unexposed	
	170	68	
	M Sd	M Sd	*p*
I. Learning and Memory			
Story 1	10.2 + 4.1	10.5 + 3.5	.57
Story 2	6.8 + 3.8	9.7 + 4.1	.0001
II. Visuospatial			
Visual reproduction	8.7 + 3.3	10.1 + 3.3	.03
III. Perceptual motor speed and manual dexterity			
Pegboard dom	76.4 + 21.1	68.9 + 11.5	.001
IV. General intelligence			
Culture Fair 2A	23.8 + 8.5	30.6 + 6.1	.0001
Block design (WAIS)	26.9 + 10.5	31.0 + 10.3	.008
B.D. % of predicted*	85.5 + 32.5	97.2 + 29.3	.001
Digit Symbol	52.4 + 14.5	56.8 + 14.9	.07
V. Attention			
Digits forward	6.2 + 1.6	6.7 + 1.5	.0001
Digits backward	4.3 + 1.5	4.7 + 1.3	.004
Trails A	38.6 + 17.6	29.4 + 9.2	.0001
Trails B	91.9 + 50.6	68.5 + 39.2	.0001
Trails B % of predicted**	135.3 + 62.5	107.7 + 48.4	.001

* *Regression equations:* Block design = 38.11 − .1636 age, r^2 = 0.03%.

B.D. % of predicted = Block design exposed/calcul. block design exposed × 100.

** Trails B = 33.31 + .7962 age, r^2 = 0.041.

compared to the unexposed, a difference that was significant ($p < 0.001$). The exposed group took longer to make trails A and B and made more errors on B than the unexposed, and these differences remained significant after adjusting for age. The error rates for the recognition of numbers written on fingertips were not different in exposed and unexposed subjects. All significant differences in scores between the groups remained so after age adjustment. Although CRT, block design, and trail making B had the largest age coefficients in the regression models, the variances attributable to age were small (adj. r^2 of 0.03 and 0.04, respectively).

Questionnaires showed no evidence of alcohol abuse; in fact, alcohol use was infrequent. No illicit drug use was reported beyond brief experimentation with marijuana. Hours of general anesthesia was not a significant determinant of any test score in regression models. Medically diagnosed degenerative neurologic diseases and emotional disorders were absent. There were no occupational exposures to neurotoxins except for several subjects who cleaned metal with TCE at the plant that contaminated the wells.

Neurobehavioral test scores were not correlated with any TCE exposure parameter, including duration of residence, life average, life maximum (year), and life cumulative (average × duration), in linear regression analyses. Also, the mean test scores for the highest quartile of exposure group compared to the scores for lowest quartile group showed no significant differences (t-test).

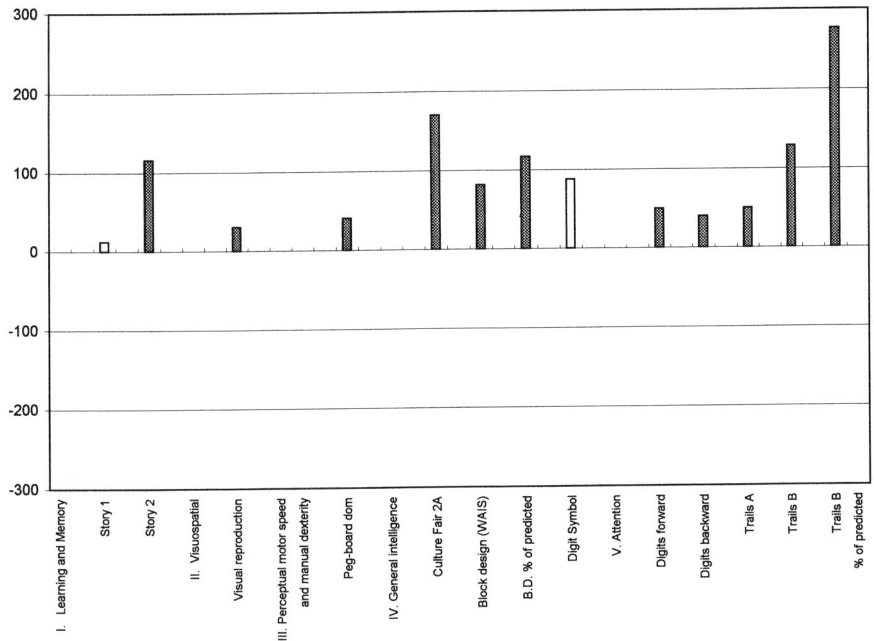

FIGURE 11.11. Comparison of neurobehavioral tests in 170 exposed adults (Tucson) and 68 unexposed adults by ANOVA. Hatched bars are statistically significant.

Summary and Conclusions

Subjects with long-term exposure to TCE, trichloroethane, chromium, and other chemicals in southwest Tucson well water showed uniformly lower scores on neurophysiological and neuropsychological testing as compared to unexposed combined residential unexposed and subsequently to Arizona (regional) unexposed. The lower scores were not attributable to differences in age or educational level. Although there is no evidence that the subjects studied were not representative of the entire resident population, no claim can be made from this preliminary investigation for the tested residents. However, three large groups were studied, and impairment of function was not explained by occupational exposures, lifestyle factors including illicit drug use, unconsciousness from head trauma, therapeutic drugs including anesthetic agents, or emotional disorders. Regression modeling of many neurobehavioral functions, including CRT, block design, and trail making B, showed that they decreased with aging. Furthermore, the age coefficients of many tests in the exposed group exceeded the age coefficients of the unexposed group. ''Accelerated aging'' was attributed to duration and cumulation of exposure running concurrently with age.

High POMS scores, which were due to elevated scores for anger, tension, confusion, and depression in the exposed group, were associated with exposure to chemicals. However, in regression models high adverse POMS scores did not influence the score on any other test significantly. It appears that the direct effects of chemicals on the limbic system may well disturb mood states or emotions. Alternately one's perception of disordered cognitive and neurological function (caused by chemicals) may disturb one's emotions. The ''emotional trauma construct'' is an unlikely cause of impairment in exposed subjects because POMS scores did not influence or predict performance scores in the models.

TCE doses were modeled for exposed subjects from accumulated water sampling data, the outputs of wells into the delivery system grid, and detailed residential site duration, but neither concentration estimates nor their surrogates were correlated in regression analyses with impairment of neurobehavioral tests, nor did subjects in the upper and lower quartiles of exposure have significantly different neurobehavioral test scores. Nevertheless, overall there was abnormal slowing of eye closure and blink latency (R-1), previously associated with residential (5) and occupational (16) exposure to TCE.

Why there were no TCE dose gradients on the tests is unclear. Possible explanations include the following: the dose surrogates were unsatisfactory; the lowest doses and duration may have exceeded the thresholds for neurobehavioral impairment; and greater doses may not increase impairment in a linear fashion. Also, there are large variations in the innate abilities of subjects, including those exposed. However, preliminary evidence showed that sway speed and reaction time do increase linearly in human volunteers during increasing doses of TCE and ethanol, and that this combination is synergistic (34).

The most attractive of these possibilities is that neurobehavioral impairment thresholds were exceeded after protracted, nearly continuous, exposure at comparatively low doses, and that such cumulative decay is nonlinear (35). An assumption of a linear dose–response for human subjects has no precedents in community exposure to solvents (10, 11). Furthermore, the Tucson mixture of several solvents and other chemicals may have been synergistic, more than additive. Supporting this possibility are synergistic effects of xylene and ethanol on human volunteers (34) and experiments showing that pairs of solvents have synergistic effects on nerve cells such as the giant axon of the squid (35). Although neurobehavioral test scores are linearly related to blood lead in children exposed environmentally (27), dose–response has been investigated for only a few occupational chemical exposures with variable results (36). However, protracted or chronic encephalopathies from occupational TCE exposure have been reported for individuals and in epidemiological studies (36, 37), although some authors have not been able to demonstrate such changes (38).

Comparing a population's mean test scores after chemical exposures to those before the exposures would provide the strongest evidence for causation, but baseline data are rarely available. Next best is comparison of the exposed group's scores to those of an unexposed population, which was used here. The unexposed were similar in all relevant ways to the exposed except for locality. These are conservative comparisons, as histology technicians exposed to low levels of formaldehyde and solvents may have had their eye closure and blink reflex somewhat slowed, which decreased their difference from the exposed group and thus our ability to detect an effect (6, 31). The Southwest

Tucson residents' daily doses of TCE were probably 1/100 to 1/1000 as large as those found in most occupational or experimental studies, and resemble those in Woburn, Massachusetts (14, 19). Although at first glance larger doses at work argue for cumulative occupational exposures being much greater than residential ones (36, 39), the fourfold greater time spent at home may be most important. Assuming that the observations of residents of Woburn and Tucson are confirmed, their greater susceptibility may relate to their being not as healthy as workers and their not being ''selected for resistance by attrition from exposure at work.'' Environmental exposure differs from occupational in affording much less ''time away'' for elimination of TCE. The almost uninterrupted dosing may be a crucial factor in cumulative effects, such as in chronic encephalopathy, which has not been considered in studies of workers (37). These points add to the plausibility of the conclusion that chronic low level exposures, which are effectively continuous, facilitate chronic damage in the brain and other susceptible organs.

STUDY 3: OCCUPATIONAL EXPOSURE AT TINKER AIR FORCE BASE AND ENVIRONS NEAR OKLAHOMA CITY, OKLAHOMA

This investigation illustrates how the initial focus of a study on the lung had to be changed to the brain. Jet engine repair includes welding, smelting, and grinding of jet engine fans, which are made of stainless steel composed of cobalt, nickel, chromium, and manganese as well as iron. Fans are worked with hard metal tools made of tungsten carbide sintered with cobalt. Air monitoring of the work areas showed elevated levels of 11 metals including those just listed and beryllium, titanium, and aluminum. Engine parts had been cleaned with chlorinated solvents, including tetrachloroethylene, trichloroethylene (TCE), 1,1,1-trichloroethane, and ethanol, methanol, toluene, ethylacetate, and acidic sodium chromates, for the past 15 years. Adhesives were made pliable with 1,1,1-trichloroethane.

Tinker Air Force Base (AFB) is centered on the Gerber-Wellington aquifer, which supplies well water to central Oklahoma (Figure 11.12). It extends about 88 km north and south and 56 km east and west. Contamination of soil and water with solvents (TCE was measured as the sentinel) resulted in the designation of Tinker AFB as a group 9 Superfund site in 1987 (40). Solvents such as those listed above had been used on the site, especially in building 3001, for over 50 years, and surface drainage was via Soldier Creek to the North Canadian River. Aircraft metals were cleaned by immersion in 70 large vats in building 3001. Some solvents, such as freon 113, were heated.

Workers used dust masks and canister respirators infrequently, and none wore air supply respirators. Other exposures in the work areas were to noise, acetylene, freon (trichlorotrifluoroethane), and radiation from nickel–thorium. Workers complained of nose, throat, and airway irritation, phlegm production, shortness of breath, and depression and rheumatic symptoms. Our hypothesis was that workplace exposures to solvents and metals had adversely affected neurobehavioral and pulmonary function.

In July 1993, 154 jet engine repair workers from Tinker AFB were studied by using the neurobehavioral test battery, chest X-rays and pulmonary function tests, a profile of mood states, and extensive questionnaires. They were compared to 112 of the workers' friends and associates who did not work at Tinker AFB.

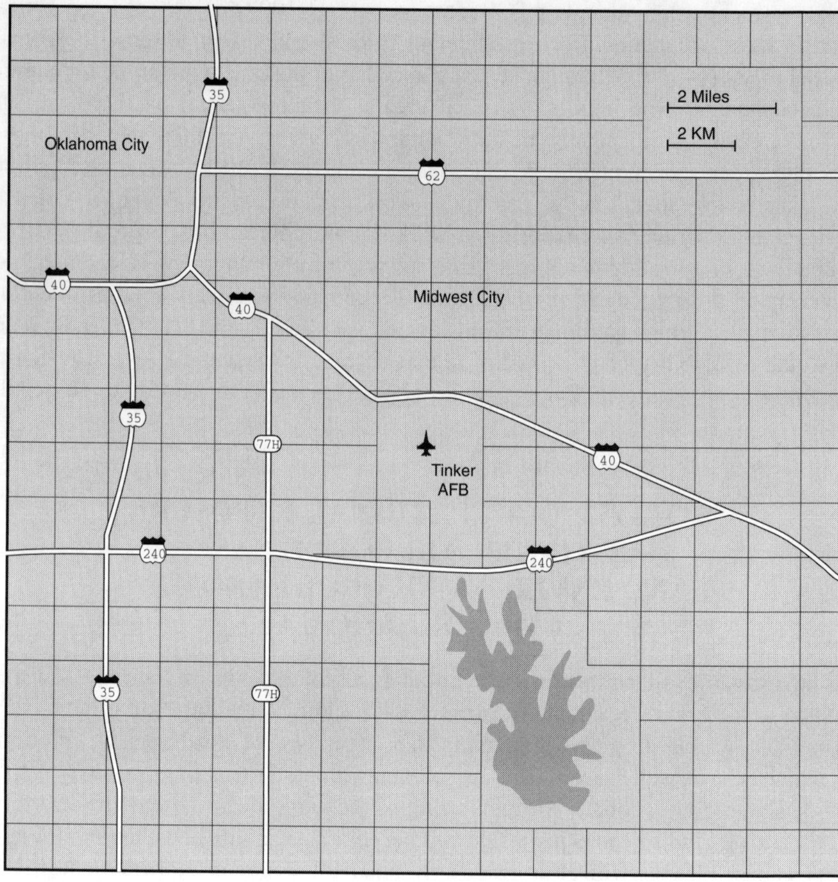

FIGURE 11.12. Tinker Air Force Base, Oklahoma and environs.

Exposed Population

One hundred fifty-four workers volunteered and came for study from a total of approximately 500 who were invited. They included 51 women and 103 men, 27 of them African-American and 127 Caucasian (Table 11.12). Workers contacted proposed matched unexposed subjects, who called our office and were accepted if they met the criteria for age, education, and absence of Tinker-type exposures. The local match group included 46 women and 66 men, of whom 21 were African-American and 91 were Caucasian. Forty-two workers failed to find an unexposed subject. Gender had no influence on tests except for grip strength; so the sexes were pooled for analyses. To verify unexposed status, we compared the exposed group to 117 distant unexposed, 68 women and 49 men, recruited from the election rolls of Wickenburg, Arizona, as

TABLE 11.12 Demographic information for Tinker and unexposed populations

	Exposed			Unexposed		
		154			112	
	Mean		Sd	Mean		Sd
Age	42.7		8.8	41.9		8.2
Education	12.4		1.4	12.9		2.1
Grade Point Average	3.4		0.6	3.6		0.7
Sex Male %		67			59	
Race Caucasian		114			87	
African-American		27			21	
Alcohol (breathalyzer)	0.0008		0.003	0.0024		0.014
Height	171.8		8.0	170.7		9.0
Weight	96.7		20.3	81.2		20.9
Pulse	74		13	70		13

already described. Our staff at Tinker were blinded as to the exposed or unexposed status of subjects.

Testing of Subjects

Tests included simple and choice reaction times, speed of sway with eyes open and with eyes closed, and color hue discrimination. Blink reflex latency was measured because of the major use of TCE at Tinker. The staff and methods for testing blink were identical to those used in the Arizona unexposed. Neuropsychological tests including Culture Fair A, peg placement in a grooved pegboard, trail making A and B, and the profile of mood states (POMS), which, as completed by all subjects, was shortened from that used previously. Alcohol was measured in expired air with a breathalyzer.

Analysis of results showed that the mean age of 42.7 years for the 154 exposed and the mean of 41.9 years for the 112 unexposed did not differ, nor did family income (see Table 11.12). Educational attainments were 12.4 and 12.9 years, respectively (although statistically significant, the difference was of small magnitude); and school grade point averages were not different, 3.4 and 3.6 (C+). An additional exposed man who was legally intoxicated (with alcohol >0.1 μg/dl) was dropped from analysis.

Simple and choice reaction times were significantly longer in the exposed subjects, by 60 ms ($p < .0001$) and 96 ms ($p < .0000$) (Table 11.13, Figure 11.13). Sway speed with the eyes open was significantly different, 0.92 vs. 0.76 cm/s ($p < .0001$), as was sway speed with the eyes closed, 1.60 vs. 1.30 cm/s ($p < .0001$). Color discrimination was impaired in the exposed group. Blink reflex latencies after glabellar stimulation were the same, 15.8 ms, on the right in both groups; but on the left, 15.9 ms vs. 15.3 ms, they were significantly different from Oklahoma City unexposed. After supraorbital taps BRL R-1's were not different from those of local unexposed (Table 11.13). However, latencies after glabellar and supraorbital taps were both statistically significantly different from those of the Arizona unexposed (Table 11.14).

In contrast, cognitive function tested by Culture Fair and vocabulary was not different in exposed compared to unexposed subjects. Perceptual motor function was also not different for grooved pegboard and trail making B. Trail making A was different, but of little importance, as it is a familiarization drill for trail making B.

TABLE 11.13 Neurophysiological and neuropsychological function in Tinker exposed workers and unexposed subjects

	Exposed		Unexposed		
	154		112		
	Mean	Sd	Mean	Sd	*p*
Neurophysiological					
Simple Reaction Time ms	349	145	289	87	0.000
Choice Reaction Time #2 ms	628	165	532	95	0.000
Balance, Sway Speed cm/s					
Eyes Open #2	0.92	0.36	0.76	0.16	0.000
Eyes Closed #2	1.60	.76	1.30	0.38	0.000
Color Vision Score	12.2	1.5	11.8	1.1	0.022
Blink Reflex Rt ms	15.8	2.1	15.8	1.5	0.771
Glabellar Lft ms	15.9	1.8	15.3	1.8	0.024
Supraorbital Rt ms	13.8	1.8	13.5	1.8	0.353
Lft ms	13.8	1.8	13.8	1.8	0.974
Neuropsychological					
Cognitive Function					
Culture Fair A	27.8	6.6	27.0	6.8	0.381
Vocabulary	20.3	8.3	19.0	8.4	0.214
Perceptual Motor Speed					
Pegboard Dominant sec	75.0	18.4	72.0	18.2	0.193
Trail Making A	37.5	14.0	33.2	11.3	0.008
Trail Making B	79.9	28.4	79.7	35.8	0.951

Profile of mood states score for exposed subjects was 83 (mean) and more than four times higher than for unexposed subjects (Table 11.15, Figure 11.14). Their anger, tension, confusion, depression, and fatigue were all significantly elevated, and vigor was depressed. The POMS scores were examined for interaction with neurobehavioral test scores in a correlation matrix for exposed subjects and in one for unexposed. All coefficients were insignificant (<.16) in the unexposed group. Exposed subjects had low-order coefficients (.19–.26) of borderline significance, which suggest little interaction with the abnormal neurophysiological functions.

Symptom frequencies were higher for exposed subjects than for unexposed for all 35 complaints. Neurobehavioral, irritative–respiratory, and general–vegetative symptoms were all statistically significant.

Large differences in respiratory symptoms between the groups were exemplified by 58% of the exposed subjects producing phlegm compared to 11.6% of unexposed. In addition, chronic bronchitis, shortness of breath at rest, walking, and climbing stairs, and wheezing and shortness of breath with wheezing were all significantly more frequent in the exposed subjects.

The rheumatic complaints that comprise the American Rheumatism Association's criteria for lupus erythematosus were all significantly more frequent in the exposed than in the unexposed except for seizures. Nearly 72% of the exposed groups had numb fingers, 44% had had pleurisy (pain on breathing), 38% had anemia, and 32% had had rheumatic pain. Comparison of numbers of exposed and unexposed subjects with five or more symptoms showed 18% vs. 0%, and with four symptoms 34% vs. 0.9% ($p < .0001$). Four or more symptoms comprise a presumptive diagnosis of lupus erythematosus (10, 41).

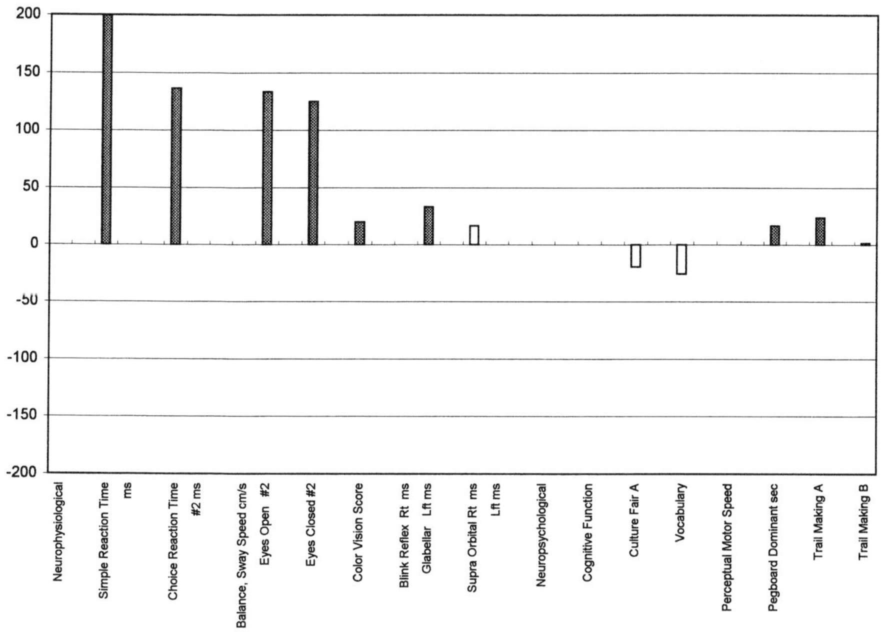

FIGURE 11.13. Comparison of 154 exposed adults and 112 unexposed adults (Oklahoma City) by ANOVA. Hatched bars are statistically significant.

TABLE 11.14 Comparison of blink reflex latency after glabellar and supraorbital tap of Tinker workers, Oklahoma City unexposed, and Arizona unexposed

	Exposed	Unexposed			
		Oklahoma	Arizona	p_1	p_2
Number	154	112	117	118	32
Glabellar Tap					
Right	15.8 ± 2.1	15.8 ± 1.5	14.5 ± 1.9	.77	.0000
Left	15.9 ± 1.8	15.3 ± 1.8	15.1 ± 1.8	.024	.0000
Supraorbital Tap					
Right	13.8 ± 1.8	13.5 ± 1.8	12.8 ± 2.1	.35	.0003
Left	13.8 ± 1.8	13.8 ± 1.8	12.9 ± 2.1	.97	.0000

p_1 values for comparison of exposed to unexposed.

p_2 values for comparison of both exposed and unexposed to AZ unexposed.

TABLE 11.15 Affective status as measured by the profile of mood states for Tinker workers and unexposed

	Exposed		Unexposed		
	154		112		
	Mean	Sd	Mean	Sd	*p*
POMS Score	83.0	42.4	14.5	28.2	0.000
Anger	20.0	11.3	7.3	7.0	0.000
Tension	19.3	7.9	7.7	5.6	0.000
Vigor	9.7	6.0	18.7	5.5	0.000
Confusion	13.8	6.1	4.9	3.5	0.000
Depression	21.2	13.3	6.2	7.9	0.000
Fatigue	18.3	6.4	7.2	5.6	0.000

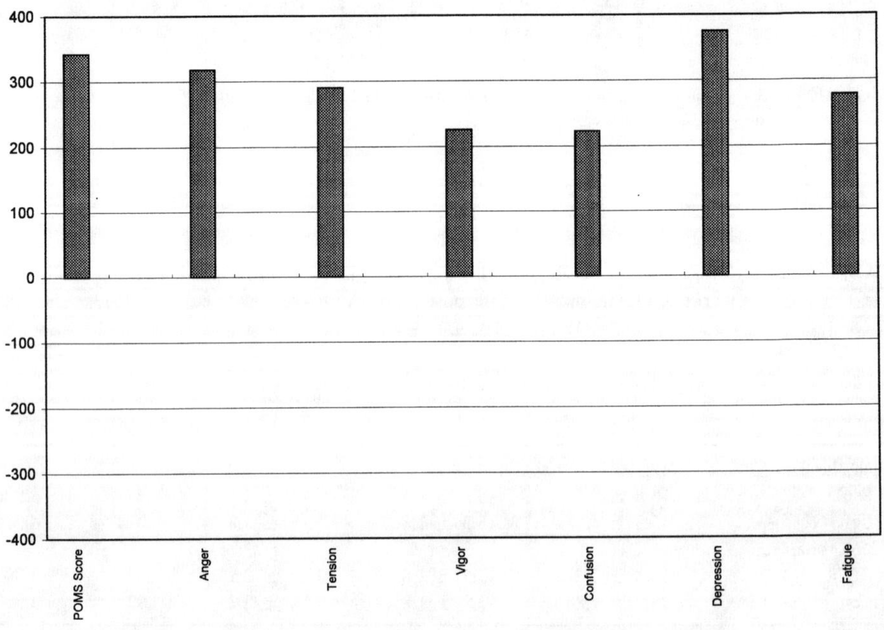

FIGURE 11.14. Profile of mood states for 154 exposed adults and 112 unexposed adults by ANOVA. Hatched bars are statistically significant.

Confounding

The prevalence of respiratory disorders, medical diseases, and the use of medication showed only small differences between the exposed and the unexposed subjects. Only angina pectoris was more common in the exposed. In contrast, use of alcohol, overdose with alcohol or with drugs, and use of marijuana and LSD were low and equal for the two groups. Comparison of the frequency of other historical factors that could possibly influence neurobehavioral performance, such as head injury, unconsciousness, hours of anesthesia, heart bypass surgery, and neurological illnesses, revealed that they were infrequent and not different between the groups. However, there were significant differences in past psychiatric illness, found in 13.6% of exposed vs. 4.5% of unexposed, and the prevalence of depression, in 12.3% of exposed and in 3.6% of unexposed; and 30.5% of exposed vs. 15.1% of unexposed had used tranquilizers. Tranquilizer use was examined as a possible confounder of neurobehavioral tests, but there were no significant differences between group mean values of tranquilizer users and nonusers in either exposed or unexposed subjects. Depression also showed no significant effects on neurobehavioral test scores and symptoms.

The exposed group had significantly more occupational exposures to metal refining solvents, aerospace adhesives, asbestos, and vibrating tools; but as these exposures reflected regular work assignments at Tinker, they were not confounders. Only one other exposure, to herbicides, was more prevalent in exposed, 4.5%, than in unexposed, 0.6%, but was so infrequent as not to affect analyses.

The finding of abnormally long blink reflex latencies in the Tinker AFB workers and in the local unexposed group was unexpected. This shows the usefulness of comparisons outside the region. The difference was appreciated by comparison to the Wickenburg, Arizona reference group. Blink was examined further by subdividing all subjects based on their city of residence. Thus, blink reflex latency, R-1, response times to a right supraorbital tap as mean values were compared by analysis of variance (ANOVA) for exposed and unexposed subjects in ten communities surrounding Tinker AFB. In Oklahoma City and Shawnee exposed subjects' R-1's were slower than those of unexposed, whereas in Del City, located immediately west of Tinker, the opposite was found; unexposed were significantly slower than exposed subjects. Only in Moore did unexposed and exposed subjects match with entirely normal latencies of 12.5 ms, which were statistically significantly lower than those in Oklahoma City, Del City, and Midwest City. This suggested either that Tinker workers from Moore had little exposure to chlorinated solvents, particularly TCE, and that Moore was away from environmental exposure to these chemicals; or that if all relevant chemical exposure was from environmental sources, Moore was not in the TCE exposure zone of the G-W aquifer.

Discussion

Jet engine repair workers had neurobehavioral impairment measured. In addition, they had excess prevalences of chronic bronchitis, shortness of breath, and other respiratory complaints. Also, their rheumatic and neurobehavioral symptoms and POMS scores exceeded those of unexposed subjects. Balance, simple and choice reaction time, blink reflex latency, and color discrimination were impaired in exposed subjects. Blink reflex latency, R-1, delay from chemicals usually indicates TCE toxicity (3, 5, 16). Psychiatric disorders, principally depression and the use of tranquilizer drugs, were significantly more common in the exposed subjects than the unexposed, and so are tentatively attributed to solvents because individual causes for them were absent.

The excessive frequency of chronic bronchitis, shortness of breath, and other respiratory symptoms, together with a reduced vital capacity, were diagnostic of industrial bronchitis. This diagnosis was made more plausible by the absence of radiographic evidence of parenchymal pulmonary diseases from hard metal (cobalt) (42, 43), manganese steel welding (44), or asbestos (45).

Excessive symptoms of a lupus-like rheumatic disorder were the third abnormality of the exposed group. One-third of them had four or more of these symptoms (20, 41). In the previous study of environmental trichloroethylene exposure in Tucson, symptomatic subjects also had greatly increased antinuclear antibody titers (7), thus fulfilling the ARA diagnostic criteria for lupus erythematosus (41). This aggregation of features of a lupus–scleroderma disorder has been identified previously in subjects exposed occupationally to TCE (46), vinyl chloride (47), and silicone breast implants (48) and after residential exposure to TCE (6).

Bias

Tester bias was minimized by withholding the exposure status of test subjects from the staff doing the examinations. That the tested subjects were volunteers has been thought possibly to bias questionnaire responses such as symptom frequencies and mood state scores; but as all subjects were volunteers, including those in reference group, such volunteer effects would be expected to cancel each other. Also, it is implausible that volunteer status would alter performance of balance, blink, and reaction time. It is unlikely that groupwide bias affects subconscious and automatic responses such as blink and balance. Also, it is nearly impossible to fake impairment of performance of physiological tests. Being plaintiffs in a lawsuit has been considered by some (23, 28, 29, 49) to increase the frequency of symptoms and of negative moods; but this conjecture was based on instructed responses of college students in introductory psychology courses to imaginary situations, not the responses of chemically exposed workers or bystanders.

Instead, consider the plausibly of increased depression, other psychiatric illnesses, and tranquilizer use as effects of chemicals. This idea is more logical than believing that an unknown nonchemical stimulus had operated in parallel and impinged only on the chemically exposed individuals to impair them and produce complaints. Absence of stressful events in their individual work or personal histories effectively ruled out post-traumatic stress syndrome. Thus, frequent psychological disorders, neurobehavioral impairment, upset mood status, and high symptom frequencies are more plausibly associated with chemical exposures than anything else. Confounding due to seeing, hearing, or reading news media reports is also unlikely, as this problem engendered little or no publicity (49).

Conclusion

It appeared that these abnormalities were related to chlorinated solvents used in jet engine repair by the exposed subjects but not by the unexposed. These neurotoxic chemicals include trichloroethylene, tetrachloroethylene, and other metal cleaning solvents, and 1,1,1-trichloroethane, the main solvent in adhesives. The abnormalities of blink, balance, and reaction time suggest trichloroethylene as the most important neurotoxin. Hopefully, these findings will bring about monitoring of current workplace levels of solvents, historical reconstruction of exposures, and follow-up evaluations of these subjects to add to the certainty of this attribution.

In contrast to the solvent etiology of neurotoxic effects, the industrial chronic bronchitis and the shortness of breath with wheezing, especially on exertion, are tentatively attributed to welding and grinding of stainless steel, producing respirable particles containing cobalt, manganese, chromium, and nickel. Solvent inhalation can also irritate and injure airways (1).

This causal hypothesis should explain the neurophysiological impairment, the mood disorder, and the excessive frequency of symptoms. Trichloroethylene is the most powerful neurotoxic agent in this workplace and has adversely affected environmentally exposed populations (5, 14, 19). The similarity of abnormality of blink measurements in exposed workers and in local unexposed might argue against TCE exposure; but as they are both abnormal, chemical exposure of the unexposed is suggested because their blink reflex latencies were significantly prolonged as compared to all of our unexposed groups (22, 33), which have virtually identical blink measurements. Thus the blink R-1 of the Tinker exposed group and of the reference group were delayed in reference to all unexposed groups. The best explanation is that delayed blink reflex latency is due to trichloroethylene (16)-type solvents. Solvents may have migrated from the Tinker Superfund site and other sources to contaminate the Gerber-Wellington aquifer and affect blink reflexes over a broad zone. Tetrachloroethylene and 1,1,1-trichloroethane (1) are related chemically and considered together with TCE. Manganese toxicity (43) and the use of vibrating tools cannot be ruled out as contributing to the neurobehavioral impairment of these workers. Prolonged low level exposure to hydrogen sulfide from surrounding oil wells and refineries seems unlikely (33).

To narrow the choices for causal attribution, patterns of water use and of TCE concentrations in this aquifer and airborne levels of hydrogen sulfide from crude oil recovery and refining plus distributions of other chemicals should be sought. Mapping the zones of neurotoxic effects and the plumes of TCE, H_2S, and other chemicals should be a priority.

STUDY 4: COMMUNITY IN THE MUSCLE SHOALS, ALABAMA ENVIRONS

Two chemicals appeared to contribute to effects at Muscle Shoals. Neighbors living south and west of an aluminum die-casting plant that had begun operations in 1956 had noted sour well water by 1970 to 1971. Analyses of water showed volatile organic chemicals (VOCs) and hydrogen sulfide. The VOCs included methylene chloride, trichloroethylene (TCE), chloroform, toluene, dichloroethene, trichloroethene, tetrachloroethene, and bromofluorobenzene. In addition, levels of polychlorinated biphenyls (PCBs) were up to 3,500 ppm. Up to 100,000 gallons per year of PCBs had been mixed with ethylene glycol for hydraulic fluid in aluminum die-casting machines for 17 years, beginning in 1956. Multiple analyses of well water showed variable high levels of organic chemical PCBs, and solvent concentrations differing by one to two orders of magnitude among samples. Cyanide and arsenic were also detected. By 1990 many neighbors of the die-casting plant had developed headaches, numbness or tingling of the hands and feet, dizziness, blurred vision, staggering gait or loss of balance, abnormal heartbeat, excessive sweating, and depression. Such symptoms and many cancer deaths stirred the concern of residents in the neighborhood, just as they have at other toxic waste sites (10, 14, 19, 49). This pattern of symptoms led to measurements of neurobehavioral performance of an age-stratified random sample of the survivors, who included 169 men and 186 women, in June 1992. They had filed a class action lawsuit.

Exposed Population

The design matched 63 women and 54 men between the ages of 15 and 71 years in the exposed group with a recruited unexposed population of 27 women and 19 men, a ratio of 2.5 : 1. The exposed participants were an age-stratified random sample selected from over 355 residents who had furnished medical histories and were plaintiffs in a lawsuit. They and the unexposed were African-Americans. Approximately 80% of persons who resided within 2.4 km west and southwest of the site for at least 4 years were in this group. Thus the 117 study subjects were representative of the population exposed between 1956 and 1981, and most still lived there. Subgroups were defined as near (less than 1.5 km) or far from (more than 1.5 km) the plant center (Figure 11.15). Duration of exposure was calculated as years of residence for each subject. The unexposed group were persons from Russellville, Alabama (in Franklin County, 30 km distant) and surrounding towns, who were recruited to match the exposed group for sex, age, and years of educational attainment, and for absence of employment at the

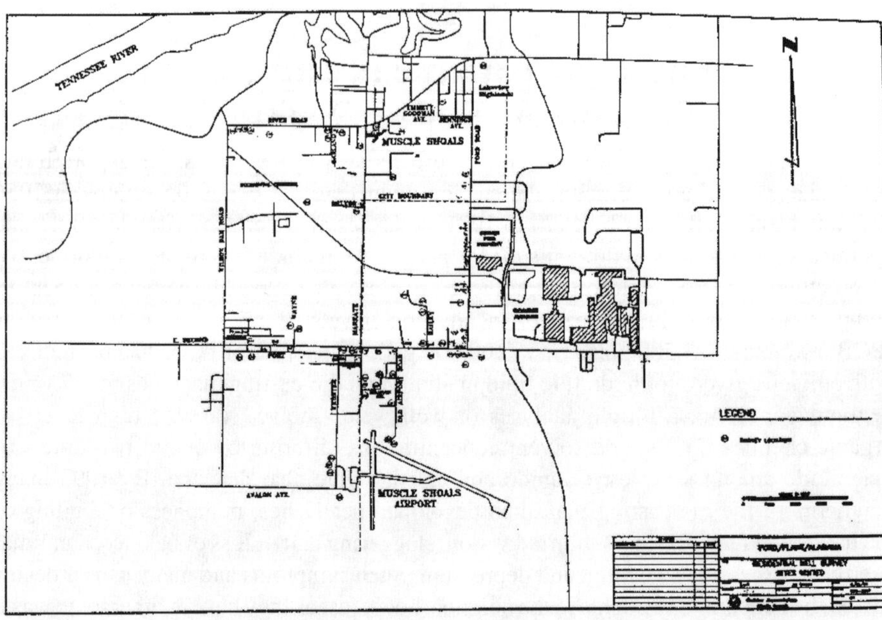

FIGURE 11.15. Muscle Shoals community. The map shows, by numbered circles, residences with wells in the vicinity of the casting plant. Most subjects lived west or southwest. Distances were measured from the center of the plant.

TABLE 11.16 Neurophysiological and neuropsychological test results and profile of mood states scores for 117 Muscle Shoals exposed and 46 unexposed subjects: means and standard deviations with t-tests

	Exposed	MS Unexposed		National Unexposed	NR-R	NR-Exp
	M Sd	M Sd	p	M Sd	p	p
NEUROPHYSIOLOGICAL						
Simple Reaction Time ms	355 ± 130	324 ± 138	NS	281 + 55	.005	.0000
Choice Reaction Time ms 1	644 ± 163	556 ± 134	.0015			
2	654 ± 149	585 ± 116	.006			
3	642 ± 155	597 ± 157	.09	524 + 86	.0002	.0000
Av	647 ± 146	579 ± 130	.007			
Sway Speed Eyes Open cm/s	1.08 ± 0.40	0.92 ± 0.25	.014	.87 + 0.22	NS	.0000
Eyes Closed cm/s	1.50 ± 0.71	1.27 ± 0.36	.034	1.31 + 0.57	NS	.02
Color (Hue) score 1st	12.8 ± 6.4	12.3 ± 6.0	NS	11.4 + 1.6	NS	NS
Best	12.9 ± 7.0	12.5 ± 6.3	NS			
Blink Reflex R-1 ms Right	15.7 ± 1.9	14.4 ± 1.9	.004	14.4 ± 1.9	NS	.0000
Left	16.7 ± 2.0	15.7 ± 1.6	.003	14.6 ± 2.1	.016	.0000
NEUROPSYCHOLOGICAL						
Cognitive						
Culture Fair A score	20.9 ± 7.3	20.8 ± 7.1	NS	29.3 ± 8.3	.0000	.0000
Block Design score	16.9 ± 10.0	16.5 ± 9.7	NS	30.0 ± 10.4	.0000	.0000
Digit Symbol score	46.7 ± 16.3	47.4 ± 16.5	NS	55.7 ± 15.1	.007	.0003
Embedded Figures	26.4 ± 6.0	26.5 ± 6.0	NS	31.2 ± 5.2	.000	.0000
Finger Writing Errors Right	4.2 ± 3.6	4.7 ± 4.0	NS	2.5 ± 2.7	.0000	.0000
Left	3.6 ± 3.6	3.6 ± 4.0	NS	2.2 ± 2.7	.002	.0007
Psychomotor Speed						
Pegboard score	82.4 ± 21.4	83.4 ± 29.3	NS	74.6 ± 20.0	.03	.005
Trails A	47.2 ± 23.0	44.2 ± 21.5	NS	33.8 ± 14.1	.0004	.0000
Errors	0.37 ± 0.69	0.39 ± 0.74	NS	0.35 ± 0.77	NS	NS
Trails B	104.6 ± 44.3	93.2 ± 42.4	NS	74.9 ± 44.3	.0175	.0000
Errors	1.38 ± 2.04	1.1 ± 1.7	NS	0.61 ± 1.13	NS	.0004
Recall (Wechsler Memory Scale)						
Story 1	9.2 ± 3.5	9.6 ± 3.3	NS	11.0 ± 3.9	.036	.0003
Story 2	9.6 ± 3.7	9.5 ± 3.2	NS	10.4 ± 3.2	NS	NS
Visual Reproduction						
Immediate	29.2 ± 6.6	29.4 ± 7.1	NS	34.6 ± 7.6	.005	.0001
Delayed	21.1 ± 9.5	23.8 ± 9.5	NS	26.2 ±		
Digits Forward	6.3 ± 1.5	6.6 ± 1.3	NS	6.7 ± 1.4	NS	.06
Backward	3.9 ± 1.2	4.0 ± 1.1	NS	4.6 ± 1.2	.005	.005
Overlearned Memory						
Information score	12.8 ± 4.6	13.2 ± 5.5	NS	17.8 ± 5.8	.0000	.0000
Picture Completion	11.1 ± 4.1	11.3 ± 3.9	NS	14.7 ± 3.3	.0000	.0000
Similarities	14.7 ± 5.9	16.0 ± 5.2	NS	20.0 ± 5.1	.0000	.0000
Profile of Mood States						
POMS score	38.3 ± 38.5	18.1 ± 24.2	.001	16.8 ± 28.4	NS	.0000
Tension	12.2 ± 7.3	8.6 ± 5.0	.002	8.9 ± 6.6		
Depression	12.0 ± 12.1	7.2 ± 7.1	.013	8.1 ± 9.7		
Anger	10.6 ± 9.9	6.4 ± 6.0	.009	9.2 ± 8.8		
Vigor	14.6 ± 5.8	17.7 ± 6.3	.003	17.8 ± 6.5		
Fatigue	9.1 ± 6.6	7.3 ± 4.9	.09	7.7 ± 6.3		
Confusion	9.0 ± 5.2	6.4 ± 4.1	.003	6.3 ± 4.5		

site or living within 8 km of the site at any time. Participants had a donation made in their name to a charity. Examiners were blinded as to the exposure status of the subjects. National unexposed were 118 subjects from the matched cohorts of investigations in Louisiana, Wyoming, and California and included Caucasian, Cajun, and Latino participants (22, 33).

Testing of Subjects

The ages, educational attainment, average high school grades, heights, and weights of exposed and unexposed men and women were similar (Table 11.16, Figures 11.16a–c). The exposed group had significantly *higher* family incomes for the past 3 years than did the unexposed. Alveolar air alcohol levels were below .03 μg/dL in all subjects of both groups. Grip strength was greater in unexposed than exposed women but not different in men. More of the unexposed group (83%) than the exposed group (69%) had been occupationally exposed to 15 potential neurotoxicants (Table 11.17), with an overall effect of narrowing the group difference and decreasing the apparent effects of

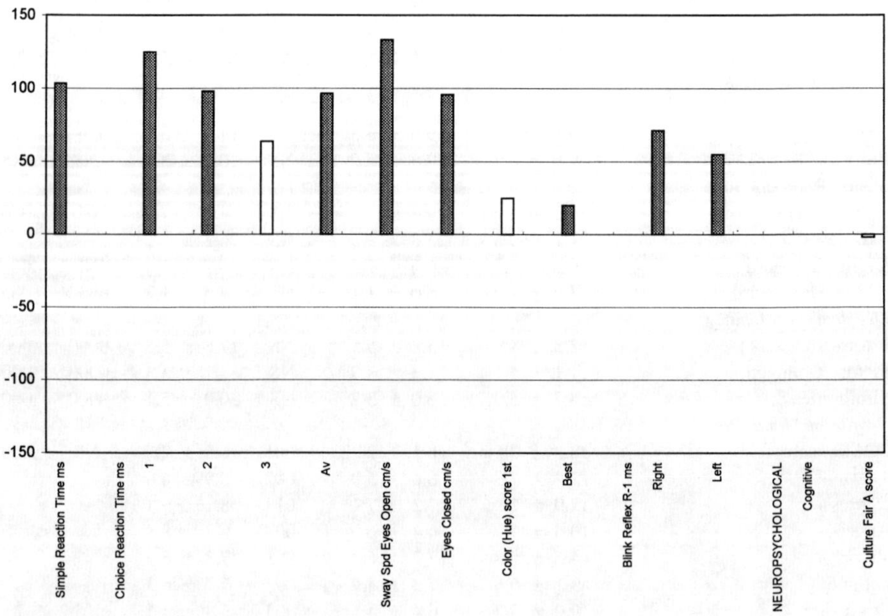

FIGURE 11.16a. Comparison of 117 exposed adults and 46 unexposed adults by ANOVA (Muscle Shoals). Hatched bars are statistically significant.

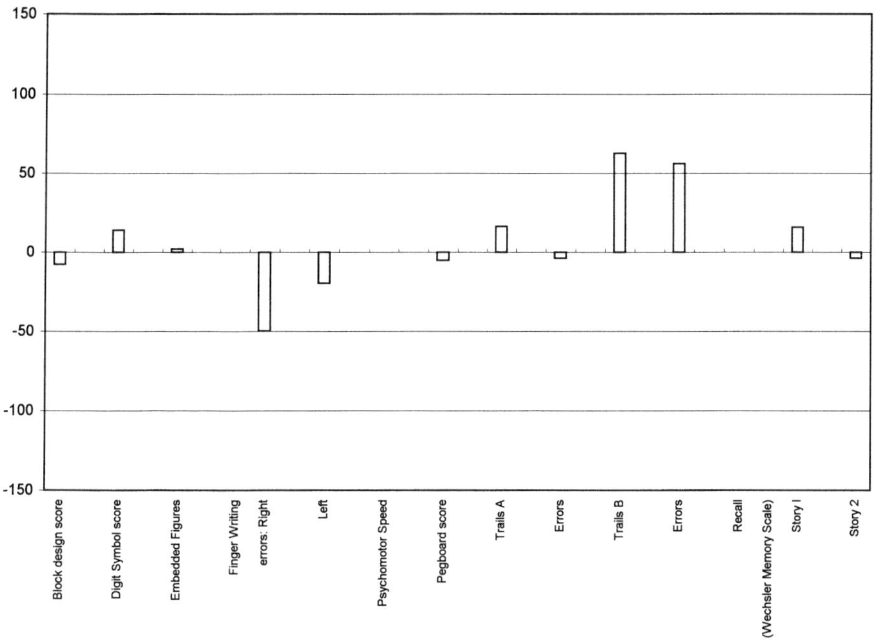

FIGURE 11.16b. Comparison of 117 exposed adults and 46 unexposed adults by ANOVA (Muscle Shoals). Hatched bars are statistically significant.

the residential exposure. Each of the 15 occupational exposure groups was too small for separate comparison, but the aggregate was too large to be eliminated from the analysis. However, elimination of subjects in each occupational exposure group from exposed and unexposed groups, in turn, did not alter significantly their differences for any neurophysiological test.

The questionnaire data showed significantly more ARA lupus erythematosus symptoms ($p < .0004$) among the exposed group than the unexposed (Table 11.18, Figure 11.17). Also, the proportions of arthritis or rheumatism lasting for more than 3 months, Raynaud's phenomena, malar rashes, photosensitive skin, and hair loss were significantly higher in the exposed, with increases in oral sores and proteinuria approaching significance. Chronic bronchitis, shortness of breath at rest and walking, wheezing alone and with dyspnea, and abnormal heart rhythm were all more frequent in the exposed subjects than the unexposed (Figure 11.18). Depression and use of tranquilizers were also more common in the exposed. In contrast, the exposed and the unexposed groups did not differ in their prevalences of cigarette smoking, use of marijuana and stimulant or depressant drugs, and use of therapeutic drugs. Slightly higher proportions

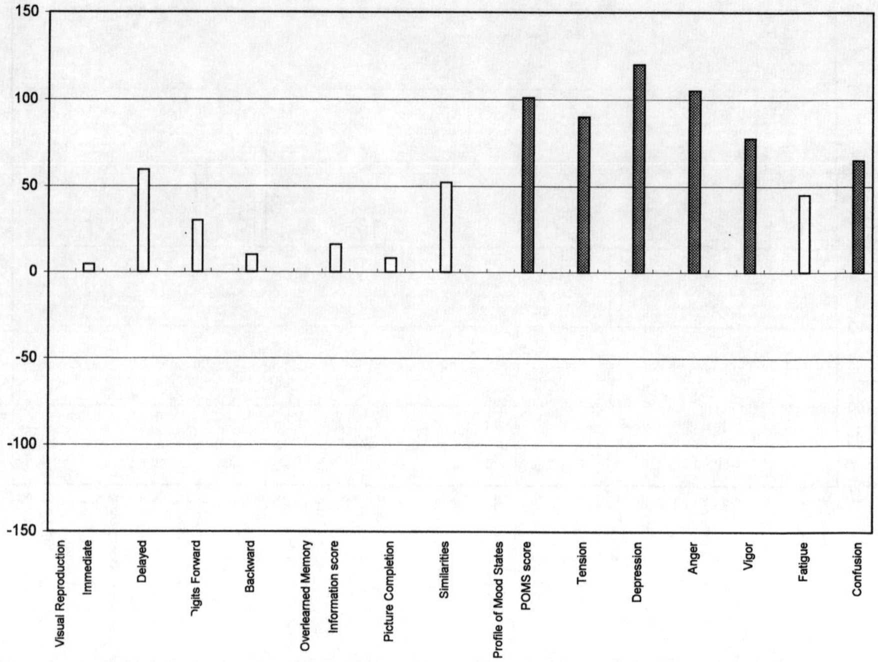

FIGURE 11.16c. Comparison of 117 exposed adults and 46 unexposed adults by ANOVA (Muscle Shoals). Hatched bars are statistically significant.

of exposed than unexposed worked in industries with exposure to chemicals. Also, prevalences of cancer, leukemia/lymphoma, allergies, and asthma were similar.

The neurophysiological tests showed that exposed compared to Muscle Shoals (local) unexposed were impaired for choice reaction time; for balance as sway speed tracked at the head and by a force platform, and thus measured at the feet, with the eyes open and with the eyes closed; and for blink reflex latency R-1 (Table 11.16). Color (hue) discrimination was different. Comparisons to national unexposed (Table 11.16), half of whom were from a small town in southeastern Louisiana, increased the apparent abnormality of the exposed subjects for choice reaction time, sway speed and force, and blink reflex latency. In addition, the test means of the Alabama *unexposed group* were abnormal for reaction time and blink reflex latency when compared to our national unexposed group (Table 11.16, Figures 11.19a–c). The neuropsychological tests showed that trail making B was significantly more impaired in exposed than unexposed women but not in men, and scores for the Muscle Shoals unexposed group were significantly worse than predictions. Comparing the exposed group to the national unexposed group also showed greater abnormality for cognitive function, tested by Culture Fair,

TABLE 11.17 Occupational exposures of Muscle Shoals exposed and unexposed groups

	Exposed 117	Unexposed 46
Power plant	9	2
Refinery	0	4
Metal refining	17	4
Explosives	6	1
Chemicals	6	6
Dyes	8	4
Rubber–plastics	9	2
Dry cleaning	6	0
Textiles	1	7
Photography lab	3	1
Solvents	6	5
Aerospace	1	0
Rocket fuel	1	1
Pesticides	3	1
Herbicides	5	0
% Exposed to 15 processes	69	83
(Vibrating tools)	18	7
(Asbestos)	10	4

block designs, and errors in fingertip number writing, than found in comparison to local unexposed subjects. Similarly there were differences for pegboard and trail making A and trail making B performances that were not seen with comparison to the local unexposed group. Also, there were significant differences between exposed subjects and local unexposed when compared to national unexposed for overlearned memory tested by information, picture completion, and similarities from the WAIS. For verbal recall (Wechsler stories 1 and 2), visual reproduction and digits forward and backward there was a consistent pattern, with the national group's performance exceeding that of both Muscle Shoals (exposed and unexposed) groups. These differences are not due to educational attainment, age, or sex when tested in regression models.

The affective status as measured by the profile of mood states showed significantly higher mean scores in the exposed than unexposed subjects (Table 11.16, Figure 11.16c). In addition, exposed subjects' individual scores for depression, anger, confusion, and tension were significantly higher and vigor significantly lower, but fatigue was not different, compared to unexposed. Scores for the local matched unexposed and the national unexposed were nearly identical in these categories. The symptom inventories showed higher frequencies of all symptoms in the exposed, and 30 of the 34 differences were statistically significant (Table 11.19, Figures 11.20a,b). These symptom frequencies confirmed and extended the symptom prevalences recorded earlier from the entire plaintiff group.

Reproductive histories showed that similar proportions of women had been pregnant and had had still births, miscarriages, and abortions (Table 11.20). The 61 exposed women reported 13 children with birth defects, compared to none in the 27 unexposed women.

TABLE 11.18 Prevalence of symptoms of lupus including arthritis, cardiopulmonary disorders, respiratory depression, smoking, drug use, and cancer in muscle shoals and unexposed groups

	Percentage		
	Exposed	Unexposed	*p*
Lupus Erythematosus Criteria	24	13	*
Arthritis or rheumatism 3 months	42	29	
Raynaud's	64	43	*
Oral sores	7	0	+
Low blood count	45	39	
Malar rash	14	2	*
Photosensitive skin	16	2	*
Pleurisy	21	11	
Proteinuria	11	2	+
Hair loss	19	2	*
Seizure	5	0	
Cardiopulmonary Disorders			
Chronic bronchitis	15.4	2	*
Shortness of breath			
Resting	24	0	*
Walking level ground	36	17.4	*
Climbing two flights	58	43.5	
Wheezing	27	6.5	*
With shortness of breath	21	10.9	*
Abnormal heart rhythm	16.2	4.1	*
Others			
Any psychiatric illness	5.1	0	
Depression	13.7	2.2	*
Tranquilizers	11	2.2	*
Leukemia, lymphoma	2.6	2.2	
Cancer	4.2	6.5	
Therapeutic drugs	6.8	0	
Cigarette smoking	44	35	
Marijuana, stimulants, depressants	8.5	4.3	

* Different by chi sq $p < 0.05$; $+p < 0.07$.

Associations of Exposure Surrogates and Effects

Neither distance from the site nor duration of residence had significant coefficients when entered as independent variables with age into regression models for tests that differed between exposed and unexposed subjects (50). Thus in this group two of the common surrogates suggested for exposure lacked discriminatory power.

Discussion

The neurophysiological tests showed solidly different (poorer) performances for the exposed, which were well below those of local unexposed and national unexposed (22, 31) including subjects from a neighboring state (22). Mood scores and symptom frequencies were significantly elevated in the exposed subjects. Only women were abnormal for trail making B, which has been the most sensitive of the neuropsychological tests for detecting the effects of exposure to solvent mixtures containing trichloroethylene (TCE) (6) and other organic solvents and to dibenzofurans (32). Women generally

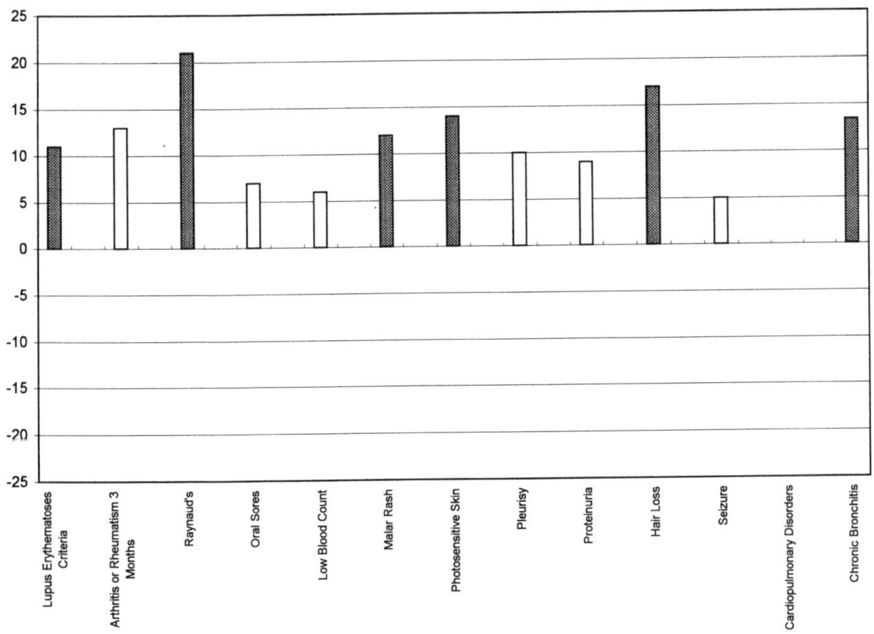

FIGURE 11.17. Comparison of symptoms of lupus erythematosus and others in 117 exposed adults and 46 unexposed adults by ANOVA (Muscle Shoals). Hatched bars are statistically significant.

spend more hours per week at their residence (because of homemaking) than do men. An abnormal blink reflex latency has been characteristic of TCE exposure, having been observed in populations so exposed at Woburn, Massachusetts (5) and Tucson, Arizona (6). The significantly higher proportion of exposed subjects with depression, with any psychiatric diagnosis, and with abnormal heart rhythms may reflect effects of exposure compared to unexposed. The most plausible interpretation of the findings is that they reflect long-term residential exposure to TCE and other organic chemicals, especially solvents, that leaked into groundwater from the die-casting plant and its evaporative ponds. Because PCBs were used in hydraulic fluid of the die-casting machines and presently contaminate exposed subjects' wells, it is highly probable that dibenzofurans are contributing to the neurotoxicity in these subjects (51). Commercial-grade PCBs such as Aroclor 1254 and 1260 contain polychlorinated dibenzofurans as impurities (52). The above PCBs and Aroclor 1248 are transformed at temperatures of 270°C to 300°C into polychlorinated dibenzofurans (51–54). These temperatures would be reached in hydraulic die machines heated by molten aluminum (660°C).

Toxic neurophysiological effects were deduced from the observation that choice

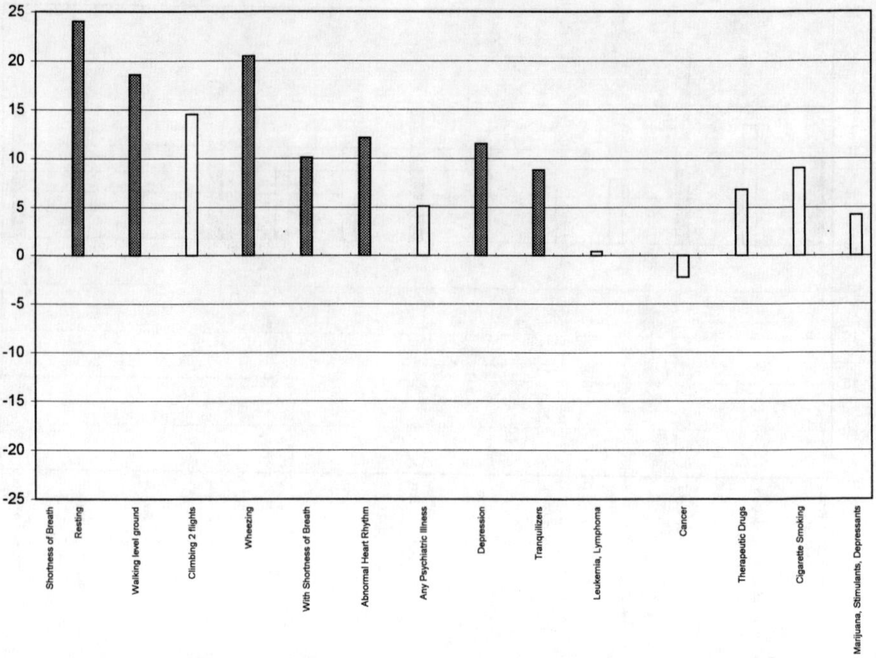

FIGURE 11.18. Comparison of respiratory symptoms and other factors in 117 exposed adults and 46 unexposed adults by ANOVA (Muscle Shoals). Hatched bars are statistically significant.

reaction time, sway speed, and blink reflex latency were impaired in exposed subjects compared to unexposed. Each of these tests reflects a major integrated performance of the central nervous system. Sway speed of the trunk, measured either at the head or as a force vector measured at the feet, depends on peripheral proprioceptors and vestibular apparatus, integrative control by the cerebellum, and eye integrative paths and is executed by balance effectors. Choice reaction time involves receptors in the eye, pathways to the optical cortex, cortical decision making, and motor (parietal cortex) effectors. Blink, in contrast, has a trigeminal receptor and afferent transmission to the pons for both uncrossed and crossed responses. The motor response is via the facial nerves. In the past, blink latency as delay of R-1 has been considered specific for TCE effects (5), but several other chemicals act similarly (see Chapter 4). Of the chemicals known to be at this site, chlorinated solvents are most probably responsible for the delay of blink R-1.

Possible confounding occupational or personal exposures to neurotoxins and the presence of neurological or systemic diseases or of brain-function-damaging influences, such as alcohol, drugs, head trauma with unconsciousness, or anesthesia, were uncom-

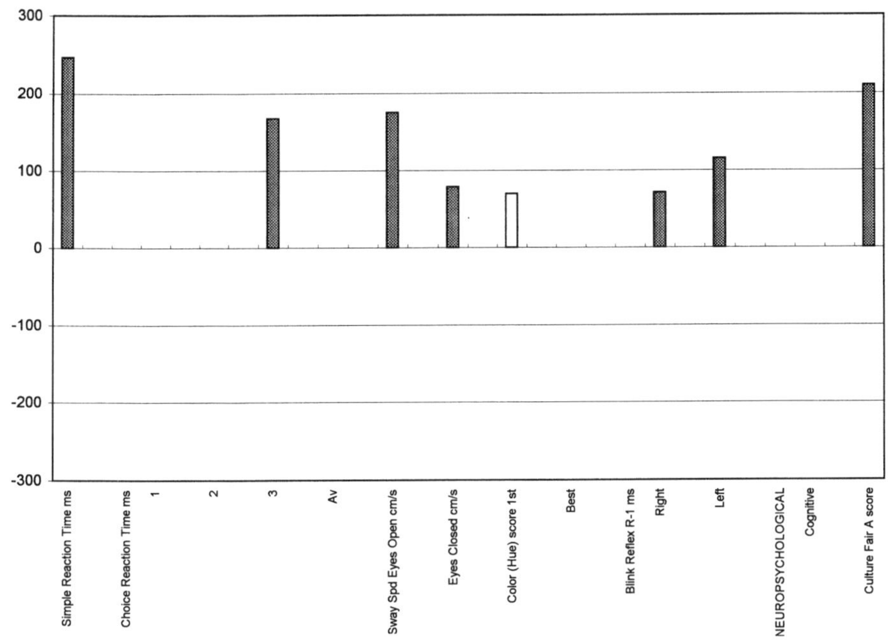

FIGURE 11.19a. Comparison of 117 exposed adults (Muscle Shoals) and 68 unexposed adults (national referents) by ANOVA. Hatched bars are statistically significant.

mon and not different between the groups. Exposures to occupational neurotoxicants were higher in the local unexposed subjects. POMS scores were higher in exposed than unexposed subjects but were not so elevated as in other exposed groups (6, 22, 31). Individual test scores were not affected by mood as measured by POMS scores.

Low scores on psychological tests and the "blunted" affect scores of both exposed and unexposed raise speculation about some overriding influence modulating the effects of exposure to index chemicals in these northwestern Alabama people. Categorization of the unexposed from Russellville as rural is questionable, as it has a population of about 4,000. Also, whether Muscle Shoals is truly urban is uncertain despite its census status of being part of a population center of 50,000. Actual "way of life" differences between these sites appear small. Jobs are much more frequently industrial than farming, but we found no evidence for a shared exposure factor that could have lowered scores of both groups. However, the fact that the unexposed group scores were below national reference scores was associated with rural residence and lower income. To ascertain whether family income was a determinant of performance scores of exposed subjects or unexposed, family incomes were inserted as independent variables with and without

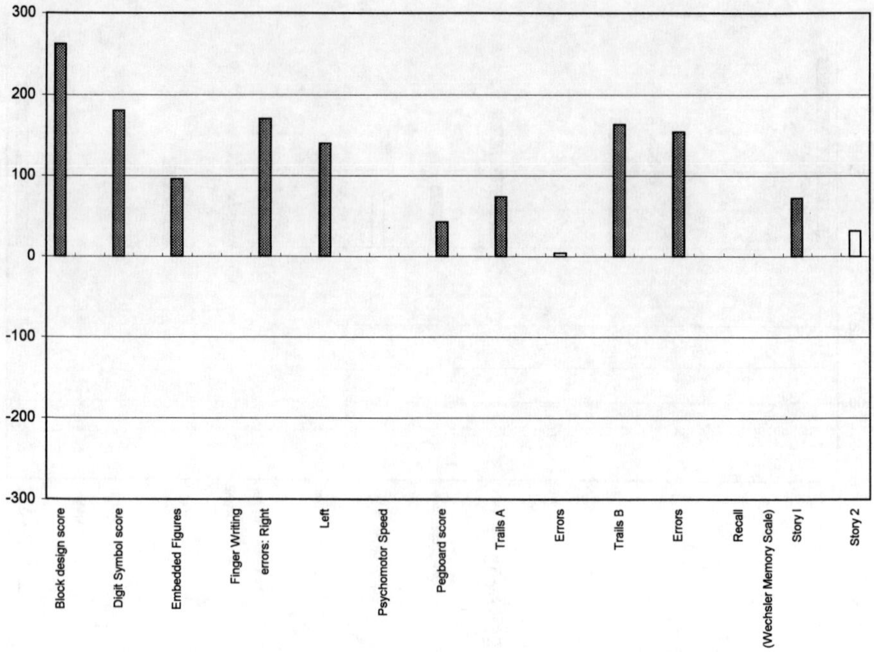

FIGURE 11.19b. Comparison of 117 exposed adults (Muscle Shoals) and 68 unexposed adults (national referents) by ANOVA. Hatched bars are statistically significant.

age in regression equations for choice reaction time, sway speed with eyes open and with eyes closed, blink reflex latency, Culture Fair A score, pegboard score, block design score, and trail making B. In no instance did income have a significant coefficient for a performance score.

A final question was, why were the rural unexposed scores on many of the standard neuropsychological tests below those of other unexposed and not different from those of the exposed group? This shift of scores downward in the local unexposed psychological tests, despite a clear separation on the neurophysiological tests, could be due to an adverse cofactor. However, there are two obvious differences: (1) the local unexposed were, by census category, rural compared to the urban status for the exposed group; (2) unlike the national unexposed, these unexposed and exposed subjects were African-Americans. Rural–urban differences on standard psychological tests that are not explained by educational attainment are well known (55, 56). Perhaps this unexposed group was the residue of selection manifested as migration north and to cities. Such differences are also attributed to poorer opportunity for education and life experience

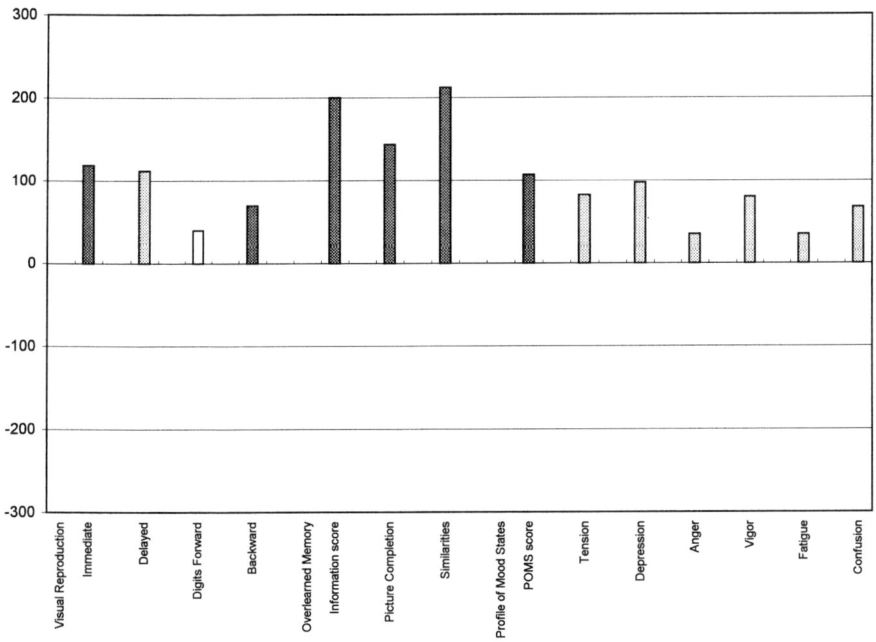

FIGURE 11.19c. Comparison of 117 exposed adults (Muscle Shoals) and 68 unexposed adults (national referents) by ANOVA. Hatched bars are statistically significant.

for those left behind, a rural population who may have less capacity to succeed in tests of mental ability (56, 57). These considerations would not be expected to affect the timed (physiological) performances of blink, balance as speed of sway, and visual two-choice reaction time, and they did not.

TRICHLOROETHYLENE: SUMMARY AND GENERAL CONCLUSIONS

1. TCE was associated with adverse effects on neurobehavioral function in four cross-sectional epidemiological investigations.

TABLE 11.19 Frequency of 34 symptoms compared by ANOVA of means in Muscle Shoals and unexposed

Symptom	Exposed (117)	Unexposed (46)	*p*
Skin	36.8 ± 29.9	23.3 ± 28.5	.0091
Fingernail changes	21.5 ± 27.8	6.9 ± 11.0	.0007
Chest tightness	25.0 ± 23.6	11.1 ± 14.3	.0003
Palpitations	17.8 ± 20.9	8.0 ± 12.7	.0036
Chest burning	23.7 ± 23.6	11.1 ± 14.2	.0009
Shortness of breath	31.9 ± 26.4	18.1 ± 20.9	.0018
Dry cough	27.0 ± 25.0	13.7 ± 17.4	.0012
Cough with mucus	27.0 ± 25.7	16.8 ± 20.1	.0172
Cough with blood	8.6 ± 13.9	5.3 ± 9.7	.1445
Dry mouth/nose/throat	25.8 ± 26.2	17.1 ± 19.5	.0422
Eye irritation	35.5 ± 30.0	19.6 ± 25.2	.0018
Reduced sense of smell	20.1 ± 23.7	11.4 ± 16.6	.0239
Headache	42.8 ± 29.8	32.3 ± 23.6	.0338
Nausea	23.7 ± 22.5	13.1 ± 14.8	.0039
Dizziness	31.9 ± 25.0	12.9 ± 16.6	.0000
Lightheadedness	28.4 ± 25.3	13.4 ± 17.1	.0003
Unusual exhilaration	10.9 ± 15.6	7.0 ± 12.5	.1400
Loss of balance	24.1 ± 23.7	14.9 ± 19.6	.0212
Loss of consciousness	9.2 ± 12.7	4.4 ± 7.9	.0183
Extreme fatigue	32.8 ± 28.0	19.8 ± 21.7	.0055
Somnolence	28.2 ± 30.2	16.5 ± 23.1	.0191
Insomnia			
Cannot fall asleep	24.1 ± 25.1	12.9 ± 16.9	.0061
Wake frequently	31.5 ± 26.2	14.8 ± 21.8	.0002
Sleep few hours	31.4 ± 28.6	13.7 ± 19.2	.0002
Irritability	39.5 ± 28.8	16.8 ± 21.5	.0000
Lack of concentration	39.0 ± 30.5	19.0 ± 22.0	.0000
Recent memory loss	33.8 ± 29.5	19.0 ± 21.4	.0023
Long-term memory loss	25.3 ± 26.5	15.0 ± 20.4	.0177
Instability of mood	27.0 ± 28.9	12.0 ± 20.1	.0016
Decreased libido	26.2 ± 28.9	16.7 ± 22.6	.0476
Dec. alcohol tolerance	17.9 ± 28.7	11.4 ± 21.3	.1705
Indigestion	31.5 ± 25.8	17.9 ± 20.9	.0018
Loss of appetite	18.9 ± 21.2	15.0 ± 18.2	.2721
Bloating			
All	29.2 ± 26.9	17.6 ± 21.9	.0098
Women	32.1 ± 27.1	18.4 ± 22.7	.0007

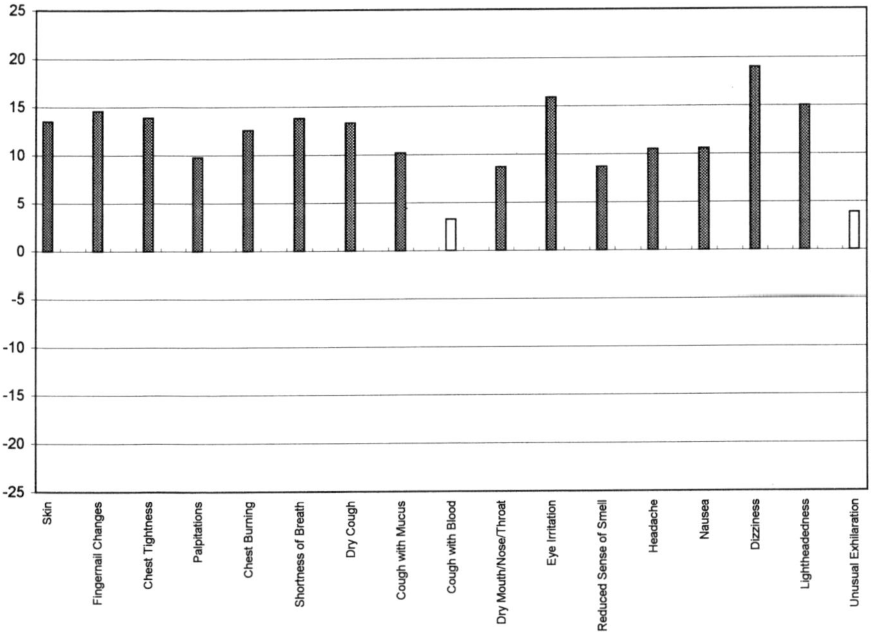

FIGURE 11.20a. Comparison of symptom frequencies of 117 exposed adults (Muscle Shoals) and 46 unexposed adults by ANOVA. Hatched bars are statistically significant.

TABLE 11.20 Reproductive histories of Muscle Shoals exposed and unexposed women

	Exposed (61)	Unexposed (27)
Ever pregnant	84%	77%
Pregnant now	.033 (2)	.037 (1)
Ever had a miscarriage, stillbirth, or abortion	18%	26%
Child with birth defect	14%	0

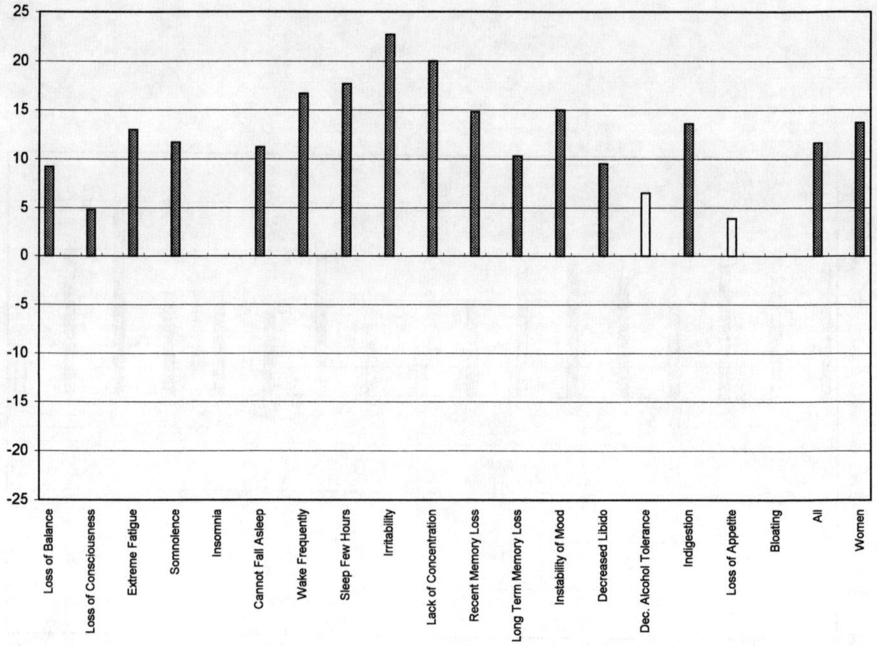

FIGURE 11.20b. Comparison of symptom frequencies of 117 exposed adults (Muscle Shoals) and 46 unexposed adults by ANOVA. Hatched bars are statistically significant.

2. Groundwater spread of TCE was the cause of human exposure and ill effects as perceived in these examples. One group had occupational TCE exposure.
3. Adverse effects have not reversed and appear to be permanent (Phoenix retest group Oct.–Dec. 1991).
4. These observations show effects from low concentrations over several years, perhaps punctuated by brief peaks of exposure.
5. Other chemicals such as PCBs or chlorinated aliphatics may contribute to the impairment that was measured and attributed mainly to TCE.
6. Amelioration, as practiced in capping wells, and diverting water in Tucson and Phoenix had no measurable beneficial benefit (Phoenix subjects in the 1957–83 exposure zone only after the 1983 amelioration still show impaired function).

Future Considerations

There are several unanswered questions:

1. Are adverse TCE effects permanent?
2. Do the adverse effects continue to worsen with aging if exposure ceases? Are they additive or synergistic to aging effects?

3. Can these effects or the course be modified by treatment?
4. Do exposures to other chemicals influence TCE effects?

References

1. Davidson IWF and Beliles RP: Consideration of the target organ toxicity of trichloroethylene in terms of metabolite toxicity and pharmacokinetics. *Drug Metab Rev* 1991;23 (5&6): 493–599.
2. Bergman K: Whole-body autoradiography and allied tracer techniques in distribution and elimination studies of some organic solvents. *Scand J Work Environ Health* 1979;5 (Suppl. 1).
3. Feldman RG: Trichlorethylene. In: *Handbook of Clinical Neurology,* PJ Vinken and GW Bruyn (eds.). New York: North-Holland Publishing Co., 1979, pp. 457–464.
4. Ruijten MWMM, Verberk MM, and Salle HJA: Nerve function in workers with long term exposure to trichloroethene. *Brit J Indust Med* 1991;48:87–92.
5. Feldman RG, Chirico-Post J, and Proctor SP: Blink reflex latency after exposure to trichloroethylene in well water. *Arch Environ Health* 1988;43:143–148.
6. Kilburn KH and Warshaw RH. Effects on neurobehavioral performance of chronic exposure to chemically contaminated well water. *Intl J Toxicol Indust Health* 1993;9:391–404.
7. Kilburn KH and Warshaw RH: Prevalence of symptoms of systemic lupus erythematosus (SLE) and of fluorescent antinuclear antibodies associated with chronic exposure to trichloroethylene and other chemicals in well water. *Environ Res* 1992;57:1–9.
8. Goldberg SJ, Lebowitz MD, Graver EJ, and Hicks S: An association of human congenital cardiac malformations and drinking water contaminants. *J Am Coll Cardiol* 1990;16: 155–164.
9. Arizona Department of Environmental Quality (ADEG): Ground water hydrology. East Washington Area, July 13, 1993. Sampled Oct.–Dec. 1992.
10. Levine R and Chitwood DD: Public health investigations of hazardous organic chemical waste disposal in the United States. *Environ Health Perspect* 1985;62:415–422.
11. Upton AC, Kneip T, and Toniolo P: Public health aspects of toxic chemical disposal sites. *Annu Rev Publ Health* 1989;10:1–25.
12. Grisham JW (ed.): *Health Aspects of the Disposal of Waste Chemicals.* New York: Pergamon Press, 1987.
13. Neutra R, Lipscomb J, Satin K, and Shusterman D: Hypotheses to explain the higher symptom rates observed around hazardous waste sites. *Environ Health Perspect* 1991;94:31–38.
14. Lagakos SW, Wessen BJ, and Zelen M: An analysis of contaminated well water and health effects in Woburn, Massachusetts. *J Am Statist Assoc* 1986;81:583–596.
15. Buffler PA, Crane M, and Key MM: Possibilities of detecting health effects by studies of populations exposed to chemicals from waste disposal sites. *Environ Health Perspect* 1985; 62:423–456.
16. Barret L, Garrel S, Dane V, and Debra JL: Chronic trichloroethylene intoxication: a new approach by trigeminal-evoked potentials? *Arch Environ Health* 1987;42:297–302.
17. Kilburn KH, Warshaw R, and Thornton JC: Formaldehyde impairs memory, equilibrium, and dexterity in histology technicians: effects which persist for days after exposure. *Arch Environ Health* 1987;42:117–120.
18. Mergler D, Huel G, Bowler R, Frenette B, and Cone J: Visual dysfunction among former microelectronics assembly workers. *Arch Environ Health* 1991;46:326–334.
19. Byers VS, Leven AS, Ozonoff DM, and Baldwin RW: Association between clinical symptoms and lymphocyte abnormalities in a population with chronic domestic exposure to industrial solvent contaminated domestic water supply and a high incidence of leukemia. *Cancer Immunol Immunother* 1988;27:77–81.
20. Levin RE, Weinstein A, Peterson M, Testa MA, and Rothfield NF: A comparison of the sensitivity of the 1971 and 1982 American Rheumatism Association criteria for the classification of lupus erythematosus. *Arthritis Rheum* 1984;27:530–538.

21. Ordy JM, Brizzee KR, and Johnson HA: *Cellular Alterations in Visual Pathways and the Limbic System: Implications for Vision and Short-Term Memory in Aging and Human Visual Function.* New York: Alan R. Liss, 1982, pp. 79–117.
22. Kilburn KH and Warshaw RH: Neurotoxic effects from residential exposure to chemicals from an oil reprocessing facility and Superfund site. *Neurotox Teratol* 1995;17:89–102.
23. Lees-Haley PR and Brown RS: Biases in perception and reporting following a perceived toxic exposure. *Percept Motor Skills* 1992;75:531–544.
24. Schaumberg NH and Spencer PS: Degeneration in central and peripheral nervous systems produced by pure *n*-hexane—an experimental study. *Brain* 1976;99:183–192.
25. Cavender FL, Casey HW, Salem H, Graham DG, Swenberg JA, and Gralla EJ: A 13-week vapor inhalation study of *n*-hexane in rats with emphasis of neurotoxic effects. *Fund Appl Toxicol* 1984;4:191–201.
26. Selikoff IJ and Seidman H: Asbestos-associated death among insulation workers in the United States and Canada 1967–1987. *Ann NY Acad Sci* 1991;643:1–14.
27. Needleman HGL, Gunnow C, and Leviton A: Deficits in psychological and classroom performance in children with elevated lead levels. *NEJM* 1970;300:689–695.
28. Shusterman D, Lipscomb J, Neutra J, and Satin K: Symptom prevalence and odor–worry interaction near hazadous waste sites. *Environ Health Perspect* 1991;94:25–30.
29. Brown RS, Williams CW, and Lees-Haley Paul R: The effect of hindsight bias on fear of future illness. *Environ Behav* 1993;25:577–585.
30. Von Lindern I and Van Braun M: Assessment of historical exposures to contaminated drinking water sources in the southside/airport area of Tucson, AZ 1952–1981. Moscow, ID: Terragraphics Environmental Engineering, 1989.
31. Kilburn KH and Warshaw RH: Neurobehavioral effects of formaldehyde and solvents on histology technicians: repeated testing across time. *Environ Res* 1992;58:134–146.
32. Kilburn KH, Warshaw RH, and Shields MG: Neurobehavioral dysfunction in firemen exposed to polychlorinated biphenyls (PCBs): possible improvement after detoxification. *Arch Environ Health* 1989;44:345–350.
33. Kilburn RH and Warshaw RH: Hydrogen sulfide and reduced sulfur gases adversely affect neurophysiological functions. *Toxicol Indust Health* 1995;11:185–197.
34. Savolainen K: Combined effects of xylene and alcohol on the central nervous system. *Acta Pharmacol Toxicol* 1980;46:366–372.
35. Narahashi T: Nerve membrane ionic channels as the target of toxicants. *Arch Toxicol* 1986; 2(Suppl.):3–13.
36. Arlien-Soborg P, Bruhn P, Gyldensted C, and Melgaard B: Chronic painters syndrome. *Acta Neurol Scand* 1979;60:149–156.
37. Arlien-Soborg P: *Solvent Neurotoxicity.* Boca Raton, FL: CRC Press, 1992.
38. Triebig G, Schaller KH, Erzigkeit H, and Valentin H: Biochemische untersuchungen und psychologische studien an chronisch trichlorathylen—belasteten personen unter berucksichtigung expositionsfreier intervalle. *Intl Arch Occup Environ Health* 1977;38:149.
39. Hane M, Axelson O, Blume J, Hogstedt C, Sundell L, and Ydreborg B: Psychological function changes among house painters. *Scand J Work Environ Health* 1977;3:91–99.
40. National priorities list, supplement lists and supporting materials, August 1990 HW-10-145. Washington, DC: U.S. Environmental Protection Agency Office of Emergency Remedial Programs.
41. Cohen AS, Reynolds WE, and Franklin EC: Preliminary criteria for the classification of systemic lupus erythematosus. *Bull Rheum Dis* 1971;21:643–648.
42. Coates EO and Watson JHL: Diffuse interstitial lung disease in tungsten carbide workers. *Ann Intern Med* 1971;75:709–716.
43. Sprince NL, Oliver LC, Eisen EA, Greene RE, and Chamberlin RI: Cobalt exposure and lung disease in tungsten carbide production. *Am Rev Respir Dis* 1988;138:1220–1226.
44. Davies TAL: Manganese pneumonitis. *Brit J Indust Med* 1946;3:111–135.
45. Kilburn KH and Warshaw RH: Pulmonary functional impairment associated with pleural asbestos disease: circumscribed and diffuse thickening. *Chest* 1990;98:965–972.

46. Lockey JE, Kelly CR, Cannon GW, Colby TV, Aldrich V, and Livingstone GK: Progressive systemic sclerosis associated with exposure to trichloroethylene. *J Occup Med* 1987;29: 493–496.
47. Ward MA, Sopsamorn U, Watkins J, Walker AF, and Darke CS: Immunological mechanisms in the pathogenesis of vinyl chloride disease. *Brit Med J* 1976;1:936–938.
48. Press RI, Peebles CL, Kumagai Y, Ochs RL, and Tan EM: Antinuclear autoantibodies in women with silicone breast implants. *Lancet* 1992;340:1304–1306.
49. Roht LH, Vernon SW, Weir FW, Pier SM, Sullivan P, and Reed LJ: Community exposure to hazardous waste disposal sites: assessing reporting bias. *Am J Epidemiol* 1985;122:418–433.
50. Kilburn KH and Warshaw RH: Neurobehavioral testing of subjects exposed residentially to ground-water contaminated from an aluminum die-casting plant and local unexposed. *J Toxicol Environ Health* 1993;39:483–496.
51. Neal RA: Mechanisms of the biological effects of PCBs, polychlorinated dibenzo-*p*-dioxins and polychlorinated dibenzofurans in experimental animals. *Environ Health Perspect* 1985; 60:41–46.
52. Buser H-R: Formation, occurrence and analysis of polychlorinated dibenzofurans, dioxins and related compounds. *Environ Health Perspect* 1985;60:259–267.
53. Hutzinger O, Choudhry GG, Chittim BG, and Johnston LE: Formation of polychlorinated dibenzofurans and dioxins during combustion, electrical equipment fires and PCB incineration. *Environ Health Perspect* 1985;60:3–9.
54. Poland A, Greenlee WF, and Kende AS: Studies on the mechanism of action of the chlorinated dibenzo-*p*-dioxins and related compounds. *Ann NY Acad Sci* 1979;320:214–229.
55. Anastasi A: *Psychological Testing.* New York: Macmillan Co., 1988.
56. Wechsler D: The IQ as an intelligence test. *The New York Times,* June 26, 1966.
57. Reitan RM: A research program on the psychological effects of brain lesions in human beings. In: *International Review of Research in Mental Retardation,* NR Ellis (ed.), New York: Academic Press, 1966.

12

Combustion—Toluene-Rich Vapor Exposure

More than 5,000 people live within a 7.0 km radius from the Combustion Superfund site east of Baton Rogue, Louisiana. As much as 9 million gallons of used motor oil and waste chemicals was processed here in 1975–76 and 3 to 4 million gallons each year from 1977 to 1983. Lesser amounts had been handled before 1975. The residents noted an apparent excess of cancers and cancer deaths, including a cluster of acute leukemia in kindergarten children, which triggered community concern by 1989. Preliminary investigation showed many cancers and a high frequency of health complaints in residents and confirmed the large throughput of neurotoxic solvents and tetraethyl lead at the site.

We hypothesized that neurotoxicity had occurred because of proximity to the site, based on the exposure and the complaints. A neurobehavioral evaluation was planned to compare a self-selected group of symptomatic residents to an unexposed group from 35 km away, outside the modeled plume of contamination. Neurobehavioral testing was appropriate because toluene and lead, known neurotoxicants, were most abundant in the chemicals that passed through the site. They were also most common in samples of sludge. Based on bills of lading and admissions of waste chemical disposed at the site during 17 years of operation, the plant is presumed to have emitted toluene, hexane, benzene, xylene, styrene, hydrocarbons, trichloroethylene, tetrachloroethylene, 1,1,1-trichloroethane, chlorobenzene, dichlorobenzene, tri(ortho)cresyl phosphate, tetraethyl and tetramethyl lead, ethylene dibromide, ethylene dichloride, carbon monoxide, PCBs, dibenzofurans, lead, cadmium, mercury, thallium, and other metals. After operations ceased in 1983, the ponds, grounds, and runoff water were contaminated with these and many other chemicals (Table 12.1); so the site was placed on state and national Superfund lists.

EXPOSURE AND EXPOSURE SURROGATES

We assumed that exposures to residents occurred mainly during active waste processing, not after the site became inactive. This assumption was mainly based on the volumes

TABLE 12.1 List of chemicals that have been identified at Combustion site and the maximum concentrations reported in various media

	Concentration (ppb)			
Chemical	Sludge	Soil	Oil	Water
Methylene chloride	51,000	8,100	2,500	5,790
Chloroform		1,700		60
1,2-Dichloroethane			1,600	1,700
1,1-Dichloroethane	78,600		3,600	940
1,1-Dichloroethylene	130			20
trans-1,2-Dichloroethylene	2,500	3,800		13
trans-1,3-Dichloropropene		93		
Trichloroethylene	53,000		20,000	300
bis (2-Chloroethyl) ether				7
2-Chloroethylvinylether	1,300			
Tetrachloroethylene	216,000	4,100	10,000	50
1,1,1-Trichloroethane	83,800			100
1,1,2-Trichloroethane	61,500			170
1,1,2,2-Tetrachloroethane				
Chlorobenzene	244,000	270		
Dichlorobenzenes (587)	37,000			68
4-Chloro-3-methylphenol	5,800			9
2-Chloronaphthalene	3,100			
PCBs	11,000	380	228,000	
Benzene	1,175,000	500,000	6,200	1,040
Toluene	1,026,000	980,000	38,000	1,250
Xylenes	560,000	35,000	48,000	102
Ethylbenzene	525,000	21,000	13,000	38
Styrene	110,000	26	8,300	
Naphthalene	280,000	38,000		130
2-Methylnaphthalene	2,300,000	19,000		
Phenanthrene	1,300,000	36,000	69,400	
Anthracene	300,000	11,000	255,000	
Pyrene	430,000	11,000		
Crysene	81,000		48,700	
Fluorene	180,000	12,000		
Fluoranthrene	520,000	13,000	101,000	
Acenaphthene	72,000	2,180		
Acenaphthalene	60,000	680		
Benzo (a) anthracene	41,000			
Benzo (b) fluoranthrene	40,000	1,300		
Benzo (k) fluoranthrene	23,000	1,100		
Ideno (1,2,3-cd) pyrene		680		
Dibenzofuran	32,000			
Methanol (unconfirmed contents of Tank 13)				36
Phenol	40,000			100
2-Methylphenol				15
4-Methylphenol				29
2,4-Dimethylphenol				18
Benzoic Acid				74
Acetone	2,000	2,400	5,400	1,400
2-Butanone	2,700			178
4-Methyl-2-Pentanone				51
2-Hexanone	130,000			910
Nitrophenol				141
3-Nitroaniline				18

(continued)

TABLE 12.1 *(continued)*

	Concentration (ppb)			
Chemical	Sludge	Soil	Oil	Water
2,4-Dinitrotoluene		37,000		39
Benzidine		14,100		
N-Nitrosodi-N-propylamine	23,000			
N-Nitrosodiphenyl amine	1,800,000			
Diphenylhydrazine	75,000			
Di-*n*-octylphthalate	770	960		
Di-*n*-butylphthalate	34,000	515		
Butylbenzophthalate	330,000	96,000	187	
bis (2-Ethylhexyl) phthalate	160,000	84,000		49
Diethylphthalate	13,100	1,480		
Dimethylphthalate	20,000			
Antimony	40,000	58,000	18,000	30,000
Arsenic	12,880	37,900	1,500	70
Barium	930,000	663,000	480,000	1,420
Beryllium	20,000	1,200		10
Cadmium	8,300	3,000	2,100	
Chromium	122,000	26,200	27,000	18,000
Cobalt	79,000	14,000	6,600	6,000
Copper	280,000	22,000	2,100	124
Lead	2,800,000	970,000	545,000	3,900
Mercury	2,420	950		1
Nickel	38,370	41,500	6,000	2,000
Selenium	23,330	2,120	500	110
Silver	7,630	500	1,400	900
Thallium	21,600	2,460		220
Vanadium	11,000	28,000		
Zinc	362,900	173,000		15,600

of chemicals known to have been received at the Combustion facility. No air or water monitoring measurements were found to have been taken for its active period. Measurements of chemicals in the site's water and soil provided us with an inventory and showed some off-site migration by water. Between 1966 and 1972 the active heat processing of chemicals increased; it peaked at 9 million gallons in 1975 and 1976, and then it gradually decreased until closure in 1983. As the proportions of chemical received did not match subsequent analysis of the site's ponds and soil, it was assumed that proportionately more volatile chemicals became airborne and less volatile ones remained as residues to be analyzed. Modeling, using toluene and benzene as the tracers and standard U.S. government assumptions (1–3), together with prevailing winds and water drainage, predicted asymmetry from a concentric 6 km dispersal eastward out to 8.5 km for airborne spread. Water drained south–southwest into the streams and rivers.

Investigations of populations exposed to chemicals from manufacturing or waste sites have focused on symptoms (4–6) and have often been inconclusive. Characteristically irritability, memory loss, inability to concentrate, lightheadedness, dizziness, disturbed sleep, headache, and excessive fatigue have been reported (4, 7–10). Symptoms are difficult to interpret, and objective data have rarely accompanied these reports (7, 8, 11). However, objectively measured functions of the human nervous system are exquisitely sensitive to noise (12), lead (13), hydrogen sulfide (14), and solvents (7, 8).

Toluene, the best-known neurotoxicant of the chemicals disposed of in quantity at the Combustion site, is a component of petroleum. Sniffing of toluene or glue (15), occupational exposures (16, 17), and human exposure experiments (16) have demonstrated adverse effects on balance, cognitive function, and color discrimination plus a high frequency of symptoms. Toluene toxicity was enhanced by simultaneous administration of methyl ethyl ketone (16), a finding that suggests possible enhancement of its toxicity by other neurotoxicants.

Lead concentrations were high at the Combustion site, and lead is an obvious candidate for cofactor neurotoxicant. It has chronic effects on cognitive function, affective (mood) status, and perceptual motor function (13). There is recent evidence that childhood lead exposure produces chronic subclinical encephalopathy (18).

Recently, we showed that living in proximity to manufacturing and refining sites or using water from wells chemically contaminated with trichloroethylene was associated with impaired balance and slowed reaction time (7).

The Subjects

The Combustion investigation compared neurophysiological and neuropsychological functions of community residents and unexposed subjects together with their self-assessed frequency of symptoms and mood states. In 1990 we studied 43 self-selected exposed subjects and 34 unexposed subjects, and we completed the Phase 1 investigation in 1991 by adding 88 randomly selected exposed and 32 unexposed subjects. Phase 2 followed closely.

Phase 2 clients, all participants in a class action lawsuit, were selected in segments defined by four concentric circles drawn around the site at 0.8 km (0.5 mile) intervals and divided into eight sectors based on compass octants. A proportional sample that averaged 13 or 14 subjects was recruited for testing from the clients in each interval-sector. Over 80% of all the residents in these sectors were clients. They were called in random order to fill the sampling matrix. Thus 114 subjects (71 new and 43 tested in 1990) were selected from 1.2 to 2.4 km, 102 from 2.41 to 3.2 km, 102 from 3.21 to 4.0 km, and 102 from 4.01 to 4.8 km. A family was skipped if not reached in two calls. Fewer than 10% of those contacted could not be studied because of conflicting schedules. Eleven of 43 previously tested subjects could not be found or rescheduled, and one did not complete the testing; so comparisons were made in 31.

TESTING OF SUBJECTS

Methods

A matched cohort design was used with 77 women and 54 men in the exposed group, between the ages of 15 and 65 years, in Phase 1. After the exposed group was chosen, a 1:2 unexposed population of 37 women and 29 men was recruited. The exposed participants, both self-selected and randomly selected, were from a roster of nearly 3,000 residents prepared during the investigation of the cancers near the site. They were plaintiffs in a class action suit against the site operators and waste contributors. Approximately 85% of persons residing within 2.4 km of the site were in this plaintiff group. They had resided near the site in Livingston Parish, Louisiana for a mean of

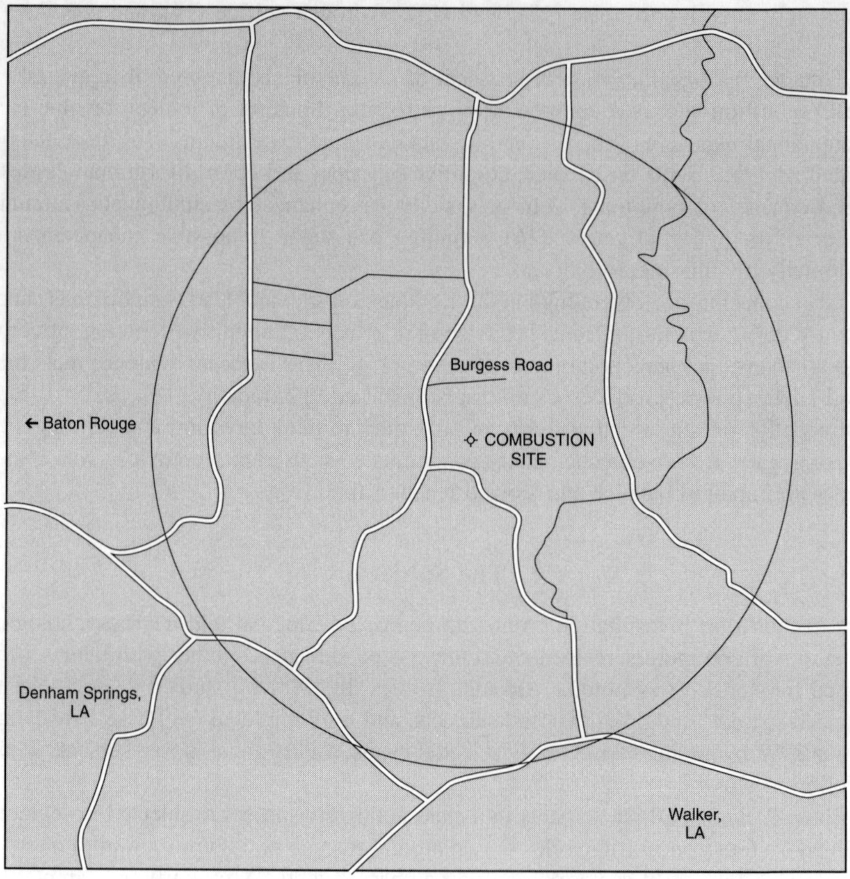

FIGURE 12.1a. The map center is midway between the process area (lower) and the ponds (to the right) of the combustion site. The homes of subjects tested in 1990–91 are shown by small black rectangles.

9.3 years (range 2–17 years) from 1966 to 1983 (Figure 12.1a). A windrose for 1975 to 1979 showed eastward movement (Figure 12.1b).

The unexposed cohort was from Springfield, Louisiana (35 km distant). They were chosen from voter registration rolls using a random numbers array and contacted by telephone to ascertain both their willingness to be tested and that they had never been employed at or resided within 10 km of the Combustion site. The plan was to match the cohorts for sex, age, and years of education (highest school grade attained). As seen in Table 12.2, the unexposed had 1.4 more years of education, and the difference was statistically significant. Over 80% of those who matched and were not excluded because of exposure were tested. They were reimbursed $25 for their participation and paid for mileage. Exposed subjects were not compensated. Exposed and unexposed

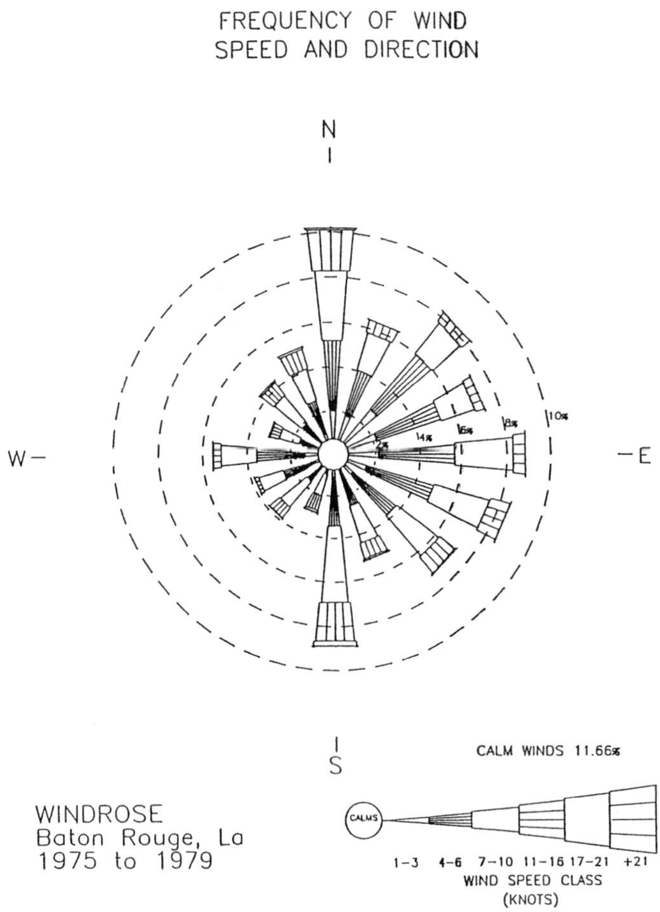

FIGURE 12.1b. The windrose for Baton Rouge, Louisiana, 33 km west of the site, showed that only up to 8% of the time were winds of Beaufort number 2 or 3, 2.5 m/s or greater, and they moved air mainly to the east. Similar virtual stagnation of the air mass was assumed for the combustion site.

subjects were studied in combined groups so that examiners were blinded as to their exposure status. The protocol was approved by the Human Studies Review Committee of the University of Southern California.

It was assumed that 75% of the concentration of VOCs in the processed oil was lost from the stacks of the four heat treatment tanks. The basic atmospheric dispersion of pollutants from the site was estimated by using the EPA Industrial Source Complex Model and 1978 continuous hourly meteorological data for Baton Rouge (surface station #13970 and upper air station #3937) (1, 19).

Each of the 24 sectors formed by eight compass directions and three distances of 0.8 km was filled by selecting 12 to 15 subjects at random from those living in that sector from the pool of 1,753 residents. These pools of subjects in a sector effectively leveled variation in scores due to individual ages, educational levels, and test performances (20). This facilitated comparison of mean scores of groups of subjects in each sector to determine the influences of distance, direction, and duration.

The major objectives of the Phase 2 study were to map the neurotoxic impairment

TABLE 12.2 Descriptive data for exposed and unexposed groups as means with standard deviations and *p* values by t-test

	Exposed		Unexposed		
	M	Sd	M	Sd	*p*
n	131		66		
Women	77		37		
Men	54		29		
Age yrs	40.5 ±	14.1	41.2 ±	15.0	NS
Range	(15–64)		(16–65)		
Education level yrs	11.1 ±	2.3	12.5 ±	2.3	.0000
Income (×$1,000)	23.7 ±	12.9*	29.6 ±	13.3	.015
Pulse rate/min	71.5 ±	13.8	71.3 ±	13.0	NS
Blood pressure Systolic	130 ±	17	131 ±	16	NS
Diastolic	80 ±	10	81 ±	11	NS
Alveolar carbon monoxide	12.1 ±	11.2	12.5 ±	11.8	NS
Alveolar alcohol ppm	4.0 ±	3.0	3.8 ±	1.2	NS
Height cm Women	162.8 ±	4.7	161.7 ±	6.8	NS
Men	174.9 ±	7.2	175.4 ±	5.8	NS
Weight kg Women	68.9 ±	22.8	68.3 ±	19.2	NS
Men	90.7 ±	15.7	83.2 ±	11.6	NS

* Based on 29 women and 14 men.

and determine its perimeter, locate the directions of maximal and minimal impairment, and determine the duration of residence needed for impairment. Previous detailed neurobehavioral testing of the 88 Phase 1 subjects showed which tests were sensitive (20), and these tests were used to screen subjects in this mapping phase. A final objective was to determine if impairment was persistent by retesting subjects who lived within 1.2 km of the site.

All subjects were studied during a period of three days by a staff of 22 examiners led by the author at a medical clinic building in Denham Springs, Louisiana, employing the same staff and site as for Phase 1. The order of tests varied, as alternate groups of subjects were first given Culture Fair and POMS, followed by individual tests in random order. Others were tested first at individual stations and then gathered for Culture Fair and POMS. Pegboard and trail making A and B were done in series for each individual by one of several examiners. Questionnaires were checked for omissions and completed by staff interviewers after completion of the testing.

Test scores were compared in 377 new and 31 retested subjects in 24 sectors within the perspective of their overall abnormality, which was established by comparison to the 66 unexposed subjects tested and compared previously (20). These unexposed subjects had been recruited by calling in random order people from the voter registration rolls of Springfield, Louisiana, which is 35 km east–southeast from the Combustion site (20). Potential unexposed were excluded if they had worked at the Combustion site or lived within 11 km of it. They matched the exposed group for age, gender, and race, but they had 1.9 years more educational attainment, a significant difference.

Results, Descriptive Data

Mean ages of 40.5 years in exposed and 41.2 years in unexposed, and the age distributions were not different. Despite efforts to match them, educational levels favored the

TABLE 12.3 Neurophysiological and neuropsychological test results and profile of mood state scores for exposed and unexposed groups: means and standard deviations with t-tests

	Exposed		Unexposed		
	M	Sd	M	Sd	*p*
NEUROPHYSIOLOGICAL					
Simple Reaction Time ms	328	± 112	288	± 53	.001
Choice Reaction Time ms 1	579	± 111	534	± 84	.003
2	575	± 108	523	± 84	.003
3	588	± 129	534	± 90	.003
Sway Speed cm/s Eyes Open 1	.96	± .31	.85	± 21	.0003
2	.97	± .34	.85	± 31	.0003
3	1.00	± .35	.83	± .21	.0003
Eyes Closed 1	1.52	± .50	1.25	± .36	.0001
2	1.49	± .58	1.22	± .34	.0001
3	1.50	± .57	1.19	± .33	.0001
Color (hue) Score	12.6	± 7.7	11.4	± 1.6	NS
Blink Reflex R-1 ms Right	14.7	± 1.9	14.4	± 2.0	NS
Left	14.9	± 1.9	14.5	± 1.8	NS
Grip Strength kg					
Women Right	27.8	± 7.4	31.0	± 6.9	NS
Left	26.6	± 6.9	30.0	± 6.4	NS
Men Right	52.1	± 10.5	57.3	± 9.8	NS
Left	51.1	± 8.4	54.3	± 10.1	NS
NEUROPSYCHOLOGICAL					
Cognitive					
Culture Fair A Score	24.3	± 8.8	28.2	± 8.3	.0002
Block Design Score	31.0	± 9.4	33.9	± 9.4	.044
Digit Symbol Score	49.9	± 15.4	52.3	± 15.1	NS
Embedded Figures	29.3	± 5.3	31.2	± 5.2	NS
Psychomotor Speed, Perception, Attention					
Finger Writing					
Errors: Right	2.4	± 2.9	2.2	± 2.0	NS
Left	2.0	± 3.2	1.8	± 2.3	NS
Pegboard Score sec.	81.0	± 26.4	71.0	± 14.2	.005
Trails A sec.	38.5	± 22.8	32.1	± 11.4	.04
Trails B sec.	86.8	± 38.4	75.0	± 40.7	.03
Recall Memory					
Story 1	9.0	± 3.8	10.1	± 3.4	.03
Story 2	8.4	± 4.3	8.9	± 3.2	NS
Visual (original)	8.6	± 4.1*	10.1	± 3.3	NS
(revised)	27.8	± 7.3**	29.0	± 7.6	NS
Digits forward	6.5	± 1.1*	6.8	± 1.5	NS
backward	4.3	± 1.6*	4.7	± 1.2	NS
15 Form Test (malingering index)	12.6	± 3.0**	12.6	± 2.9	NS
Overlearned Memory					
Information score	14.4	± 4.8*	16.9	± 5.3	.04
Picture completion	14.9	± 4.0*	15.3	± 3.1	NS
Similarities	18.6	± 6.3*	20.2	± 5.3	NS
Profile of Mood States					
POMS score	56.2	± 39.9	23.2	± 32.9	.0002
Tension	16.2	± 7.8	8.9	± 6.6	.0001
Depression	15.5	± 12.4	8.1	± 9.7	.001
Anger	13.6	± 9.7	9.2	± 8.8	.05
Vigor	13.1	± 5.7	17.8	± 6.5	.0014
Fatigue	13.1	± 6.9	7.7	± 6.3	.0002
Confusion	10.9	± 6.0	6.3	± 4.5	.0005

* Based on 43 exposed and 34 unexposed
** Based on 88 exposed and 32 unexposed

ms: milliseconds; cm/s: centimeters per second; sec: seconds.

unexposed by 1.4 years and their annual incomes were $5,900 greater than those of the exposed (Table 12.2). Prevalences of potential confounding exposures were low, including alcohol intoxication, illicit drug use, unconsciousness from head trauma or anesthesia, occupational neurotoxin exposures, and spontaneous neurological diseases and disorders, including seizures and blackouts. Moreover, these prevalences were similar in both groups. Significantly more unexposed than exposed subjects had used herbicides and pesticides. Chronic bronchitis, asthma, and myocardial infarction were significantly more prevalent in the exposed group but were not explained by cigarette smoking. Current smoking did not differ significantly between the groups, as their alveolar carbon monoxide levels were nearly identical. More unexposed, 59%, than exposed, 49%, had ever smoked. Average age of starting smoking was 17.5 years for both groups, but exposed had smoked only 18.1 cigarettes per day vs. 26.8 in unexposed. Mean pulse rates, blood pressure, height, and weight of men and of women did not differ between the groups. Because scores had only slightly different age coefficients (slopes) in women and men, which did not alter the interpretation of results, the test

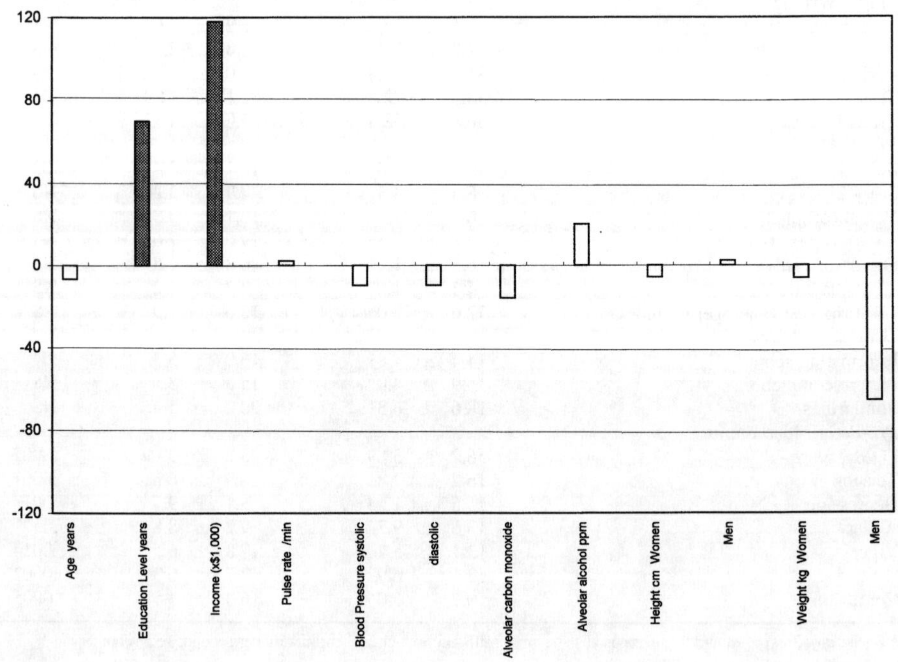

FIGURE 12.2a. Comparison of 88 exposed adults and 66 unexposed adults by ANOVA (Combustion, Livingston, LA). Hatched bars are statistically significant.

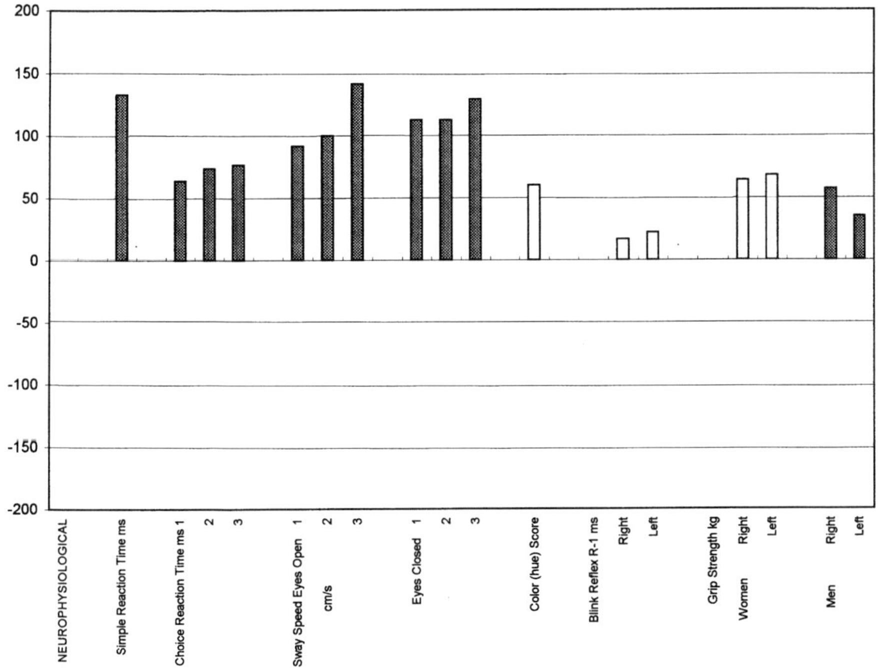

FIGURE 12.2b. Neurophysiological test comparisons of 88 exposed adults and 66 unexposed adults by ANOVA (Combustion, Livingston, LA). Hatched bars are statistically significant.

scores of women and men were analyzed together in both exposed and unexposed groups.

Neurophysiological Tests

This domain included simple reaction time, which was longer by 40 milliseconds (ms), and two-choice visual reaction time, which was longer by 54 ms in the third trial in the exposed subjects compared to unexposed, differences that were significant (Table 12.3, Figures 12.2a–d). Moreover, the group means of the individual medians of the final seven trials of three 20-trial sequences were stable. Mean speed of sway of exposed subjects with eyes open (1.00 cm/s) and that with eyes closed (1.50 cm/s) were significantly faster than the sway speeds of the unexposed, and means of both groups were stable through the three trials. Speed of sway was 25% faster, more abnormal, in exposed compared to unexposed women and men. The latency of the blink reflex R-1 was similar in exposed and unexposed subjects. Although more exposed than unexposed subjects failed to blink, this difference was not significant. Color (hue) discrimination was not different in exposed and unexposed subjects. Regression coefficients for age

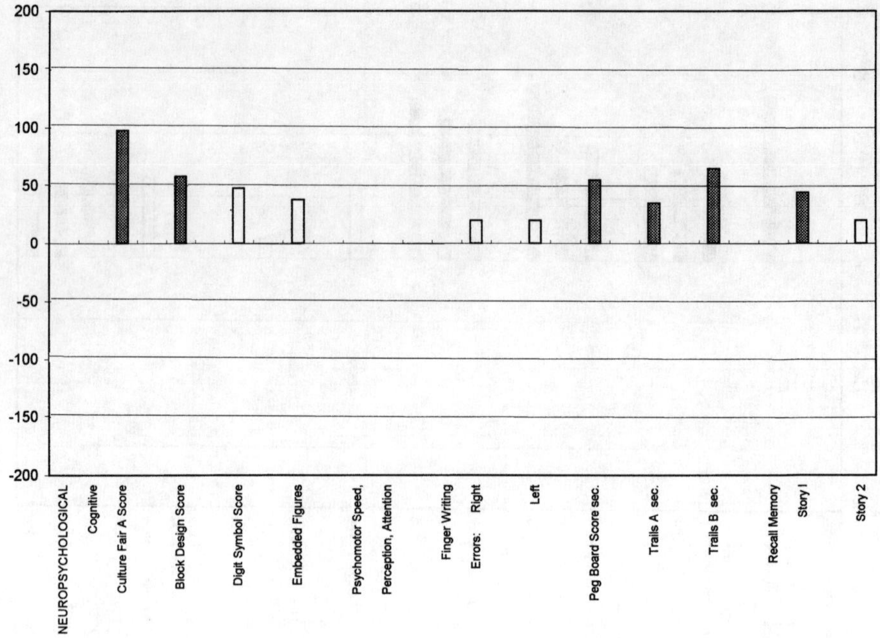

FIGURE 12.2c. Neuropsychological test comparisons of 88 exposed adults and 66 unexposed adults by ANOVA (Combustion, Livingston, LA). Hatched bars are statistically significant.

differed between exposed and unexposed subjects for these same tests (Table 12.4). The exposed subjects' physiological domain was abnormal for the two functions involving multiple brain centers (i.e., balance and reaction time) as compared to two tests of more localized CNS functions (i.e., color discrimination and blink), which were not significantly different. It was concluded that the generalized functions of this domain were affected by exposure but not the localized ones.

Neuropsychological Tests

Culture Fair score was 3.9 lower ($p<.0002$) in exposed subjects than in unexposed, and block design score was 2.9 lower ($p<.044$), but digit symbol scores and embedded figures recognition were not significantly different. Thus, the cognitive domain was different for exposed and unexposed subjects, and this was confirmed by significantly different age coefficients for Culture Fair and block design (Table 12.4).

Peg placement took longer in exposed than in unexposed subjects ($p<.005$), trail making A took 6.4 s longer in exposed than unexposed ($p<.04$) and the trail making B difference was 11.8 s ($p<.03$). For these tests, only trail making B had a significant

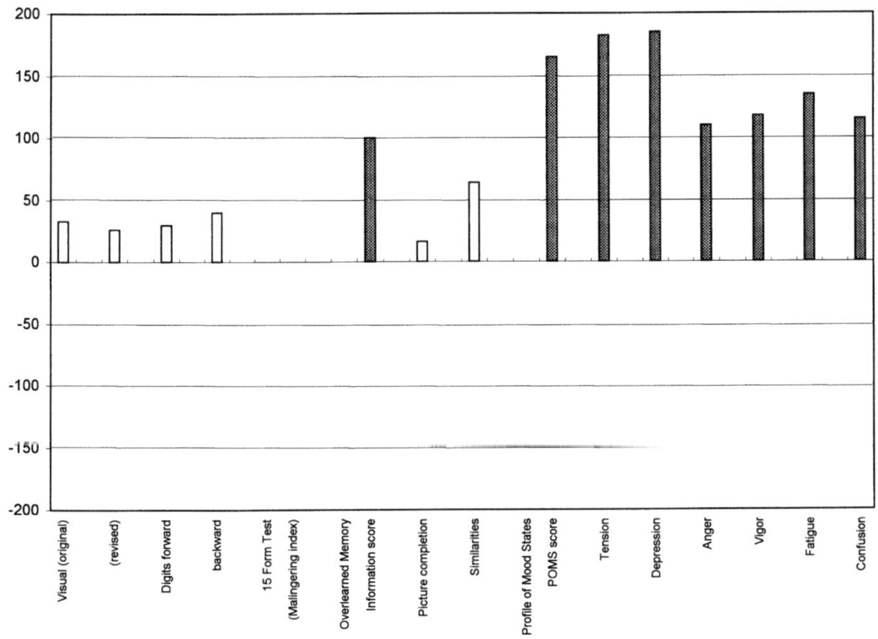

FIGURE 12.2d. Neuropsychological test comparisons of 88 exposed adults and 66 unexposed adults by ANOVA (Combustion, Livingston, LA). Hatched bars are statistically significant.

difference on age coefficients between the groups (Table 12.4). Exposed subjects made more errors in these three tests than unexposed and in fingertip writing of numbers, where the differences were not significant in exposed and unexposed. Although this domain was thought to be positive for differences between exposed subjects and unexposed (20, 21), that interpretation depends on trail making, which is the most sensitive test for chemical exposure in this domain (22).

Exposed subjects' immediate recall of story 1 was 1.1 items less than that of unexposed, a difference that was significant ($p<.03$), but the difference of 0.5 item in story 2 was not significant. The difference in visual recall of 1.5 items was not significant in the 1990 group ($p<.077$) or in 1991. Digit span, forward and backward, was not different between the groups. However, when age-adjusted coefficients were compared, story 2 and visual recall were significantly different, and the differences of story 1 and digits backward were nearly so (Table 12.4). The Rey 15 form test, used to detect malingering, had identical group means in the exposed and unexposed (12.6 items recalled) without a difference between the groups in the items missed. Thus the recall domain was equivocal for differences between exposed and unexposed subjects.

TABLE 12.4 Regression coefficients for age for unexposed and exposed subjects, differences in coefficients and significance of the differences (*p* values)

	Unexposed	*p*	Exposed	Diff. in Coeff.	*p* of Diff.	Adj. r^2
Simple React. Time ms	.059	.9	1.581	1.523	.001	.132
Choice React. Time ms	2.832	.003	5.75	2.916	.000	.410
Sway Speed cm/sec						
Eyes open	.001	.816	.010	.009	.000	.193
Eyes closed	−.003	.616	.013	.016	.004	.088
Color (Desat. hue test)	.027	.210	.055	.028	.032	.101
Blink Right R−1 ms	.038	.037	−.003	.041	.816	.043
Left R−1 ms	.043	.034	−.002	.045	.893	.045
Fingertip number writing errors Right	.040	.087	.064	.024	.106	.087
Fingertip number writing errors Left	.059	.042	.075	.016	.365	.069
Recall						
Story 1	−.015	.615	.051	.066	.064	.042
Story 2	−.011	.702	.060	.071	.008	.093
Visual	−.102	.001	.144	.246	.031	.237
Digits Forward	.0003	.982	.0111	.0111	.140	.007
Backward	−.025	.042	.040	.065	.057	.126
Overlearned Memory						
Information (ed 1)	.107	.01	.068	.034	.225	.124
Picture Completion (ed 1)	−.087	.003	.070	.157	.4	.067
Similarities (ed 1)	−.042	.5	.200	.242	.006	.108
Cognitive						
Culture Fair A (ed 1)	−.277	.000	−.392	.115	.001	.511
Block Design sc. (sex slope)	−.215	.005	−.335	.120	.013	.226
Digit Symbol sc. (ed 1, sex slope)	−.569	.000	−.578	.009	.8	.354
Embedded Figures	−.036	.443	.091	.127	.065	.051
Perceptual-Motor						
Pegboard (ed 1, sex slope)	.583	.000	.755	.172	.08	.316
Errors	.133	.131	.135	.002	.767	.004
Trails A (ed 1)	.520	.001	.545	.025	.8	.177
Trails B	1.081	.000	1.937	.856	.001	.331
Ed 1 sex slope (males)						
Ed 1 no diff. (females)						
Affective Status						
POMS Score	−.9783	.012	1.951	2.929	.000	.171

Significant *p* values are underlined. cm/sec = centimeters/second
ms = milliseconds ed 1 = educational level
sex slope—age coefficients differed for sex (difference was shown to be due to different age distributions).

Information scores were 2.5 items lower in exposed vs. unexposed subjects ($p<.038$), but scores for similarities and picture completion were not different; so the overlearned memory domain was considered unaffected by exposure. The age coefficient was significantly different for similarities, a tradeoff, which let stand this domain interpretation as unaffected (Table 12.4).

Profile of Mood States

The POMS scores were significantly higher for exposed than for unexposed subjects ($p<.0002$), as were depression, anger, tension, confusion, and fatigue scores. The vigor score was significantly lower in exposed subjects (13.1 vs. 17.8).

Symptom Frequency Scores

Frequency scores for all 32 complaints were 3 to 30 times higher in exposed compared to unexposed subjects. The only exception was decreased alcohol tolerance in men. Twenty-nine of 32 of these differences were significant after adjustment for age (age coefficients are compared in Table 12.5). The three that were not significant, cough with blood, decreased alcohol tolerance, and loss of consciousness, were rare in both groups. Each symptom frequency score was tested for the influence of age, educational level, and POMS score (independent variables). The 19 symptoms most affected by POMS score are shown in Table 12.6 for exposed and unexposed groups. In the exposed group, ten symptoms had significant correlations with POMS scores: headache, nausea, fatigue, lightheadedness, somnolence, lack of concentration, irritability, mood, long-term memory loss, and chest tightness. Only four—fatigue, somnolence, irritability, and mood swings—were significant in the reference group.

Confounding Factors

Both groups were free of neurological diseases, psychiatric disorders, and seizures. Prescription drug use, substance abuse including alcohol, hours of general anesthesia, and exposure to solvents and lead in crafts or avocations were infrequent and not different between the groups. Pesticide and herbicide use were more frequent in the unexposed group and would minimize differences between groups; so they were ignored. No subject in either group reported regular use of alcohol, nor was alcohol detected in any subject's alveolar gas. No potential confounding factor had a significant coefficient in the regression models, including occupational exposures and hours of anesthesia. The test scores of 4 male residents who had worked briefly at Combustion did not differ from those of the 50 men whose only exposure was residential. No women in the exposed group had worked at Combustion.

Exposure Indices and Test Scores

Group mean test scores of the 43 self-selected and highly symptomatic subjects within 1.2 km of the site who were studied in 1990 and the 88 randomly selected exposed subjects within 2.4 km of the site studied in 1991 were not different. There were no test score differences between subject groups who had lived within 0.8 km and those who lived from 1.6 to 2.4 km of the site. The performance was similar in the two random selections of unexposed subjects made from voter rolls a year apart. Neither duration of exposure, the reciprocal of residential distance from the Combustion site, nor distance squared, nor the reciprocal of distance duration times was a significant determinant of any neurobehavioral test score by regression modeling. All the exposed subjects had lived within 2.4 km (1.5 miles) of the Combustion Site, but distance from

TABLE 12.5 Frequency quotients for 32 complaints in exposed and unexposed women and men: group means of the subjects' scaled frequencies are compared by age coefficients with *p* values

	Women		Men		Men and Women Combined *p* of coeff	
	Unexposed	Exposed	Unexposed	Exposed	Unexposed	Exp. vs. Ref.
Skin						
Itching	5.6	33.0	21.5	50.5	.260	.000
Dryness	11.0	40.5	7.3	29.1	.457	.000
Redness	0.6	22.2	2.4	39.8	.493	.000
Chest and Irritation						
Chest tightness	3.9	32.3	9.8	33.7	.767	.000
Rapid heart rate	2.4	22.8	3.8	17.9	.33	.000
Chest pain	1.1	35.4	10.0	32.9	.046	.000
Dry cough	8.2	37.2	4.1	23.7	.274	.000
Cough with blood	0.2	3.6	0.7	3.7	.662	.107
Dry mouth	10.5	42.4	8.7	45.3	.489	.000
Throat irritation	12.3	41.1	14.9	36.2	.222	.000
Eye irritation	4.8	44.6	4.8	39.7	.026	.000
< Odor perception	5.7	18.1	0	25.6	.886	.012
General						
Headache	33.4	61.6	12.8	35.7	.000	.000
Indigestion	18.2	27.1	18.7	50.7	.807	.025
Nausea	9.2	27.4	7.0	11.5	.084	.004
< Alcohol tolerance	1.2	6.8	6.4	7.4	.255	.453
Fatigue	15.2	59.6	9.5	58.5	.120	.000
< Libido	6.6	27.4	4.6	17.5	.410	.005
Neurological and Sleep						
Dizziness	4.3	39.3	4.5	19.4	.415	.000
Lightheadedness	6.8	43.7	1.6	20.2	.032	.000
Loss of balance	3.7	33.4	1.6	24.3	.082	.000
Mood instability	3.3	32.3	5.2	14.7	.177	.001
Irritability	10.5	53.5	21.2	38.3	.001	.000
Exhilaration	0	14.2	0	3.5	.030	.05
Loss of consciousness	0	2.0	0	4.7	.900	.102
Recent memory loss	4.2	33.2	3.4	49.7	.998	.000
Long-term memory loss	7.7	16.7	0	19.4	.386	.016
Lack of concentration	8.0	51.3	4.0	34.7	.018	.000
Somnolence	4.3	44.9	5.9	23.4	.001	.000
Cannot fall asleep	11.6	28.6	1.4	27.9	.849	.004
Wake frequently	11.9	40.9	6.5	48.0	.360	.000
Sleep few hours	9.1	30.8	2.9	39.9	.948	.000

the site did not predict the degree of impairment on any test. There was no support for the notion that effect varied inversely with the square of the distance, as it does for ionizing radiation or heat.

Data Analysis

For the exposed and the unexposed groups, age was the dominant determinant of performance for most neurophysiological and neuropsychological tests (Table 12.4). Although

TABLE 12.6 Regression analysis of each symptom frequency with POMS as the independent variable for exposed and unexposed subjects, showing coefficient standard errors (SE), adjusted r^2, and significance (p values)

	Exposed				Unexposed			
	Coeff	SE	r^2	p	Coeff	SE	r^2	p
Headache	.0021	.0009	.086	.032	.0015	.0013	.0096	.259
Nausea	.0028	.0007	.2604	.000	.0011	.0006	.0457	.118
Dizziness	.0017	.0010	.0430	.097	−.0002	.0005	−.0258	.682
Lightheadedness	.0034	.0009	.2315	.000	.0004	.0006	−.0195	.548
Exhilaration	.0013	.0007	.0494	.082	.0	.0	.0	.0
Fatigue	.0041	.0010	.2830	.000	.0040	.0012	.2343	.002
Somnolence	.0030	.0011	.1226	.012	.0017	.0006	.1559	.012
Insomnia Cannot fall asleep	.0002	.001	−.0237	.865	.0012	.001	.0082	.865
Insomnia Wake frequently	.0012	.0012	−.0036	.362	.0009	.0009	.0023	.307
Insomnia Sleep only a few hours	.0017	.0011	−.0344	.122	−.0001	.0009	.0306	.885
Irritation	.0039	.0009	.2790	.000	.0040	.0009	.3449	.000
Lack of concentration	.0041	.0009	.2854	.000	.0001	.0006	.0005	.900
Recent memory loss	.0015	.0011	.0160	.202	.0002	.0004	−.0205	.566
Long-term memory loss	.0022	.0009	.1051	.019	−.0001	.0008	−.0303	.864
Mood	.0033	.0010	.1997	.002	.0016	.0005	.2324	.002
Indigestion	−.0000	.001	−.0244	.991	.0026	.0013	.0808	.057
Chest tightness	.0025	.0010	.1084	.018	.0009	.0006	.0198	.206
Palpitation	.0008	.0009	−.0030	.355	.0006	.0003	.0688	.073
Reduced sense of smell	.0007	.0011	−.0149	.540	−.0006	.0008	−.0131	.454

family income and educational attainment were significantly higher in unexposed subjects than in exposed, subjects' income alone and with educational level and age had no significant correlations with test scores, whereas educational level alone had significant coefficients for only a few psychological tests in linear regression models. Group comparisons were adjusted by using educational level coefficients when they were significant. POMS score had no significant coefficients with performance on any tests in the exposed subjects or in the unexposed group despite coefficients with symptom frequency. Gender appeared to influence the slopes for block design, digit symbol, pegboard, and trails B, but it disappeared after adjustment for age.

Regression models for scores on choice reaction time, sway with the eyes closed, and trail making B were different for the older (above age 40) and younger halves of the population. Age, distance from the site, and Culture Fair Score had significant coefficients for reaction time, sway speed, and trails B in the older half, but distance alone and distance and age did not because the older exposed people had a larger negative age coefficient for Culture Fair. Although such birth decade differences have been ascribed to cultural changes in education (23, 24), educational level did not substitute for Culture Fair score in these models, a finding suggesting that only the latter was an exposure outcome, and educational levels were obviously fixed.

The mean test scores in 408 subjects were compared to the group means of 88

TABLE 12.7 Neurophysiological and neuropsychological test results and mood state scores for exposed and unexposed, mean and standard deviations with *p* values

	Combined Unexposed	Phase 1 Exp '91		Phase 2 Exp '91	
Number ( )	M (66) Sd	M (88) Sd	*p*	M (408) Sd	*p*
Women	37	48		205	
Men	29	40		203	
Age	41.2 ± 15.0	40.5 ± 14.1	.718	40.0 ± 16.0	.807
Ed Level	12.5 ± 2.3	11.1 ± 2.3	.010	10.6 ± 2.9	.002
Neurophysiological					
SRT ms	288 ± 53	329 ± 112	.500	371 ± 172	.001
CRT ms	535 ± 91	587 ± 129	.008	621 ± 170	.007
Sway cm/s					
eyes open	0.83 ± 0.21	1.00 ± 0.35	.013	0.99 ± 0.51	.013
eyes closed	1.19 ± 0.34	1.50 ± 0.57	.001	1.50 ± 0.82	.001
Color score	11.4 ± 4.6	12.0 ± 5.2	.010	12.2 ± 1.3	.012
Blink reflex					
R-1 Right	14.3 ± 1.9	14.9 ± 1.9	.408	14.3 ± 2.4	.433
R-1 Left	14.5 ± 2.1	15.2 ± 1.6	.190	14.3 ± 2.2	.265
Neuropsychological					
Culture Fair A	28.2 ± 8.3	24.2 ± 8.9	.005	23.5 ± 8.7	.005
Pegboard sc	71.1 ± 14.2	81.0 ± 26.7	.005	82.0 ± 25.0	.008
Trail making A	32.1 ± 11.4	38.6 ± 21.5	.042	43.0 ± 24.0	.006
Trail making B	75.0 ± 39.0	89.6 ± 39.5	.002	93.7 ± 43.1	.002
POMS score	22.2 ± 32.9	53.6 ± 35.5	.001	52.3 ± 40.8	.001

exposed near-site subjects and 66 unexposed evaluated in 1991 (Table 12.7, Figures 12.3 and 12.4). The 408 exposed subjects were slightly younger (40.0 years) ($p<0.4$) and less educated (10.6 years) ($p<.007$) than the unexposed (41.2 years and 12.5 years). There were no significant differences in scores between men and women; so they constituted one group. The 88 subjects of Phase 1 and 408 subjects of Phase 2 had nearly identical test scores, which were abnormal compared to 66 unexposed subjects. In the following descriptions, means for Phase 2 subjects are compared to means of unexposed.

Simple reaction times at 371 vs. 288 milliseconds (ms) and choice reaction times at 621 vs. 535 ms were significantly prolonged (abnormal) compared to unexposed ($p<.001$). Balance as speed of sway with the eyes open was 0.99 cm/s vs. 0.83 cm/s in unexposed ($p<.013$), and with eyes closed sway speed was 1.50 cm/s vs. 1.19 cm/s in unexposed ($p<.001$). Blink reflex latency of exposed subjects was not significantly different from that of unexposed. Exposed subjects' Culture Fair (A) score of 23.5 was significantly lower than the 28.2 in unexposed. Peg placement time of 82 sec was significantly longer than 71.1 sec for unexposed; trail making A at 43.0 sec and trail making B at 93.7 sec were significantly longer (more abnormal) than the unexposed values of 32.1 sec and 75.0 sec, respectively. POMS scores of 52.3 in the exposed group and 22.2 in the unexposed were significantly different. In the exposed subjects, POMS components anxiety, depression, anger, fatigue, and confusion were increased, and vigor was decreased. Simple reaction time was more abnormal in the 408 subjects,

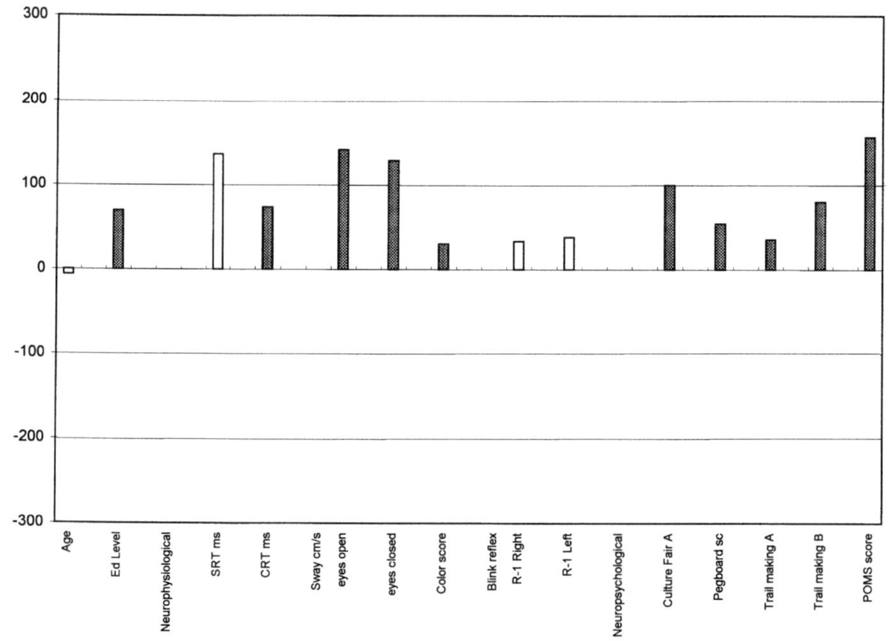

FIGURE 12.3. Comparison of initial 88 exposed adults to 66 unexposed adults by ANOVA (Combustion). Hatched bars are statistically significant.

but otherwise mean scores in this study were not different from those of the earlier 88-subject sample of this exposed cohort.

Comparisons of mean test scores for the 31 retested exposed subjects were similar (Table 12.8) (11 of the original 43 could not return, and one did not complete the retesting). Interval variations were not statistically significant, including small improvements in Culture Fair and color discrimination and longer simple and choice reaction times, faster sway speeds, and increased POMS scores.

Distance

The two-choice visual reaction time (CRT) and balance as sway speed with eyes closed (SC3) as dependent variables were examined in regression models with distance from the site alone and within the eight compass octants as independent variables (Table 12.9). Distance from the site had no significant coefficients for predicting CRT or SC3. Analyses of grouped data also showed no trends. The CRT of the 30 subjects who resided less than 0.4 km (0.25 mile) from the site was 669 ms, compared to an average 612 ms mean in the 370 subjects who resided beyond 1.6 km. Sway speed showed

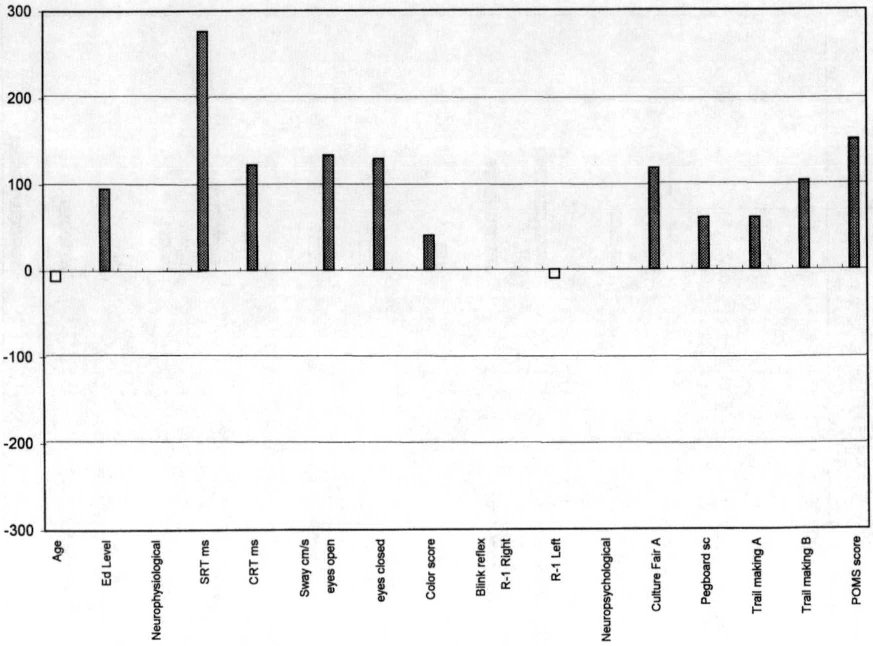

FIGURE 12.4. Comparison of 408 exposed adults to 66 unexposed adults by ANOVA (Combustion). Hatched bars are statistically significant.

similar variation without improving with distance. Simple reaction time for those residents under 0.4 km had similar relative differences, being 415 ms vs. 282 ms in unexposed and 365 ms for residents beyond 0.4 km, but the differences were not significant. All of the other test scores were analyzed for distance, and none showed significant coefficients. Whether age was included or excluded as an independent variable, distance and duration coefficients were insignificant (lower portion of Table 12.9).

Direction

The test scores of all subjects within the eight major compass octants (N, NE, E, SE, S, SW, W, NW) were examined in regression models against distance. The regression analyses for CRT, balance, sway with eyes open and eyes closed, and trail making B in the eight directions for distance and duration are summarized in Table 12.10. The only consistent trend was to the north. All abnormal test scores were examined similarly, including sway speed, color score, Culture Fair, POMS, peg placement, trail making A, and trail making B. None showed significant relationships to direction in compass octants, to distance within octants, or to direction, distance, and duration of residence.

TABLE 12.8 Comparison of retest in 31 combustion exposed subjects tested November 1990 and December 1991

	1990		1990		1991		
	M	Sd	M	Sd	M	Sd	*p*
n	All 43		Match 31		Match 31		
Age	37.8	± 14.1	39.4	± 15.5	40.4	+ 15.4	N
Ed Level	11.0	± 2.3	10.0	± 2.5	10.4	± 2.5	N
Reaction Time ms							
SRT1	347	± 98	368	± 99	429	± 197	N
CRT3	601	± 155	635	± 157	709	± 204	N
Balance-Sway							
SO3	1.17	± 0.46	1.20	± .45	1.33	± 1.04	N
SC3	1.65	± 0.75	1.65	± .69	2.09	± 1.34	N
Glab R-1 Tap ms							
Right	14.3	± 1.7	14.2	± 2.07	14.2	± 2.38	N
Left	14.3	± 2.1	14.7	± 2.14	14.5	± 2.15	N
Color score	13.1	± 2.8	13.9	± 3.0	12.2	± 1.4	.002
CFA score	24.4	± 8.6	22.7	± 8.7	24.4	± 9.1	N
POMS score	61.6	± 47.7	54.6	± 45.9	73.8	± 43.2	N
Peg D sec	80.9	± 12.6	83.5	± 28.9	81.5	± 28.3	N
Trail A sec	38.0	± 10.1	41.1	± 29.9	44.6	± 29.6	N
Trail B sec	80.4	± 30.7	86.5	± 41.4	86.4	± 43.7	N
Grip Right	35.3	± 14.5	35.4	± 14.6	35.9	± 15.0	N
Left	34.2	± 13.6	34.1	± 13.8	32.4	± 14.2	N

N = Not significant

Latency of the first component of blink (R-1) was also unrelated to these approximations of exposure.

Duration

The effect of duration of exposure is shown in tabular form in Table 12.11 and was assessed by regression models of each test score. Duration had no significant influence on any test score (not shown). However, examination by comparison by t-test of scores for the shortest vs. the long durations showed a tendency toward normality at 2 years (25 subjects) and under 2 years (8 subjects). These numbers were small, which limited the statistical power of the comparisons. Nevertheless, mean values for sway speed with eyes open and with eyes closed appeared normal at under 2 years pegs and trails making A were nearly so, while for trail making B the differences compared to those exposed for 17 years were statistically significant. POMS score, Culture Fair A, and pegs tended toward normal, but CRT remained definitely abnormal at under 2 years. The trends were consistent with lesser impairment with shorter durations, but only trails B were statistically significantly different compared to scores of subjects exposed for 17 years. The average duration of residence was significantly shorter, 5.4 years (5.9 years in 31 retest subjects and 5.3 years in 88 original subjects) within 2.4 km of the Combustion site, which may be a confounding factor; but as the means exceeded the 2 years "threshold," this is less likely.

Combined Dose Surrogate

Further analyses of duration and derivatives of distance, including natural logarithm (ln), reciprocal, square, and square root, did not produce significant coefficients with any of the test scores.

TABLE 12.9 Choice reaction time CRT3 and sway speed with eyes closed SC3, mean and standard deviation at distances outward from the Combustion site

Number of Subjects	Distance km	CRT3 Mean	CRT3 Std Dev	Sway Speed Eyes Closed Mean	Sway Speed Eyes Closed Std Dev
9	.02–.14	653	136	1.78	.57
21	.16–.40	677	209	1.79	1.23
35	.41–1.6	588	43	1.40	.70
27	1.6–2.4	651	134	1.49	.65
28	2.4–2.8	617	250	1.34	.68
93	2.8–3.2	604	160	1.48	.63
15	3.2–3.6	648	183	1.31	.47
91	3.6–4.0	628	159	1.53	.98
20	4.0–4.4	614	147	1.06	.40
61	4.4–4.8	595	144	1.50	.63
TOTAL 400	0–4.8	618	165	1.50	.83

As an example, regression models for choice reaction time show that distance and duration coefficients are not statistically significant; only age is significant:

CRT	Coefficient	t	p	Adjusted r^2
Equation 1				
Age	2.664	4.95	.000	
Distance	−10.928	−1.04	.300	.0614
Duration	−.8915	−0.53	.599	
Equation 2				
Distance	−16.628	−1.54	.124	.0010
Duration	.935	0.55	.584	

TABLE 12.10 Regression analysis in eight directions for distance and direction on neurobehavioral tests

Direction	# of Subjects	Average Distance	Reaction Time	Balance Eyes Open	Balance Eyes Closed	Trail Making B Alone	Trail Making B Plus Age
N	79	1.33	0	dis	dis	dur	dur
NE	37	2.57	dis	0	0	0	0
E	12	1.32	0	0	0	0	0
SE	96	2.40	0	0	0	age	0
S	30	1.60	0	0	0	age	0
SW	28	1.69	0	0	dis	age	0
W	38	1.89	0	0	0	dis	dis
NW	51	2.51	0	0	0	age	0

dur = interaction with duration
age = interaction with age
dis = interaction with distance

TABLE 12.11 Scores for selected tests (means) by duration of exposure at Combustion (1966 to 1983) (compared by t-test for unequal-size groups)*

Duration yrs	1.5 or less	2 or less	4 or less	5–17	17
Number	(8)	(25)	(56)	(346)	(105)
Age yrs	39.0	38.7	37.4	40.8	45.1
p	N	N	N	N	
CRT3 ms	693	671	641	619	646
p	N	N	N	N	
Sway Speed cm/s					
Eyes Open	.84	.89	.97	1.00	1.01
p	N	N	N	N	
Eyes Closed	1.19	1.32	1.48	1.51	1.51
p	N	N	N	N	
Pegs sec	83	78.4	78.6	83.1	88.1
p	N	0.14	N	N	
Trails A	34	36.1	38.3	43.8	47.4
p	N	0.72	N	N	
Trails B	68.7*	73.1*	82.9	95.1	98.9
p	.07	.01	N	N	
Culture Fair A	26.1	27.1	26.8	22.7	21.0
p	N	N	N	N	
POMS	42.2?	52.8	54.4	51.9	51.4
p	N	N	N	N	

* All comparisons to 17 years group
N = Not significant
? = Borderline significance

DISCUSSION

Residents' neurobehavioral impairment did not vary with distance out to 4.8 km from the chemical processing site using regression analysis of each test. It was surprising to find an equal extent of neurobehavioral impairment in all of the subgroups defined by distance from Combustion; this differed from the predicted cancer risk for the site, which was based on an air dispersal model (19). As to direction, the scores of subjects in all segments of the compass octant samples were similar to those of the the initial study. Duration alone showed a trend, suggesting a gradient of effect below 2.5 years of exposure but no gradient between 3 and 17 years. Therefore, alternate questions were examined: (1) whether the effects could be spurious, and (2) whether there could be causal factors other than the Combustion exposure.

Were Effects Based on Inappropriate Comparisons?

The test performance of this population was significantly impaired compared to unexposed from Springfield, Louisiana. Also they were impaired compared to Shreveport, Louisiana firefighters (21), whose performance matched that of the Springfield, Louisiana unexposed (20). These unexposed population test scores matched those of a national study group (25), a group of California unexposed (14), two reference groups from Louisiana, and one from Arizona (Table 12.12). Because the Springfield unexposed test scores matched other unexposed groups, we rejected the hypothesis that exposed

TABLE 12.12 Comparison of neurobehavioral test scores of six reference groups in various sections of the United States

	Natl/350		WY/50		LA/14		CA/32		AZ/117		LA/66	
Site/#	22		21		20		14		21		21	
Reference	M	Sd	M	Sd	M	Sd	M	Sd	M	Sd	M	Sd
Age yrs	40.4/10		50.4/20.1		35.0/8.5		38.9/12.5		42.4/15.4		41.2/15.	
Ed Level yrs	14.3/1.1		12.4/2.4		12.5/3.4		12.2/2.4		13.2/2.1		12.5/2.3	
SRT ms	—/—		280/59		—/—		266/50		285/64		288/53	
CRT3 ms	577/118⁺		539/94		572/81⁺		527/88		528/85		534/90	
SO3 cm/s	1.12/.48		.94/.21		1.3/.33*		.80/.19		.78/.18		.83/.2	
SC3 cm/s	1.14/.41		1.40/.41⁺⁺		1.55/.86*		1.16/.31		1.26/.39		1.19/.31	
Cul Fair A	31.2/7.8		27.6/7.9		26.7/6.3		30.3/6.39		29.7/7.5		28.2/8.3	
Block Des	30.2/7.6		28.7/10.6		31.9/6.0		30.2/11.5		31.3/9.7		33.9/9.4	
Peg s	66.9/16.2		82.7/25.8		70.4/6.6		69.7/10.3		71.3/18.1		71.0/14.1	
Trails A	27.8/8.8		39.8/12.1		27.8/6.5		29.3/8.3		31.0/8.8		32.1/11.4	
Trails B	63.8/28.6		83.8/33.8		66.4/17.3		68.3/25.6		71.0/27.0		75.0/40.7	
Story 1	13.2/3.1		11.7/4.4		13.6/2.8		10.8/3.8		12.2/3.9		10.1/3.4	
Story 2	8.4/3.2		11.4/3.6		9.6/4.1		1.6/4.3		11.1/4.2		10.1/3.3	
Finger Rt	2.5/2.4		2.6/3.0		1.7/1.5		3.1/3.4		1.9/1.9		2.2/2.0	
Errors Lt	2.2/2.1		2.3/2.7		2.3/1.9		2.4/3.2		1.1/1.4		1.8/2.3	
Information	ND		17.7/5.5		ND		19.0/6.2		18.5/5.8		16.9/5.3	
Pic Comp	ND		15.3/2.9		ND		24.0/5.7		15.0/3.0		15.3/3.1	
Similarities	ND		21.4/6.4		ND		14.7/3.2		20.9/4.6		20.2/5.3	

⁺ Systematic 45 ms keyboard delay.
⁺⁺ Abnormal from hydrogen sulfide exposure.
* Firemen judged abnormal from hazardous material exposures.

ms = milliseconds
S = seconds
ND = Not done

subjects' lower scores resulted from comparison to unexposed whose scores were atypically high.

Bias by testers was an unlikely explanation because in the studies just summarized, the testers were blinded as to the exposure and comparison status of subjects, who were always tested at the same time. Another important point is that the 22 testers did not know in which residential sector any of these 408 subjects lived. Although duration of residence near the site was a crude surrogate for cumulative dose, there was evidence of less effect at under 2 years of residence in the circle. Subjects at distances under 1.6 km had shorter durations of residence than others, but this difference was not significant and was well over the 2.5 years threshold.

Were There Other Causal Factors?

Could other factors alone or in combination explain these low scores? Questionnaires showed exposures to other neurotoxic factors, but these were usually more frequent in unexposed than exposed subjects, with alcohol and drug use equally unusual, and more unexposed had used pesticides and herbicides. The most common exposure, hours of general anesthesia (a solvent exposure) was not a significant independent variable in regression models for any test score. Occupational exposures to solvents, neurotoxic metals, and spontaneous neurological and medical diseases were unusual in both groups and were not more frequent in the Combustion residents than in nonresidents.

Neurophysiological and neuropsychological test scores are cumulatively reduced by aging (23), head trauma (22), and chemical exposures (14, 25). Accelerated functional impairment with advancing age may reflect cumulative exposure to agents and can be detected after making careful comparisons to aging effects in an unexposed population (14, 25). A major confounding factor, differences in speed of development, applies only to children, but no children were examined. No occupational or other exposure factors appeared as reasonable alternatives to exposure to air, water, and soil at the Combustion site. Water drained to the south–southeast, but no test score gradient was seen in this direction; so adverse effects from water drainage are unlikely. Soil contaminated by chemicals should remain near the site unless migration rates exceed current estimates by 10 to 100 times (19, 26).

A most germane alternative explanation was proximity of the exposed subjects to hydrogen sulfide (H_2S) and other reduced sulfur gases from gas and oil wells and oil collection hubs (14). This exposure was shared by unexposed; so it seems unimportant. There have been two other major chemical exposures in the Combustion (Livingston–Walker, LA) area. First, was a 1982 train derailment, which scattered 21 carloads of toxic chemicals in Livingston Parish on the southeast edge of the study perimeter. Second, there is exposure in another Superfund site (CECOS) south of Livingston, which also impinges on the southeast portion of the Combustion study circle. However, it is not considered as hazardous as Combustion, and its proximity and that of the derailment were considered indirectly in the octant analyses. They were dismissed when the populations in the south–southeast compass segments that contained these sites did not show greater effects than other exposed subjects.

Potential Weaknesses

That the severity of neurobehavioral impairment is proportional to the cumulative effect of toxic chemicals is a reasonable assumption, but there are almost no neurobehavioral dose–response curves for single neurotoxins (5, 26, 27); so assumptions of linear effects should be considered first approximations. Combustion (20) and most real-world situations involve exposures to many agents (5, 27, 28), which are likely to have synergistic effects on the brain (29). It is also possible that less than 2 ½ years' residential exposure to volatile organic chemicals measurably impairs nervous system performance, but subsequent deterioration is not linear.

This site's contamination effect zone as judged from neurobehavioral impairment was widespread and uniform out to 4.8 km. Thermal spread of volatile neurotoxic chemicals distilled into a stagnant air mass during Combustion's operating years has been postulated, in part because other possibilities do not seem plausible. Ordinarily prevailing winds, temperature, and thermal inversions and other meteorological conditions modify the primary emissions from hot processes such as distillation. However, the nearly stagnant air at the Combustion site appeared to have produced a largely invisible, chemically rich, ground fog. This exposure was for up to 24 hours per day for 1 to 17 years for subjects nearby. After distillation ceased, air dispersal probably was reduced to evaporation of chemicals from surface water.

Thirty-one subjects retested after one year showed no improvement; in fact, they showed a worsening trend for simple and choice reaction time, sway speed with eyes open and eyes closed, and POMS score. Continuing deterioration could be due to ongoing neurotoxic effects of body burdens of chemicals, to aging processes that unmask or accentuate damage due to loss of neurons (23, 24, 30), and to lower levels of continuing exposures due to volatilization after distillation ceased in 1983.

Impairment of Exposed Subjects Compared to Unexposed

The exposed and the unexposed groups were closely matched, as shown by memory for ''overlearned'' information, the ''hold'' functions (tested by information, picture completion, and similarities (31)), which supported the assumption that they had been similar prior to being exposed. Sixty-six unexposed subjects provided adequate statistical power. The difference in the recall domain was borderline, suggesting that it is less sensitive to the mix of chemicals at Combustion. The groups remained different after scores in the cognitive, perceptual motor, and overlearned memory domains were adjusted for age and for 1.4 more years of education in the unexposed, by using coefficients from regression models. Reaction time, sway speed, color, and blink had no significant coefficients for education. The test results for four men who had worked and resided at the site were not different from results for those who only resided there.

The matter of adjusting *p*-values for simultaneous inference (31) because of multiple comparisons was carefully considered because 28 tests (including left and right performance of blink, grip, and fingertip writing) were compared. The solution appeared to be conceptual rather than statistical. Seven domains of function or performance were tested, with three to seven tests each. Tests within a domain were not equal in sensitivity; so the plausibility of associations was based on past experience (7, 8, 11, 20, 25, 28). Clearly tests in the physiological domain measure distinct central nervous system functions so that prolonged simple and choice reaction times reflect eye–cerebral–hand pathways (eye, perceptive decision making, and effector pathways) (33), and balance dysfunction measures proprioceptive, vestibular, cerebellar, eye, and effector pathways (11).

Cognitive function for ''fluid'' or problem-solving and constructional tasks, measured by Culture Fair and block design, was adversely affected, but ''hold,'' overlearned, or crystallized functions of language and memory (31) (information, picture completion, and similarities) were not. Culture Fair and block design impairment has accompanied abnormal balance and reaction time in previous studies, implying that slowing of problem-solving ability and delays of automatic responses are associated. Previous studies showed that educational level, which is a fixed achievement measure, predicts scores for the ''hold'' functions, which are least affected by exposure. Fingertip number writing was more resistant to damage than ''fluid'' tasks, suggesting that parietal lobe areas were unaffected (22). Despite its relative insensitivity as compared to self-appraisal, the recall domain was probably affected because several of its test score differences were significant when tested by regression analyses.

The absence of correlation of Culture Fair with the embedded memory–intelligence tests (information, picture completion, and similarities) and its association with choice reaction time and trail making A and B suggest that impaired Culture Fair and impaired block design are effects of exposure. Furthermore the more traditional interpretation of scaling factors for premorbid intelligence applied only to the reference group.

Age-Related Differences in Exposed and Unexposed Subjects

Age was a major independent variable and had a negative coefficient for Culture Fair and for block design after adjustment for the covariant of educational level in exposed and unexposed subjects. The age coefficients of exposed subjects were significantly higher than those of unexposed (Table 12.4). Culture Fair was correlated with the Raven Progressive Matrices, with a coefficient of .95 in a direct comparison of 18 subjects exposed environmentally to trichloroethylene (personal observation). The Raven test has been highly regarded as a sensitive cognitive test for neurotoxic effects in occupational studies (34). Both it and Culture Fair are strongly correlated with perceptual motor performance, as in trail making A and B, and to a lesser extent with recall.

Self-selection

Self-selection bias was eliminated by finding that the bellweather subjects who were tested in the first group because they had many complaints in 1990 and those randomly selected in 1991 were not different. If self-selection were a bias, the ''complainers'' should have scored lower than the ''random'' group, but they did not. A small proportion, only 15% of area residents, were not in the client pool. They would have had to be greatly impaired to have decreased the outcome scores significantly, and conversely they would have to be unusually good performers to raise the mean scores of the exposed and thereby reduce the differences from unexposed. However, the standard deviations were not so large as to indicate any anomaly. Neither possibility seems likely. Also exposed and unexposed subjects had identical malingering indices, and the mean scores across three repetitive measurements of balance, blink, and choice reaction time were nearly identical in exposed and unexposed groups. Furthermore, examination of three trial sequences in all these individuals did not show erratic results from trial to trial, as occurs with faking in the absence of profound insight and training (35). Clients have not been awarded or compensated in this class action because it has not yet come to trial, though most dependents have settled. Thus any possible secondary gain is unrealized after three to four years and seems unlikely to have affected these tests although it could have raised symptom frequency or POMS score.

Confounding Factors

The exposure of both exposed and unexposed groups to possible confounding factors, including drugs, trauma, pesticides, occupational chemicals, and spontaneous neurological or psychiatric diseases, were similar. When they differed, more unexposed than exposed subjects had confounders. Both groups shared exposure to oil and natural gas drilling, pumping, collecting, and refining of southern Louisiana. The factor consistently associated with impairment of neurobehavioral performance was proximity to the Combustion site, which we suggest is responsible for it.

The test scores of those exposed at the Combustion site could have been made to appear low if the local unexposed group's scores were systematically better than other unexposed values. This is highly unlikely because these unexposed scores matched those of several other unexposed groups including Louisiana unexposed firemen (21), our national unexposed group (25), and unexposed in other studies that are being prepared for publication (Table 12.12). The similar test scores among these reference groups selected for freedom from exposure show good test consistency in people without known chemical exposures.

The greatly elevated mood disorder (POMS) total and component scores in the exposed suggested chemical effects on the limbic system, which includes the amygdala, the cingulate gyrus, and the hippocampus. These centers control emotion and drive cortical and brain stem centers for avoidance or self-preservation (i.e., for fight or flight) (33). There is no evidence that an emotional pathway influencing test responses as POMS scores did not correlate with any test. We suggest that chemical exposures elevated the POMS scores as yet another manifestation of organic brain damage. Insidious impairment and symptoms without a triggering event and with no disturbing memories made unlikely a post-traumatic stress or somatization disorder (36).

Reconstructing the Chemical Exposures at This Site

Vaporization from lubricating oils during remanufacturing at the Combustion site liberated toluene, tri(ortho)cresyl phosphate, tetraethyl lead, ethylene dibromide, ethylene dichloride, benzene, and related aromatics and polyaromatics (26, 37), based on lists of chemicals delivered to the site, the operations performed, and pond and sludge analyses after many years (Don Rosebrook, Endoenvironment Inc., Prairieville, LA, 1992). In addition, this site received polychlorinated biphenyls, tetraethyl lead, chlorinated hydrocarbons, and chlorinated aliphatic solvents, including trichloroethylene and tetrachloroethylene. This waste oil operation was never monitored for chemical releases during 1966 to 1983; thus there were no measurements of chemicals (38). Analysis of chemicals in ponds, wells, and boreholes confirmed the above residues after modification by leaching, evaporation, combination, and interaction with soil, water, and plants across time (5, 27). Although effluent air and water from existing waste oil reclaiming facilities could be measured, the absence of chemical wastes not related to crankcase oil in such operations would limit comparability. Therefore, surrogates for exposure (dose) were examined.

One possibility to explain finding no gradient of effects with distance is the model of atmospheric air inversion in a nearly stagnant air mass as depicted in the windrose pattern (Figure 12.1b). As the heated vessels boiled off some chemicals and combustion products were produced from others consumed in heat production, these chemicals would mix and spread by convection into the stagnant air mass and extend beyond 2.4 km, where our most peripheral of tested subjects resided.

Exposure duration of 1 to 17 years was not a dose surrogate in regression analyses, suggesting that adverse effects were produced within 2 years. Other explanations should be considered such as greater sensitivity in older subjects, because the older half of the population in several tests showed adverse effects from nearness to the site that were not shared by the younger half or by the entire group. However, in these analyses, age, distance, and Culture Fair score related to educational level, with all influencing the tests contributing to the poorer performance observed in older exposed subjects.

The surrogates for exposure were distance from the site's center, the reciprocal of distance ($1/D$), the square of distance from the site center and other transformations including the ln of distance. Neither these factors nor duration of exposure (DE), taken separately and then as a product ($1/D \times DE$), correlated with mean test scores of the exposed subjects. The center of the Combustion site was large and irregular because the oil reprocessing boilers were 100 yards from the waste ponds (Figure 12.1a), so the measurements of residential distance from the estimated center were somewhat imprecise. Also the windrose (Figure 12.1b) suggested that the polluted air mass would drift east and south, and this could not be defined in the 2.4 km circle of human effects sampling. This imprecision did not appear to be responsible for the absence of correlations of neurobehavioral performance and distance or with the reciprocal of the product of duration and distance. Because the test scores of quartiles of subjects who were nearest and farthest from the center were identical, testing of subjects farther from the site are needed to define the boundary of effects from Combustion.

Residential Exposures Differ from Occupational Ones

Although residential chemical exposures have been assumed to be lower than occupational ones, in fact almost none have been measured; and frequently by the time a problem is identified, conditions have changed. The mixture of chemicals at Combustion provided opportunities for additive or synergistic interactions, which have been observed in model systems (39) and in acute human testing (29). In several of the residential populations studied (4–6, 9, 40), excessive frequency of symptoms and complaints about odors have justified objective (neurobehavioral) testing. At Combustion physiological abnormalities accompanied high frequencies of many symptoms; so this study joins investigations of trichloroethylene (7) and hydrogen sulfide (Chapter 5). A difference between studies was that in subjects environmentally exposed to TCE-rich solvents (7), blink reflex latency was also abnormal. TCE is toxic for the trigeminal nerve (41).

Confirmation that cumulative residential chemical exposures impair functions of the human central nervous system should stimulate protective strategies for public health (13, 26, 42). These strategies cannot wait for (unavailable) dose–response data (5). Effects on unselected populations of virtually continuous chemical exposures for many years (4, 7, 18) appear to exceed those from usual occupational exposures (16, 17, 43).

References

1. Air/Superfund National Technical Guidance Study series, Vol. 1, Application of air pathway analyses for Superfund activities. PB 90–113374.
2. Health Assessment Summary Tables (Third Quarter FY 1990), U.S. Environmental Protection Agency PB 90–921103.
3. Industrial Source Complex (ISC) Dispersion Model User's Guide (2nd ed., revised), Vol. 1. U.S. Environmental Protection Agency PB 88–171475 (Dec. 1987).
4. Byers VS, Leven AS, Ozonoff DM, and Baldwin RW: Association between clinical symptoms and lymphocyte abnormalities in a population with chronic domestic exposure to industrial solvent-contaminated domestic water supply and a high incidence of leukemia. *Cancer Immunol Immunother* 1988;27:77–81.
5. Levine R and Chitwood DD: Public health investigations of hazardous organic chemical waste disposal in the United States. *Environ Health Perspect* 1985;62:415–422.
6. Roht LH, Vernon SW, Weir FW, Pier SM, Sullivan P, and Reed LJ: Community exposure to hazardous waste disposal sites: assessing reporting bias. *Am J Epidemiol* 1985;122:418–433.
7. Kilburn KH and Warshaw RH: Effects on neurobehavioral performance of chronic exposure to chemically contaminated well water. *Intl J Toxicol Environ Health* 1993;9:391–404.
8. Kilburn KH and Warshaw RH: Neurobehavioral effects of formaldehyde and solvents on histology technicians: repeated observations across time. *Environ Res* 1992;58:134–146.
9. Lagakos SW, Wessen BJ, and Zelen M: An analysis of contaminated well water and health effects in Woburn, Massachusetts. *J Am Statist Assoc* 1986;81:583–596.
10. Ozonoff DM, Colten ME, Cupples A, Heeren T, Schatzkin A, Mangione T, Dresner M, and Colton T: Health problems reported by residents of a neighborhood contaminated by a hazardous waste facility. *Am J Indust Med* 1987;11:581–597.
11. Kilburn KH, Warshaw RH, and Hanscom B: Are hearing loss and balance dysfunction linked in construction iron workers? *Brit J Indust Med* 1992;49:138–141.
12. Juntunen J, Ylikoski J, Ojala M, Matikainen E, Ylikoski M, and Vaheri E: Postural body sway and exposure to high-energy noise. *Lancet* 1989;2:261–264.

13. Needleman HL: What can the study of lead teach us about toxicants? *Environ Health Perspect* 1990;86:183–189.
14. Kilburn KH and Warshaw RH: Neurobehavioral impairment downwind from a petroleum refinery with a desulfurization unit: low dose hydrogen sulfide exposure. *Toxicol Occup Health* 1995;11:185–197.
15. Grabski DA: Toluene sniffing producing cerebellar degeneration. *Am J Psychiatry* 1961; 118:461–462.
16. Deek RB, Setzer JV, Wait R, Hayden MB, Taylor BJ, Tolos B, and Putz-Anderson V: Effects of acute exposure to toluene and methyl ethyl ketone on psychomotor performance. *Intl Arch Occup Environ Health* 1984;54:91–99.
17. Larsen F and Leira HL: Organic brain syndrome and long-term exposure to toluene: a clinical psychiatric study of vocationally active printing workers. *J Occup Med* 1988;30:875–878.
18. White RF, Diamond R, Proctor S, Morey C, and Hu H: Residual cognitive defects 50 years after lead poisoning during childhood. *Brit J Indust Med* 1993;50:613–622.
19. Coerr S: Geographical extent of health risk from air pollutant emissions of the Combustion site. Chapel Hill, NC: Stanton Coerr Consulting, 1990.
20. Kilburn KH and Warshaw RH: Neurotoxic effects from residential exposure to chemicals from an oil reprocessing facility and Superfund site. *Neurotoxicol Teratol* 1995;17:89–102.
21. Kilburn KH, Warshaw RH, and Shields MG: Neurobehavioral dysfunction in fireman exposed to polychlorinated biphenyls (PCBs): possible improvement after detoxification. *Arch Environ Health* 1989;44:345–350.
22. Reitan RM: A research program on the psychological effects of brain lesions in human beings. In: *International Review of Research in Mental Retardation*, NR Ellis (ed.). New York: Academic Press, 1966.
23. Potvin AR, Syndulko K, Tourtellotte WW, Lemmon JA, and Potvin JH: Human neurologic function and the aging process. *J Am Geriatr Soc* 1980;28:1–9.
24. Cattell RB, Feingold SN, and Sarason SB: A culture free intelligence test II evaluation of cultural influences on performance. *J Educ Psych* 1941;32:81–100.
25. Kilburn KH, Warshaw R, and Thornton JC: Formaldehyde impairs memory, equilibrium, and dexterity in histology technicians: effects which persist for days after exposure. *Arch Environ Health* 1987;42:117–120.
26. Greisham JW: *Health Aspects of the Disposal of Waste Chemicals.* New York: Pergamon Press, 1986.
27. Gamberale F and Kjellberg A: Behavioral performance assessment as a biological control of occupational exposure to neurotoxic substances in neurobehavioral methods in occupational health. *Adv Biosci* 1983;41:137–144.
28. Kilburn KH: Evidence that the human nervous system is most sensitive to chemical toxins. *J Environ Sci Health* 1991;C8(2):327–337.
29. Savolainen K: Combined effects of xylene and alcohol on the central nervous system. *Acta Phamacol Toxicol* 1980;46:366–372.
30. Brizzee KR: Gross morphometric analyses and quantitative histology of the aging brain. In: *Neurobiology of Aging: An Interdisciplinary Life-Span Approach*, JM Ordy and KR Brizzee (eds.). New York: Plenum Press, 1975.
31. Ryan CM, Morrow LA, Bromet EJ, and Parkinson DK: Assessment of neuropsychological dysfunction in the workplace: normative data from the Pittsburgh occupational exposures test battery. *J Clin Exper Neuropsych* 1987;9:665–679.
32. Wright SP: Adjust *p* values for simultaneous inference. *Biometrics* 1992;48:1005–1013.
33. Brodal P: *The Central Nervous System, Structure and Function.* New York: Oxford University Press, 1992.
34. Anger WK: Work site behavioral research: results, sensitive methods, test batteries and the transition from laboratory data to human health. *Neurotoxicology* 1990;11:629–720.
35. Reitan RM: Validity of the trail-making test as an indicator of organic brain damage. *Percept Motor Skills* 1958;8:271–276.

36. McFarlane AC: The phenomenology of posttraumatic stress disorders following a natural disaster. *J Nerv Ment Dis* 1988;176:22–29.
37. Terrill JB, Montgomery RR, and Reinhardt CF: Toxic gases from fires. *Science* 1978;200: 1343–1347.
38. Lawrence RD: Combustion, Inc. site, Livingston Parish, Louisiana. Department of Environmental Quality, Solid and Hazardous Waste, Inactive and Abandoned Sites Division.
39. Narahashi T: Nerve membrane channels as the target of toxicants. *Arch Toxicol* Suppl. 1986; 2:3–13.
40. Shusterman D, Lipscomb J, Neutra J, and Satin K: Symptom prevalence and odor–worry interaction near hazardous waste sites. *Environ Health Perspect* 1991;94:25–30.
41. Feldman RG, Chirico-Post J, and Proctor SP: Blink reflex latency after exposure to trichloroethylene in well water. *Arch Environ Health* 1988;43:143–148.
42. Neutra R, Lipscomb J, Satin K, and Shusterman D: Hypotheses to explain the higher symptom rates observed around hazardous waste sites. *Environ Health Perspect* 1991;94:31–38.
43. Kilburn KH and Warshaw RH: Neurobehavioral effects of formaldehyde and solvents in histology technicians: repeated testing across time. *Environ Res* 1992;58:134–146.

13

Aluminum Recycling: Vinyl Chloride and Other Contaminants

The Alabama Reclamation aluminum remelt facility of Reynolds Aluminum (in Muscle Shoals, AL) consists of six large-capacity furnaces made of fire brick and insulated with asbestos. Ordinarily five are in operation and one is being rebuilt at any given time. The facility was opened in 1968 on the west side of an aluminum refinery, which had been built in the 1940s and had six pot rooms in operation until 1986, when electrolytic refining of virgin aluminum ceased. Metal scrap includes engine blocks and heads from automobiles, borings and turnings from industrial operations, aluminum siding, and aluminum containers, particularly beer and soft drink cans coated inside with polyvinyl chloride. Less well-characterized scrap contains copper, iron, and other metals along with rubber, plastics, and polyvinyl electrical insulation.

The scrap is dumped into a metal shredder, a seven-story structure that reduces it to pieces under 10 centimeters on a side that can be fed into the furnace. The remelting is a continuous operation in which dross is removed by additives including manganese, chlorine, and chryolite. The remelt operation generates a sweet, irritating chemical odor that can be perceived throughout the plant. Large amounts of glistening black, slick dust are produced, and are caught in a baghouse. Workers describe the baghouse as an area having treacherous footing, where they work up to their waists in loose, slick, shiny, black, greasy dust. The usual protective equipment is a dust mask or two and sometimes a paper suit, but never a full suit and air supply respirator. Air supply masks are only occasionally available. Characteristically, after emerging from the dust house or finishing a shift, workers need to scrub their skin with baby oil to remove adherent black dust.

The furnace fumes cause coughing, shortness of breath, tightness of the chest, and chest burning, together with eye irritation, which are particularly severe after a furnace has been charged. The removal of dross, the nonaluminum or aluminum pour contaminants, is a major process. Some dross floats and is skimmed off; the rest falls to the bottom and is removed after the aluminum has been drawn off. The heavier portion characteristically is shipped to a hazardous waste site in Emelle, Alabama.

The electrolytic aluminum refinery, which used the Hall-Heroult process, opened in the 1940s and ceased operation in 1986 when much aluminum became available for remelting. In 1988 we studied 670 aluminum workers at this plant and compared them with 659 pipefitters from Muscle Shoals (1). We excluded from the pipefitter group anyone who had worked in the aluminum refinery. As the pot rooms had been closed for two years, this was a study of remelt workers, some of whom had worked previously in pot rooms. Irregular opacities, X-ray findings similar to asbestosis, were found in 20.7% of workers who had been employed for 20 years. Among the notable differences from usual asbestos-exposed workers were that the remelt workers had more fine s/s opacities of a low degree of profusion, mostly 1/1, and almost no pleural abnormalities (2.1%). In contrast 12% of the pipefitters had pleural abnormalities only, and 6.7% had pulmonary and pleural asbestosis vs. 2.8% in the aluminum workers. Aluminum workers also had worse small airways disease than the pipefitters. A Monday across-a-work-shift study of 57 aluminum workers showed that 32% had more than a 15% decrement in FEF_{27-75} or 5% decrement in FEV_1.

Many ex-workers complained of difficulties with balance, and some were in wheelchairs. Choice reaction time, balance using the head tracker, time required to place pegs in a slotted pegboard, and scores for trail making A and B and digit symbol were significantly different in 28 current and ex-workers from results obtained in resident or worker unexposed groups, including Louisiana firemen (2) and Louisiana and California resident reference groups (3). In 1993 a pilot study was focused on aluminum remelt workers from this plant who had neurobehavioral and pulmonary complaints and were plaintiffs in a lawsuit. They were compared to local reference subjects.

TESTING OF SUBJECTS

Subjects

A cohort comparison design was used. All 146 current workers were invited, and 14 women and 27 men volunteered for this pilot study. Each of these subjects invited an unexposed relative or friend as her or his local comparison subject. The 14 women and 18 men comparison subjects matched the educational level of workers (Table 13.1a, Figure 13.1), but were almost 6 years younger, a significant difference. Also more exposed than unexposed subjects were African-Americans. Unexposed and workers resided in the Muscle Shoals–Florence, Alabama area. We excluded as unexposed those ever employed at the remelt plant or at chemical plants, and those who had lived within 8 km of the site.

The 66 regional unexposed from Springfield, Louisiana (aged 18–68 years) had no evidence of having experienced chemical contamination of air or of water and matched the sex, age, and educational attainment of a previously studied exposed cohort (4) (Figure 13.2). Selected at random from voter registration rolls, they had been interviewed for matching criteria and willingness to be tested. They were reimbursed for their time and mileage.

Muscle Shoals subjects' exposure was not known to the testers, and the Springfield unexposed subjects' testing had also been blind. After a complete explanation of the testing, all subjects gave their informed consent. The protocol was approved by the Human Studies Research Committee of the University of Southern California School of Medicine. The testers had been trained before previous studies, were given a 4-hour refresher, and did not attempt to differentiate workers and unexposed subjects when testing them.

TABLE 13.1a Demographic, neurophysiological, cognitive, and perceptual motor speed scores in aluminum remelt exposed and (local and regional) unexposed subjects compared by analysis of variance

	A Exposed	B Local Unexposed	A to B	C Regional Unexposed	C to B
	n = 41	n = 32	p	n = 66	p
	mean Sd	mean Sd	value	mean Sd	value
Age yrs	45.4 ± 6.1	39.6 ± 8.5	.001*	41.2 ± 15.0	.25
Education Level yrs	12.0 ± 1.6	12.7 ± 2.1	.08	12.6 ± 2.1	.34
Neurophysiological					
Simple Reaction Time s	334 ± 85	257 ± 45	.0001*	288 ± 53	.09
Choice Reaction Time s	637 ± 113	500 ± 76	.0001*	523 ± 84	.40
	637 ± 113	523 ± 24**	.0001*	534 ± 90	.50
Balance Sway Speed cm/s					
Eyes Open	1.03 ± .36	.80 ± .14	.001*	0.83 ± 0.21	.32
Eyes Closed	1.62 ± .53	1.30 ± .35	.005*	1.19 ± 0.33	.56
Blink Reflex Latency ms					
Glabellar Tap					
Right	14.9 ± 1.7	14.4 ± 1.7	.250	14.4 ± 2.0	.09
Left	15.9 ± 1.5	15.1 ± 1.3	.045*	14.5 ± 2.0	.44
Color					
Discrimination sc	12.4 ± 6.0	11.3 ± 3.9	.0001*	11.4 ± 2.0	.56
Visual Acuity score					
Right	3.1 ± 1.8	2.4 ± 1.0	.050*		
Left	3.2 ± 2.1	2.4 ± 1.0	.044*		
Cognitive					
Culture Fair A sc	20.4 ± 7.5	28.7 ± 5.4	.0001*	28.2 ± 8.3	.42
Perceptual Motor Speed					
Pegboard s	75.1 ± 12.9	66.6 ± 13.8	.008*	71.0 ± 14.2	.83
Trail Making s A	45.3 ± 18.9	32.7 ± 11.2	.001*	32.1 ± 11.4	.34
B	114.1 ± 40.5	64.5 ± 21.0	.0001*	75.0 ± 40.7	.41

* = significant differences ** Age-adjusted unexposed.
ms = milliseconds sc = score
s = seconds sd = standard deviation

Results

Exposed and reference groups were not significantly different for educational attainment, alcohol use, past smoking of cigarettes, and alveolar carbon monoxide, but their ages differed significantly (Table 13.1a). Blood alcohol levels were all below .01 deciliter/ml (dl/ml) except in one unexposed subject (.026 dl/ml); the means did not differ, and alcohol use was not different between the groups. Alveolar carbon monoxide levels as evidence of cigarette smoking were lower in exposed than unexposed subjects (Table 13.2a).

All of the neurophysiological tests showed significant differences between the groups (Table 13.1a). Simple reaction time differed by 77 ms ($p<.0001$), and two-choice visual reaction time was different by 137 ms ($p<.0001$). Balance (sway speed) with eyes open in the exposed group was 1.03 cm/s and thus different from the 0.80 cm/s in the unexposed ($p<.001$). Balance with eyes closed was 1.62 cm/s in the exposed group, significantly faster than the 1.30 cm/s in the unexposed ($p<.0005$). Color discrimination was also different ($p<.0001$). Blink reflex latency of R-1 was significantly

TABLE 13.1b POMS scores and medical histories

	Exposed		Local Unexposed		A to B	Regional Unexposed		C to B
	mean	Sd	mean	Sd	*p* value	mean	Sd	*p* value
POMS score	82.2 ±	40.6	20.3 ±	35.2	.0001*	23.2 ±	32.9	.35
Tension	20.0 ±	8.0	9.5 ±	7.7	.0001*	8.9 ±	6.6	.44
Depression	23.6 ±	13.6	8.6 ±	9.0	.0001*	8.1 ±	9.7	.57
Anger	19.5 ±	11.4	6.4 ±	6.2	.0001*	9.2 ±	8.8	.43
Vigor	11.4 ±	5.1	19.0 ±	6.0	.0001*	17.8 ±	6.5	.54
Fatigue	15.2 ±	6.3	8.9 ±	6.8	.0001*	7.7 ±	6.3	.72
Confusion	15.2 ±	4.9	6.0 ±	4.9	.0001*	6.3 ±	4.5	.91

	Exposed %	Local Unexposed	*p* % Value*
Psychiatric illness (depression)	19.5	3.1	.035
Neurological disease	4.9	0	.793
Stroke	4.9	0	.764
Angina pectoris	19.5	9.4	.459
Diabetes mellitus	7.3	3.1	.374
Allergies	31.7	21.9	.289

* By chi square.

longer on the left side but not on the right. Color discrimination and visual acuity were significantly poorer in exposed subjects. Contrast sensitivity was significantly less for the exposed in the more discriminatory ranges of C, D, and E.

Cognitive function as measured by Culture Fair was significantly lower, 20.4 in exposed and 28.7 in unexposed subjects ($p<.0001$). Trail making A at 45.3 s in exposed vs. 32.7 s in unexposed was different ($p<.0013$), as was trail making B at 114 s in exposed vs. 64.5 in unexposed ($p<.0001$). Putting pegs in the slotted pegboard took almost 9 s longer in exposed than in unexposed ($p<.008$).

POMS score averaged 82.2 in exposed subjects, four times that of unexposed subjects, a significant difference (Table 13.1b). All of the adverse moods were significantly elevated, with decreased vigor, in exposed workers compared to unexposed. Despite these elevations, POMS score was not predictive of other tests in regression models. The local unexposed group showed no statistically significant differences (Tables 13.1a and 13.1b) from regional unexposed (4).

Past diseases prevalences were similar, except that the exposed group had significantly more chronic bronchitis by questionnaire criteria. Respiratory symptoms were 3 to 12 times more prevalent in the exposed than the unexposed (Table 13.2a). The forced vital capacities and flows of aluminum workers were slightly lower than those of the unexposed, but these differences were not statistically significant, nor were workers different from regional unexposed (Table 13.2b). Function in all groups was significantly below predicted (national) values (5).

Sources of drinking water did not differ between the groups; so confounding from chemicals in water is unlikely. Group differences in occupational exposures, including asbestos and work in power plants, metal reduction, plastics, and use of vibrating tools, were explained by aluminum remelting (Table 13.3). Otherwise, unexposed had more

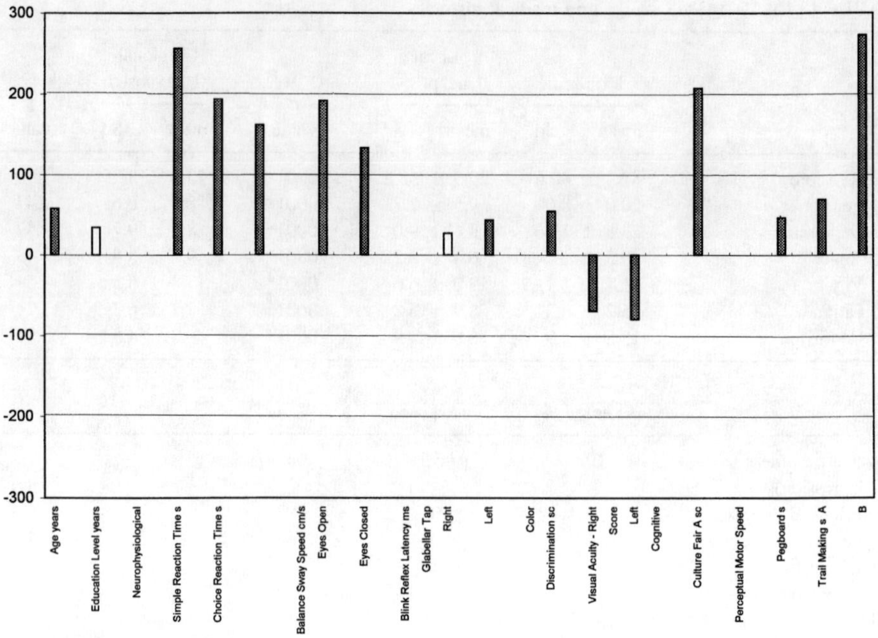

FIGURE 13.1. Comparison of 41 exposed adults to 32 unexposed adults by ANOVA (aluminum workers). Hatched bars are statistically significant.

adverse occupational exposures than exposed subjects, which would be expected to decrease differences between the groups. On the 11-part ARA rheumatism questionnaire (6), twice as many exposed subjects as unexposed had numbness of the fingers, seven times as many had sun-related rashes, pleural pain was four times higher, and three times as many had had unexplained hair loss (Table 13.4). Only one subject had a diagnosed neurological disease, which was a mild stroke. However, a diagnosis of depression was six times more frequent in exposed workers than in unexposed (Table 13.1b).

Workers had significantly higher frequencies than the unexposed for 32 of the 35 symptoms, particularly in the respiratory–irritative group and the neurological category, including loss of balance, irritability, unstable moods, recent and long-term memory loss, lack of concentration, extreme fatigue, and shortened sleep periods (Table 13.5, Figures 13.3a, b). Differences for chest tightness, chest burning, shortness of breath, and palpitations were also large. Only three infrequent symptoms, loss of consciousness, bloody sputum, and inability to fall asleep, were not different.

Because the age difference of 5.8 years was significant, age coefficients were calcu-

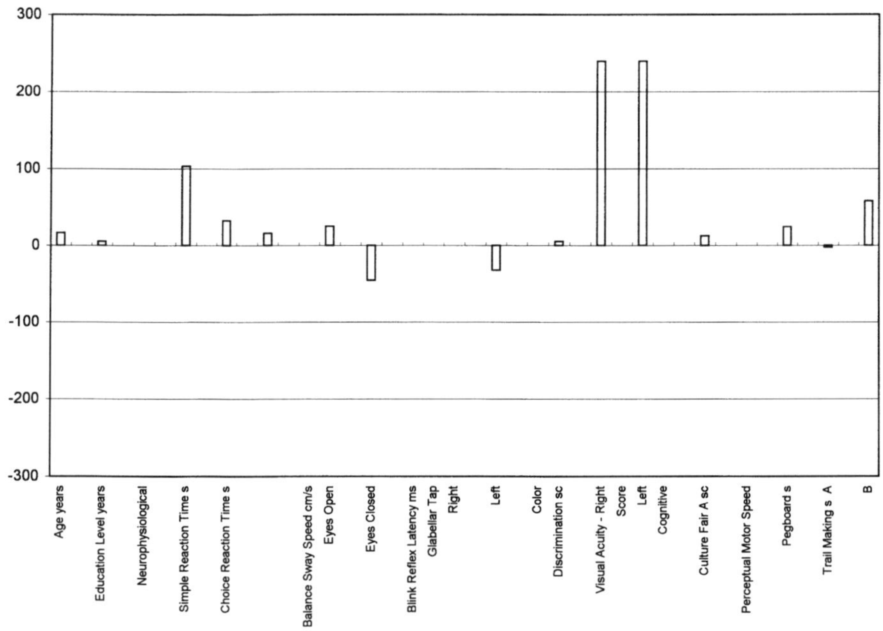

FIGURE 13.2. Comparison of 32 local unexposed adults to 66 national unexposed adults by ANOVA. Hatched bars are statistically significant.

TABLE 13.2a Prevalences of respiratory symptoms and other illnesses in exposed subjects and unexposed as percentage, compared by analysis of variance

	Exposed	Unexposed	*p*
Ever smoked	52.5	40.6	.384
Carbon monoxide level ppm (in alveolar gas by consumptive meter)	7.8	10.5	.753
Chronic bronchitis diagnosed previously	9.8	3.1	.153
Phlegm	56.1	12.5	.0005*
Chronic bronchitis by criteria	41.5	6.3	.0005*
Short of breath			
At rest	36.6	3.1	.0004*
Walking	53.7	6.3	.0003*
Climbing	78.0	28.1	.00005*
Wheezing	39.0	9.4	.0037*
Wheezing with shortness of breath	41.5	9.4	.0037*

* Significantly different $p < 0.05$.

TABLE 13.2b Pulmonary function tests in exposed vs. unexposed

	A Exposed		B Unexposed		A to B	C Regional Unexposed		A to C
	Mean	Sd	Mean	Sd	p Value	Mean	Sd	p value
FVC % pred*	95.9 ±	11.7	100.7 ±	11.7	.082	109.8 ±	18.0	.005
FEV_1 % pred	93.6 ±	13.9	98.0 ±	14.3	.134	94.2 ±	13.1	.767
FEV_{25-75} % pred	87.9 ±	28.8	88.8 ±	24.5	.889	92.2 ±	30.2	.154
FEV_{75-85} % pred	74.9 ±	28.2	82.6 ±	30.7	.270	82.6 ±	51.1	.867
FEV_1/FVC	78.1 ±	6.2	79.7 ±	5.3	.269	74.7 ±	9.3	.547

* % Predicted adjusts for height, sex, age, and years of cigarette smoking.

lated for each test for the reference groups. When the coefficient was statistically significant, mean test scores of unexposed were adjusted for age before comparison to exposed scores. The choice reaction time age coefficient was 3.88 ms per year, which multiplied by 6 years, the age difference, subtracted 23 ms from the difference of 137 ms, but this reduced difference remained statistically significant ($p<.0001$) (Table 13.1a). Balance function had no significant age coefficients and so did not need correction. After Culture Fair and trails B scores were age-adjusted, groups remained significantly different. No other test required age adjustment, and ethnic differences were insignificant.

TABLE 13.3 Occupational exposures of exposed and local unexposed subjects as percent of group

	Exposed	Unexposed
Power plant	17.1*	9.4
Refinery	0	0
Metal reduction	26.8*	6.2
Explosives	7.3	3.1
Chemical or pharmaceutical industries	12.2	9.4
Dyes	4.9	9.4
Plastics	14.6*	6.3
Dry cleaning	2.4	9.4
Textiles	12.2	18.8
Photography	0	3.1
Solvents	14.6	12.5
Printing	0	3.1
Electronics	2.4	6.4
Aerospace	4.9	0
Rocket fuel	0	0
Vibrating tools	39.0*	21.9
Adhesives	24.4	16.7
Spray painting	7.3	9.4
Pesticides	2.4	9.4
Herbicides	0	6.2
Asbestos	39.0*	9.7

* Significantly different.

TABLE 13.4 Prevalence of American Rheumatism Association symptoms of lupus erythematosus compared in exposed and unexposed subjects by analysis of variance (one-way)

	% Exposed	% Local Unexposed	*p*
Rheumatism	25	19	.0001
Numb fingers	50	28	.000
Mouth sores	20	0	.007
Anemia	28	31	.122
Rash on cheeks	8	0	.117
Sun rash	20	3	.004
Painful breathing	49	12	.001
Protein in urine	13	9	.653
Hair loss	24	9	.099
Seizures	2	3	.874

DISCUSSION

Balance, simple and choice reaction time, color discrimination, cognitive function, and perceptual motor speed were definitely impaired, and blink reflex latency and visual contrast sensitivity were probably impaired in aluminum remelt workers as compared to local unexposed. These findings in the absence of confounding factors strongly suggest workplace exposure to neurotoxins. The elevated symptom frequencies and depression were also consistent with toxic exposures in these young workers. Adverse neurobehavioral effects were definitely associated with remelting aluminum (7). The functional disabilities are more severe than those associated with potroom palsy or encephalopathy (8–10) found in workers refining virgin aluminum.

Pulmonary function of exposed subjects was impaired when compared to standard unexposed groups (5), but the differences between Muscle Shoals exposed and unexposed groups and regional unexposed subjects were also not significant; so ambient air pollution in Muscle Shoals did not need to be considered.

Although aluminum is an obvious first choice for impairing neurobehavioral performance and increasing the frequency of neurobehavioral, rheumatic, and respiratory symptoms (7), an exclusive attribution is not possible because of exposures to manganese, fluorine, chlorine, and other process chemicals (8) and to contaminants such as vinyl chloride monomer released from polyvinyl coatings on aluminum siding or insulation on electrical wire in the remelt process. Future studies should measure these chemicals in workplace air and use internal dose markers such as elevated serum aluminum, manganese, and vinyl chloride in workers.

An alternate explanation for the differences between workers and unexposed subjects was not found in careful scrutiny of occupational exposures, medical diseases, neurological disease, or other possible confounders. Although workers were self-selected, they in fact opposed both the company and the union in order to be studied. A venturesome spirit is not predictive of impaired function, but even if they were worst cases, a problem has been demonstrated by their test scores. Even if their anger and despair might elevate mood status scores or exaggerate questionnaire symptom frequencies, no mechanism has been demonstrated by which chronic anger could impair performance on involuntary

TABLE 13.5 Comparison of frequency of 35 symptoms on scale of 11 in exposed and unexposed subjects using analysis of variance

	Exposed	Unexposed	
	Mean Sd	Mean Sd	*p* Value
Skin itching	5.54 ± 3.35	3.56 ± 3.37	.0138
Fingernails abnormal	3.03 ± 3.03	1.53 ± 1.48	.0199
Chest tightness	4.78 ± 2.83	1.72 ± 1.20	.00005
Palpitations	3.68 ± 2.73	2.13 ± 2.25	.00005
Burning chest	4.27 ± 2.88	1.65 ± 1.17	.00005
Shortness of breath	5.68 ± 2.89	2.16 ± 1.80	.00005
Dry cough	4.53 ± 2.81	2.23 ± 1.43	.0001
Cough with mucus	5.30 ± 3.15	2.60 ± 2.25	.0002
Cough with blood	1.83 ± 1.71	1.23 ± 0.82	.0845*
Dry mouth	5.70 ± 3.15	2.97 ± 2.50	.0002
Throat irritation	5.23 ± 2.76	2.87 ± 2.45	.0004
Eye irritation	5.15 ± 3.22	3.53 ± 2.99	.0364
Reduced smell	4.62 ± 3.68	2.20 ± 2.52	.0030
Headache	6.43 ± 3.09	4.23 ± 2.79	.0031
Nausea	3.15 ± 2.51	2.13 ± 1.22	.0449
Dizziness	3.90 ± 2.79	1.8 ± 1.22	.0004
Lightheadedness	3.75 ± 2.64	1.83 ± 1.09	.0004
Exhilaration	2.20 ± 2.19	1.28 ± 0.58	.0249
Loss of balance	4.07 ± 3.09	1.63 ± 1.31	.00005
Loss of consciousness	1.68 ± 1.49	1.41 ± 0.91	.3590*
Extreme fatigue	6.32 ± 3.42	3.28 ± 2.36	.00005
Somnolence	4.58 ± 3.50	2.78 ± 2.55	.017
Insomnia:			
Cannot fall asleep	4.10 ± 2.76	3.03 ± 2.43	.0892*
Wake frequently	4.85 ± 3.10	3.16 ± 2.44	.0132
Sleep few hours	5.73 ± 3.25	2.88 ± 1.81	.00005
Irritability	6.51 ± 3.31	3.31 ± 2.60	.00005
Lack of concentration	7.46 ± 3.17	3.81 ± 2.95	.00005
Recent memory loss	8.02 ± 3.20	3.53 ± 3.04	.00005
Long-term memory loss	6.23 ± 3.92	2.66 ± 2.89	.00005
Mood instability	5.95 ± 3.84	2.50 ± 2.17	.00005
Decreased libido	5.53 ± 3.39	2.78 ± 2.90	.0005
Dec. alcohol tolerance	2.92 ± 3.08	1.62 ± 1.08	.0336
Indigestion	5.85 ± 2.85	3.31 ± 2.62	.0002
Loss of appetite	3.30 ± 2.07	1.97 ± 1.60	.0038
Stomach bloats	5.55 ± 3.36	2.28 ± 2.05	.00005

* Not statistically significant.

tests such as balance and blink or even reaction time, color discrimination, visual acuity, Culture Fair, and pegboard and trail making. Manipulating these test outcomes presupposes knowledge of expected results for many different tests, which seemed unlikely in these workers.

Also, since the purpose of this preliminary investigation was to determine whether a problem existed and to generate hypotheses rather than survey the average worker's status, this consideration is not crucial. Selection of an unexposed reference subject by each worker could have biased the comparison, but it is unlikely that workers, naive as they were to the tests, had the insight to pick superior performers. More important, if selection had been biased, the hand-picked local unexposed should have performed

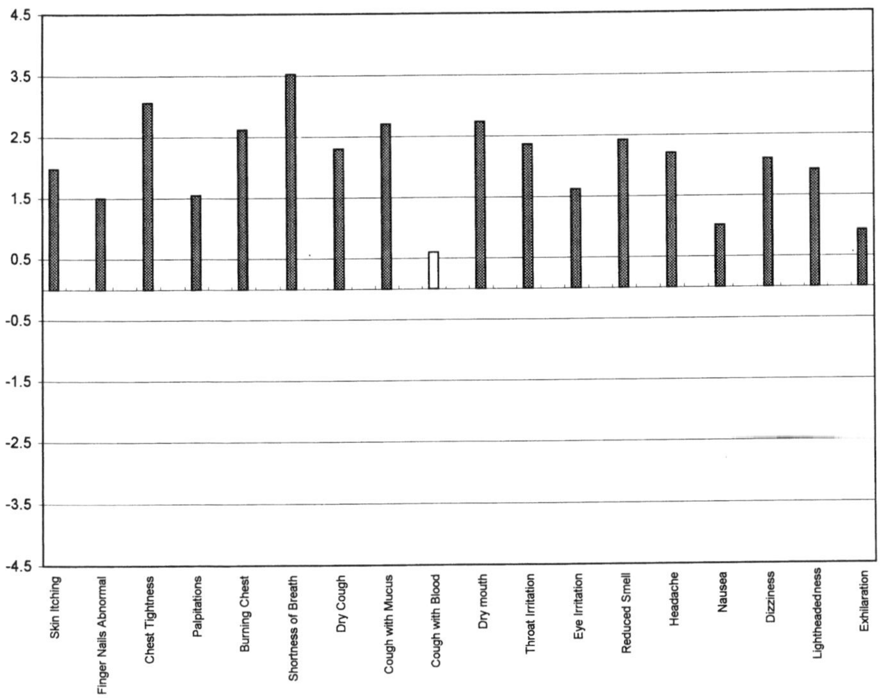

FIGURE 13.3a. Comparison of symptom frequencies in 41 exposed adults and 32 unexposed adults by ANOVA (aluminum remelting workers). Hatched bars are statistically significant.

better than regional and other unexposed groups, and they did not do so (3, 4). Examiner bias was avoided by concealing the exposure status of all subjects from the examiners. Ethnicity did not influence the comparisons.

Elimination of these factors suggested that the differences in function should be attributed to the subjects' inhaling chemicals while working remelt aluminum furnaces, which was the remaining difference between workers and reference subjects. (At this plant, the cooperation needed for further characterization of this airborne exposure was denied us.) Inhalation exposure is also invoked to explain these workers' high frequencies of symptoms for elevated mood (POMS) scores as compared to the unexposed populations. The small airways obstruction predicted in these workers from earlier studies (1, 7) was found, but its attribution to aluminum is equivocal because they did not differ from unexposed in the impairment.

Aluminum is neurotoxic and produced rapidly progressive encephalopathy after more than a decade of exposure in an aluminum ball mill worker over 30 years ago (8). Subsequently, potroom palsy, consisting of incoordination, intention tremor, and spastic paraparesis, was described in longstanding aluminum refinery workers exposed

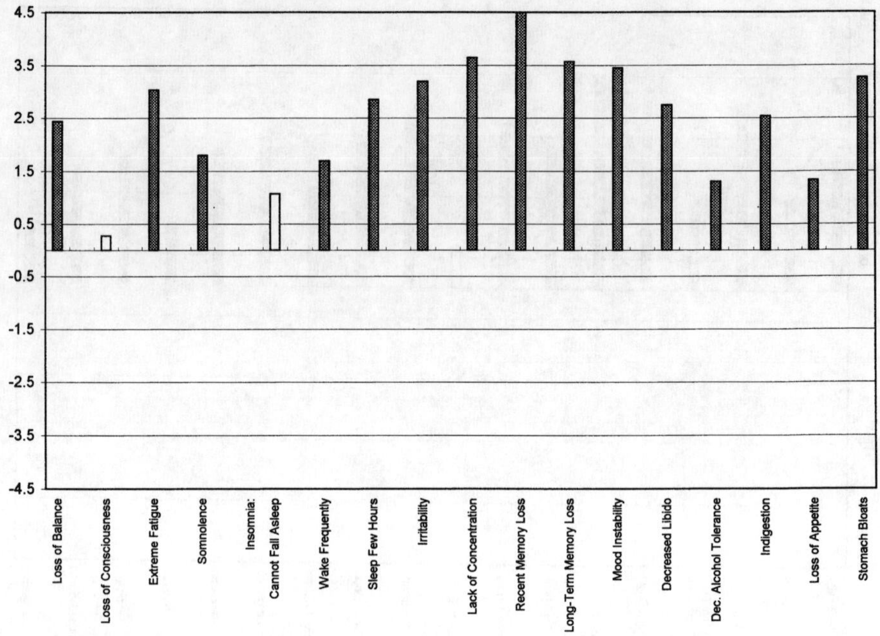

FIGURE 13.3b. Comparison of symptom frequencies in 41 exposed adults and 32 unexposed adults by ANOVA (aluminum remelting workers). Hatched bars are statistically significant.

to manganese, chrysolite, chlorine, fluorine, and other process chemicals including coal tar (9)—who also showed poor short-term memory on testing. Curiously, their Halstead-Reitan impairment index was normal, but it is a battery of 1950-era tests. The addition of 22 current and retired workers confirmed these findings (10). Renal dialysis patients using aluminum-enriched water and aluminum-hydroxide antacids had deficient performance on block design, digit symbol, and picture arrangement from Wechsler's battery (11). Manganese, which is added to aluminum during remelting, causes a movement disorder resembling Parkinson's disease (12), and chlorinated solvents—particularly vinyl chloride, the metabolite of many of them—are known neurotoxins (3). Vinyl chloride monomer, a thermal degradation product of polyvinyl chloride, causes asthma and is probably neurotoxic, based upon Veltman et al.'s report (13) and personal observations.

The next logical step would be to extend this study to other groups, where the chemicals in the workplace air could be characterized and linked to the neurological impairment, symptoms, and depression. Repeated sampling under various furnace conditions may be needed to characterize workers' exposures in further study of this hazardous process.

Meanwhile, workers should be protected by enclosing the remelt process. Such "closed retorting" greatly reduced hydrocarbon emissions from the Sodeberg cells in the primary aluminum Hall-Heroult refining process (7). Furthermore, workers in dust-catching areas such as the baghouse should wear air supply respirators and chemically resistant suits.

References

1. Kilburn KH and Warshaw RH: Irregular opacities in the lung, occupational asthma, and airways dysfunction in aluminum workers. *Am J Indust Med* 1992;21:845–853.
2. Kilburn KH, Warshaw RH, and Thornton JC: Formaldehyde impairs memory, equilibrium, and dexterity in histology technicians: effects which persist for days after exposure. *Arch Environ Health* 1987;42:117–120.
3. Kilburn KH and Warshaw RH: Effects of chronic exposure to trichloroethylene and other chemicals in well water on neurobehavioral performance. *Toxicol Indust Health* 1992;9: 391–404.
4. Kilburn KH and Warshaw RH: Neurotoxic effects from residential exposure to chemicals from an oil reprocessing facility and Superfund site. *Neurotox Teratol* 1995;17:89–102.
5. Miller A, Thornton JC, Warshaw R, Bernstein J, Selikoff IJ, and Teirstein AS: Mean and instantaneous expiratory flows, FVC and FEV_1: prediction equations from a probability sample of Michigan, a large industrial state. *Bull Eur Physiopath Respir* 1986;589–597.
6. Levin RE, Weinstein A, Peterson M, Testa MA, and Rothfield NF: A comparison of the sensitivity of the 1971 and 1982 American Rheumatism Association criteria for the classification of lupus erythematosus. *Arthritis Rheum Dis* 1978;118:7–54.
7. Kilburn KH: Pulmonary neurobehavioral impairment from aluminum. In: *Environmental and Occupational Disease* (2nd ed.), W Rom (ed.). Boston: Little, Brown and Co., 1992, pp. 470–473.
8. McLaughlin AIG, Kazantzis G, King E, Teare D, Porter RJ, and Owen R: Pulmonary fibrosis and encephalopathy associated with the inhalation of aluminum dust. *Brit J Indust Med* 1962;19:253–263.
9. Longstreth WT, Rosenstock L, and Heyer NJ: Potroom palsy? neurologic disorder in three aluminum smelter workers. *Arch Intern Med* 1985;145:1972–1975.
10. White DM, Longstreth WT, Rosenstock L, Claypoole KHJ, Brodkin CA, and Townes BD: Neurologic syndrome in 25 workers from an aluminum smelting plant. *Arch Int Med* 1992; 152:1443–1448.
11. Wills MR and Savory J: Aluminum poisoning: dialysis encephalopathy, osteomalacia and anaemia. *Lancet* 1983;2:29–34.
12. Mena I, Marin O, Fuenzalida S, and Cotzias GC: Chronic manganese poisoning: clinical picture and manganese turnover. *Neurology* 1967;17:128–136.
13. Veltman G, Gange GE, Juke S, Stein G, and Backner U: Clinical manifestations and course of vinyl chloride disease. *Ann NY Acad Sci* 1975;246:6–17.

14

Diesel Exhaust

Slowness of response, memory loss, and disordered sleep in ten railroad workers and in six electricians referred for shortness of breath suggested that diesel exhaust affected the brain. Neurobehavioral and pulmonary testing was done on seven diesel mechanics and three train crewmen, and on six electricians who were wiring nine substations as part of a new shopping mall became a 0.4 km tunnel. These 16 men performed significantly less well than did reference men for reaction time, balance, blink reflex latency R-1, Culture Fair, peg placement, trail making, and verbal and visual recall. Visual fields were abnormal in 13, with constriction in both eyes in 11. Nine men, including four who had never smoked, had small airways obstruction. No confounding factor or bias accounted for these differences. The severity of neurobehavioral impairment in diesel-exposed workers appeared related to the type of work and its duration. Other cohorts should be studied to confirm these findings.

BACKGROUND

Air pollution from diesel engine exhaust has been a major respiratory problem in underground mines and occasionally in the holds of ships. Symptoms of productive cough and frequent respiratory infections were found, but spirometric abnormalities were not found in an iron ore mine that was studied (1). However, asthma has recently been diagnosed in train crews (2). Guinea pigs, rabbits, and mice exposed experimentally to atmospheres in which diesel engines were running under varying conditions showed irritation of the eyes with lachrymation and deaths from severe lung damage within 5 hours. Guinea pigs were most sensitive, showing bronchiolitis. Lung edema was attributed to nitrogen dioxide, but lachrymation was attributed to formaldehyde and acrolein (3). Concern for deaths from lung cancer among railroad workers has emerged since 1959, when relative odds were 1.41, 95% confidence interval (CI) = 1.06–1.88, and the latter figure has been revised to 1.57, 95% CI = 1.19–2.05 (4, 5).

Adverse central nervous system effects from diesel exhaust have not been reported and may not have been considered previously. However, inhalation of petroleum combustion mists, similar to diesel exhaust, produced encephalopathy and vestibulopathy (abnormal balance) in three welders while they were welding steel patches on an oil storage tank insulated with fiberglass (6); and in six welders who were dismantling oil tank cars with oxyacetylene cutting torches (unpublished) exposure to the fumes produced encephalopathy and vestibulopathy. Difficulties with recall and concentration, sleeping disorders, and clumsiness in the dark in 16 diesel-exposed workers led to neurobehavioral evaluations, assessments of symptom frequencies and profile of mood states, and pulmonary function testing. This test battery had been used in subjects with other chemical exposures (7–11).

TESTING OF SUBJECTS

Methods

The subjects included 10 diesel mechanics and trainmen and 6 electricians exposed to diesel exhaust, all of them men, and 13 people exposed to smoke and fumes from a diesel fire and a subsequent gasoline fire. Of the 16 occupationally exposed men studied, 10 had worked 15 to 40 years as diesel train crew men, as mechanics or electricians; and the other 6 were electricians exposed for approximately a year to diesel and gasoline exhaust gases while building a large shopping mall. The 10 railroad workers, aged 43 to 60 years, were being evaluated for asbestosis and the pulmonary effects of diesel exposure. Seven came from a diesel engine repair yard, and three were train crew members; two drove locomotives. Seven had lived in the Los Angeles area and worked in diesel repair at Southern Pacific Railroad for 15 to 40 years (see Table 14.1). Crew members were stationed at Needles, California and worked for the Santa Fe Railroad. The lifelong diesel mechanics worked indoors during the period before 1988, when diesel engines were run indoors during servicing and tuning. Exposures to chlorinated solvents, aqueous cleaning fluids, paints, detergents, glues, and mastics were occurring weekly. Burning of mucous membranes, shortness of breath, and coughing were frequent, but loss of recall or recent memory and of concentration shifted focus from asbestosis and respiratory problems to impaired neurobehavioral performance and its association with diesel exposure.

The six electricians were wiring the nine electrical substations for a large shopping mall in New Jersey while the work site, approximately 0.4 km long, was converted to a tunnel by roofing it over with multiple concrete decks. Ready-mix concrete trucks ran diesel engines at idle constantly. Combustion from other diesel and gasoline delivery vehicles made the space a smoky tunnel. Patients' eyes teared; noses, throats, and chests burned; and headache and nausea were common during exposures of 7 to 18 months, with symptoms leading to emergency room visits. Carbon monoxide levels were measured in alveolar air but did not exceed 50 ppm.

The 13 environmentally exposed test subjects were representative of over 1,000 plaintiffs who lived near a train derailment site in San Bernardino, California, and were exposed to a diesel fire and a subsequent gasoline fire on May 12 and May 25, 1989. A train of 6 locomotives and 69 hopper cars derailed and spilled 6,258 metric tons (6,900 tons) of trona, a mineral salt mixture of sodium sulfate and bicarbonate, and 45,420 liters (12,000 gallons) of diesel fuel. About two weeks later an underground gasoline pipeline, nearly under the derailment, burst, and over 151,400 liters (40,000 gallons) of gasoline burned for 8 hours. No air monitoring equipment was functioning; so neither concentration nor the plume extent was measured.

The 159 unexposed comparison subjects, from Wickenburg, Arizona, were recruited at random from voter registration rolls to match in sex, age, and years of educational attainment (highest school grade completed) an exposed group of subjects studied in Phoenix for effects of chemicals (manuscript submitted). They have been compared to other exposed groups because they appear representative of unexposed subjects from other parts of the United States. They were contacted to ascertain whether they met the matching criteria and would permit testing. They were reimbursed for their time and mileage. The Wickenburg subjects' unexposed status was known to the testers.

TABLE 14.1 Demographic data, exposure duration, and major symptoms

Age (yrs)	Ed Level (yrs)	Smoking (yrs)	Occupation	Duration	Average Frequency of 35 Symptoms Mean	POMS Score Mean	Abnor-malities	Major Symptoms
60	12	N	Welder	40 (yrs.)	1.9	−22	16	Fatigue, memory loss
60	14	N	Machinist	31	6.5	62	16	Shortness of breath, nausea
60	12	C28	Boilermaker	23	3.5	33	12	Shortness of breath, memory loss
58	13	N	Electrician (railroad)	22	5.9	25	11	Memory loss, decreased libido
60	14	C31	Electrician (railroad)	20	3.7	111	17	Chest tightness, cough with mucus
52	13	C6	Boilermaker	17	4.8	52	16	Chest pain, shortness of breath
45	12	N	Boilermaker	15	3.9	25	6	Memory loss, sleepiness
55	12	X20	Engine driver	34	2.1	−12	5	Shortness of breath, wheezing on exertion
46	12	N	Brakeman, conductor	20	6.3	55	11	Hives, memory loss, productive cough, irritability
43	14	N	Engine driver	19	7.0	30	14	Hives, anaphylaxtoid reactions, shortness of breath, memory loss
49	14	C22	Electrician	15 (mos.)	4.4	37	4	Extreme fatigue, tremor, impaired recall and memory
56	12	X31	Electrician	7	5.5	87	18	Extreme fatigue, irritability, disturbed sleep
49	12	N	Electrician	18	5.3	16	13	Headache, disturbed sleep, loss of recent memory
47	14	C30	Electrician	11	3.3	41	7	Headache, short-term memory loss, extreme fatigue
44	12	C28	Electrician	11	4.5	49	5	Recent memory loss, extreme fatigue, loss of libido
42	12	X2	Electrician	12	4.5	93	15	Reduced sense of smell, headache, extreme fatigue, lack concentration
					Means			
53.9	12.8			23.5	4.5	35.7	12.3	

C = Current smoker
N = Never smoked
X = Ex-smoker

All subjects gave their informed consent, and the protocol was approved by the Human Studies Research Committee of the University of Southern California School of Medicine.

Results

For train mechanics and crews, ages averaged 53.9 years, mean educational level was 12.8 years, and average exposure was 23.5 years. The electricians' mean age was 47.8 years, educational levels averaged 12.7 years, and exposures were for 18 months or less as the mall's lower floors were completed. Both symptom frequencies (means) and profiles of mood state (means) were elevated (Table 14.1). Respiratory symptoms, loss of recall memory, headache, sleepiness, and loss of libido were frequent. The exposed men's ages and adjusted educational levels were not different from those of unexposed (Table 14.2). Balance, with eyes open but particularly with eyes closed, simple and choice reaction time, and blink reflex latency showed statistically significant differences from results for unexposed. Also scores for cognitive functions (Culture Fair and vocabulary), perceptual motor functions (pegboard, trails A and B), and recall (verbal and visual) were significantly different from the mean scores for the population-based unexposed.

TABLE 14.2 Neurobehavioral performance of patients compared to unexposed means

	Unexposed		Exposed		
	159		16		*P*
	Mean	Sd	Mean	Sd	Value
Age yrs	50.7	20.0	51.6	5.8	.328
Educational Level yrs	13.2	2.4	12.8	0.9	.541
Balance cm/sec					
Eyes Open	0.83	0.2	1.03	0.5	.02
Eyes Closed	1.34	0.46	1.87	0.59	.01
Simple Reaction Time ms	282	62	369	71	.01
Choice Reaction Time ms	543	90	673	136	.001
Blink Reflex Latency					
Supraorbital Tap					
Right ms	13.3	2.2	14.0	1.4	.001
Left ms	13.3	2.2	14.2	1.3	.01
Culture Fair score	26.7	7.0	20.6	3.0	.0001
Pegboard score	82.0	28.9	93.7	36.0	.001
Trails A score	37.8	23.5	44.1	11.4	.05
Trails B score	82.2	35.3	123.2	48.7	.02
Fingertip Writing errors sc	3.7	1.9	8.8	3.4	.03
Recall score					
Verbal Immediate	22.1	7.2	10.2	2.1	.0001
Delayed	17.7	6.4	6.3	2.3	.0001
Visual	35.6	4.7	15.6	3.2/2.6	.0001
Vocabulary score	24.4	8.9	14.1	3.6	.001

ms = milliseconds
n = normal

TABLE 14.3a Neurobehavioral performance of diesel mechanics and trainmen compared to unexposed means

	1	2	3	4	5	6	7	8	9	10	% Abnormal
Balance cm/s											
Eyes Open	0.86	1.37*	0.95	0.77	2.06*	1.00	0.53	0.74	0.92	0.87	20
Eyes Closed	1.56	1.75*	1.66*	1.17	2.62*	1.66*	0.68	1.44	1.84*	1.97*	60
Simple Reaction Time ms	403*	279	219	374*	343*	364*	241	337	530*	760*	60
Choice Reaction Time ms	603*	626*	496	722*	619*	893*	506	554	756*	918*	70
Grip Strength (kg)	49	41*	59	48	15*	48	62	40*	72	52	30
Right											
Left	44*	43*	64	43*	10*	46	55	40*	60	36	50
Blink Reflex Latency											
Supraorbital Tap ms											
Right	12.5	16.2*	15.5*	16.2*	14.0	NR*	15*	12.4	12.9	14.9*	60
Left	17.0*	17*	14.5	15.1*	13.7	NR*	15*	11.3	12.4	14.9*	60
Color Discrimination	Abn	Abn	Abn	Abn	N	Abn	N	Abn	Abn	N	70
Visual Fields	Nerve fiber defect L	Con	Scotoma L	Con	Con	Con	N	N	Abn	Sev Con	80
Vibration	Dec	Dec	Dec	Dec	Dec	Dec	N	Dec	Dec	Dec	90
Hearing	ND	ND	ND	ND	Dec	Dec	Dec	Dec	Dec	Sdec	100
Culture Fair sc	11*	9*	8*	16*	14*	14*	18*	26	19	30	70
Pegboard s	100*	81	102*	77	179*	86*	79	81	113*	119*	60
Trails A sc	51*	38	56*	47	61*	44*	27	38	43	78*	50
Trails B sc	170*	151*	239*	77	175*	269*	70	74	107	145*	60
Fingertip Writing errors	22*	—	—	—	22*	—	8*	0	19*	12*	83
Recall											
Verbal I/D	3/2*	2/1*	4/4*	5/2*	8/6*	5/1*	7/6*	25/18	19/10*	4/3*	90
Visual I/D	1/7*	7/4*	11/10*	4/4*	8/6*	3/2*	5/4*	29/28	25/12*	30/10*	90
Vocabulary	10*	8*	3*	11*	11*	3*	10*	31	19	27	70
Pulmonary Function											
FEV_1/FVC	74	74	73	78	74	85	86	59*	83	75	76.3
FEF_{25-75} L/S	78	79	57*	95	71*	119	124	23*	96	92	83.4
FEF_{75-85} L/S	92	56*	29*	55*	34*	101	100	84	81	66	70

ms = milliseconds; I/D = immediate/30 min. delay; N = normal; L/S = Liters per second
s = seconds; Sdec = slightly decreased; * = abnormal; ND = not done
sc = score; Con = constriction

TABLE 14.3b Neurobehavioral performance of six electricians exposed to engine exhaust compared to unexposed means

	11	12	13	14	15	16	% Ab-normal	Composite of Abnormal
Balance cm/sec								
Eyes Open	0.70	1.38*	1.00*	1.09	1.21	1.03	33	25
Eyes Closed	1.34	2.38*	2.43*	2.60*	2.54*	2.23*	83	69
Simple Reaction Time ms	225	366*	373*	230	294	560*	50	56
Choice Reaction Time ms	549	782*	745*	576	416	1011*	60	63
Grip Strength (kg)								
Right	74	35*	60	50	65	28*	33	31
Left	74	40*	50	50	69	24*	33	44
Blink Reflex Latency								
Supraorbital Tap ms								
Right	13.9	15.2*	12.9	12.2	13.1	12.1	17	44
Left	13.0	16.8*	13.0	12.1	13.3	12.4	17	44
Color Discrimination	N	Abn	Abn	Abn	N	Abn	67	56
Visual Fields	scotoma > blind spot	scotoma Rt Lft	bil upper hemisphere loss	upper hemisphere	normal	4 quadrant loss R>L	83	81
Vibration	Dec	Dec	Dec	Dec	Dec abs	Dec	100	94
Hearing Right and Left	dec	dec	dec	dec	dec	dec	100	100
Culture Fair sc	27	18*	20	28	33	18	17	50
Pegboard s	78	104*	69	74	82	70	17	44
Trails A sc	32	33	53*	39	27	50*	33	44
Trails B sc	88	215*	88	72	59	119*	17	50
Fingertip Writing errors	4	14*	4	1	5*	40*	50	58
Recall								
Verbal I/D	12/11*	14/7*	16/5*	12/6*	15/14*	12/4*	100	94
Visual I/D	36/26	16/0*	18/14*	18/16*	28/24	10/7*	67	81
Vocabulary	20	14*	7*	30	18	6*	50	63
Pulmonary Function								
FEV_1/FVC	66*	76	79	71*	86	81	33	19
FEF_{25-75} L/S	40*	93	91	82	52*	103	33	31
FEF_{75-85} L/S	30*	100	56*	51*	40*	76	83	56

ms = milliseconds N = normal I/D = immediate/30 min. delay
s = seconds Abn = abnormal D = decreased
sc = score Con = constricted L/S = Liters per second

Comparison of subjects exposed throughout their working years to those exposed for a year showed similar effects. The railroad group showed abnormalities of visual fields in 80%, of hearing in 100% of those measured (6 of 10), of vibration in 90%, of verbal recall in 90% and visual recall in 90%, of fingertip number writing (errors) in 5 of 6 tested, of balance with eyes closed in 60%, of choice reaction time in 70%, and of Culture Fair in 70% (Table 14.3a). Also frequent were delayed blink reflex latency in 60%, abnormal color discrimination in 70%, slowed trail making A in 50% and B in 60%, and decreased vocabulary in 70%. One had airway obstruction, and six had small airways obstruction. The ten men chronically exposed to diesel fumes during locomotive repair or on train crews showed reductions in neurobehavioral function, including visual fields and blink reflex latency through balance, and in reaction time, including cognitive, perceptual motor speed, and recall functions, all of which apparently were impaired. Their degree of impairment for many tests increased with years of diesel exposure (Table 14.1). Of the six construction electricians, five had abnormal sway speeds, six had decreased hearing, five had abnormal visual fields, and four had

TABLE 14.4 Abnormalities found in 13 test clients from San Bernardino train derailment and fire

	Exposed Average	Expected
Ages 14 to 77 yrs	45.6	42.4
Educational Level 6–14 yrs	10.2	
Simple Reaction Time	354	295
Choice Reaction Time	675	500
Balance Eyes Open	0.96	0.82
Closed	1.63	1.18
Culture Fair A	21.5	30.9
Verbal Recall	14.5	24
Finger Writing Errors Right	6.5	2
Left	4.8	2
Pegboard	93.2	68
Trail Making A	65.8	29.7
Trail Making B	116.3	62.0
Information	11.0	16.9
Picture Completion	11.7	15.3
Similarities	15.3	15.3
POMS	38	52

abnormal color discrimination (Table 14.3b). All six had decreased immediate verbal recall, which worsened at 30 minutes, four had diminished visual recall, and three had excessive errors for fingertip number writing; whereas cognitive functions (Culture Fair and vocabulary), pegboard, and trail making were impaired in three or fewer of them.

The gasoline–diesel-fire-exposed subjects had simple and choice reaction times increased compared to national unexposed, and these differences were statistically significant (Table 14.4). Balance measured as sway with eyes open and balance as sway with eyes closed were also significantly increased. BRL R-1 was abnormally long on both right and left sides, and four of six measured had abnormal visual fields (Table 14.5). Culture Fair and verbal recall results were significantly below expected (Table 14.4). Peg placement and performance of trail making A and B were impaired significantly. The prevalences of abnormality were consistent with the differences in means.

Pulmonary function tests of long-time diesel workers showed that three men had decreased flows and volume, and thus airways obstruction, 20% had air trapping 10% and another 50% had small airways obstruction, after the data were adjusted for age and cigarette smoking (Table 14.3a). Ten of ten longtime workers had chronic bronchitis with chest pain and tightness and hyperreactive reaction airways, which confirmed the respiratory ill effects of breathing diesel exhaust. Methacholine challenges were all reported as positive. Chest radiographs showed no evidence of asbestosis or of other pulmonary disease.

Pulmonary function tests were abnormal in 11 of 13 fire-exposed subjects, shown by airways obstruction in 5 and small airways obstruction in 6 (Table 14.5).

In another study discussed here, 13 subjects were tested after a train derailment and diesel fire, followed by a gasoline fire a few days later. Neurobehavioral and pulmonary abnormalities were observed (Tables 14.4 and 14.5) in these exposed subjects, which appear to underscore the risk that diesel combustion presents to the public as well as to workers.

TABLE 14.5 Prevalences of abnormal tests in the San Bernardino train derailment and fire-exposed subjects

	Abnormal Tests	Clients Tested
Blink Reflex Latency	6	6
Verbal Recall	11	13
Vibration Sense	9	13
Profile of Mood States	9	13
Finger Writing Errors	8	12
Balance	8	13
Choice Reaction Time	8	13
Visual Field Defects	4	6
Grip Strength	7	13
Color Discrimination	7	13
Abnormal Pulmonary Function	11	13
Airways Obstruction	5	13
Small Airways Obstruction	6	13
Normal	2	13

DISCUSSION

This report shifts the focus of diesel health effects to the central nervous system (CNS), including visual field constriction, reflecting dysfunction of the retina and/or optical cortices; deafness; delayed blink reflex latency, indicating dysfunction of the circuit of trigeminal nerve, pons, and facial nerve; and balance impairment from defects in vestibular, cerebellar, and associative pathways as well as afferent pathways (as reduced vibration sense) and efferent posture control nerves. Thus, functions of cranial nerves II, V, and VIII seem particularly susceptible to the effects of diesel exhaust. Impaired recall-memory, problem solving, and perceptual motor speed reflect cortical dysfunction, especially of the parietal lobe. None of these effects appears to be caused by inhaled particles of diesel exhaust, which cause the pulmonary toxicity. Respiratory symptoms in railroad workers, particularly bronchitis in four men and small airways obstruction in five, including four who had smoked for up to 28 years, suggest that pulmonary toxicity is second in importance to CNS dysfunction. All six electricians had respiratory complaints and positive methacholine challenges, and four had small airways obstruction so that they had occupational asthma. High prevalences of airways obstruction after the diesel–gasoline fire incident also supported the conclusion of induced asthma.

What chemicals in diesel exhaust might impair the CNS? Acrolein, a three-carbon aldehyde and an important product of diesel fuel combustion, irritates the mucous membranes (3) and like formaldehyde has adverse CNS effects (12). Toluene and xylene, the most neurotoxic diesel fuel components, must be considered. Chlorinated solvents used in metal cleaning, especially trichloroethylene and 1,1,1-trichloroethane, which are used in diesel locomotive repair and refitting, adversely affect CNS function (7) and slow blink reflex latency R-1 (13, 14). Methyl terbutyl ether (MTBE), a gasoline additive yielding formaldehyde and methanol on combustion, may have contributed to the exposure of the electricians building the shopping mall. Carbon monoxide seems unlikely as a cause of impairment, as no workers, even in the mall, had levels above those of smokers of 40 cigarettes per day.

This pilot study has observed abnormalities, probably from high diesel exhaust exposures, in four environments. It is hoped that the study will stimulate further observations and help to generate hypotheses. For instance, the increased latency of blink reflex R-1 in the mechanics with years of exposure but not in electricians exposed for one year suggests either that prolonged diesel exposure was needed for the effect or that chlorinated solvents contributed to impairment in the mechanics, one trainman, and one electrician. Only diesel mechanics were exposed to solvents, not the electricians or the train crewmen. Aldehydes or methanol may be responsible for abnormalities. Methanol is the most plausible explanation of the losses of visual fields. However, MTBE and manganese are added to gasoline, not to diesel fuel; so only the construction electricians could have been exposed to them. Additionally, the fact that abnormal BRL R-1 was found in all six subjects who were exposed downwind to a diesel fire followed 10 days later by a gasoline fire supports fuel combustion products, perhaps the aldehydes, as causal. It is also possible that hydrogen sulfide or other reduced sulfur gases volatilize from diesel fuel, as it frequently contains more sulfur than does gasoline, which is desulfurized (15).

These risks to the brain from large diesel fume exposures indoors and downwind recommend better work policies for locomotive maintenance workers and train crews. The implications are even more serious for the electricians, representing construction workers, whose exposure of only one year impaired them similarly to railroad workers who were exposed for 15 to 40 years. Further studies should be linked to air monitoring for neurotoxic organic chemicals in locomotive cabs, in train repair sheds, and in tunnel-like construction sites. Impaired crews cannot be expected to operate trains safely; so diesel-exposed train crews should be monitored for neurobehavioral status. The recent prohibition of combustion of diesel fuel indoors, whether in locomotives or in trucks in mines, is supported by this new evidence. Now this question must be raised: is burning diesel outdoors in locomotives or trucks without appropriate pollution control devices too risky for engine drivers, train crews, and the public, particularly in air basins such as those of Los Angeles, Las Vegas, Phoenix, and Salt Lake City?

References

1. Jorgensen H and Svensson A: Studies on pulmonary function and respiratory tract symptoms of workers in an iron ore mine where diesel trucks are used underground. *J Occup Med* 1970;12:348–354.
2. Wade JF and Newman LS: Diesel asthma: reactive airways disease following overexposure to locomotive exhaust. *J Occup Med* 1993;35:149–154.
3. Pattle RE, Stretch H, Burgess F, Sinclair K, and Edginton JAG: The toxicity of fumes from a diesel engine under four different running conditions. *Brit J Indust Med* 1957;14:47–55.
4. Garshick E, Schenker MB, Munoz A, Segal M, Smith TJ, Woskie SR, Hammond SK, and Speizer FE: A case-control study of lung cancer and diesel exhaust exposure in railroad workers. *Am Rev Respir Dis* 1987;135:1242–1248.
5. Garshick E, Schenker MB, Munoz A, Segal M, Smith TJ, Woskie SR, Hammond SK, and Speizer FE: A retrospective cohort study of lung cancer and diesel exhaust exposure in railroad workers. *Am Rev Respir Dis* 1988;137:820–825.
6. Hodgson MJ, Furman J, Ryan C, Durrant J, and Kern E: Encephalopathy and vestibulopathy following short term hydrocarbon exposure. *JOM* 1989;31:51–54.
7. Kilburn KH and Warshaw RH: Effects on neurobehavioral performance of chronic exposure to chemically contaminated well water. *Intl J Toxicol Indust Health* 1993;39:391–404.
8. Kilburn KH and Warshaw RH: Neurobehavioral effects of formaldehyde and solvents on histology technicians: repeated testing across time. *Environ Res* 1992;58:134–146.
9. Kilburn KH, Warshaw RH, and Shields MG: Neurobehavioral dysfunction in firemen ex-

posed to polychlorinated biphenyls (PCBs): possible improvement after detoxification. *Arch Environ Health* 1989;44:345–350.
10. Miller JA, Cohen GS, Warshaw R, et al.: Choice (CRT) and simple reaction times (SRT) compared in laboratory technicians: factors influencing reaction times and a predictive model. *Am J Indust Med* 1989;15:687–697.
11. Kilburn KH and Warshaw RH: Are hearing loss and balance dysfunction linked in construction iron workers? *Brit J Indust Med* 1992;49:138–141.
12. Kilburn KH, Warshaw RH, and Thornton JC: Formaldehyde impairs memory, equilibrium, and dexterity in histology technicians: effects which persist for days after exposure. *Arch Environ Health* 1987;42:117–120.
13. Feldman RG, Chirico-Post J, and Proctor SP: Blink reflex latency after exposure to trichloroethylene in well water. *Arch Environ Health* 1988;43:143–148.
14. Barret L, Garrel S, Danel V, and Debru JL: Chronic trichloroethylene intoxication: a new approach by trigeminal-evoked potentials? *Arch Environ Health* 1987;42:297–302.
15. Kilburn KH and Warshaw RH: Hydrogen sulfide and reduced sulfur gases adversely affect neurophysiological functions. *Toxicol Indust Health* 1995;11:185–197.

15

Pervasiveness of Impaired Brains: Implications from ''Controls'' Being Abnormal

There were 25 epidemiological studies conducted over a decade (Table 15.1), of which 15 were complete matched studies that had control groups. Ten were pilot studies with comparisons to available referent groups (Histotech; Shreveport firefighters; San Luis Obispo; Springfield, LA; etc.). Of the 15 studies with control groups, 2 were of children only and limited in number, and so are not included in this summary.

Four of the ''control'' groups were found to be highly similar so that they were accepted as unexposed controls (Springfield, LA; San Luis Obispo, CA; Wickenburg, AZ and Tennessee). Test results were modeled to develop prediction equations and to verify the equations (see Chapter 3). Three groups comprised volunteers from voter registration lists (VRL). One of these had a secondary church group whose tests were identical to those of the VRL group.

The other control groups were recruited through public appeal and advertisement (SE Houston), a church group (Russellville, AL), and community networking (Casper, WY), with two others using workers selected by matching analyzed groups as comparison groups (Muscle Shoals aluminum remelting and Tinker Air Force Base workers). The Shreveport firefighters' incident fire had exposed them to PCBs and pyrolysis products such as dibenzofurans; controls were firefighters not involved in the incident. Also an appeal was made to Abbeville (LA) residents living in manufactured homes similar to those exposed to a truck that leaked hydrochloric acid during transport; and a community sample was obtained, in the same state, of individuals who were without *known* chemical exposure (south central Phoenix for Southwest Tucson TCE). Lastly, there was a matching community in the same state some 30 miles from an exposure site community (Superior, MT).

Study-by-study analyses showed that test results for these nine groups fell between the better scores shown by the four unexposed groups and the scores of the exposed groups the nine groups had been recruited to match. Usually, this approach had permitted the detection of an exposure effect; however, the nine groups had function in a midrange, not as good as that of unexposed controls. We recommend one explanation

TABLE 15.1. Summary of 25 epidemiologic investigations

Population	Exposure	Abnormal	Control	Conclusion
Histotech	(B-LV)	No	None	
Stringfellow, CA	Acid pits	Yes	None (Pilot)	
Tucson, AZ	TCE	Yes	Phoenix, AZ (?)	
Morrison, CO	TCE suspected	No	None (Pilot)	
Nipoma, CA	H_2S	Yes	San Luis Obispo, CA	Unexposed
Shreveport, LA	DBF fire	Yes	Firefighters not in fire	
Combustion, LA	Toluene	Yes	Springfield, LA	Unexposed
Biloxi, MS	Polyurethane	No	Biloxi (C)	
Muscle Shoals, AL	PCB	Yes	Russellville (R)	
Bergholtz, OH	Fires	No	Steubenville (C)	
Muscle Shoals, AL	Aluminum	Yes	Muscle Shoals	
Bryan, TX	Arsenic	Yes	None (pilot)	
Phoenix, AZ	TCE	Yes	Wickenburg, AZ	Unexposed
Joplin, MO	TCE	Yes	None (pilot)	
Tinker AFB, OK	TCE	Yes	Oklahoma City (TCE)	
Houston, TX	Chlordane	Yes	SE Houston (H_2S)	
Abbeville, LA	HCl	Yes	Abbeville (MH)	
Odessa, TX	Chem fire	Yes	None (pilot)	
Seymour, IN	MNBE	Yes	None (pilot)	
San Bonito, TX	Arsenic	Yes	None (pilot)	
Lobelville, TN	PCB	Yes	SH & HM, TN	Unexposed
Wilmington, CA	H_2S	Yes	None (pilot)	
Alberton, MT	Cl_2	Yes	Superior (?)	
Casper, WY	Chemicals	Yes	Casper (H_2S)	
Oak Ridge, TN	Incinerator	Yes	None (pilot)	

B-LV = Boston, Anaheim, Little Rock, Washington, Las Vegas
TCE = Trichloroethylene
DBF = Dibenzofurans
PCB = Polychlorinated biphenyls
R = Rural
C = Children not included in analysis
AFB = Air Force Base
HCl = Hydrochloric acid—road spill
H_2S = Hydrogen sulfide—oil refinery
MH = Manufactured homes, indoor air
MNBE = Methyl *n*-butylether—refinery
SH & HM = Springhill and Hurricane Mills
Cl_2 = Chlorine cresylate rail spill

rather than individual ones for these nine intermediate results; the single explanation is that these nine groups had been exposed to chemicals *without being aware* of the exposure, as described in the following paragraphs.

1. One such control group was Shreveport, Louisiana nonincident firefighters not engaged in fighting or cleanup of the fire, in which transformers containing PCBs boiled and exploded. *Conclusion*: All firefighters have been chemically exposed.

2. In Abbeville, Louisiana many control people were living in manufactured, that is, factory-built, homes about 10 miles from the hydrochloric acid spill (Chapter 7), which exposed a group with similar housing. These controls were recruited to match in age and educational level those exposed to hydrochloric acid, and they showed differences from the exposed group; but they also differed from unexposed controls (Chapter 3). *Conclusions*: Indoor air exposure from factory-built homes includes formaldehyde, organic solvents, and other volatile organic chemicals. Intermediate results for this control group were similar to those of the 26 people exposed to indoor air, who comprised the largest exposure category of patients seen in consultation (Chapter 4).

3–4. Two groups, Houston (chlordane, Chapter 9) and Casper controls (Chapter 11), lived in immediate vicinities of oil refineries. These zones were downwind from hydrogen sulfide and other gases and hydrocarbons. *Conclusion*: Hydrogen sulfide exposure probably impaired neurobehavioral function in Nipoma and Wilmington, California as described in Chapter 5.

5. Muscle Shoals, Alabama aluminum remelt workers were a small group whose study members selected matched subjects who were analyzed as a group. This community has numerous chemical plants and has been heavily polluted for 60 years. *Conclusion*: The chemical exposure of controls cannot be excluded.

6. Superior, Montana controls for Alberton were recruited from and through the patients of a local medical practitioner. Also many had driven through the site of a derailment spill (Chapter 6) to reach the nearest trading and supply area in Missoula. *Conclusion*: The doctor's practice had some people who were chemically sensitive, and all controls had some exposure to chlorine, cresylate, and other chemicals as they traveled the canyon to shop and trade. Thus they were unlikely to be normal.

7. The Tucson exposed group original control subjects were from south central Phoenix. The mean scores for their functions were not different from those of the Tucson group. *Conclusion*: Upon examination of this Phoenix group, they were not on the TCE plume and not in Marysville. However, later information showed that 4 or 5 of the other 33 Superfund sites in Phoenix may have contaminated their homes. They lived west and south of the airport, south of the Salt River aquifer, and were studied in 1987, five years before TCE contamination of the aquifer east of them was shown by analysis of water wells.

8. The Tinker Air Force Base exposed group and controls each had about equal proportions of African-American and Caucasian people, including some subjects with Spanish surnames. The ethnic subgroups' test results were not different in exposed or controls. However, the results of test of these controls were more abnormal than those of the tests of the four groups of unexposed standard subjects. *Conclusion*: As blink reflex latency was delayed in both exposed and control groups, an off-site migration of TCE into the Eaton-Wellington aquifer could have spread the effect so that blink, the most sensitive effect of TCE exposure, was abnormal. Tinker workers showed increased abnormalities from adding occupational to residential exposure.

9. In another study, the Russellville, Alabama controls were rural, but the Muscle Shoals group exposed to PCBs were considered to live in urban census tracts. Physiological test outcomes of the controls were identical to the predicted values of unexposed control people, but psychological functions and intelligence tests were low. *Conclusion*: Being born and living in a rural area seemed to affect some tests in the same way as did chemicals.

The implication of these studies is that chemicals adversely affected 9 of 13, just over two-thirds, of the control groups. Although this conclusion may surprise readers, its gradual emergence did not impact the author until after this summary showed that *to be unimpaired was unusual.* Fortunately, four virtually identical groups from different sections of the country define the performance on these tests for subjects exposed to chemicals minimally or not at all. As the methods of measurement were uniform, the groups' differences were identified by checking distributions of age, educational level, and other factors so that each difference in test score means could be reliably detected. After prediction equations were developed, predicted values were used for every test for each individual; so the comparisons were as a percentage of predicted.

Thus, one must assume that exposure to chemicals is widespread in the United States so that four populations with equal function share either no exposure or minimal exposures. Therefore, a problem that at first makes the comparisons more difficult appears to enhance the main message, that *chemical causes should be sought* when evidence of neurotoxic effects is identified. It suggests that the strategy used in this series of studies can and should be extended. The steps should be: to identify impaired neurobehavioral performance in populations or individuals first triggered by symptoms, indicating distress, and then to look for exposure factors. *The conclusion is unavoidable that chemicals have injured human brains in the United States in many people who are not aware that they have been chemically exposed. Unless this pandemic is stopped, it threatens our existence.*

16

Mechanisms of Brain Damage from Chemicals

A SPECULATIVE OVERVIEW

Possible mechanisms of neurotoxicity are varied. The challenge is to explain how chemicals, coming through the lungs from inhaled ammonia, cyanide, hydrogen sulfide, chlorine, or other chemicals, produce *lesions that become progressively worse over an incubation time of months to years.* Putting chronic exposures aside, how can a single dose of a chemical that is not lethal cause progressive impairment of function so that performance deteriorates, and the brain be progressively destroyed? Mechanically the situation resembles the progressive contamination of a computer's hard drive and operating system so that more and more nonsense is circuiting the board and the machine.

My speculation is that astrocytes have been stimulated to relinquish their nurturing duties, the fostering and protection of the neurons. For neurons rapidly fail and die (apoptosis) when supplies of growth factors and amino acids (i.e., glutamate and cysteine) from astrocytes are curtailed. Neurons also die when the phagocytic and digestive functions of the astrocytes are unregulated by foreign chemicals. Neurons appear to starve but also may be eaten. However, since astrocytes remove or store the toxic and undigestible debris produced by cell death (i.e., cholesterol, fatty acids, and insoluble protein fragments) and produce the lipoproteins (Apo E) required for transport out of the brain of these cellular toxic residues, it is not surprising that overwhelming of astrocytes by foreign chemicals causes progressive losses of neurons.

The idea is that the astrocytic (phagocytic) helper cells are the principal target, and that neural death is the end result. This idea explains slowing of neurotransmission and incapacitating symptoms: fatigue, headache, memory loss, lack of concentration, and loss of interest in sex. The neurons are starving. The limbic system, which controls memory, emotion, and sex drive, is overdriven. The limbic system is peculiarly susceptible to impulses coming into the nasal passages, from molecules landing on the olfactory bulbs and with access to the cingulate gyrus, the amygdala, the hippocampus, and the rest of the limbic circuit. With daily exposure to low doses of hydrogen sulfide in refinery workers, energy production and utilization by astrocytes may be compromised, and the astrocytes may also begin to starve. Thus, cells in the brain falter and die.

This situation is somewhat comparable to the use of a war machine, specifically the one used in the invasion of Europe in World War II. Although it included armies, navies, and air forces, and night planes, day planes, and a whole series of complex maneuvers on the terrain of the Continent, the destruction was basically due to explosives.

ENTRY OF CHEMICALS INTO THE CNS

Lung to Blood to Blood–Brain Barrier Route

Chemicals reach the brain by crossing the blood–brain (b-b) barrier and enter nerves across the blood–nerve barrier (1). From inhaled air they cross the lung's alveolo-capillary barrier, enter arterialized blood, and circulate to the brain. However, all brain is not equal; in some areas, the median eminence of the hypothalamus and the fourth ventricle's capillaries lack glial processes and pass chemicals more readily than do other parts of the brain (2). Only small molecules in the blood pass freely through capillaries of the choroid plexus, whose endothelial cells, the choroidal epithelium, have circumferential seals by tight junctions to prevent free diffusion (3). Brain capillaries also have complete rings of tight junctions.

Astrocytes, which also function as permeability regulators and maintain normal brain water and electrocyte distributions rapidly swell when damaged by foreign chemicals. This swelling, if severe, further compromises neurons by impinging on their matrix territory (4). Again, neuronal function fails.

Lipid-soluble materials such as oxygen and carbon dioxide, and nonpolar solvents such as ether, ethanol, and trichloroethylene pass the b-b barrier easily. In addition, certain proteins or peptides that are receptor-mediated (insulin, transferrin, and growth factor) or absorptive-mediated (polycationic proteins: histone, cationized albumin) trancytose through the blood–brain barrier. Another mechanism is to ''open the barrier'' with chemical agents such as leukotrienes, which selectively pass through the endothelial tight junction barrier in brain tumors without affecting this barrier in normal brain (5). Thus, in truth, the brain capillaries are a regulatory interface. A blood–nerve barrier was demonstrated a quarter century after the blood–brain barrier by using the dye trypan blue. Schwann cells and the nerves within remained unstained, while epineural and perineural connective macrophages and some ganglion cells in dorsal root ganglia absorbed trypan blue.

Cerebrospinal fluid is secreted by the epithelial cells of the choroid plexus, circulates in the ventricles and subarachnoid space, and is in equilibrium with fluid (1) in the extracellular space. This extracellular space constitutes 15 to 25% of the brain (4). Lead and cadmium damage vascular endothelial cells, causing edema and hemorrhage, increased cell death, delayed synaptogenesis, and reduced dendritic fields (1). Triethyltin (an organotin) and hexachlorophene (a phenol) cause brain edema, localized to white matter and myelin sheaths, by splitting myelin lamellae at intraperiod lines and causing vacuolation of the sheaths. The effects of hexachlorophene are most severe in premature infants of low birth weight and resemble the experimental effects of triethyltin (4).

The Olfactory Route

The other pathway into the brain for chemicals, including odorants, leads into the nasal olfactory bulb (made up of olfactory cells of the brain), by crossing the cribriform plate of the nose and entering olfactory nerves for access to the brain's limbic pathways. The subarachnoid space continues along the olfactory nerves from the olfactory bulb into the mucous membrane of the nose (6). Thus, odor stimuli are detected by nerves and not receptors, such as those for visual stimuli in the eye. These nerves and the surrounding subarachnoid space filled with cerebrospinal fluid provide a path for entry into the brain of bacteria, viruses, metals such as cadmium and aluminum, and some chemicals.

The finding of transmission of chemicals, including viruses, through the nasal mucosa into the olfactory nerves or into the cerebrospinal fluid followed observations that bacterial infection took this path. In swine the Aujeszky disease virus antigen has been detected in nasal epithelial cells, gland cells, olfactory nerve cells, and neurons of the olfactory bulb (7) (see Figure 16.1). The herpes simplex encephalitis virus (HSV1), inoculated intranasally in mice, was detected 4 days later at the olfactory bulbs and the trigeminal root entry zone in the brain stem. From the olfactory bulbs the virus spread to the anterior olfactory nucleus, lateral olfactory tract, septal nuclei, temporal lobe, hippocampus, and cingulate cortex (8). Aluminum and cadmium have been observed in the nasal-olfactory reflections as well. Rabbits given aluminum lactate and aluminum chloride intranasally showed lesions in the olfactory bulb, pyriform cortex, and hippocampus (9). Yellow staining of olfactory bulbs, anosmia, and yellow incisors and front teeth was observed in a tool setter in a battery factory exposed to cadmium for 11 years (10). Similar yellow staining of the olfactory bulb has been produced experimentally in rats (11). Fifty-five cadmium-exposed workers who brazed with cadmium alloys had hyposmia (44% mild and 13% moderate or severe) to butanol, which was associated with high urinary cadmium levels and tubular proteinuria (12). Anosmia and disorders of balance and movement were the most notable neurobehavioral deficits observed in two men who were exposed to fumes from a NiCd battery fire (13).

Many olfactory fibers discharge into a single mitral cell of the bulb, olfactory bipolarneuron (Figure 16.2) which amplifies the stimulus, and this helps explain the low threshold for detecting odors. The second-order neurons separate into three strands, lateral to the amygdaloid nucleus, intermediate to the anterior perforated substance, and medial to the subcallosal gyres and part of the head of the caudate nucleus (Figure 16.1). From these three centers the fibers converge to form the olfactotegmental tract (14). Neurophysiological exploration of smell began relatively late; by the 1930s, Adrian showed from multiple unit recordings that odorants could be categorized by the site of their maximal stimulation of the bulb. Water-soluble substances excited the anterior portion and lipid-soluble ones the posterior portion. Individual cells were specific, some responding to only one odor, others to more; but the neuronal units were categorized into four or five main groups: aromatic hydrocarbons, esters, alkanes, terpenes and terpenoids, and sulfur compounds. Later, in 1963, single olfactory receptor recordings confirmed Adrian's concept (15). Powell et al. showed that the pyriform cortex sent substantial projections to the hypothalamus and to the dorsomedial and lateral habenular nuclei of the thalamus, connecting the ''smell brain'' to sites of emotional and reproductive behavior (16).

Thus, there is a likelihood that the odor entry pathway that helped protect evolving small (smell-reliant) mammals persists as a breach in brain defenses against chemicals. It appears that olfactory stimulation, orders of magnitude above threshold, occurs from human exposure to inhaled chemicals, gases, vapors, and fumes (17, 18).

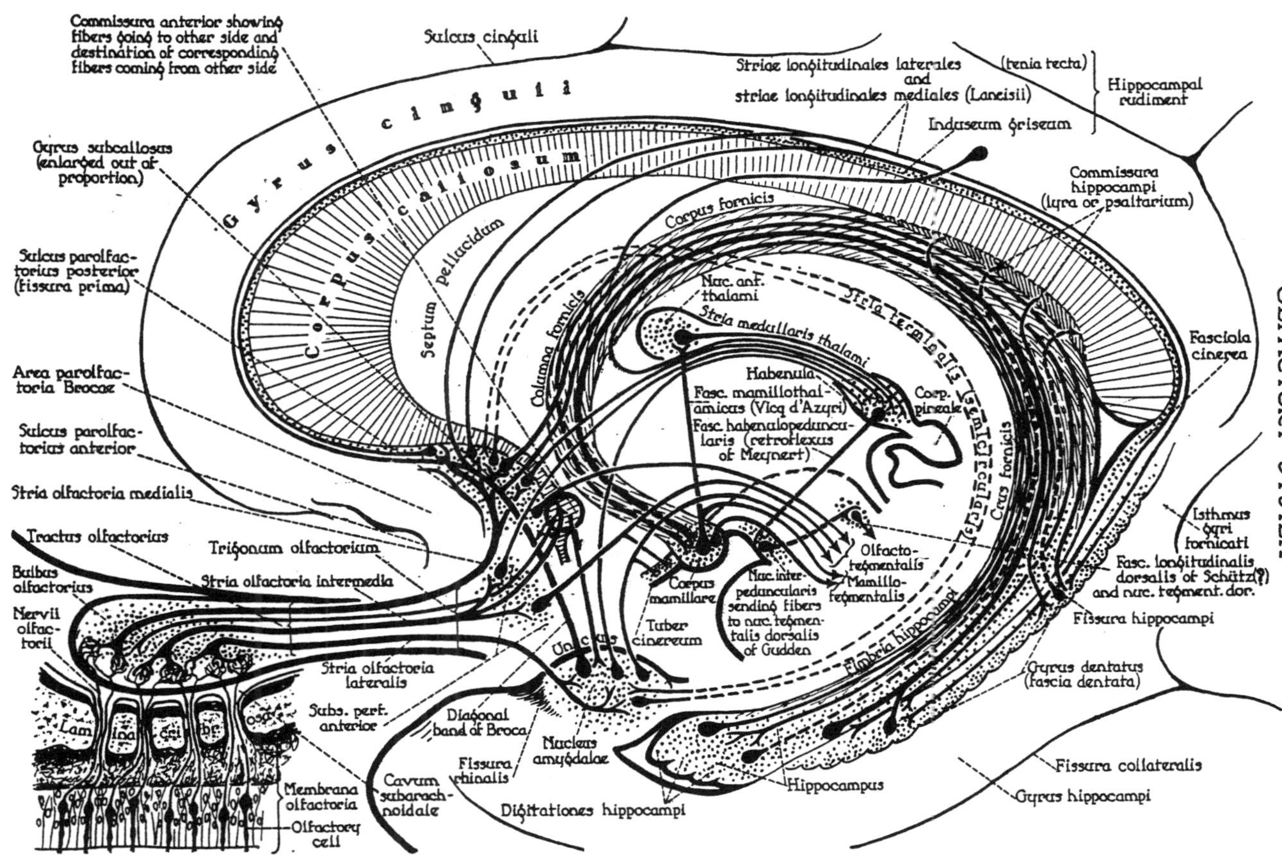

FIGURE 16.1. No one has improved upon Rasmussen's 1935 drawing for emphasizing the connections of olfactory sense apparatus (shown left bottom) to the brain's limbic system: the gyrus cinguli, corpus fornicis, and nucleus amygdalae to the hippocampus, hypothalamus, and pituitary. (From A. T. Rasmussen *The Principal Nervous Pathways*. New York: Macmillan, 1935.)

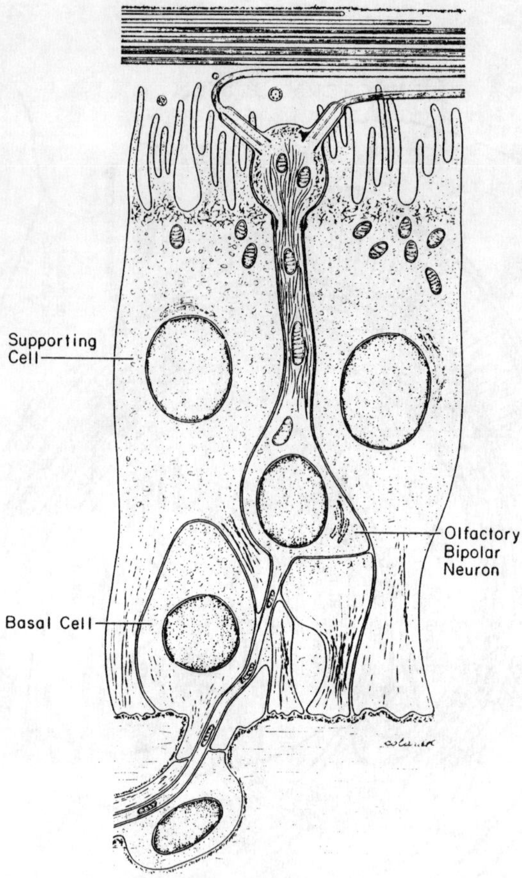

FIGURE 16.2. The details of the olfactory epithelium have been enhanced, as shown in this drawing based on an electron-microscope picture, to show the olfactory nerve cell with dendrites facing the environment through a layer of mucus below and extended through the cribriform plate to the olfactory stalk above. (From W. Bloom and D. Fawcett, *A Textbook of Histology*, 9th ed., Philadelphia: W. B. Saunders, 1969, page 633. With permission from Chapman & Hall, New York.)

Mechanisms of Amplification

Large doses of chemicals may enter via the lungs as in an ammonia or hydrogen sulfide cloud. Alternately, an amplification of the effects of a chemical acting on the brain could explain responses to orders-of-magnitude smaller doses, such as occur in drug idiosyncrasy (a name, not a mechanism) and the exaggerated response of a sensitized subject to a bee sting.

There are several possible mechanisms for amplification. The anaphylatic reaction exemplifies immune amplification. Enzymes induced in the liver hasten drug processing, amplifying detoxification. The sympathetic nervous–endocrine system amplifies by secretion of epinephrine or norepinephrine. Pharmacologic amplification can also alter base settings to exaggerate responses to cocaine, lidocaine, amphetamine, or apomorphine (19). ''Habituation.'' diminishes these responses. In epilepsy a neurocircuit appears to resonate, and because of electrical or electrochemical pulsing (timing) it

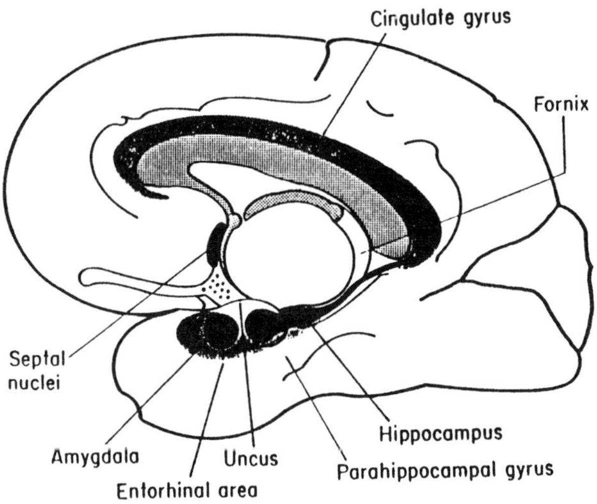

FIGURE 16.3. The limbic system connections are shown shaded. The rhincephalon or smell brain has internal, short pathways to activate practically the entire brain. (From P. Brodal, *The Central Nervous System*, Oxford University Press, 1992. With permission.)

ascends in power, amplifies (kindles) such that seizures are induced by progressively smaller stimuli (20). It is logical to assume that other neurophenomena may kindle the limbic system (Figure 16.3) chemically or electrochemically. After being induced by chemicals, from the olfactory bulb or generalized absorption from the lung, the amplitude builds somewhat like a pulsed laser. This amplification could explain the exaggerated responses shown by some patients to odorants or other chemicals (18, 21) (Figure 16.4).

Rate of Damage Determines Effect

A neural lesion produced in divided stages causes far less functional impairment than a lesion of equal size or extent from a single insult (22, 23). The intrinsic compensatory mechanisms of the brain adjust to damage at a slow pace, sometimes over decades, so that functional deficits can be concealed until a vast amount of capacity has been destroyed. The rate of damage may also determine the threshold for detecting a functional effect (24).

Quantitative measurements of performance may transcend the event threshold, when the loss of functional reserve by the neural system produces clinical manifestations (25) or those recognizable by relatively crude bedside or office neurologic testing. Thus, although Parkinson's disease is not clinically manifest until 80% of cells in the substantia nigra are lost, physiological testing alone or combined with brain imaging might detect it considerably earlier, as has been shown for chemical Parkinson's disease in MPTP-exposed subjects by positron emission tomography (26). Brain atrophy has been identified in patients with CNS involvement in systemic lupus erythematosus by proton magnetic resonance spectroscopy using *n*-acetylaspartate (27).

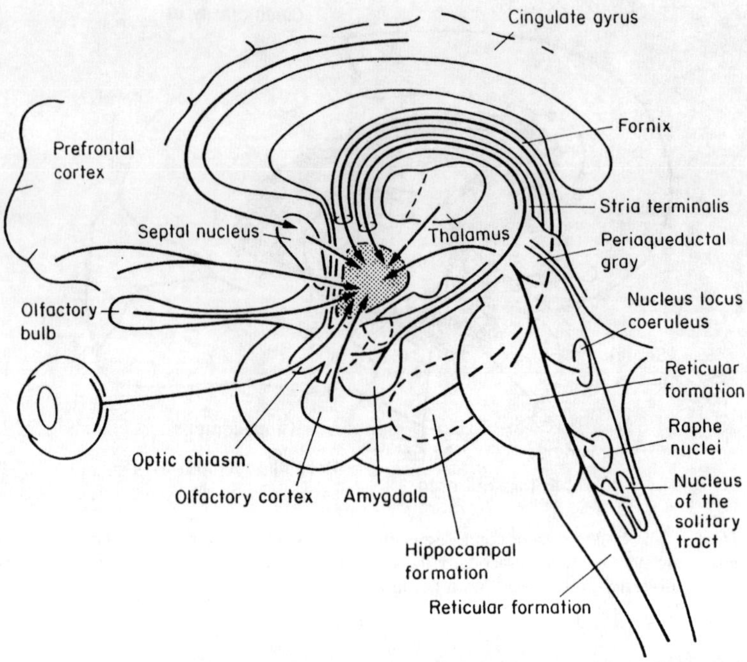

FIGURE 16.4. The pivotal position of the hypothalamus (shaded) for information gathering puts it in a key position to facilitate rapid responses as in fight or flight or release of neuromediators and pretropic hormones. (From P. Brodal, *The Central Nervous System*, Oxford University Press, 1992. With permission.)

LESSONS FROM TRAUMATIC BRAIN DAMAGE

Automobile Accidents

Traumatic brain damage provides clues that may be applied to chemical brain damage (i.e., types of performance deficits and their relative severity). Brain damage from blunt trauma has been studied extensively to chart its patterns to estimate its rate or completeness of recovery, to assist in rehabilitation, and to help the patient and his or her family in coping (28). Amnesia and aphasia follow blunt head trauma. Patients frequently complain of memory loss, and losses are perceived by relatives. Objective memory assessment showed deficits (29), measured by using vocal digit span and free recall of 20 lists of ten common words. Long-term memory assessed by word lists was much more abnormal than short-term memory in head-injured patients. This finding contrasts with chemical brain injury patients whose long-term memory is usually intact. Further studies of 82 patients compared to 34 normal subjects using the Wechsler memory scale showed logical memory (verbal recall) and associative learning (word pairs) were most impaired in the brain-damaged patients. These deficits were related to severity of head injury and increasing age but not to persisting neurological deficits, dysphasia, and skull fracture (30). Regarding memory function after head trauma, Schacter and Crovitz (31) had three recommendations: (1) test other cognitive deficits; (2) make finer discrimination between events prior to and following post-traumatic amnesia; and (3) explore deliberate efforts to improve the memory of patients with memory deficits after closed-head injury.

A sharp dichotomy between the lower scores on performance subtests vs. the verbal subtests of the Wechsler Adult Intelligence Scale (WAIS) was demonstrated in brain-damaged subjects in an early study (32), in contrast to an unexposed group classified as neurotic. In a subsequent study, verbal subtests from the WAIS showed less initial impairment with more rapid recovery than performance subtests (33) in 40 severely head-injured adults compared to 40 uninjured men. These differences were confirmed by serial testings.

Comparison of similar tested subjects with brain damage from the same center, using Raven matrices, verbal recall, associative learning, Mill-Hill vocabulary, and Rey figure with clinical data, showed that the outcome of intellectual function was related to the duration of post-traumatic amnesia and had little relation to duration of coma and other clinical measures. Measures of focal damage to the brain, presence of hematoma and age, dividing patients at age 30, were not predictive (34).

Improved studies of the events surrounding post-traumatic amnesia have not elucidated whether they are predictive except to show that more head-injury patients requiring hospitalization had previously ingested alcohol, which is a plausible finding and counters the folk wisdom that drunks escape serious injury in accidents, regardless of causation, involving motor vehicles, falls, or assaults (35).

Psychosocial characterization shows that slowness in 85% and tiredness in 82% are the most important problems in brain-injured patients at 3 months after injury, but at 12 months irritability in 71%, impatience in 71%, and poor memory and tiredness each in 69% led the list (28). A further follow-up study of 40 patients at 10 to 15 years showed permanent psychosocial change in two-thirds, led by poor memory in 75%, changes in personality and emotion in 65%, loss of social contact in 68%, and "sensitivity distress" in 68% (36). Another model group for study has been patients with the Korsakoff syndrome from alcohol, in whom confusion, disorientation, and memory deficits abound. Imagery worked better in aiding them than cueing or rote learning, but cueing aided recall of items (37).

Memory retraining methods, or mnemonic techniques using "memory pegs," have been tried in blunt trauma head injury patients, with considerable improvement in their ability to perform test sequences such as learning word lists (38). Of these methods, the most plausible for real-life situations is visual imagery, which is a paired associative technique often using absurd mental pictures (39). The purported "universal" success of these methods might argue for their trial in chemically brain-injured subjects although these individuals' long-term memory seems relatively resistant to chemical damage, just as it is to damage from blunt head trauma.

The general features of neurobehavioral impairment in patients who have suffered traumatic blunt brain damage are analogous to those in patients with chemical encephalopathy, although limited to evaluation by standard psychometric tests and thus not encompassing neurophysiological effects such as those of balance, blink reflex latency, or choice reaction time. The performance tests, such as block design, digit symbol, and Raven matrices, were more sensitive to damage and showed slower, often incomplete, restoration than did tests of verbal recall, visual reproduction, or associative learning. These blunt trauma brain-damaged patients have symptoms and psychosocial dysfunctions similar to those observed with chemical encephalopathy. Fatigue, memory loss, and difficulty in concentrating are most frequent. The apparent success with memory training using mnemonics, especially (absurd) imagery, in several groups of brain-damaged patients suggests that training more broadly directed to performance functions might aid patients with chemical encephalopathy.

Neurological Ill Effects of Open-Heart Surgery

"Neurological and intellectual disturbances after extracorporeal circulation" have always been dreaded complications, which sometimes mar an otherwise successful operation (40–42). The incidence of such effects in operated-on subjects is as high as 53% (2) with a low of 15% (40). Finer intellectual functions were compared in 144 patients (including 48 aortic valve, 36 with mitral, 27 with coronary, 15 with mitral and aortic, 16 with congenital heart disease and 2 with other diseases) subjected to extracorporeal circulation (ECC), and 53 thoracic surgery patients without ECC. Test I was done preoperatively, test II postoperatively (usually within a week of surgery), test III after two months, and test IV after one year, using a six-test battery consisting of synonyms, figure classification, a block (design) test with 16 blocks, Thurston's picture memory test, figure rotation, and figure identification. Of the 144 patients, 14 died within one month after surgery and 8 after one month without being tested further, and 9 did not complete the protocol. Of the 113 remaining, 14 had obvious postoperative cerebral complications (group B), whereas the other 99 (group A) did not. These complications included hemiplegia, unconsciousness, seizures, slow awakening, unusual lethargy, confusion, hallucinations, and vertigo. Of the 53 unexposed, 7 had the test program discontinued mainly because they were too ill to continue. For the 99 group A patients, five tests were significantly worse than the 46 without ECC at test II, and two remained different at test III. Group B was significantly different from A on five tests at the test III interval. There were minor differences between the diagnostic subgroups of group A. Perfusion times in excess of 140 minutes increased the test II deficits of patients. Reducing opportunities for microembolization by the insertion of an ultrapore filter in the ECC system during surgery reduced impairment at test II and increased improvement at test III. From 11 to 23% of patients did not achieve their preoperative performance level at test III and so were considered to have permanent residual effects of ECC. In another series, factors considered responsible for a 53% prevalence of neurological complications in 100 open-heart surgery patients included hypotension, advanced age, and prolonged bypass. Major causes were air embolism from within the heart and particle microembolism, which were most frequent after surgery on calcified valves (43). Hill et al. (44), in reviewing 215 autopsies of patients who died after ECC, found fat emboli in 80% vs. 48% in nonoperated patients, whereas 31% had nonfat emboli compared to 8% in the nonoperated group. An additional marker for damage to the brain is release of adenylate kinase (AK) into cerebrospinal fluid during open-heart surgery, which was correlated with the tests of intellectual function (45) as described before (40). Such elevated enzyme levels are thought to reflect metabolic disturbances of brain cells, probably related to poor oxygenation. High AK levels together with increased lactate and glutathione concentrations appear to correlate with irreversible injury and may be due to microembolism.

Follow-up physical evaluations and psychiatric interviews in 70 of 142 survivors one year after operation (46) showed that 90% had improved in physical condition compared to their preoperative status, psychological adjustment had declined across the operation, and one-third of patients were significantly impaired psychologically.

A Conceptual Level Analogy Test (CLAT) was administered *preoperatively* to 100 patients who underwent open-heart surgery, and showed low scores indicating impaired ability to abstract. Such preoperative brain dysfunction was associated with poor postoperative outcome. Thus, the authors added preexisting brain damage to a list of intraoperative mischances causing adverse effects (47). Follow-up, postoperatively and at 18 months, showed that long-term outcome depended upon the medical diagnosis and the surgical procedure, but was also highly significantly related to preoperative CLAT scores (48). These were better predictors than ten other variables, including medical and surgical factors, in-hospital outcome, demographic measures, and vocabulary and digit symbol from the WAIS.

Autopsy studies have shown ischemic lesions along cerebral artery boundary zones. These were demonstrated when an electroencephalographic monitor measuring microvolts peak to peak to assay cerebral function showed major depression of activity in patients undergoing open-heart surgery (49). Clearly the "sensitivity" of tests affects the incidence of postoperative neurological and psychological impairment. Thus, reliance on visual reproduction and verbal recall (50), relatively resistant measures as compared to Raven matrices, Culture Fair, or neurophysiological measurements, underestimates postoperative incidence and severity of impairment. That the patients have resumed economic and social function (51) does not guarantee that their intelligence was unaffected (52).

Whatever one believes concerning the benefits of open-heart surgery, coronary artery bypass operations were done in over 1 million Americans, in some of them two or three times, from 1967 to 1978 (53). In the 1983–93 period, 1 million coronary revascularizations were done each year at an estimated cost of $15 billion (54). Many of these patients incurred obvious temporary neurobehavioral impairment. Some of them have permanent deficits, the percentage estimated depending on the sensitivity of the evaluative methods. Agents associated with cerebral injury from surgical bypass procedures include not only air and particle embolism but outgassing monomers from polyvinyl chloride tubing (vinyl chloride), ethylene oxide from sterilants, heparin stimulation of platelet aggregation, and diversion of blood away from intact brain areas to damaged ones by artificially high oxygen and low carbon dioxide partial pressures in arterial blood (55). Therapeutic drugs may also be responsible for cerebral impairment (56).

THEORIES FOR CHEMICAL BRAIN DAMAGE

Diverse Effects of Chemicals

A single, or unifying, theory may be premature because the central nervous system is complex, and many diverse chemicals disturb it. The theories were reviewed to suggest themes (56). Targets for chemicals include the neuronal cell body, axons, myelin, neural vessels, astroglia, and all membranes. Using this breakdown of targets, Spencer and Schumberg classified neurotoxins in 1980 (Table 16.1).

Central nervous system effects of chemicals vary, including: beneficial and reversible toxicity (reduction of pain and awareness by anesthetics and soporifics); seizure control by phenytoin phenobarbital, and carbamazepine and stimulation of seizures by picrotoxin, metrazol, and chlorinated hydrocarbon pesticides lindane and dieldrin (in rodents); microfibrillar aggregation with dying back and axonal cell death (57) (models from *n*-hexane and epoxides); demyelination from Thuler's murine encephalo-myelitis virus and in multiple sclerosis; altered astrocyte metabolism (58) (in lead and mercury poisoning); cell death from pyridine, beta-oxalonaminoalanine and beta-methyl-

TABLE 16.1 Classification of neurotoxins according to cellular target site

Neuron	Myelinating Cell	Astrocyte	Endothelial Cell
Somal disease or neuronopathy:	Somal disease or myelin gliopathy	Hepatic dysfunction	Lead
A. Cytoplasmic	A. Ethidium bromide	Ouabain	Cadmium
Mercury	B. Actinomycin		
Aluminum	C. Cuprizone		
B. Nuclear			
Doxorubicin			
C. Postsynaptic			
Glutamate			
Process disease or axonopathy:	Process disease or myelinopathy:		
A. Proximal	A. Hexachlorophene		
$\beta\beta$-Iminodiproplonitrile	B. Triethyltin		
B. Distal	C. Acetyl ethyl tetramethyl tetralin		
1. Central			
Clioquinol			
2. Central-peripheral			
Filamentous:			
Carbon disulfide			
Acrylamide			
Hexacarbons and 1,4-diketones			
Tuboluvesicular:			
Tri-o-cresyl phosphate			
Zinc pyridinethione			

Adapted from Spencer and Shaumberg (1980), Chap. 7 (56).

aminoalanine, 2,5-hexanedione, manganese, and aluminum; and endothelial vascular effects from cadmium and lead (56). In addition to these associations, we have a rapidly expanding knowledge of neurotransmitters and their roles [including the effects of gases: nitric oxide, NO (59, 60) and carbon monoxide, CO (61, 62)], as well as other vulnerabilities related to the production, transmission, and effects of chemicals. For many neurotoxic agents no mechanism has been identified.

Adverse metabolic effects on neurons, such as are unleashed by head trauma and stroke, constitute a cascade proceeding inexorably to cell death (62). Some chemical injuries may trigger this cascade, which begins by a voltage gate in cell walls bursting open and releasing excitatory amino acids, particularly glutamate. Glutamate receptors are of two major types: ionotropic receptors, coupled directly to the membrane ion channel, and metabotropic, coupled to G proteins, which modulate intracellular secondary messengers, including calcium, inositol triphosphate, and cyclic nucleotides (63). The ionotrophic receptors are of three types, named for their selective agonists: N-methyl D-asparate (NMDA), α-amino-3-hydroxy-5-methyl-4-isoxazolepropionate (AMPA), and kainate. Excesses of glutamate open the ion channels of calcium and sodium, and their massive influx combined with potassium loss steps up glycolysis to fuel ion pumping across cell membranes to restore the milieu interieur of the cells. As energy balance shifts, protein synthesis is slowed, and excessive lactic acid forms, proteases and lipases are activated, and proteolysis and lipolysis break down cell membranes (64). If this process continues long, cell death is inevitable.

General processes that damage the brain include reduced oxygenation or reduced energy metabolism and decreased blood flow in general or in localized areas, which cause decreased brain function (62); free radical or epoxide formation (59–62); delipidation; accumulation of metals and pigments in cells, including in astrocytes, to alter nerve cell micro-environments (58); and depletion or exhaustion of neurotransmitter production by neuroexcitants, additional ''over''-stimulation (65, 66), or other means. Excessive stimulation of surviving cells may cause their death (64). Hypoxia, irrespective of the cause, induces swelling of the neuron and its organelles, dispersion of the rough endoplasmic reticulum, swelling of the nucleus, increased hydrogen ion concentration, and inactivation of cellular oxidative enzymes (62, 67). Neurons consume ten times as much oxygen as glia and have no anaerobic metabolism; so their general vulnerability to anoxia is high whether it is due to inadequate blood flow, reduced oxygen-carrying capacity of the blood (as in carbon monoxide poisoning), ischemia, or cytotoxic effects of cyanide, sodium azide, hydrogen sulfide, or nitrogen trichloride (62).

A molecule formerly famous as a toxin in smog and acid rain, nitric oxide, serves multiple roles in the human body (59, 60). It is the first gas known to act as a biological messenger in mammals, a neurotransmitter, a sexual excitant, and an information conveyor and to reduce high blood pressure. Two types of the formative enzymes that comprise NO synthase, which are both constitutive and inductive (increase 1,000-fold for cellular defense), inhibit key pathways to block growth or to kill cells directly.

Carbon monoxide appears important in stimulating guanylyl cyclase in the brain, and it is made indigenously by hemeoxygenase, which is concentrated in the olfactory pathway (limbic system) and other areas, including vessel walls. Carbon monoxide may raise intercellular cyclic guanosine monophosphate (GMP) in the olfactory bulb and in smooth muscle cells of capillaries and other blood vessels (61, 62).

Neurodegeneration, or progressive neuronal death, often selective for functionally related pathways, has been proposed as the mechanism for Alzheimer's dementia, Parkinson's disease, and amyotrophic lateral sclerosis (68). There are two types of toxic damage, due to extrinsic chemicals, as discussed below, and to intrinsic chemicals; two of these are excitatory amino acids, notably glutamate, and the free radicals just described. Other mechanisms may fit within these major classes, including failure of DNA repair, autoimmunity, failure of a vital (mitochondrial) energy function, and late expression of a lethal gene. One fascinating parallel is that of Dopa-responsive dystonia and dystonia due to manganism (66), which simulates Parkinsonism.

MPTP (N-methyl-4-phenyl-1,2,3,6-tetrahydropyridine) is a neurotoxin that also induces Parkinsonism (69, 70). An MPTP metabolite, 1-methyl-4-phenylpyridine, selectively destroys nigrostriatal dopamine neurons to produce the clinical signs of Parkinson's disease (71). An analogous causal relationship, illustrating the role of analytical epidemiology, was found in Guam, Japan, and other Pacific islands where ALS and Parkinson's disease occur in excess (72). In Guam, it is attributed to a neuroexcitant toxin from the cycad-breadfruit-tree (β-N-methylamino-L-alanine (73). In Japan, a different species of cycad yields the same toxin (74). Lathyrism is another example of a serious neurological disease from a plant-derived amino acid (75), related to β-amino proprionitrile.

Some patients with a genetic neurological disorder known as olivopontocerebellar atrophy or degeneration of adult onset have a partial deficiency of the brain enzyme glutamate dehydrogenase. These adults show typical signs of progressive atrophy of the brain stem areas, spinal cord, cerebellum, and substantia nigra with extrapyramidal signs associated with decreased glutamate metabolism (76).

Excitotoxic nerve cell death has been linked to tryptophan metabolites, endogenous factors for excitation exemplified by quinolinic acid, which acts at very low concentrations to cause axon-sparing cell death (77). Kynurenic acid, in contrast, acts as a broad spectrum antagonist of quinolinic acid and has anticonvulsive and other antineurotoxic properties.

Solvents are exogenous neurotoxic chemicals for workers exposed to them in manufacturing, use, and waste handling. In the leather shoe industry, for example, excesses of motor neuron disease, amyotrophic lateral sclerosis, were noted by 1981, together with excess risk of perinatal mortality, congenital malformation, and trisomy 18 (78). Axonal neuropathy from a 2-diketone, which cross-links proteins after entering neurons as 2-5 hexanedione, may be responsible for this neurotoxicity (79). The "focused" trigeminal toxicity of trichloroethylene is still puzzling and the subject of speculations (78), but TCE appears to form epoxides (80) and to initiate axonal swelling neuropathy as one mechanism for widespread toxicity for the brain (see Chapter 11).

Many drugs imitate spontaneous neurodegenerative diseases, especially in elderly patients (81). Phenothiazines, butyrophenones, and even thioridazine (Melleril) are notorious for inducing extrapyramidal disorders (82).

Altered heme synthesis has been incriminated in chemical injury to the nervous system. Clues have come from clinical similarities in neurologic and psychiatric symptoms and impairments in acquired and inherited porphyrinopathies (83). An unfortunate problem is that chemicals causing acquired porphyrinopathy, such as lead and polychlorinated hydrocarbons, are also directly neurotoxic, so a clean separation of mechanisms is difficult. The spectrum of clinical problems porphyrinopathy ranges from weakness, fatigue, muscle and joint pain with slowed conduction velocity, and gait disturbances to quadriplegia and mild to severe disturbances of mood, diagnosed as dementia and psychosis. Learning ability and intelligence are impaired, and grand mal seizures have been reported in acute intermittent porphyria. The consistent histological finding is demyelinization in peripheral nerves and in the CNS. In vitro glia and Schwann cells can convert delta-aminolevulinic acid to porphyrins.

The metabolism of 2,5-substituted hexacarbon solvents (*n*-hexane) produces 2,5-dimethyl pyrrole (84). This pyrrole cross-links microtubules irreversibly, thus inhibiting axonal transport, and gradually produces focal axonopathy (84, 85). Furthermore, heme is essential in maintaining CNS cells in culture, and inhibition of porphyrin metabolism by lead causes demyelination, which is reversed by adding heme. Thus, both axons and glia are targets for damage in inherited porphyrinopathy (86).

Astroglia May Have a Central Role

Most cells of the central nervous system in vertebrates, some 90% in humans, are astrocytes. Astrocytes and neurons are both derived from the neuroepithelial cells of the neural tube, and why a particular neuronal or glial cell differentiates in its pattern is unknown. Much has been learned from culturing neuronal cells and glial cells from mature rat brains in vitro without exposure to neuronal cells (87). The glial cells grown alone do not form fibrils, but in a medium that has been bathed by neuronal cells—both in cell cultures growing on plastic and in those separated by a 1 millimeter glass rod—fibrillar structures develop. The glial cells act as a potassium buffer, and have the ability to take up neurotransmitters and to metabolize them; thus they have receptors for neuropeptides and also are able to synthesize proteins, which they release into the culture medium (87). A number of animal models have been used to show that reactive gliosis varies in duration, hyperplasia, and the expression of glial fibrillar acidic protein (GFAP) staining, and in messenger RNA. Gliosis can be induced by trimethyltin, which damages neurons and limbic structures, and MPTP, which targets the nigrostriatal dopamine energic pathway.

One of the most outstanding examples of gliosis is adrenoleukodystrophy, a genetic defect in which long chain fatty acids accumulate because of a defect in the long chain fatty acid transporter. Rodent models of gene defects, including the twitcher mouse, the Gunn rat, and the brindled mouse, show high levels of GFAP and continuous gliosis during their reduced life span. The common inflammatory human demyelinating disease, multiple sclerosis (MS), also has extensive gliosis. The best model of MS is experimental autoimmune encephalomyelitis in the guinea pig and the mouse.

Norton et al. (88) emphasized that there is considerable plasticity in response to injury, that this varies from region to region of the brain, but that the GFAP expression is always elevated. The effect of glia on axon growth vs. inhibition is complex.

Along with GFAP, the "S-100 protein," named for its solubility in saturated ammonium sulfate in glial cells, is related to calcium-binding proteins (89). It is generally distributed in the same pattern as GFAP, and its presence has been confirmed with mynoclonal antibodies. GFAP and "S-100" provide useful markers for the astrocytic response to injury and to establish the histogenic origin of brain tumors (90). Practically all gliomas contain GFAP positive cells, which suggest differentiation even in anaplastic tumors. There are also GFAP positive cells in oligodendroglioma and ependymoma, which suggest the mixed origin for these tumors. This has also been seen in the malignant neural tumors of infancy, retinoblastoma, and neuroblastoma. Glutamine synthetase, an enzyme that catalyzes the amidation of glutamate to glutamine, is a useful marker of astrocyte differentiation and is a marker of gliomas that is not seen in other brain tumors (91).

Alzheimer 2 cells are large astrocytes with enlarged rounded vacuolated nuclei and cytoplasmic vacuoles, scant cytoplasm, and frequently excessive amounts of lipofuscin granules (92). Hepatic encephalopathy produced Alzheimer 2 cells, a morphologic abnormality seen 20 years ago. Sometimes these cells were lobulated and found mostly in gray matter. In those instances of hepatic encephalopathy that reverse, these cells disappear. Electron microscopic and histochemical studies show a decrease in GFAP content and an increase in glutamic dehydrogenase activity. These changes are most strongly associated with circulating ammonia levels. Ammonia is a neurotoxin at high concentrations that causes seizures, stupor, and coma. In animal models, raising the ammonia level produced brain histopathologic changes similar, if not identical, to those of the hepatorenal syndrome. Ammonia affects the bioenergetics of the cell membrane to cause depolarization and a uniform depression in blood glutamate, and affects neurotransmitters. Also short chain fatty acids and phenol levels are elevated in hepatic encephalopathy (92). These concentrations are correlated with the severity of encephalopathy. Thus, ammonia and phenol appear to affect astrocytes in a specific detrimental way that produces a neuronal disorder characterized by stupor and coma. When these materials are removed, both the clinical and the histopathological effects reverse.

Regeneration in the adult mammalian central nervous system is limited although it remains unclear whether adult neurons have the potency for axonal growth but are frustrated in reestablishing connections, either by a glial-derived inhibitory factor or by the loss of appropriate levels of astrocyte-derived neurotropic factors and matrix (93). Clearly astroglial cells have an important role, both in providing neuronal growth factors and in maintaining an environment conducive to neuronal growth. Perhaps the most practical outcome of the recent development of primary cultures from the cerebral cortex of neonatal rats was finding that the alpha-1-adrenoreceptors regulate the uptake of glutamate, followed by glutamic oxaloacetate transaminase activation. Beta-adrenergic receptors regulate the uptake of GABA, followed by activation of gamma-aminobutyric acid and alpha-ketoglutarate transaminase, which are the fast signaling agents (94). Astrocytes also possess glutamate-sensitive ion channels. Glutamate induces increased cytoplasmic free calcium, which propagates in waves within the cytoplasm of astrocytes and between adjacent astrocytes so that networks of astrocytes could constitute a long-range signaling system within the brain (95).

The Limbic System as a Target for Chemicals

A promising hypothesis is that neurotoxicity is induced by chemicals that enter the brain via the olfactory tracts or across the blood–brain barrier to stimulate, activate, or derange functions, including emotions, that are controlled by the limbic system, especially the hypothalamus (Figures 16.5, 16.6). Abundant connections from the hypothalamus radiate into the brain via the limbic system, which has variously been called the paleomammalian brain or the rhinocephalon (smell brain). The limbic system is composed of the amygdala, hippocampus, hypothalamus, cingulate gyrus, dentate gyrus, basolateral, mesopallidal and anterior temporal circuits, and so forth (14). Odors may *stimulate* electrical activity in the amygdala and hippocampal areas of the limbic system. The amygdala is concerned with self-preservation, with feelings, and with activities usually considered to be emotional responses, such as the flight-provoking amplification of information from hearing the growl of a bear when walking in the woods (96). Its other major domains are concerned with audiovisual communication for child bearing and nursing and playing behaviors. The amygdala responds by electrical discharge to electrical or chemical stimulation, and a decrease in its content of acetylcholine esterase parallels the increase in hypersensitivity to stimuli. The hippocampus is also involved with the amygdala in making and encoding memories, and is thus essential for learning (97). From this it is concluded that decrements in learning and memory could be consequences of exposure to chemical toxins. In contrast to deficits of function, limbic derangement appears due to overstimulation or to loss of modulation or governor function.

Clues as to the varied role of limbic structures are provided in patients with emotional disturbances, psychiatric symptoms, and tumors of limbic structures or the area of the third ventricle (hypothalamus). Seizures are frequent with temporal lobe tumors (98). Also, of 2,484 patients with psychomotor epilepsy, 50% had psychiatric symptoms, which were, in order of decreasing frequency, personality disturbances, mental deficiency, unclassified psychosis, memory defects, paranoid tendencies, and schizophrenia (99). Viral encephalitis frequently presents as schizophrenia, hysteria, or depression, thus producing diagnostic confusion, as limbic structures malfunction when cells are irritated or destroyed (100). Fifty-seven percent of habitual aggressor prisoners had abnormal electroencephalograms, and 80% had abnormalities of the temporal lobe (101), even after those with mental retardation, epilepsy, and head injuries were removed from analysis. These observations led neurologists to conclude that human violence may be organically determined, as violent aggressiveness requires extensive collaboration among many parts of the brain (102).

A model for responses to chemicals involving the olfactory–limbic system, built upon Post's kindling model for affective disorders (19), suggests that amplification of response to low levels of environmental chemicals could occur by kindling and initiate persistent affective, cognitive, and somatic symptoms (18). Such kindling may be facultatively unmasked and then enhanced by neuronal damage due to unrelated chemicals. The hypothalamus governs body temperature, reproductive behavior, feeding and drinking, aggressive behavior, and fight or flight. The limbic system is the major control center of the sympathetic and parasympathetic nervous system and also produces hormones that influence the pituitary gland. Its major information inputs are from the limbic and the olfactory areas (103). Widely different chemicals appear to have remarkably similar effects on the limbic system.

Bidirectional interplay between biological phenomena leading to physiological stress is often represented vividly as emotional responses. The concept of Papez (104) that emotion has evolved as "a physiologic process which depends on anatomic mechanism" requires a structural location. Since Papez's insightful proposal in 1937, much evidence has localized emotion in the visceral brain, specifically in the limbic system, where not only is control exerted on feeding, breathing, and heart rate, but awareness of bodily order and disorder resides (105). Therefore, the argument that heightened emotional activity (tension–anxiety, anger) can speed performance related to arousal and vigilance is logically based, and is consistent with Cannon's fight-or-flight hypothesis (106).

Fear conditioning in the rat has been studied as a quantitative model for the observed increase in startle when afraid, reported in humans (107). The acoustic startle reflex measured electromyographically is 6 ms in the foreleg and 8 ms in the hind leg. It is so fast that only a few synapses could be involved when an electric foot shock is the conditioning (fear) stimulus. The pathway length can be shortened by implanting recording electrodes in neck muscles. A light flash is synchronized with the shock for conditioning. After light-shock conditioning, rats were operated on to transect bilaterally the cerebellar peduncles, the red nucleus, or the central nucleus of the amygdala. Only the latter lesions blocked the potentiated startle. The pathway is in the caudal levels of the ventral amygdalofugal pathway; lesions here blocked potentiated startle without affecting baseline startle. Electrical stimulation of the amygdala potentiates startle.

Because receptors for N-methyl-D-aspartate (NMDA) have a critical role in synaptic plasticity, NMDA antagonists such as AP5 (DL-2-amino-5-phosphonopentanoic acid) or AP7 (DL-2-amino-7-phosphonopentanoic acid) prevent induction of long-term potentiation. When rats were infused with AP5 or AP7 via implanted basolateral amygdaloid nuclei cannulae, the acquisition of but not the expression of conditioned fear-potentiated startle was blocked (108). This did not result from permanent disruption of amygdaloid function or from decreased sensitivity of the animals to the conditioning stimulus. Intra-amygdaloid infusion of a non-NMDA antagonist, 6-cyano-7-nitroguinoxaline-2,3-dione, did not block extinction of conditioned fear (109).

Follow-up experiments found that the mediator was probably N-methyl-D-aspartate NMDA (110). Infusions of corticotropin-releasing factor (CRF), a 41 amino acid peptide, has behavior-activating and anxiogenic effects in rats, demonstrated by the Porsolt swim test (110). Direct injection into the locus coeruleus of a 10 ng dose of CRF produced significant behavioral activation (decreased floating in the swim test), whereas a 500 ng dose was needed for the same effect when injected in the lateral ventricle. Bilateral infusions of CRF into nucleus locus coeruleus caused significant increases of 3,4-dehydroxyphenylglycol, a norepinephrine metabolite, into the amygdala and posterior hypothalamus.

These experiments reinforce the probable role of the limbic system in the excessive frequency of symptoms in chemically exposed subjects, and begin to bridge the gap to direct chemical inhibition of CNS pathways, which may enhance and inhibit reactivity and performance of such seemingly diverse functions as balance, blink, and choice reaction time.

This logic suggests that enhanced emotional responses due to limbic hyperactivity would improve performance on neurobehavioral tests such as choice reaction time, pegboard, trail making, and digit symbol, not impair it. The reverse argument, that depression, particularly if accompanied by confusion and fatigue, could impair performance, makes intuitive sense (111). However, applying these concepts to the interpretation of testing of chemically exposed subjects is difficult, as in almost all instances when tension and anger scores were elevated, the depression, confusion, and fatigue scores were also elevated in the profile of mood states (POMS), which could cancel stimulating effects.

Furthermore, linear regression analysis showed that the POMS score or its components rarely had significant coefficients for any neurobehavioral test score, whether physiological or psychological (Chapter 3). Even errors (on CRT, trail making B, or finger writing) that increased with blood levels of ethanol were unaffected. In contrast, greatly elevated POMS scores were almost invariably associated with impairment of neurophysiological and neuropsychological tests. However, blink reflex latency and color discrimination, which reflect relatively circumscribed or localized brain functions, were notable exceptions.

Epilepsy from Chemicals as Limbic Kindling

Seizures are related to structural alterations of the hippocampus characterized as sclerosis and identified macroscopically. This is the most consistent pathology in the brains of epileptic patients. The hippocampus, amygdala, and parahippocampal gyrus comprise major parts of the limbic system (112) (Figures 16.5 and 16.6). As the hippocampus is also involved in making and encoding memory, it is not surprising that epileptic seizures disturb memory. The complex partial seizures of the temporal lobe on the left, but not on the right, have the greatest effect on verbal learning, immediate memory, and retrieval of verbal material from memory (113).

Seizures are not rare although their causes have been identified in less than a quarter of epileptic patients (114). Seizures have numerous causes, but hypoxia is most common, followed by brain tumors, diseases of other organ systems (particularly of the endocrine glands), drugs, environmental chemicals, and electrical and traumatic events (115). Classes of drugs that commonly cause seizures include antibiotics, anticholinergics, antidepressants, antihistaminics, antipsychotics, bronchodilators, sympathiomimetics, and local anesthetics (113). The environmental chemical causes begin with lead and include most of the chlorinated hydrocarbon insecticides (112). Tonic myoclonus has been induced by bismuth, methyl bromide, toxic cooking (rapeseed) oil, gasoline sniffing, and chloralose (116). A Swedish case-control study of 104 epileptic patients in jobs using organic solvents and 312 unexposed found an eightfold higher relative risk in the solvent-exposed group, which increased through three steps of increased dose (117). Two of four patients with neurobehavioral impairment after extensive exposure to formaldehyde developed grand mal seizures, which were poorly controlled with anticonvulsants (118). Returning to myoclonus, a prospective study of Alzheimer's disease showed that myoclonus, extrapyramidal signs, and psychosis were cumulative in 72 patients who were followed for an average of 5 years from age 64. Myoclonus

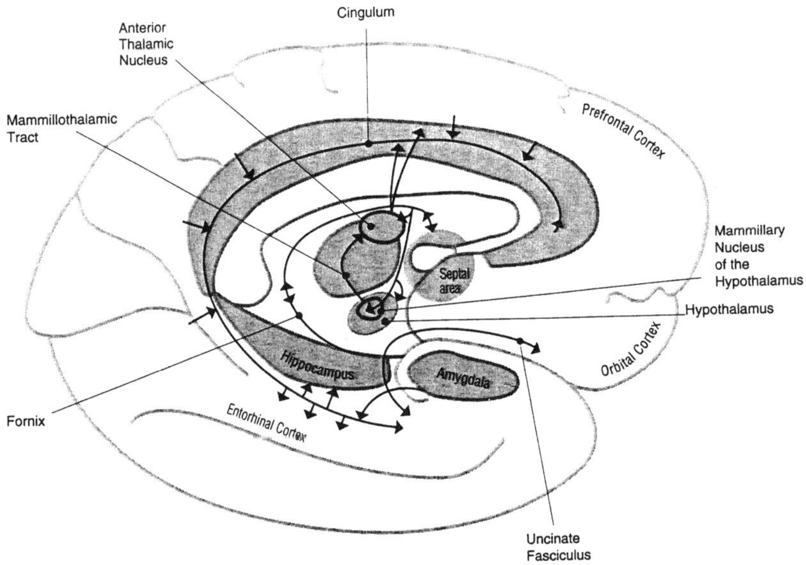

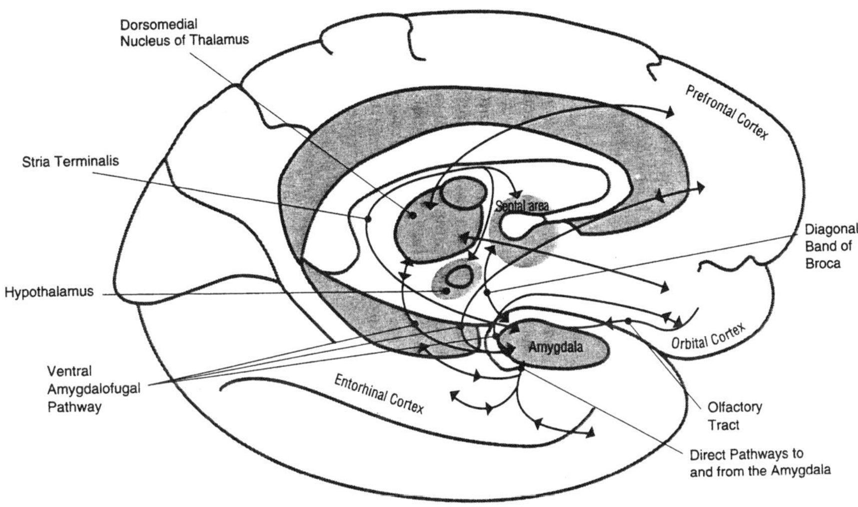

FIGURE 16.5 and 16.6. The hippocampal connections (Figure 16.5) via the cingulum and those of the amygdala (Figure 16.6) serve as short interval pathways for recall memory and emotion and equally for seizures of the partial motor (also called temporal lobe) type. (Figures from D. Reeves and D. Wedding, *The Clinical Assessment of Memory*, New York: Springer-Verlag. Used with permission.)

was present in 7% of patients in the first evaluation and increased to 34% of them in the follow-up (119).

The rat hippocampal slice preparation has been used to study, in vitro, the relationship between kindling in the limbic system and seizure activity (120–123). In fact, if such slices are depleted of magnesium, pertussis toxin, penicillin, and baclofen cause seizure discharges that are of long duration and complex morphology and have a stereotyped temporal evolution. Cycling of electrical stimulation in these slices causes hyperexcitability with spontaneous bursts of spikes and after discharges in trains. These observations narrow the gap between the mechanisms of kindling phenomena and spontaneous seizure discharges. A lowering of cerebral calcium often precedes seizures induced by pentylentrazal, penicillin, or electrical stimulation, which may reflect an inward current in presynaptic afferent fiber terminals, perhaps because of spontaneous release of transmitter substance and giant excitatory postsynaptic potentials (124). Glia cells may act to mediate these ion shifts.

In the hippocampal neurons the paroxysmal depolarizing shift (PDS) is a network-driven burst arising from a giant excitatory postsynaptic potential from the many individual cells of the network, to bring about a nearly synchronous discharge of action potentials that can be recorded extracellularly. These are probably synaptic currents (125).

In light of these observations, the occurrence of the polycystic ovarian syndrome in 5 of 20 women selected randomly from a group with temporal lobe epilepsy or complex partial seizures is instructive (126). A follow-up study showed that polycystic ovarian syndrome was associated with predominantly left-sided lateralization of epileptic discharges, whereas hypogonadotropic hypogonadism was more common when discharges were right-sided (127). Three possible explanations were offered: (1) epileptic discharges in medial temporal limbic structures may disrupt hypothalamic regulations of pituitary gonadotropin release, (2) anovulatory cycles of reproductive endocrine disorders may promote epileptic discharges, or (3) temporal lobe epilepsy and these associated reproduction disorders may represent parallel effects on prenatal development of the brain and the reproductive system.

The observations summarized in this section suggest causal connections between the exposure to chemicals and seizures. These occurrences probably do not have a single pathway or mechanism, but there is evidence of prenatal effects on the one hand and of major disruption of seizure inhibition on the other. Clearly the inquiry about seizures and their investigation in subjects with neurobehavioral symptoms and performance deficits should continue. Seizures may manifest another link between chemically triggered emotional-memory, learning and performance deficits, and the limbic dysfunction. Certainly seizures as a CNS discharge are the model of kindling. However, it is possible that they are an epiphenomenon. Additional investigation is needed.

References

1. Jacobs JM: Vascular permeability and neural injury. In: *Experimental and Clinical Neurotoxicology*, PS Spencer and HH Schaumburg (eds.). Baltimore: Williams & Wilkins, 1980, pp. 102–117.
2. Norton S: Toxic responses of the central nervous system. In: *Casarett and Doull's Toxicology: The Basic Science of Poisons* (3rd ed.), CD Klassen, MD Amdur, and J Doull (eds.). New York: Macmillan Co., 1986, pp. 359–386.
3. Rowland LP: Blood–brain barrier, cerebrospinal fluid, brain edema. In: *Principles of Neural Science*, ER Kandel and JH Schwartz (eds.). New York: Elsevier/North-Holland, 1981, pp. 650–672.
4. Powell HC, Myers RR, and Lampert PW: Edema in neurotoxic injury. In: *Experimental and Clinical Neurotoxicology*, PS Spencer and HH Schaumburg (eds.). Baltimore: Williams & Wilkins, 1980, pp. 102–117.
5. Partridge WM, Boado RJ, Black KL, and Cancilla PA: Blood–brain barrier and new approaches to brain drug delivery. *West J Med* 1992;156:218–286.
6. Rasmussen AT: *The Principal Nervous Pathways.* New York: Macmillan Co., 1935.
7. Narita M, Imada T, and Haritani M: Immunohistological demonstration of spread of Aujeszky's disease virus via the olfactory pathway in HPCD pigs. *J Comp Path* 1991;105:141–145.

8. Tomlinson AH and Esiri MM: Herpes simplex encephalitis. *J Neurol Sci* 1983;60:473–484.
9. Perl DP and Good PF: Uptake of aluminum into central nervous system along nasal-olfactory pathways. *Lancet* 1987;2:1028.
10. Baader EW: Chronic cadmium poisoning. *Indust Med Surg* 1952;21:427–430.
11. Arvidson B: Retrograde axonal transport of cadmium in the rat hypoglossal nerve. *Neurosci Lett* 1985;62:45–49.
12. Rose CS, Heywood PG, and Costanzo RM: Olfactory impairment after chronic occupational cadmium exposure. *JOM* 1992;34:600–605.
13. Kilburn KH and Warshaw RH: Persistent neurotoxicity from a battery fire: is cadmium the culprit? *Southern Med J* 1996;89:693–698.
14. Peele TL: *The Neuroanatomic Basis for Clinical Neurology* (3rd ed.). New York: McGraw-Hill, 1976, pp. 535–566.
15. Cain WS: History of research on smell. In: *Handbook of Perception*, Vol. VIA, *Tasting and Smelling*, EC Carterette and MP Friedman (eds.), New York: Academic Press, 1978, pp. 197–229.
16. Powell TPS, Cowan WM, and Raisman G: Olfactory relationships of the diencephalon. *Nature* 1963;199:710–712.
17. Ordy JM, Brizzee KR, and Johnson HA: Cellular alterations in visual pathways and the limbic system: implications for vision and short-term memory. In: *Aging and Human Visual Function*. New York: Alan R. Liss, 1982, pp. 79–114.
18. Bell IR, Miller CS, and Schwartz GE: An olfactory–limbic model of multiple chemical sensitivity syndrome: possible relationships to kindling and affective spectrum disorders. *Biol Psychiatry* 1992;32:218–242.
19. Post RM, Rubinow DR, and Ballenger JC: Conditioning, sensitization, and kindling: implications for the course of affective illness. In: *Neurobiology of Mood Disorders*, R Post and J Ballenger (eds.). Baltimore: Williams & Wilkins, 1984, pp. 432–466.
20. Goddard GV, McIntyre D, and Leech CK: A permanent change in brain function resulting from daily electrical stimulation. *Exper Neurol* 1969;25:295–330.
21. Post RM: Transduction of psychosocial stress into the neurobiology of recurrent affective disorder. *Am J Psychiatry* 1992;149:999–1010.
22. Finger S: *Recovery from Brain Damage*. New York: Plenum Press, 1978.
23. Weiss B: Neurobehavioral toxicity as a basis for risk assessment. *Trends Pharm Sci* 1988; 9:59–62.
24. Weiss B: Cancer and dynamics of neurodegenerative processes. *Neurotoxicology* 1991;12: 379–386.
25. Reuhl KR: Delayed expression of neurotoxicity: the problem of silent damage. *Neurotoxicology* 1991;12:341–346.
26. Calne DB, Langston JW, Martin WRW, et al.: Positron emission tomography after MPTP: observations relating to the cause of Parkinson's disease. *Nature* 1985;317:246–248.
27. Sibbitt WL, Griffey RH, Haseler LJ, Sibbitt RR, and Matwiyoff NA: Analysis of cerebral structural changes in systemic lupus erythematosus by proton magnetic resonance spectroscopy. *Clin Res* 1993;41:42A.
28. Bond MR: Neurobehavioral sequelae of closed head injury. In: *Neuropsychological Assessment of Neuropsychiatric Disorders*, I Grant and KM Adams (eds.). New York: Oxford University Press, 1986, pp. 347–373.
29. Brooks DN: Long and short term memory in head injured patients. *Cortex* 1975;11: 329–340.
30. Brooks DN: Wechsler Memory Scale performance and its relationship to brain damage after severe closed head injury. *J Neurol Neurosurg Psychiatry* 1976;39:593–598.
31. Schacter DL and Crovitz HF: Memory function after closed head injury: a review of the quantitative research. *Cortex* 1977;13:150–176.
32. Ladd CE: WAIS performance of brain damaged and neurotic patients. *J Clin Psychol* 1964; 20:114–121.

33. Mandleberg IA and Brooks DN: Cognitive recovery after severe head injury: 1. serial testing on the Wechsler Adult Intelligence Scale. *J Neurol Psychiatry* 1975;38:1121–1126.
34. Brooks DN, Aughton ME, Bond MR, Jones P, and Rizvi S: Cognitive sequelae in relationship to the early indices of severity of brain damage after severe blunt head injury. *J Neurol Neurosurg Psychiatry* 1980;43:529–534.
35. Jennett B and Teasdale G: Management of head injuries. *Contemporary Neurology Series*, Vol. 20, F Plum (ed.). Philadelphia: F.A. Davis Co., pp. 10–11.
36. Thomsen IV: Late outcome of very severe blunt head trauma: a 10–15 year second follow-up. *J Neurol Neurosurg Psychiatry* 1984;47:260–268.
37. Cermak L: Imagery as an aid to retrieval for Korsakoff patients. *Cortex* 1975;11:163–169.
38. Patten BM: The ancient art of memory. *Arch Neurol* 1972;26:2–31.
39. Jones MK: Imagery as a mnemonic aid after left temporal lobectomy: contrast between material-specific and generalized memory disorders. *Neuropsychologia* 1974;12:21–30.
40. Aberg T: Effect of open-heart surgery on intellectual function. *Scand J Thorac Cardiovasc Surg* 1974 (Suppl. 15).
41. Bjork VO and Hultquist G: Brain damage in children after deep hypothermia for open-heart surgery. *Thorax* 1960;15:284–292.
42. Tufo HM, Ostfeld AM, and Shekelle R: Central nervous system dysfunction following open-heart surgery. *JAMA* 1970;212:1333–1340.
43. Javid H, Tufo HM, Najafi H, Dye WD, Hunter JA, and Julian OC: Neurological abnormality following open-heart surgery. *J Thorac Cardiovasc Surg* 1969;58:502–509.
44. Hill JD, Aguilar MJ, Baranco A, Lanerolle P, and Gerbode F: Neuropathological manifestations of cardiac surgery. *Ann Thorac Surg* 1969;7:409–419.
45. Aberg T, Ronquist G, Tyden H, Ahlund P, and Bergstrom K: Release of adenylate kinase into cerebrospinal fluid during open-heart surgery and its relation to postoperative intellectual function. *Lancet* 1982;1:1139–1142.
46. Heller SS, Frank KA, Kornfeld DS, et al.: Psychological outcome following open-heart surgery. *Arch Intern Med* 1974;34:908–914.
47. Willner AE, Rabiner CJ, Wissoff BG, Hartstein M, Struve FA, and Klein DF: Analogical reasoning and post-operative outcome. Predictions for patients scheduled for open-heart surgery. *Arch Gen Psychiatry* 1976;33:255–259.
48. Willner AE, Rabiner CJ, Wissoff BG, Fishman F, Rosen B, Harstein M, and Klein DF: Analogy tests and psychopathology at follow-up after open-heart surgery. *Biol Psychiatry* 1976;11:687–696.
49. Malone M, Prior P, and Scholtz CL: Brain damage after cardiopulmonary bypass: correlations between neurophysiological and neuropathological findings. *J Neurol Neurosurg Psychiatry* 1981;44:924–931.
50. Savageau JA, Stanton BA, Jenkins CD, et al.: Neuropsychological dysfunction following elective cardiac operation: II. a six-month reassessment. *J Thorac Cardiovasc Surg* 1982; 84:595–600.
51. Jenkins CD, Stanton BA, Savageau JA, Kenlinger P, and Klein MD: Coronary artery bypass surgery. *JAMA* 1983;250:782–788.
52. Ross JK, Diwell AE, Marsh J, Monro JL, and Barker DJP: Wessex cardiac surgery follow-up survey: the quality of life after operation. *Thorax* 1978;33:3–9.
53. Braunwald E: Evaluation of the efficacy of coronary bypass surgery: II. *Am J Cardiol* 1978;42:161–162.
54. National Center for Health Statistics: Detailed diagnosis and procedures, National Hospital Discharge Survey, 1993. Vital and Health Statistics Series 13, No. 122. Washington, DC: U.S. Government Printing Office, 1995 DHHS publication no. (PHS)95-1783.
55. Editorial: Brain damage after open-heart surgery. *Lancet* 1982;1:1161–1163.
56. Spencer PS and Schaumberg HH: Classification of neurotoxic disease: a morphological approach. In: *Experimental and Clinical Neurotoxicology*, PS Spencer and HH Schaumburg (eds.). Baltimore: Williams & Wilkins, 1980.

57. Mendell JR and Sahenk Z: Interference of neuronal processing and axoplasmic transport by toxic chemicals. In: *Experimental and Clinical Neurotoxicology*, PS Spencer and HH Schaumburg (eds.). Baltimore: Williams & Wilkins 1980, pp. 139–160.
58. Ronnback L and Hansson E: Chronic encephalopathies induced by mercury or lead: aspects of underlying cellular and molecular mechanism. *Brit J Indust Med* 1992;49:233–240.
59. Culotta E and Koshland DE: NO news is good news. *Science* 1992;258:1861–1865.
60. Stamler JS, Singel DJ, and Loscalzo J: Biochemistry of nitric oxide and its redox-activated forms. *Science* 1992;258:1898–1902.
61. Barinaga M: Carbon monoxide: killer to brain messenger in one step. *Science* 1993;259: 309.
62. Verma A, Hirsch DJ, Glatt CE, Ronnett GV, and Snyder SH: Carbon monoxide: a putative neural messenger. *Science* 1993;259:381–384.
63. Lipton SA and Rosenberg PA: Excitatory amino acids as a final common pathway for neurologic disorders. *NEJM* 1994;330:613–622.
64. Bloom FE: Neurotransmitters: past, present, and future directions. *FASEB J* 1988;2:32–41.
65. Taylor R: A lot of "excitement" about neurodegeneration. *Science* 1991;252:1380–1381.
66. Appel SH: A unifying hypothesis for the cause of amyotrophic lateral sclerosis, Parkinsonism, and Alzheimer disease. *Ann Neurol* 1981;10:499–505.
67. O'Dell BL and Prohaska JR: Biochemical aspects of copper deficiency in the nervous system. In: *Neurobiology of the Trace Elements*, Vol. 1, IE Dreosti and RM Smith (eds.). Clifton, NJ: Humana Press 1983, pp. 41–81.
68. Calne DB, Hochberg FH, Snow BJ, and Nygaard T: Theories of neurodegeneration. *Ann NY Acad Sci* 1992;648:1–5.
69. Uhl GR, Javitch JA, and Snyder SH: Normal MPTP binding in Parkinsonian substantia nigra: evidence for extraneuronal toxin conversion in human brain. *Lancet* 1985;1:956–957.
70. Langston JW, Ballard P, Tetrud JW, and Irwin I: Chronic Parkinsonism in humans due to a product of meperidine-analog synthesis. *Science* 1983;219:979–980.
71. Synder SH and D'Amato RJ: MPTP: a neurotoxin relevant to the pathophysiology of Parkinson's disease. *Neurology* 1986;36:250–258.
72. Rodgers-Johnson P, Garruto RM, Yanagihara R, et al.: Amyotrophic lateral sclerosis and Parkinsonism–dementia on Guam. *Neurology* 1986;36:7–13.
73. Spencer PS, Nunn PB, Hugon J, et al.: Guam amyotrophic lateral sclerosis–Parkinsonism–dementia linked to a plant excitant neurotoxin. *Science* 1987;237:517–522.
74. Spencer PS, Ohta M, and Palmer VS: Cycad use and motor neurone disease in KII peninsula of Japan. *Lancet* 1987;Dec. 19:1462–1463.
75. Ludolph AC, Hugon J, Dwivedi MP, Schaumburg HH, and Spencer PS: Studies on the aetiology and pathogenesis of motor neuron disease. *Brain* 1987;110:149–165.
76. Plaitakis A, Berl S, and Yahr MD: Abnormal glutamate metabolism in an adult-onset degenerative neurological disorder. *Science* 1982;216:193–196.
77. Schwarcz R, Whetsell WO, and Turski WA: Kynurenines and nerve cell death. In: *Neurodegenerative Disorders: The Role Played by Endotoxins and Xenobiotics*, G Nappi et al. (eds.). New York: Raven Press, 1988, pp. 7–21.
78. Hawkes CH, Cavanagh JB, and Fox AJ: Motoneuron disease: a disorder secondary to solvent exposure? *Lancet* 1989;1:73–76.
79. Cavanagh JB: Solvent neurotoxicity. *Brit J Indust Med* 1985;42:433–434.
80. Muller G, Spassowski M, and Henschler D: Metabolism of trichloroethylene in man. *Arch Toxicol* 1975;33:173–189.
81. Sterman AB and Schaumburg HH: Neurotoxicity of selected drugs. In: *Experimental and Clinical Neurotoxicology*, PS Spencer and HH Schaumburg (eds.). Baltimore: Williams & Wilkins, 1980, pp. 593–612.
82. Murdoch PS and Williamson J: A danger in making the diagnosis of Parkinson's disease. *Lancet* 1982;1:1212–1213.
83. Silbergeld EK: Role of altered heme synthesis in chemical injury to the nervous system. *Ann NY Acad Sci* 1987;514:297–308.

84. DeCaprio AP and O'Neill EA: Alterations in rat axonal cytoskeletal proteins induced by in vitro and in vivo 2,5-hexanedione exposure. *Toxicol Appl Pharmacol* 1985;78:235–247.
85. Graham DG, Anthony DC, Boekelherde K, Maschmann NA, Richards RG, Wolfram JW, and Shaw BR: Studies of the molecular pathogenesis of hexane neuropathy. *Toxicol Appl Pharmacol* 1982;64:415–422.
86. Cavanagh J and Ridley AR: The nature of the neuropathy complicating acute intermittent porphyria. *Lancet* 1967;2:1023–1024.
87. Hansson E: Astroglia from defined brain regions as studied with primary cultures. *Prog Neurobiol* 1988;30:369–397.
88. Norton WT, Aquino DA, Hozumi I, Chiu FC, and Brosnan CF: Quantitative aspects of reactive gliosis: a review. *Neurochem Res* 1992;17:877–885.
89. Eng LF, Vanderhaeghen JJ, Bignami A, and Gerstl B: An acidic protein isolated from fibrous astrocytes (short communication). *Brain Res* 1971;28:351–354.
90. Hatten ME, Liem RKH, Shelanski ML, and Mason CA: Astroglia in CNS injury. *Glia* 1991;4:233–243.
91. Dahl D, Bjorklund H, and Bignami A: Immunological markers in astrocytes. In: *Astrocytes: Cell Biology and Pathology of Astrocytes*, Vol. 3, S Fedoroff and A Vernadakis (eds.). New York: Academic Press, 1986, pp. 1–25.
92. Norenberg MD: Hepatic encephalopathy: a disorder of astrocytes. In: *Astrocytes: Cell Biology and Pathology of Astrocytes*, Vol. 3, S Fedoroff and A Vernadakis (eds.). New York: Academic Press, 1986, pp. 425–460.
93. Lindsay RM: Reactive gliosis. In: *Astrocytes: Cell Biology and Pathology of Astrocytes*, Vol. 3, S Fedoroff and A Vernadakis (eds.). New York: Academic Press, 1986, pp. 231–233.
94. Hansson E and Ronnback L: Regulation of glutamate and GABA transport by adrenoceptors in primary astroglial cell cultures. *Life Sci* 1989;44:27–34.
95. Cornell-Bell AH, Finkbeiner SM, Cooper MS, and Smith SJ: Glutamate induces calcium waves in cultured astrocytes: long-range glial signaling. *Science* 1990;24:470–473.
96. McLean PD: Some psychiatric implications of physiological studies on the front temporal portion of the limbic system. *Electroenceph Clin Neurophysiol* 1952;4:407–418.
97. Ordy JM, Brizzee KR, and Johnson HA: Cellular alterations in visual pathways and the limbic system: implications for vision and short-term memory. In: *Aging and Human Visual Function.* New York: Alan R. Liss, 1982.
98. Malamud N: Psychiatric disorder with intracranial tumors of limbic system. *Arch Neurol* 1967;17:113–123.
99. Gibbs FA and Gibbs EL: *Atlas of Electroencephalography*, Vol. 2. Cambridge, MA: Addison Wesley, 1952.
100. Pincus JH and Tucker GJ: Limbic system and violence. In: *Behavioral Neurology.* New York: Oxford University Press, 1985, pp. 70–100.
101. William DT: Neural factors related to habitual aggression. *Brain* 1969;92:503–513.
102. Brodal A: *Neurological Anatomy in Relation to Clinical Medicine* (3rd ed.). New York: Oxford University Press, 1981.
103. Herrick JG: The function of the olfactory parts of the cerebral cortex. *Proc Natl Acad Sci USA* 1933;18:7–14.
104. Papez JW: A proposed mechanism of emotion. *Arch Neurol Psychiatry* 1937;38:725–743.
105. Smith WK: Function signs of the rostral cingulate cortex as revealed by its responses to electrical excitation. *J Neurophysiol* 1945;8:241–253.
106. Yakovlev PI: Motility, behavior and the brain; sterodynamic organization and neural coordinates of behavior. *J Nerv Ment Dis* 1948;107:313–335.
107. Davis M: Pharmacological and anatomical analysis of fear conditioning using the fear-potentiated startle paradigm. *Behav Neurosci* 1986;100:814–824.
108. Miserendino MJD, Sananes CB, Melia KR, and Davis M: Blocking of acquisition but not expression of conditioned fear-potentiated startle by NMDA antagonists in the amygdala. *Nature* 1990;345:716–718.

109. Falls WA, Miserendino MJD, and Davis M: Extinction of fear-potentiated startle: blockade by infusion of an NMDA antagonist into the amygdala. *J Neurosci* 1992;12:854–863.
110. Butler PD, Weiss JM, Stout JC, and Nemeroff CB: Corticotropin-releasing factor produces fear-enhancing and behavioral activating effects following infusion into the locus coeruleus. *J Neurosci* 1990;10:176–183.
111. Magoum HW: The ascending reticular system. *Res Publ A, Nerv Ment Dis* 1952;30: 480–502.
112. Engel J: *Seizures and Epilepsy*. Philadelphia: F. A. Davis Co., 1989.
113. Chen JY, Stern Y, Sano M, and Mayeux R: Cumulative risks of developing extrapyramidal signs, psychosis, or myoclonus in the course of Alzheimer's disease. *Arch Neurol* 1991; 48:1141–1143.
114. Hauser WA and Kurland LT: The epidemiology of epilepsy in Rochester, Minnesota, 1935 through 1967. *Epilepsia* 1975;16:1–66.
115. Messing RO, Closson RG, and Simon RP: Drug-induced seizures: a 10-year experience. *Neurology* 1984;34:1582–1586.
116. Obeso JA, Viteri C, Martinez Lage JM, and Marsden CD: Toxic myoclonus. *Adv Neurol* 1986;43:225–230.
117. Littorin ME, Fehling C, Attewell RG, and Skerfving S: Focal epilepsy and exposure to organic solvents: a case-referent study. *J Occup Med* 1988;30:805–808.
118. Kilburn KH: Neurobehavioral impairment and seizures from formaldehyde. *Arch Environ Health* 1993;49:37–44.
119. Hermann BP, Wyler AR, Richey ET, and Rea JM: Memory function and verbal learning ability in patients with complex partial seizures of temporal lobe origin. *Epilepsia* 1987; 28:547–554.
120. Lewis DV and Wilson WA: Spontaneous electrographic seizures in the hippocampal slice: an in vitro model for the study of the transition from interictal bursting to ictal activity. In: *Kindling 4*, JA Wada (ed.). New York: Plenum Press, 1990, pp. 11–19.
121. Hoffer BJ, Seiger A, Taylor D, Olson L, and Freedman R: Seizures and related epileptiform activity in hippocampus transplanted to the anterior chamber of the eye. *Exper Neurol* 1977;54:233–250.
122. Dichter M, Herman C, and Seltzer M: Penicillin epilepsy in isolated islands of hippocampus. *Electroenceph Clin Neurophysiol* 1973;34:631–638.
123. Anderson WW, Lewis DV, Swartzwelder HS, and Wilson WA: Magnesium-free medium activates seizure-like events in the rat hippocampal slice. *Brain Res* 1986;58:215–219.
124. Somjen GG: Interstitial ion concentration and the role of neuroglia in seizures. In: *Electrophysiology of Epilepsy*, PA Schwartzkroin and HV Wheal (eds.). New York: Academic Press, 1984, pp. 304–341.
125. Johnston D and Brown TH: Mechanisms of neuronal burst generation. In: *Electrophysiology of Epilepsy*, PA Schwartzkroin and HV Wheal (eds.). New York: Academic Press, 1984, pp. 277–301.
126. Herzog AG, Seibel MM, Schomer D, Vaitukaitis J, and Geschwind N: Temporal lobe epilepsy: an extrahypothalamic pathogenesis for polycystic ovarian syndrome? *Neurology* 1984;34:1389–1393.
127. Herzog AG, Seibel MM, Schomer DL, Vaitukaitis JL, and Geschwind N: Reproductive endocrine disorders in women with partial seizures of temporal lobe origin. *Arch Neurol* 1986;43:341–346.

17

Prognosis and Therapy

PROGNOSIS OF CHEMICAL ENCEPHALOPATHY

Lacking the essential long-term follow-up studies of groups of chemically brain-injured subjects, the limited and preliminary impressions of prognosis given here reflect short follow-ups of from 3 to 30 months in five groups. All of these subjects were thought to be less exposed (one was unexposed) during the follow-up interval than at peak periods, but none was unexposed, as they remained in the same jobs or residences. These impressions are supplemented by follow-ups of individual patients after their removal from exposure.

Groups Show No Improvement on Retesting

Results in five groups of chemically exposed subjects are consistent with irreversible neurotoxicity. Many of the histology technicians in the first group (1) had decreased or ceased exposure to formaldehyde and solvents, but their test scores did not improve although they remained stable across 4 years (Tables 17.1 and 17.2) with appropriate small decrements attributable to age in most tested functions. In the second group (Table 17.3), 18 subjects who were exposed environmentally via air and culinary water to trichloroethylene and other solvents showed small familiarity on learning effects when retested at 2 months. The third group, 31 subjects (Table 17.4) who were exposed residentially before 1983 to toluene and other chemicals, showed minor variation without significant changes in any test except color discrimination when retested after one year (2). A fourth group, exposed to hydrogen sulfide and reduced sulfur gases (3), was stable across 30 months during which exposure may have decreased (Table 17.4). A fifth group, subjects exposed as residents to a hydrochloric acid roadside spill, showed normalization of blink reflex latency in the interval of 12 months, but other functions remained impaired (Table 17.5).

TABLE 17.1 Description and neurobehavioral tests (group means) and standard deviations for 19 histology technicians retested yearly

	Year							
	1982		1983		1985		1986	
	Mean	Sd	Mean	Sd	Mean	Sd	Mean	Sd
Age yrs	46	10.6	47	10.6	49	10.6	50	10
Education yrs	14.4	0.9	14.4	0.9	14.4	0.9	14.4	0.9
Memory (Wechsler Memory Scale)								
Story 1 Immed. Recall	13.0	3.6	15.1	2.7*	14.3	3.9	14.9	3.9
Story 2 Immed. Recall	8.8	2.9	10.8	3.1*	11.7	3.3	11.2	4.8
Visual Immed. Recall	9.9	3.4	10.6	2.2	11.1	2.6	11.8	2.0
Digits Forward	6.5	1.3	6.4	1.2	6.6	1.1	6.3	1.1
Backward	4.7	1.4	4.7	1.2	4.7	0.8	4.9	1.2
Cognitive Function								
Block score (WAIS)	32.2	7.3	35.4	9.3	35.6	7.7	35.7	9.7
Perceptual Motor Speed								
Slotted Pegboard sec	67.5	15.5	68.4	9.3	72.3	16.0	70.5	15.5
Choice Reaction Time msec	571	89	545	59	655	134	620	105
Trails A sec	28.2	7.6	30.2	13.0	34.2	12.8	28.9	9.0
Trails B sec	64.3	25.1	65.2	29.3	69.6	39.5	61.8	23.3
Peripheral Sensory								
Fingers Right	1.8	2.0	1.7	1.8	1.7	1.7	1.5	1.8
Left	1.4	1.5	1.6	1.6	1.3	1.6	1.7	2.4
Balance (sway) Distance								
Eyes Open cm/sec					1.12	0.52	1.22	.42
Eyes Closed cm/sec					1.12	0.52	1.19	.38
POMS score					39	14	13	6

Group tested: 19 Histology technicians tested four times (1982–1986).
* $p < 0.05$.

Consistency and Patterns in Patients Restudied

Individual patients who were studied two or more times over intervals showed three patterns (see Chapter 4). One was virtual stability, with small improvements in scores on those tests known to be improved by familiarity and learning, as described above for the histology technicians. This pattern characterized most of the patients. Another pattern was of continuing deterioration of function, as exemplified by two male railroad conductors who were seen three times—immediately, 6 months, and 12 months after exposure to a nickel–cadmium battery fire. This pattern also was seen in three men heavily exposed to chemicals such as vinyl chloride, styrene, tetraethyl lead, solvents, and others. One was a highway patrolman exposed at the site of a train derailment and fires, another did hazardous material cleanup, and two of the three injected hazardous waste chemicals into pumped-out oil wells. The third and least common pattern was improvement during 3 to 27 months after moderately severe impairment. There were 3 implications: First, a pulse of exposure caused limited but permanent damage so that there was stability after the exposure stopped. Second, for continued adverse effects, agents such as cadmium, vinyl chloride monomer, styrene monomer, and ethylene dichloride may kill cells and be released, to be absorbed by new cells and kill them as the cycle continues. Third, either recovery of injured cells or restitution of damaged

TABLE 17.2 Description and neurobehavioral tests (group means) and standard deviations for 299 retested histology technicians

	Year							
	1982		1983		1985		1986	
	Mean (*N* = 47)	Sd	Mean (*N* = 98)	Sd	Mean (*N* = 91)	Sd	Mean (*N* = 63)	Sd
Age yrs	44.0	10.2	45.0	10.1	46.1	10.1	47.9	10.2
Education yrs	14.1	1.7	14.1	1.8	14.1	1.7	14.6	1.8
Memory (Wechsler Memory Scale)								
Story 1 Immed. Recall	13.9	3.5	14.4	2.6	14.4	3.4	15.4	3.7
Story 2 Immed. Recall	8.4	3.1	10.2	2.6	11.2	3.0	10.6	4.4
Visual Immed. Recall	9.0	3.3	12.2	3.0	11.0	2.4	11.3	2.1
Digits Forward	6.1	1.2	6.5	1.1	6.6	1.1	6.4	1.2
Backward	4.6	1.3	4.8	1.13	4.9	1.0	4.6	1.2
Cognitive Function								
Block score (WAIS)	31.6	7.5	34.2	8.6	33.0	8.4	34.0	9.7
Perceptual Motor Speed								
Slotted Pegboard sec	71.7	18.5	69.9	11.8	76.5	18.6	75.1	18.6
Choice Reaction Time msec	562	86	558	63	623	152	606	101
Trails A sec	28.0	7.8	34.6	15.7	34.5	12.6	29.9	9.2
Trails B sec	69.4	28.4	69.4	34.8	69.2	39.1	69.2	28.7
Peripheral Sensory								
Fingers Right	2.4	2.4	2.3	2.1	1.4	1.4	2.3	2.5
Left	1.5	1.5	1.7	1.6	1.1	1.7	2.3	3.2
Balance (sway) Distance								
Eyes Open cm/sec					1.04	0.42	1.04	0.36
Eyes Closed cm/sec					1.17	0.45	1.17	0.38
POMS score					34	8.0	11	5.4

Group tested: 299 Histology technicians tested 2 to 3 times.

circuits by the brain's functional redundancy and rebuilding (recruiting) restored function.

Test Reproducibility–Stability

The neurophysiological tests and psychometric techniques we use help evaluate improvement or progression of impairment. Each test category or domain must be examined because improvement may continue by learning or familiarity after the first testing. It follows that repeated testing to a best performance, or to a reproducible one initially, avoids misinterpretation of testing across an interval. Such virtual stability was shown by histology technicians tested at 1- or 2-year intervals for 4 years (1). Neurobehavioral measures such as choice reaction time, slotted pegboard, and balance generally reached reproducible scores within the first training period, and thereafter remained stable (2, 3).

Recall

As some psychometric tests have novel verbal or visual recall features, as in the Wechsler stories or recall of figures in visual reproduction, there may be improvement in

TABLE 17.3 Cognitive, perceptive, and motor speed tests compared across 2 months and to unexposed from Phoenix

	Phoenix (n = 18)				Combined Unexposed (n = 118)		
	Oct 14		Dec 21				
	Mean	Sd	Mean	Sd	Mean	Sd	p
Culture Fair A (intelligence nonverbal)	25.1	10.0	25.2	11.8	29.3	7.1	.07
Block Design (construction)	24.8	12.7	25.8	14.7	30.0	10.4	.05
Digit Symbol (coding)	49.6	15.4	51.8	19.4	55.7	15.4	.17
Recall	4.5	2.2	—	—			
Embedded Figures (recognition in complex array)	28.6	7.0	—	—	31.2	5.2	.088
Pegboard Grooved (dexterity) dom.	87.6	30.2	83.5	31.2	74.6	20.0	.03
Trail Making A (perceptual motor)	42.1	16.0	33.9	16.0	33.8	14.1	.003
Trail Making B (perceptual motor and decision making)	108.7	53.5	83.8	44.5	74.9	44.3	.043
Errors	1.1	1.4	1.7	2.0	0.6	1.0	NS

TABLE 17.4 Hydrogen sulfide exposure, 1989 testing compared to 1991

		1989		1991		
		Mean	Sd	Mean	Sd	p
Age yrs		38.2	9.7	39.7	12.0	N
Ed Level yrs		11.8	1.9	11.7	2.2	N
Simple Reaction Time		323	73	336	145	N
Choice Reaction Time		566	118	593	106	N
Balance—Sway	Eyes Open	1.12	0.35	0.92	0.28	N
	Eyes Closed	1.32	0.52	1.47	0.81	N
Cognitive						
Culture Fair A sc		28.4	6.8	28.6	6.5	N
Block Design score sc		31.8	8.8	30.8	9.2	N
Digit Symbol sec		49.9	13.5	50.6	13.3	N
Perceptual Motor Speed						
Pegboard sec		69.7	10.3	74.8	21.3	N
Trails A sec		37.7	12.4	35.4	15.4	N
Trails B sec		93.2	50.4	85.1	24.0	N
Memory						
Recall Story		16.9	3.2	17.5	3.8	N
Remote Information		16.6	5.5	06.8	5.7	N
Picture Completion		15.2	2.5	15.4	2.3	N
Similarities		20.2	4.2	19.5	5.0	N
POMS Score		103.3	39.4	70.9	40.7	N

SD = Standard deviation
N = Not significant

TABLE 17.5 Hydrogen chloride exposure, 1996 testing compared to 1995

	1995		1996			
	Mean	Sd	Mean	Sd	*p*	Change
Age yrs	35.4	13.2	36.7	13.6	0.665	
Ed Level yrs	10.7	2.5	10.5	2.2	0.812	
Simple Reaction Time	394	177	410	176	0.694	w
Choice Reaction Time msec	624	196	670	201	0.303	w
Balance—Sway Eyes Open	0.81	0.33	0.88	0.38	0.338	w
Eyes Closed	1.64	1.12	1.74	0.98	0.708	w
Supraorbital Tap Right	13.5	2.3	11.1	1.6	0.000*	b
Left	13.2	2.0	11.4	1.8	0.0001*	b
Color score	12.0	1.4	12.8	1.7	0.037*	w
Pegboard sec	77.0	22.3	76.2	16.2	0.854	b
Trail Making A sec	46.6	25.4	46.3	27.7	0.971	o
Trail Making B sec	91.6	44.8	90.3	40.5	0.887	b
Culture Fair A score	25.5	8.1	24.7	7.8	0.647	b
Digit Symbol score	46.4	15.7	45.9	16.4	0.908	w
Vocabulary score	15.7	7.9	16.0	7.1	0.868	b
Information score	12.6	5.1	12.9	4.5	0.722	b
Picture Completion score	12.6	4.1	14.4	4.2	0.066	o
Similarities score	16.1	5.4	15.9	6.4	0.925	w
Finger Writing Right	4.8	4.5	3.8	5.1	0.378	b
Left	4.1	4.2	3.6	4.6	0.586	b
Story 1 Immediate	9.4	3.8	9.7	4.4	0.730	b
Delayed			7.4	4.3		
Story 2 Immediate	9.2	4.2	9.6	4.1	0.722	b
Delayed			7.5	4.3		
Grip Strength						
Females Right	26.5	9.2	30.0	6.4	0.156	b
Left	23.2	8.7	27.1	6.6	0.12	b
Males Right	48.8	11.0	50.1	14.7	0.77	b
Left	44.4	10.4	47.3	12.5	0.46	b

* = significant difference
b = better
w = worse
o = no change

performance from familiarity or learning (1). Such improvements would reduce the apparent impact of cumulative adverse effects of exposure and of aging (3). Memory-scanning (a reaction time variant) was tested in 26 mercury cell chlor-alkali workers on two occasions. Performance took longer when workers' urinary mercury levels were higher, as 12-month averages. Thus, memory-scanning appeared to be a reliable indicator of changes in exposure (4).

Establishing Baselines

The clear usefulness of baseline testing of workers before they begin jobs exposing them to neurotoxic agents, and of follow-up measurements during exposure, was realized nearly two decades ago, and this procedure was recommended as a sensitive way to monitor workers for adverse effects (5). Xintaras et al. emphasized physiological measurements such as eye movement (saccades) and auditory evoked potentials in 1979, which was rather early in such studies of neurotoxicity.

Twenty-six house painters who were restudied 2 years after exposure ceased showed no change in neurological status, neuropsychological impairment, and cerebral atrophy at a mean age of 42 years (6). However, 3 of the 26 showed further deterioration later.

Brain Trauma and Chemical Injury

Can analogies to patients with brain trauma be helpful? The follow-up of 67 patients who underwent craniotomy and surgical exploration after brain trauma, mostly associated with traffic accidents in Northern England, showed that 35 had died in hospital (7). The 32 survivors were studied for 6 years. Six patients died between 3½ and 5 years after the procedure. Of the 23 patients employed at the time of the injury, 12 suffered no financial loss, 7 had reduced earning capacity, and 4 were unable to work 6 years later. Only 8 patients, one-third, were without neurological signs. Difficulties with memory, concentration, and temperament, which were called psychiatric problems, actually explained most of the reduced earning capacity (7). Another study of 27 patients with severe head injuries between the ages of 16 and 50, who had not had preceding alcoholism, drug abuse, or psychiatric disorders, showed that all had recovered conversational speech (8). However, one-third exhibited a deficit in memory storage and retrieval, and these linguistic defects were most common in those with the greatest early impairment. Patients with nystagmus or other oculo-vestibular defects had the greatest chance of showing residual defects of cognitive function, and even in those judged only moderately affected there were neuropsychiatric problems as well as reduced performance IQ, memory, and retrieval of names, as well as behavioral changes. Looked at through the eyes of relatives at 3, 6, and 12 months later, most of 55 severely head-injured adults with post-traumatic amnesia for 2 days or more had emotional disturbances, poor memory, and subjective symptoms. These deficits were uninfluenced by whether a compensation claim was pending (8). Subjective symptoms included slowness, tiredness, poor concentration, headaches, and loss of emotional control. Characteristically, the family was disrupted by a brain-injured member in that almost all family members showed depression (9–11), but the most common manifestations were denial of a problem by the family members and unrealistic expectations for the patient. These difficulties are attributed to the patient's dependency, cognitive inefficiency, emotional disturbances, and disorders of executive functions, particularly impaired (emotional) control and inability to learn from experience (12).

Head Injury Analogy

Bond's (13) careful review of neuropsychological changes after head injury concluded that the more performance-oriented parts of the testing showed the greatest degree of impairment, although others (14) found that if memory function is impaired, it is restored more slowly than perception, intelligence, or language (13, 15). Why so little research has been devoted to sequelae of head injury is not clear. It has been estimated that there are 7 million head injuries per year in the United States, and half a million require hospital admissions (13). Earlier calculations (14) estimated a quarter of a million survivors each year with some degree of persistent damage.

Mechanisms of Recovery from Brain Injury

Much thought and investigation have been given to recovery from brain damage. Certainly the concepts of redundant representation of a function and of its multiple control imply alternate pathways, and either or both of them could explain why functions return after localized trauma. To apply these concepts to chemical brain damage postulates reduced susceptibility to poisoning in the brain zones responsible for alternate pathways, compared to primary pathways, which is an oddly conceived and thus less attractive brain model (16). Recovery could be explained by ''taking over of function'' or ''functional substitution,'' using a secondary instead of a primary area when the former is injured or destroyed. Plasticity (17, 18), radical reorganization, and reorganizational compensation have been invoked to explain recovery or return of function as a result of global changes in neuro organization (17). These concepts suggest axonal sprouting, formation of new normal or unique synapses, and, in general, the performance of tasks in a different and less efficient (more time-consuming) manner (17). Tentative and collateral sprouting after trans-sectioned nerves, or after intact cells responded to a denervated area, deactivated relatively inefficient synapses in experiments on rats (16). Combined with denervation hypersensitivity, all of these are mechanisms by which intact areas can substitute functions for those lost or injured (18).

Retraining

The classic experiments done on cats by P. D. Wall (19, 20) showed that some cells responded to afferent nerve impulses after an interval during which the cell appeared to have lost all inputs. Curiously, in 1979 Teruber (21) concluded that these observations do not apply to chemical injury. Sectioning of the spinal cord or other discrete physical injuries, including those from small arms fire and auto accidents, tended to be discrete and localized, and their distal effects related to the central dying back, whereas in chemical injury usually the whole brain was affected. Monoclonal antibodies to block brain cell growth inhibitors have been demonstrated, as well as the seeking of optic tracts by optic neurons transplanted into long tracts (22). Such exciting concepts may explain regeneration in spinal cord or peripheral nerve after injuries. However, little would be expected from localized regeneration in generalized brain injury such as from chemicals. Recently the transplantation of fetal striatal cells from rats has reduced abnormal movements in baboons (23). Similarly, fetal human cells from the substantia nigra implanted in humans have reduced symptoms in Parkinson's disease patients (24). Lastly, multipotent neural cells can participate in specialized development, as in the cerebellum (25).

Thus, we have come full circle in consideration of the prognosis of chemical injury. There is insufficient experience on which to estimate prognosis. The limited observations of subjects with chemically injured brains lead to practically the same conclusion that one would extrapolate from the literature on human brain damage from inadvertent wounds and deliberate sectioning in experimental animals. Much of the damage as reported appears permanent, but the information available for prognosis is too limited to predict outcomes for individuals.

POSSIBLE THERAPEUTIC INTERVENTIONS

Avoidance

Only the most plausible and harmless possible approaches can be advised. The tested one is actually preventive, for the keystone of all therapy in 1997 is intelligent *avoid-*

ance. A daily/hourly diary type of inventory of chemical exposures and symptoms should help to identify noxious exposures and situations causing minimal symptoms. Asymptomatic or minimally symptomatic periods should be related to differences in exposure by appropriate time offsets or latent periods. Avoidance of exposures that cause symptoms should be carefully and systematically pursued. Daily schedules should be designed to minimize symptoms. Dilution of indoor air with outdoor air (i.e., having more air turnovers) is usually helpful (26–28), as it is likely that sunlight and oxygen (photooxidation) detoxify harmful hydrocarbons. The next logical step is removal of particulate hydrocarbons from the airborne environment by air filters or precipitators using particle charges. Gaseous hydrocarbons and other organic chemicals can be adsorbed on carbon. Even the removal of chlorine from water before showering is practical and reported by some patients to avoid triggering of airway hyperresponse and of difficulties with recall and concentration.

Dietary Possibilities

Removal from exposure may involve dietary as well as airborne avoidance. Whether the important factors are all synthetic chemicals is not clear. Children having epilepsy with migraine, or hyperkinetic behavior, or both had no seizures or fewer seizures when treated with an oligoantigenic diet and substitutions, as compared to no effect of the diet on children with epilepsy alone (29). The most symptom-provoking substance was cow's milk, followed by tartazine, benzoic acid, chocolate, citric fruits, and wheat (29). One proposed explanation is that milk provides, in an easily assimilated form, the short chain fatty acids that were shown to be neurotoxic in studies of hepatic encephalopathy, especially when combined with ammonia and phenols (30, 31).

Removal of Toxicants

Chelation

Rational therapy, in contrast to prevention, like that for other organs, depends on an understanding of the mechanisms of toxicity, at least in models. These models permit choices to be proposed to interfere with the mechanism. Some agents may be removed from body burdens, whether circulating or stored. When toxic effects are associated with excessive body burdens of lead or mercury, removal by chelation is rational, and it works in practice (32, 33). Chelation therapy requires medical monitoring to demonstrate its effects and to prevent unwanted outcomes. Metals (Pb, Cd, Zn, Cu) can be removed by ethylene diamine tetraacetic acid (EDTA), British Anti-Lewisite (2,3-dimercapto 1-propanol), penicillamine, and newer agents such as dimercaptosuccinic acid.

Sweating

In contrast to chelation, bodily detoxification of PCBs, solvents, and pesticides by exercise, sauna (at 160–180°F for 15–20 minutes), and hot showers is not supported by convincing evidence; "storage is hypothetical" (34–38). Probably solvents and other chemicals stored in body fat, such as chlorinated insecticides, chlordane, heptachlor, DDT, and chlorinated biphenyls, can be mobilized from fat and muscle by exercise and excreted by sweating. An empirical approach has been employed that attempts to reduce body burdens of chemicals, particularly those stored in fats. The aim is to mobilize fat and to stimulate sweating and thus skin excretion, by exercise, sauna, and hot tub combined with injection of vasodilators such as niacin or thiamine and the administration of large amounts of vitamins, antioxidants, or other potential detoxifying agents such as glutathione (34). Evidence of a therapeutic effect from any of these treatments is marginal (34–38). No controlled clinical trials have been published. Nevertheless, belief in them ranges from operational skepticism to catholic fervor.

Scientific evaluation requires carefully designed clinical trials, which have adequate numbers of subjects carefully cataloged by objective and neurobehavioral testing because of the variability in descriptions of the human disorder. Because profound body compositional and compartmental changes can be induced, monitoring of the composition of fluid and fat compartments during the treatment is prudent for safety. Furthermore, such data could be helpful in attributing any effects.

The frequently recommended procedures are (34):

1. Aerobic exercise to mobilize fat.
2. Low temperature sauna (140–180°F) to induce sweating.
3. Nutritional supplements of niacin, a vasodilator, and thiamine, the vitamin effective in Werneckie's syndrome.
4. Water, salt, and potassium replacement.
5. Polyunsaturated oil, 2 to 8 tablespoons/day, to replace lost saturated fats and perhaps bind to chemicals.
6. Calcium and magnesium replacement as required.
7. Combining the above with balanced meals, adequate rest, and no drugs, alcohol, or medications.

Logic would suggest that supplying key factors that might be missing, starting with oxygen and dextrose and including ions such as potassium, calcium, magnesium, or zinc, as well as thiamine and vitamin E and vitamin A as antioxidants, might be useful, but no trials of these supplements have been reported (37, 38).

Diet

The diet should provide good nutrition, with a high fiber, low fat content with minimal chemical additives; the fat and protein elements should be grown and prepared so as to contain minimal chemical (pesticide and herbicide) residues from agricultural practices and processing. One should avoid (a) triggers or precipitants of symptoms identified by hourly diary; (b) precursors of neurotoxic molecules, such as short chain saturated fatty acids. Allowable additives include vitamins, minerals, unsaturated vegetable oils, and ingredients of all-organic diets. Medications and supplements suggested include niacin, thiamine, antioxidants, and others, including herbs.

Neutralization

The provocation–neutralization (37, 38) approach is analogous to allergic desensitization, a therapy that is poorly justified by well-designed studies. It consists of the administration of doses of chemicals smaller than those that elicit adverse response, given sublingually as in the neutralization therapy of classic allergens or cutaneously to stimulate IgG antibodies and suppress or overwhelm IgE antibodies. Whether most of the organic chemicals considered to be causal stimulate antibodies, especially of the IgE type, remains controversial, despite outstanding examples (picric acid, tartazine, toluene diisocyanate, and perhaps formaldehyde).

Cerebroactive Drugs

A possible approach to curtailing potential hazards would be the administration of brain-directed drugs, including neurotransmitters and psychotropic agents, which appear to accelerate or slow cerebral activity (39, 40) and have been used to treat symptoms such as depression, overeating, obesity, and schizophrenia. One might consider, on the other hand, prescribing psychotropic agents, for instance, antidepressants, to speed up and enhance activity. It can only be speculated at present whether such agents, when prescribed as drugs or taken as psychedelic agents independently (street drugs) (e.g., lysergic acid diethylamine or ergotamine derivatives), have beneficial effects. There have been no clinical trials. Despite this negativity, nicotine has been helpful in Alzheimer's disease patients subjected to limited, controlled clinical trials (41–43).

Augmentation of hepatic detoxification mechanisms, including conjugations, thiosolation, or the inhibition of product activation, which converts relatively nontoxic agents to toxic metabolites (e.g., through the p-450 microsomal enzyme system), might be considered. Unfortunately, it appears probable that most active chemicals, especially those inhaled, reach their target or are metabolized well before hepatic detoxification could ensue. Thus, this approach is less attractive than others. To postulate removal of activated metabolites further "begs the question." The assumption that the lowering of body burdens of volatile organic chemicals helps patients with chemical brain damage depends upon intoxication models as from ether or alcohol. A model of reversible inhibition of brain function, this theory postulates long durations of activity from chemicals stored in body fat. As the brain, viewed chemically, is fat, the theory is flawed. Further problems arise in assuming that organic chemicals stored in fat could be "sweated out" without reintoxicating the brain.

Rehabilitation

Rehabilitation should be considered, with provision of retraining and of providing sheltered workshops. Such efforts should be aimed at redirection of the patient's efforts, both conscious and subconscious, and encouraging surviving brain function into pathways known to improve performances. This is analogous to the use of speech therapy techniques to improve swallowing in patients who have lost pharyngeal function after strokes. The aim may be as modest as the restoration of independent living, or it might range to application of alternate processing, such as "machine memory" or problem solving (17, 43). If neurons have been destroyed, then rehabilitation or retraining is the only plausible approach. It presupposes that directed training has benefits in selecting alternative processing and speed above the injured brain's own efforts. Whether this is so remains to be seen. Optimal timing of the effort and the question of combining it with chemicals (psychotropic drugs) should be explored.

Psychotherapy

Psychotherapy, such as biofeedback, is clearly related to rehabilitation or retraining, and it also needs deliberate and controlled clinical trials with well-designed protocols, including objective testing of neurobehavioral performance of subjects. Concordance was higher between "patients diagnosed with environmental illness" in a plastics shop and prior diagnoses of anxiety, depression (recent or remote), and somatization disorder than in those without the illness (44). It is probable that this finding simply reflects psychiatric presentation of what was recognized later as environmentally induced neuropsychiatric disorders due to solvents (45), but certainty is not possible from these data.

Drugs

Although comparisons of chemical encephalopathy to Alzheimer's disease are only partly justified, the analogy has been made to suggest using pharmacological agents (chemically) to treat the cognitive defect (40). Nicotine has been reported to have improved the attentional deficits in Alzheimer's disease (41) and has been tried in other cognitive deficit states (42). Before endorsement of this ''added chemical'' approach, carefully controlled trials are essential, with awareness of the seemingly paradoxically devastating effects of L-dopa in Parkinson's disease following awakening, which were beautifully chronicled by Oliver Sacks (46).

References

1. Kilburn KH and Warshaw RH: Neurobehavioral effects of formaldehyde and solvents on histology technicians: repeated testing across time. *Environ Res* 1992;58:134–146.
2. Kilburn KH and Warshaw RH: Neurotoxic effects from residential exposure to chemicals from an oil reprocessing facility and Superfund site. *Neurotox Teratol* 1995;17:89–102.
3. Kilburn KH and Warshaw RH: Hydrogen sulfide and reduced-sulfur gases adversely affect neurophysiological functions. *Toxicol Indust Health* 1995;11:185–197.
4. Smith PJ and Langolf GD: The use of Sternberg's memory-scanning paradigm in assessing effects of chemical exposure. *Human Factors* 1981;23:701–708.
5. Xintaras C, Burg JR, Johnson BL, Tanaka S, Lee ST, and Bender J: Neurotoxic effects of exposed chemical workers. *Ann NY Acad Sci* 1979;329:30–38.
6. Bruhn P, Arlien-Soborg P, Gyldensted C, and Christensen EL: Prognosis in chronic toxic encephalopathy. *Acta Neurol Scand* 1981;64:259–272.
7. Fahy TJ, Irving MH, and Millac P: Severe head injuries: a six-year follow-up. *Lancet* 1967; 1:475–479.
8. Levin HS, Grossman RG, Rose JE, and Teasdale G: Long-term neuropsychological outcome of closed head injury. *J Neurosurg* 1979;50:412–422.
9. McKinlay WW, Brooks DN, Bond MR, Martinage DP, and Marshall MM: The short-term outcome of severe blunt head injury as reported by relatives of the injured persons. *J Neurol Neurosurg Psychiatry* 1981;44:527–533.
10. Romano MD: Family response to traumatic head injury. *Scand J Rehab Med* 1974;6:1–4.
11. Lezak MD: Living with the characterologically altered brain injured patient. *J Clin Psychiatry* 1978;39:592–598.
12. Lezak MD: Brain damage is a family affair. *J Clin Exper Neuropsych* 1988;10:111–123.
13. Bond MR: Neurobehavioral sequelae of closed head injury. In: *Neuropsychological Assessment of Neuropsychiatric Disorders*, I Grant and KM Adams (eds.). New York: Oxford University Press, 1986, pp. 348–373.
14. Brooks DN, Aughton ME, Bond MR, Jones P, and Rizvi S: Cognitive sequelae in relationship to the early indices of brain damage after severe blunt head trauma. *J Neurol Neurosurg Psychiatry* 1980;43:529–534.
15. Jennett B and Teasdale G: Management of head injuries. In: *Contemporary Neurology Series*, Vol. 20, F Plum (ed.). Philadelphia: F. A. Davis Co., 1981, pp. 10–11.
16. Laurence S and Stein DG: Recovery after brain damage and the concept of localization of function. In: *Recovery from Brain Damage: Research and Theory*, S Finger (ed.). New York: Plenum Press, 1978, pp. 369–407.
17. Dobkin BH: Neuroplasticity, key to recovery after central nervous system injury. *West J Med* 1993;159:56–60.

18. Zohary E, Celebrini S, Britten KH, and Newsome WT: Neuronal plasticity that underlies improvement in perceptual performance. *Science* 1994;263:1289–1292.
19. Wall PD and Eggers MD: Formation of new connections in adult rat brains after partial differentiation. *Nature* 1971;232:542–545.
20. Wall PD: Signs of plasticity and reconnection in spinal damage. In: *Recovery from Brain Damage: Research and Theory*, S Finger (ed.). New York: Plenum Press, 1978, pp. 35–63.
21. Teuber HL: Recovery of function after brain injury in man. In: *Recovery from Brain Damage: Research and Theory*, S Finger (ed.). New York: Plenum Press, 1978, pp. 159–190.
22. Schnell L and Schwab ME: Axonal regeneration in rat spinal cord produced by an antibody against myelin-associated neurite growth inhibitors. *Nature* 1990;343:269–272.
23. Hantraye P, Riche D, Maziere M, and Isacson O: Intrastraital transplantation of cross species fetal striatal cells reduces abnormal movements in a primate model of Huntington disease. *Proc Natl Acad Sci USA* 1992;89:4187–4191.
24. Lindvall O, Wedner H, and Rechncrona S: Transplantation of fetal dopamine neurons in Parkinson's disease: one year clinical and neurophysiological observations in two patients with putaminal implants. *Ann Neurol* 1992;31:155–165.
25. Snyder EY, Deitchn DL, Walsh C, Arnold-Aidea S, Hartwieg EA, and Capko CL: Mullipontent neural cell lines can engraft and participate in development of mouse cerebellum. *Cell* 1992;68:33–51.
26. Johansson I: Determination of organic compounds in indoor air with potential reference to air quality. *Atmospheric Environ* 1978;12:1371–1377.
27. Hollowell CD and Miksch RR: Sources and concentrations of organic compounds in indoor environments. *Bull NY Acad Med* 1981;57:962–977.
28. Norback D, Torgen M, and Edling C: Volatile organic compounds, respirable dust, and personal factors related to prevalence and incidence of sick building syndrome in primary schools. *Brit J Indust Med* 1990;47:733–741.
29. Egger J, Carter CM, Soothill JF, and Wilson J: Oligoantigenic diet treatment of children with epilepsy and migraine. *J Pediatr* 1989;114:51–58.
30. Zieve L: Synergism among toxic factors and other endogenous abnormalities in hepatic encephalopathy. In: *Artificial Liver Support*, G Brunner and FW Schmidt (eds.). New York: Springer-Verlag, 1981, pp. 18–24.
31. Norenberg MD: Hepatic encephalopathy: a disorder of astrocytes. In: *Astrocytes; Cell Biology and Pathology of Astrocytes*, Vol. 3, S Fedoroff and A Vernadakis (eds.). New York: Academic Press, 1986, pp. 425–460.
32. Linz DH, Barrett ET, Pflaumer JE, and Keith RE: Neuropsychologic and postural sway improvement after Ca^{++}-EDTA chelation for mild lead intoxication. *JOM* 1992;34:638–641.
33. Grandjean P, Jacobsen IA, and Jorgensen PJ: Chronic lead poisoning treated with dimercaptosuccinic acid. *Pharm Toxicol* 1991;68:266–269.
34. Schnare DW, Ben M, and Shields MG: Body burden reduction of PCBs, PBBs and chlorinated pesticides in human subjects. *AMBIO* 1984;13:378–380.
35. Kilburn KH, Warshaw RH, and Shields MG: Neurobehavioral dysfunction in firemen exposed to polychlorinated biphenyls (PCBs): possible improvement after detoxification. *Arch Environ Health* 1989;44:345–350.
36. Tretjak Z, Shields M, and Beckmann SL: PCB reduction and clinical improvement by detoxification: an unexploited approach? *Human Exper Toxicol* 1990;9:235–244.
37. Ashford NA and Miller CS: *Chemical Exposures: Low Levels and High Stakes*. New York: Van Nostrand Reinhold, 1991.
38. Rea WJ: *Clinical Manifestations of Pollutant Overload*. Boca Raton, FL: Lewis Publishers, 1995.
39. Hessl SM: Management of patients with multiple chemical sensitivities at occupational health clinics. *Occup Med* 1987;2:779–781.
40. Levin ED: Development of treatments for toxicant-induced cognitive deficits. *Neurotox Teratol* 1993;15:203–206.

41. Jones GMM, Sahakian BJ, Levy R, Warburton DM, and Gray JA: Effects of acute subcutaneous nicotine on attention information processing and short-term memory in Alzheimer's disease. *Psychopharmacology* 1992;108:485–494.
42. Levin ED: Nicotinic involvement in cognitive function: possible therapeutic applications. *Medicinal Chem Res* 1993;2:612–627.
43. Patten BM: The ancient art of memory: usefulness in treatment. *Arch Neurol* 1972;26:25–31.
44. Simon GE, Katon WJ, and Sparks PJ: Allergic to life: psychological factors in environmental illness. *Am J Psychiatry* 1990;147:901–906.
45. Vanliet C, Swan GMH, Volovics A, Tweehysen M, Mujers JMM, deBoorder T, and Stumans F: Neuropsychiatric disorders among solvent exposed workers. *Intl Arch Occup Environ Health* 1990;62:127–132.
46. Sacks O: *Awakenings.* New York: Summit Books, 1987.

18

The Future of Neurotoxicology: Needs and Responsibilities

Just as the performance of an electronic computer can be described without familiarity with the chemical composition of its wiring and housing, so can useful knowledge of the organism's responses be gained without understanding of the make-up and operation of its submicroscopic parts.

—Rene Dubos, *Man Adapting* (1963)

Although the origins of neurotoxicity are lost in prehistory, systematic observations of palsy and colic due to lead were made by Benjamin Franklin; and erethism (irritation), tremor, and cachexia were observed in mirror silverers exposed to mercury and amalgams, as noted by Ramazzini and Kussmaul and immortalized in descriptions of "hatter's shakes" and madness by Lewis Carroll. Despite this extensive history, there has been a belated focus on neurotoxins and an apparent lack of unifying concepts concerning their recognition and mechanisms of action.

In attempting to rectify these deficiencies, I suggest that the human nervous system, with its special senses, is a highly evolved apparatus for apprehending and perceiving the environment. However, this sensitivity may be its undoing. The intuitive hypothesis is advanced that the nervous system is the most liable of the body's systems to damage from environmental toxins. An appreciation of the damage may be precluded because of subremarkable redundancy and substitution of function, or it may be overlooked in clinical evaluations, which are usually only qualitative. Unless various functions are appraised quantitatively, dysfunction may be attributed to anxiety, tension, aging, or a deficient endowment of intelligence.

ISSUES IN TESTING

The keys to understanding neurotoxicity are quantitative measurements of diverse functions, which can be compared to past performance, to predicted scores, or to the test results of unexposed individuals or populations.

The menu of measurements is a subtle blend from the affective and the symptomatic through conscious cognitive evaluations that require the subject's cooperation to the measurement of unconscious or automatic functions that previously were explored and used by neurophysiologists.

Altered affective states, manifested as symptoms, are common in everyday human experience, particularly fatigue, headache, irritability, and depression. The application of quantitative methods, such as the Minnesota Multiphasic Personality Inventory (MMPI) or the profile of mood states (POMS), to the appraisal of affective status and the correlation of these results with the outcome of psychological tests for cognitive functions, such as perceptual motor speed, sensory motor reaction time, verbal and visual-spatial memory, and design analysis, have begun to provide insights into relationships of environmental toxins to cognitive and neurological functions.

Studies of alcoholism, procedures for selection of recruits for pilot training, explorations of effects of aging, and tests originally evolved to estimate educability for placement of children in schools, as well as analyses of the toxicity of materials in workplaces, have provided methods applied to assessing the effects of environmental toxins on the human nervous system.

I would be remiss in proceeding further without crediting the contributions of David Wechsler, who devised a broadly applied immediate learning (memory) scale and an adult intelligence scale (1, 2). Wechsler cautioned that ''the information obtained from intelligence tests is relevant to the extent that it establishes and reflects whatever it is one finds is overall capacity for intelligent behavior.'' The tests used to measure intelligence served primarily as a means to an end. ''In this respect, the tests do not differ essentially from devices employed by physicists to measure heat by the use of thermometers or thermoelectric couples,'' he wrote. Wechsler combined 11 tests in his adult intelligence scale (WAIS) (2) and standardized each. The verbal scale included information, digit span, vocabulary, arithmetic, comprehension, and similarities. The performance scale included picture completion, picture arrangement, block design, object assembly, and digit symbol. These were pencil and paper tests suited for literate and language-aware individuals. Other investigators, such as Cattell (3), devised Culture Fair, which consists of four groups of designs to be solved for: logical series, maximal difference, design completion, and definition establishment and application.

Investigators applying tests to environmental or occupational groups should appreciate Wechsler's scepticism that the abilities measured broadly characterize human behavior, intelligence is multiphasic and multidetermined with a judgment of overall competency, and, finally, test scores and competency in coping effectively with the environment are not necessarily closely related. Testing at the conscious level, nevertheless, requires the subject's cooperation, is strongly dependent on the subject's understanding of language and capacity to handle numbers, and also is somewhat sensitive to the subject's attitude and feeling state.

An attempt to reduce the dependency on intelligence, vigilance, cooperation, and feeling state, and, in another sense, to encompass other CNS processes, has led to the evolution of measurements of automatic neurophysiological functions. Examples include nerve conduction, the blink reflex, body balance, visual and auditory evoked potentials, and peripheral vibration and temperature senses. Traditionally, these measurements have been restricted to specialized laboratories, have required large investments of time, and so have seldom been employed for epidemiological or even clinical studies. Their use has been limited to confirmation rather than detection. This situation is unfortunate because there is evidence that balance is reversibly affected by ethanol

(4); that blink, particularly the initial motor response, is reduced by trichloroethylene (5); that nerve conduction is reduced by lead (6); and that visual evoked potentials, the responses to flash vs. pattern, are significantly altered in aluminum intoxication (7). All of these methods extend clinical neurology's qualitative estimates with quantitative ones, to detect subtle differences across time or delays in function induced by exposures.

Maximal investigator certainty or "comfort" is achieved when the automatic or neurophysiological tests show abnormality or dysfunction in concert with the tests requiring subject cooperation, and when these results also track with affective scores and symptoms.

Clearly, the first application of testing for the affective–symptomatic area (the conscious, cooperative cognitive and the subconscious, automatic neurophysiological) is to understand a single patient and relate his or her impairment or dysfunction to toxic exposures. Extending testing beyond this subject to many individuals in a group produces an epidemiological study. Sensitivity of testing in the latter situation may be greater than that of single-patient study because small differences in suitable comparison populations may be statistically significant, whereas the individual must be viewed in terms of 95% confidence intervals or deviations from a measured or an estimated prior level of function.

Among the vital issues is the question of how to create a surrogate for previous levels of function when they are absent. For some tests, educational level is the key predictor; for most, age is a major determinant. Functions such as balance tend to have U-shaped curves with age, showing improvement during growth and development, a plateau during adulthood, and progressive impairment in advanced age. For balance, as an example, poor performance also relates to frailty and occurs in the eighth or ninth decade (8).

Subjects exposed to both occupational and environmental chemicals can be studied by using these methods. Workers are at direct risk from airborne chemicals and metals, whereas environmental neighbors receive diluted doses downstream or downwind from industrial processes or their dump sites. Although studies of painters with exposure to lead and solvents and of rayon workers exposed to carbon sulfide have produced quantitative data for exploring these problems, it is now clear that exposure to chemicals in dumps and chemical exposure during hazardous material cleanup (particularly with the use of ingenious disposal methods such as incineration and injection into exhausted petroleum wells) are new exposures, which offer opportunities for investigation. Thus, toxic cleanup workers, HAZMAT teams, well-head injectors, and perhaps firemen are at the greatest risk of exposure.

Much remains to be done in the field of testing. Despite its long history, many branches of its developmental tree are underdeveloped or missing. It would be helpful to standardize the descriptive language and not only to group the tests but to standardize them, to increase the comparability of the work of various investigators on the same toxic substance or on similar occupationally or environmentally exposed populations. Then what is needed is a clear understanding of the relationships between major axes or components: mood inventories/frequencies of symptoms recall (mostly subjective), conscious cognitive or perceptual testing requiring cooperation (so somewhat subjective), and subconscious automatic or neurophysiological performance tests (mostly objective). As additional objective tests, portable yet robust enough for field use, are standardized and applied by many investigators, progress should accelerate. Comparisons across these three axes should profile dysfunctions of the nervous system associated with specific chemicals and mixes and their interrelationships. Quantitative comparisons should increase test specificity and predictive capacity. They will provide opportunities to add biochemical and biological markers in epidemiological studies of chemical exposure (9). Then the field will mature, as suggested in foregoing chapters, far beyond its substantial, but somewhat incoordinated, beginnings.

RECOMMENDATIONS

To move into the twenty-first century, neurotoxicology needs direction. An example of strategic decisions was provided by the Nordic Council of Ministers in evaluating existing data on occupational neurotoxicity in 1990 (10). In contrast to their look backward, we must grasp the future. In order of ascending importance, six recommendations would focus on advances in neurotoxicology:

1. Standardize names for tests and functions so that communication is clear and logical, free of mystery and jargon. Follow the example of John Pappenheimer's committee in rationalizing pulmonary physiology in 1953 (11). Criteria for the selection of tests to characterize brain function need to be expressed clearly. *Benefit:* Communication would be improved, to propose clear questions for investigation.
2. Based upon demonstrated sensitivity, describe standard measurement methods for testing balance, simple and choice reaction time, color discrimination, visual fields, hearing, blink reflex latency, H (Hoffmann) reflex, vibration, and so on, so that values can be compared between laboratories. Among the criteria are sensitivity, consistency or reproducibility, dependable portable apparatus for field use, and ease of adaptability of methods for comparison among investigators and laboratories worldwide. For example, more than 30 choice reaction time procedures should be reduced to one or two. *Benefits:* Investigators heading "rapid response units" should be able to take technically simple apparatus to sites of human exposure such as "spills" for measurements. Actual testing would replace impressions derived from extended symptoms lists or clinical guesses.
3. Create reference values to permit testing across groups of human subjects of different demographic features, to define expectations and statistical variation, extending and perfecting those begun in Chapter 3. *Benefits:* Deviations from normal can then be recognized earlier and with more certainty, and effects of age, educational attainment, mood status, ethnicity, sex, and socioeconomic level on scores for these standardized tests can be determined to make suitable adjustments of these data, as formalized in prediction equations. Such equations, by adjusting for effects of age and other factors, define test expectations and thus help us to discern whether data from new study groups are different from older data and possibly abnormal.
4. Use testing with standard batteries periodically to reassess the status of exposed subjects—individuals and populations—as a measure of efforts to ameliorate and mitigate exposure effects. *Benefit:* Investigators can determine rapidly and precisely the effects of duration and intensity of exposure in the context of aging.
5. Encourage the new epidemiology of the brain function as related to environmental exposures to chemicals. As brain functions are measured in more people, make efforts to define and understand differences between environmental neurotoxicology and occupational neurotoxicology, which have already been shown to depend greatly upon vagaries of biological selectivity within workers and progressive weeding out of the chemically sensitive from them. Then experimental models of brain function should be devised at physiological and molecular levels. *Benefits:* Success in this

area could move the assaying of chemicals for safety progressively to simpler biological systems, to the cellular or the molecular level.

6. Produce more general conceptual models of how chemical exposures damage brain cells, neurons, glia, endothelial cells, and transients such as macrophages. *Benefit:* This effort would help investigators predict real-world exposures and determine how chemical mixtures, which typify many real-world exposures, interact to damage and destroy brain function. Investigators, including toxicologists and chemists, would start a list of "incompatible mixtures," so that opportunities for such combinations would be prevented by engineering in chemical manufacturing, transportation, and waste prevention/management. Numerous examples of exposure prevention exist in the home, such as avoiding mixing chlorine and ammonia products for cleaning purposes or mixing chlorine tablets and hydrochloric acid for swimming pool maintenance.

References

1. Wechsler D and Stone CP: *Wechsler Memory Scale Manual.* New York: Psychological Corporation, 1987.
2. Wechsler D: Wechsler Adult Intelligence Scale—revised. In: *The WAIS-R Manual.* New York: Psychological Corporation (Harcourt Brace Jovanovich Publishers), 1981.
3. Cattell RB: A culture free intelligence test. *J Educ Psych* 1940;31:161–180.
4. Savolainen K: Combined effects of xylene and alcohol on the central nervous system. *Acta Pharmacol Toxicol* 1980;46:366–372.
5. Feldman RG, Hayes MK, Younes R, and Aldrich FD: Lead neuropathy in adults and children. *Arch Neurol* 1977;34:481–488.
6. Feldman RG, Chirico-Post J, and Proctor SP: Blink reflex latency after exposure to trichloroethylene in well water. *Arch Environ Health* 1988;43:143–148.
7. Altmann P, Hamon C, Blair J, Dhanesha U, Cunningham J, and Marsh F: Disturbance of cerebral function by aluminum in haemodialysis patients without overt aluminum toxicity. *Lancet* 1989;2:7–12.
8. Era P and Heikkinen E: Postural sway during standing and unexpected disturbance of balance in random samples of men of different ages. *J Gerontol* 1985;40:287–295.
9. Griffith J, Duncan RC, and Hulka BS: Biochemical and biological markers: implications for epidemiologic studies. *Arch Environ Health* 1989;44:375–381.
10. Action for a common future (Report on the Regional Conference at Ministerial Level on the Follow-up to the Report of the World Commission on Environment and Development in the ECE Region). Oslo Ministry of Environment, 1990.
11. Pappenheimer JR: Standardization of definitions and symbols in respiratory physiology. *Fed Proc* 1950;9:602–605.

19

Legal Proceedings

Our society must reduce people's chemical exposures to save their brains. Can the legal system force the needed changes? Because the investigations that led to the conclusions about brain damage from chemicals were sponsored to a major extent by lawyers, the first question to ask is, did legal redress work for people vs. corporations? The brief case descriptions that follow provide detailed answers. Despite inequalities and injustice, the legal scorecard shows both wins and losses. Regrettably the overall corporate response has been to settle few of these cases and to spend millions of dollars on a defense in which delay is a major tactic. Thus, expectations of making chemical pollution too expensive for corporations so that they will stop their releases are slow to be realized and these efforts seem almost hopeless.

Civil law applies monetary values to damages to persons or to property and relies upon juries to decide the liability and the recompense. Although litigation is thought to be a search for truth and justice, it is usually simply a contest of power, and frequently purchasing power buys the verdict. As a potential instrument of social change, civil law proceedings are too rarely effective to be taken seriously, as proclaimed by the outcomes of litigation on the study populations. They are rather like an epilogue, a statement of what has happened that ''rounds out'' the story. Therefore, I appeal to the court of last resort, public opinion, organized and galvanized by individuals who collectively can wield power to change governments and small-to-giant corporations.

Funding for the studies that made this book possible came in part from plaintiffs' law firms, for diagnosis and investigation for people who knew or suspected that they were injured by chemicals in the environment, their workplaces, and their homes. Thus, the motivation for the studies, from the legal point of view, was to find data that would prove in a court of law that chemical exposure caused adverse health effects in these individuals and populations. However, some individuals who came to us for diagnosis and understanding had not instituted legal proceedings. For three of the populations studied—Phoenix, Lobelville, and Alberton—nonclients were recruited as partners, family members, and neighbors from the same exposure area and were tested simultaneously with the clients. All people tested had remarkably similar results (see Chapters 6 and 11). These deliberate test cases confirmed my impression from patients seen in consultation that the person's status as a client or a nonclient in legal proceedings did not affect the measurements.

Their persistence of symptoms and impairments and worsening of health problems, coupled with their failure to find help and understanding from physicians and departments of public health, led the chemically injured people to lawyers. Lawyers seek redress through monetary awards, as compensation for loss of health, loss of peace of mind, or denial of property, by pursuing civil lawsuits against polluters. Some of these lawsuits were for health effects; but more often, perhaps because the proof of property damage was less complex, contentious, and expensive and could be translated more readily to dollar loss than the proof of chemically injured and impaired brains, the suits were for property damage alone. Their "ironic" basis was the loss of value of their homes, or of land on the plume of chemical contamination for further commercial development—property above health.

Often both property damage and health effects were litigated. Polluters' neighbors and attorneys representing them connected the health problems with nearness to chemicals and their use or release, and established plausible cause on a "more-likely-than-not" basis, the legal standard for a decision. This societal standard of proof is less stringent than the standard typically applied in laboratory science. If this sounds contrary to medical decision making, just consider that most medical diagnosis is made to a plausible standard of "most likely." Their doubts about which standard to apply to societal, chemical attribution, problems may be responsible for scientists' and medical teams' initial uncertainty and their failure to attribute effects to chemicals. For example, "more likely than not" is represented by 50.01% certainty not the 95% certainty required for scientific publication.

Redress of injury and disease by economic compensation is different from and alien to the goals of medical or scientific teams, who focus on treatment and amelioration of disease. It is also at odds with the public health objective of preventing or reducing adverse health effects. The legal solution fixes an estimated price on damages and assesses it to the wrongdoer, frequently adding punishment in "punitive damages" (additional compensation) awarded to the victim.

Typically a jury (of peers) is asked to judge the facts of the case, thereby providing collective common sense for deciding difficult and sometimes scientifically insoluble problems of attributing effects. Despite the legal system's many imperfections, this procedure has made exposure to asbestos too expensive for Johns Manville and other companies to continue putting those mineral fibers in insulation and construction products. It "fined" Hughes Aircraft for contaminating the water wells of southwest Tucson, providing $70,000 on average to 1,200 people in the suit while over 25,000 of their neighbors learned a hard lesson. Shell paid over $1 billion for its Louisiana refinery explosions. Corning, 3M, and DOW have been ordered to pay for breast implant–related sickness. Eventually Union Carbide may be paying people in India for hundreds of deaths and thousands of damaged lungs and brains in Bhopal.

Often fugitive losses or "spills," such as 43 tons of chlorine at Henderson, Nevada in February 1991, have stimulated immediate settlement payments from the polluter to buy off potential litigants before they have experienced or even anticipated the extent of their health damage.

The steeper penalties, in criminal proceedings that pit the government against corporate CEOs with jail terms as punishment, have rarely been assessed, even in "wrongful

TABLE 19.1 Legal proceedings

Case Name	Chap. #	Jurisdiction	Major Chemical	Plaintiffs' Firm	Location	Defense Firm	Outcome
Newman vs. Stringfellow	4	State	Acid	Milberg	San Diego, CA	McCutchen, Doyle, Brown, Emersen	Jury verdict for plaintiffs
Valenzuela vs. Hughes Aircraft	11	State	TCE	Baron & Budd	Dallas, TX	Kirkland & Ellis	Multiple settlements $100 M
Aiken vs. Unocal	5	State	H_2S	Sinsheimer, Schiebelhut & Baggett	San Luis Obispo, CA	Landels, Ripley & Diamond	Settlement
Albertson vs. Dow Chemical Co.	5	State	H_2S	Spence, Moriarity & Schuster	Jackson, WY	Mike Montgomery, Nick Murdock	Settlement
Janice Jarmon et al. vs. Ford Motor Co.	10, 11	State	TCE, PCB	Steven Murray	New Orleans, LA	Bradley, Arant, Rose & White (J. Bird), Birmingham, AL	Settlement
Alexander vs. Rust Engineering Co. (AL Reclamation)	13	State	Cl_2, F_2	Corley Moncus & Ward	Birmingham, AL	Lightfoot & Franklin	Settlement
Thomas vs. FAG Bearings	11	U.S.–MO	TCE	Humphrey, Farrington & McClain	Kansas City, MO	Hostetler & Assoc., Shawnee Mission, KS	Disallowed
Hayden vs. Atochem No. America	8	U.S.	Ar	Reich & Binstock	Houston, TX	Baker & Botts	Multiple settlements
Glen & Debra Hess vs. Texas Eastern	5	State	Refinery	Pardick	Seymour, IN	Kieg, Denault, Alexander	Settlement

Livingston Parish Police Jury vs. Arcadia Shipyard	12	State–U.S.	Toluene	Unglesby & Fayard	Baton Rouge, LA	Kean, Miller et al.	Multiple settlements
McIntire vs. Motorola	11	U.S.	TCE	O'Quinn	Houston, TX	Kirkland & Ellis	Filed
Janice Akin et al. vs. Big Three Industries et al.	11	U.S.	TCE	Weller, Green, Toups & McGown	Beaumont, TX	Thomas, Gould, Nix	Settlements
Charles vs. Kings Park Apartments (Velsicol & Dow Chemical)	9	U.S.	Chlordane	Weller, Green, Toups & McGown	Beaumont, TX	Baker & Botts CMS-Daw & Ran, Houston	Multiple settlements
Touchet vs. Baker-Hughes Chemical Co.	7	State	HCl	Morrow, Morrow, Ryan & Bassett	Abbeville, LA	Hill & Beyer	Filed
Bell et al. vs. Tenneco TPC	10	U.S. District East TN	PCBs	Davis, Jenkins	Los Angeles CA	Tenneco	Filed
Consolidated Texaco Refinery litigation	5	State (special master)	H_2S	Davis, Sareen, Fries	Los Angeles CA	Texaco McCloud	Filed
Alberton Citizens vs. Montana Rail Link and Burlington–Santa Fe Railroad	6	State	Cl_2	Mueller, Rossbach & Connell	Austin, TX Missoula, MT	Boone, Karlberg & Haddon	Not yet filed
Gutierrez et al. vs. Electric Gin Co. of San Benito	8	State	As, pest.	Jim Ragan	McAllen, TX	Thornton, Summers, Biechlin et al.	Settlement
Hill et al. vs. Oak Ridge Lockheed-Marietta	6	State	Cl_2, F_2, cyanide	Rowland & Rowland	Knoxville, TN	Hill-Oak Ridge	Not yet filed

deaths,'' and rarely have corporate officers been imprisoned. However, consideration of prosecution with such punishment is increasing. In the decade ending in 1995, criminal prosecutions by EPA increased threefold (300%), with fines of $260 million and prison sentences totaling 446 years. Even giants such as Rockwell International have been considered for ''civil and criminal prosecution'' although that corporation paid fines in the deaths of two physicists (*Los Angeles Times*, April 6, 1996).

Unfortunately many physicians and scientists, and quite a few judges and jurors, believe that human beings who initiate legal action (sue) become so self-interested in the economic outcome (or secondary gain) that their symptoms, feelings, and even measured test results are unreliable, even ''unbelievable.'' Further, they consider that the plaintiffs' participation in epidemiological studies produces unreliable or at best ''suspect'' data. This line of attack, from defense attorneys and their ''scientific experts,'' maintains that such persons have exaggerated their symptoms, magnified their disorders, and manufactured their deficits. There is little support for these contentions, nor do my own observations confirm that neurophysiological function studies, psychological tests, or mood state assays can be manipulated by the persons being tested, for their personal gain, or that most plaintiffs do so.

THE CASES

Over ten years, 22 communities were studied and analyzed in our investigations. As this book was completed, nine of the associated legal cases had been resolved, one by jury verdict and twelve by settlements. (Settlement dollars first pay the expenses of the case, and then 25 to 40% is paid to the attorneys who ''sponsored'' the case; the remaining money is divided among the injured.) Three of our investigations were scientifically negative, showing no measurable adverse health effects; so there was no legal action. Science served to preclude an action. Among the unresolved cases, four, including several of the largest populations, are bogged down in the legal system (meaning that they are 4 to 6 years into proceedings that have been variously or partially resolved), and four have not yet entered into settlement or litigation and so are without conclusions. These cases are shown as Table 19.1, and they are described individually below.

Penny Newman et al. vs. J. B. Stringfellow, Jr.— Riverside Superior Court, CA, No. 165994MF, 1985–95

The Stringfellow acid pit pilot study was not described in detail in this book. It was done on 16 adults and 6 children in 1986 prior to the full development of the test battery. The firm Milberg, Weiss, Bershad, Specthrie and Lerach of San Diego was almost ten years in litigation for the plaintiffs. A jury trial judgment was based on immunologic disorders, fear of cancer, and psychological injury. Evidence of neurobehavioral impairment was not impressive, as small numbers of persons were studied, several had preexisting neurological diseases, and other health effects outweighed these. The outcome was considered a success by the plaintiffs' attorneys, but as the community of Ribideoux and environs in Riverside County California include several hundred people, the settlement seemed small.

Valenzuela et al. vs. Hughes Aircraft, Filed in Tucson, Pima County, AZ (State) Court, 1987

First, as evidence of adverse health effects and TCE exposure from contaminated water wells was gathered (see Chapter 11), the institutions with relatively small indemnity, including the Tucson Airport Authority, Arizona's Environmental Protection Agency, and the City of Tucson Water Board, settled for several million dollars each, or rather their insurance companies did so. Then a major effort was directed at Hughes Aircraft, the main polluter. Neurobehavioral impairments were compared to calculations of individual peak doses, durations (years), averages doses, and cumulative doses. Depositions taken on the medical effects lasted over two weeks. The case came to settlement under the guidance of a court appointed ''master'' from the University of Oklahoma Law School, who guided plaintiffs' attorneys Jane Saginaw and Fred Baron and defense attorney Helen Witt of Kirkland and Ellis. The settlement-agreed value of the case was $84.5 million; with other settlements the total value approximated $100 million and was divided among approximately 1,200 plaintiffs in the action, of whom 600 had medical studies.

Subsequently separate suits were filed in federal and state courts on behalf of several thousand people from the same exposure area. They are unresolved. A major scientific study to look into neurobehavioral impairment is being planned. Approximately 25,000 people were exposed to trichloroethylene from 1951 to 1987 northwest of the south Tucson airport, at a substantial Superfund site.

Aiken et al. vs. Unocal, Filed in San Luis Obispo, CA in 1991

A Unocal refinery near San Luis Obispo, California had for several years released hydrogen sulfide and other reduced sulfur gases into a small community, Calle Bendita, downwind. This area of Arroyo Grande or Nipoma (Chapter 5) often surpasses Riverside, California in having the county's highest levels of air pollution. The releases followed refitting of the refinery's desulfurization unit using a vanadium pentoxide catalyst. The probands of the study were 13 workers, and the other major complainants were the neighbors downwind. Major questions were raised about the primary attribution of the effects on human reaction time and balance to hydrogen sulfide and similar gases. Absence of visible external signs of brain damage and only a beginning literature about these effects resulted in settlement by the plaintiffs' attorneys, instead of a trial. The settlement amount was not revealed. Sulfur dioxide, hydrogen chloride, and chromium were the major chemicals known to be released into ambient air, but the inventory overlooked reduced sulfur gases such as hydrogen sulfide and mercaptans.

Norman Scott Albertson et al. vs. Dow Chemical Company et al. Civil Action 65212 Natrona County, WY 1991–93

This suit against six chemical factories in the Brookhurst area of Casper, Wyoming, which was briefly discussed in Chapter 5, is of interest because the unexposed group, which had neurobehavioral abnormalities, was exposed to hydrogen sulfide from a large refinery located in the center of town. Thus, the unexposed group performed considerably less well on the test than would be expected for an unexposed group, so that the differences between them and Brookhurst residents were less than expected. The case was concluded by a negotiated settlement with Dow Chemical and KN Energy.

Jarman et al. vs. Ford Motor Company State Court, Muscle Shoals, AL

Neighbors surrounding the Ford Motor Company's engine block and head casting plant in Muscle Shoals, Alabama showed neurobehavioral impairment attributed to PCBs and trichloroethylene (Chapter 11). Residents on two sides of the plant had well water contaminated with effluents from the metal casting operation. TCE was used in metal cleaning, but PCBs were used in the hydraulic fluid of the casting machines. This case settled for an unrevealed amount.

Alexander vs. Rust Engineering Company, State of Alabama

The aluminum workers from Alabama Metal Reclaiming of Reynolds Aluminum in Muscle Shoals, Alabama sued for an unreasonably dangerous workplace, and they utilized scientific data produced in the study of aluminum remelting (Chapter 13). These young workers, ages in their thirties on average, had had exposures to aluminum remelting and previously to aluminum reduction from bauxite. The contaminants from aluminum remelting are to a large extent from polyvinyl chloride, which on heating yields vinyl chloride monomer. The case was called by the state court, but settlement went on before there was extensive discovery; some depositions were given, and a partial settlement was concluded. The amounts of the settlement are not known. The case continues.

Thomas vs. FAG Bearings, U.S. District Court for Missouri, Springfield

The TCE exposure in Joplin, Missouri from the FAG bearing plant was ruled immune from further legal processes concerning adverse health effects because of legal technicalities in the filing (Chapter 11). These people were exposed in neighborhoods of a bearing plant using TCE in cleaning metal. The cleanup began when a new plant director found too much loss of TCE and set about rectifying the situation by recycling the TCE. Loss had produced TCE residues in the wells of Silver Creek, Missouri. There has been legal redress of property damage, cancer risk, and fear of cancer in this case.

Lillian Hayden et al. vs. Atochem NA, U.S. District Court in Texas

In the center of Bryan, Texas arsenic trioxide was used by Atochem North America, Inc. for many years to make arsenic acid to use as a defoliant and a pesticide and to treat wood used to make playground equipment (Chapter 8). The case was filed in U.S. District Court for the Southern District of Texas, Houston Division, on behalf of Lillian Hayden et al. for about 5,000 members as a class action against Atochem, which was to be expanded. A settlement was negotiated under a special master before depositions were taken, However, there were complications in the settlement, including the provisions for monitoring the neighbors who had been substantially damaged. Our testing is shown in Chapter 8. The case, therefore, has not been resolved by trials, nor has the settlement process been concluded.

Glen and Debra Hess vs. Texas Eastern Corporation, Indiana State Court

The Seymour, Indiana refinery study, which would have fit into Chapter 5, was deleted because of its recency and to conserve space, and because of uncertainty about the role of methyl *n*-butyl ether. Action was filed against ESSO, depositions were given, and, after demonstration of substantial pulmonary injury as well as a neurological impairment, a settlement was reached.

Livingston Parish Police Jury vs. Arcadia Shipyard, U.S. District Court for Western Louisiana, Baton Rouge, LA

The most complex exposure is the one of Combustion, in Livingston parish near Baton Rouge (Chapter 12). For many years toluene-rich industrial waste from over 100 sources was processed by distilling it in the name of motor oil recycling, a cunning method of waste disposal. Surrounding this site are the homes of over 5,000 people within 4.8 km. Hearings and testimony in state court were interrupted by a defense motion that remanded the case to federal court. There was a Daubert hearing (named for the U.S. Supreme Court ruling in the Bendixin trial and obligating the presiding judge to determine the scientific credibility of expert testimony before its presentation to the jury) before Judge Haik in the U.S. District Court for Western Louisiana, challenging the scientific credibility of test results that showed adverse health effects in over 500 people. Hearings were held in March and May of 1995, but Judge Haik has not ruled. Two weeks later settlements began, which accured over $120 million for the plaintiffs by the end of 1996. Depositions of other witnesses have been taken, and it appears that this case may settle completely.

McIntire vs. Motorola, Inc., U.S. District Court for Arizona, 1991

Another complex and difficult case is Maurice L. McIntire et al. vs. Motorola, Inc. in the U.S. District Court for Arizona. Motorola is Arizona's largest employer. The plaintiffs' contention, as described in Chapter 11, is that chlorinated alipathic solvents, rich in trichloroethylene, were lost into the air, soil, and groundwater over a period of years beginning in 1956. Trial of this case has been delayed several times. The principal problem seems to be in identifying exclusivity for Motorola pollution vs. other sources. This ''defense'' does not speak well for the central eastern part of Phoenix, Arizona; nevertheless the scientific evidence, as reviewed in Chapter 11, is strong. As far as is known, no settlements have been achieved, and the case is set for trial in 1998.

Janice Akin et al. vs. Big Three Industries et al., U.S. District Court, District of Oklahoma, 1993

This case, filed for the workers at Tinker U.S. Air Force Base in Oklahoma City, focuses on trichloroethylene (Chapter 11) although originally it was thought that grinding compounds (aluminum magnesium silicates), hard metal (tungsten carbide), cleaning materials, welding of high manganese stainless steel, and so forth were responsible. After tests of the workers showed abnormal blink and other signs, this was concluded to be a trichloroethylene problem. The case has gone through several settlement conferences without resolution. The nature and the extent of government vs. private contractor involvement have entered into this matter.

Eura Charles et al. vs. Kings Park Apartments (Velsicol and Dow Chemical), State of Texas, Harris County, 1993–1997

The chlordane exposure in southeast Houston produced this suit. Neurobehavioral findings were reviewed (Chapter 9) and have been published. After taking of depositions, the exterminator settled, and the case was resolved by settlements with Velsicol in 1997.

Touchet vs. Baker-Hughes Chemical Company Louisiana State Court, 1995

The exposure in Abbeville, Louisiana concerning hydrochloric acid spilled by a Baker-Hughes Chemical truck into the environs of a mobile home court with some permanent homes is now pending in state court (Chapter 7). The lead plaintiffs include the sheriff's officers who led the evacuation and warned the people. The medical work-up has been completed, including a follow-up study that showed no improvement in function.

Bell vs. Tenneco (Tennessee Pipeline Company), U.S. District Court, Eastern District of Tennessee, 1995

A case involving exposure to polychlorinated biphenyls, pydrol, from a chemical pipeline in Lobelville, Tennessee has been filed on behalf of the people who were tested in the community (Chapter 10) against Tenneco (Tennessee Pipeline Company). Trial has been scheduled, and 10 to 15 test plaintiffs have been selected.

Consolidated Texaco Refinery Litigation, Superior Court in State of California, 1992, Case No. NC010588

A major hydrogen sulfide exposure occurred in Wilmington, California in 1992 when a Texaco refineries cracker unit exploded as hydrogen was being added to crack higher molecular weight petroleum. This major explosion exposed over 10,000 people, perhaps as many as 20,000 to 25,000, to hydrogen sulfide and reduced sulfur gases (Chapter 5). This group of people had been doubted and disbelieved before a definitive work-up was started; but the study, done in January 1996, showed brain injury beyond the orthopedic and psychic scars, affecting balance, visual fields, and recall memory and such indirect sensors as increased school-dropout rates. This case is being pursued under a special master prior to trial.

Alberton Citizens vs. Montana Rail Link, State of Montana

The chlorine spill of Alberton, Montana that occurred in April 1996 was investigated by examining 97 people in June 1996 (Chapter 6). Exposure was complex as the chlorine simultaneously spilled and mixed with ''spent'' potassium cresolate. The major potential defendants in this case are the Montana Rail Link and Burlington Northern–Santa Fe Railroad and, of course, the chlorine shipper and supplier. The demonstration, after only 7 weeks, of measurable functional impairment makes this an important case. Filing has been delayed by a Montana Supreme Court ruling in a similar case.

Gutierrez et al. vs. Electric Gin Co., State Court, McAllen, TX, 1996

In San Benito, Texas a small investigation was undertaken to see if people surrounding Electric Gin, which ginned cotton, had byssinosis, the cotton dust disease. While the gin was not operating, evidence of pulmonary impairment was absent, but reaction time and balance testing showed impairments, particularly in the adults. Examination of the records found that the cotton being ginned had been defoliated with arsenic. Arsenic is a plausible explanation for impaired function. This case settled in 1996.

Hill et al. vs. Lockheed-Marietta, State Court

The last preliminary investigation was at Oak Ridge, Tennessee, where employees at the Oak Ridge National Laboratory were found to have very abnormal balance, abnormal visual fields, and other neuromuscular impairment, more neurophysiological than neuropsychological. This is of interest because the Oak Ridge uranium refinery used amalgams and had a lithium-mercury project (thus mercury exposure) and cyanide extraction, and produced uranium compounds, including uranium hexafluoride and uranium tetrachloride, for separation of U-235 for U-237 by gaseous diffusion. Probably these employees had long-term low-grade exposure to mercury, cyanide, chlorine, and fluorine. Community exposure is likely also. Conclusions, both scientific and legal, will require further investigation.

The Low Effect or Negative Cases

The three cases with an absence of or minimal (i.e., below the limit of detection) adverse health effects included one in Mississippi, where a new polyurethane roof was put on a school and a home economics teacher showed neurobehavioral damage, one of the patients discussed in Chapter 4. The school children, who were tested and compared to unexposed subjects from a nearby school, showed no effects; so only the teacher's case was tried.

The second low effect study was in Bergholtz, Ohio. Children at an elementary school were exposed downwind from a metal reclaiming operation in which six welders had shown pulmonary and neurological impairment from cutting up the double-skinned rail tankers. The downwind exposed children were more (quantitatively) symptomatic compared to unexposed children from Steubenville, the referent Ohio town; but the test results were identical, and there were no adverse health effects, so a legal case was not pursued.

The last negative is from Morrison, Colorado, where TCE had been allegedly leaked into a water reservoir by Westinghouse. The situation had gone on for several years, and from time to time residents were symptomatic. The testing showed that they were, however, not hurt, and the case was dropped.

CONCLUSIONS

It is evident that few of these cases, particularly against major chemical companies, go to trial. Frequently small (but sometimes substantive) settlements that are attractive and without risk are accepted. Clearly, if there is no injury, the case can be cleared without major large investments. The delays in many of these cases have lasted for years. Part of this delay must be attributed to inexactitude and false starts experienced in doing the science (called the learning curve); another cause is delaying tactics by the defense, used to exhaust the plaintiffs' resources, usually contingency-fee-funded attorneys. While the clock ticks, the defense attorneys are well paid.

It appears that there will be future opportunities for studies of this sort, and that they will be of considerable aid in drawing conclusions about adverse health effects. It is peculiar that there is such a high tolerance for cruelty in industrial America, reminiscent of that in Jack London's *The Iron Heel* and Upton Sinclair's *The Jungle*. The legal proceedings become complex. They challenge the new/old science of neurotoxicology with Daubert-type hearings and ''junk science'' accusations that discourage most scientists. Defense attorneys have co-opted some scientists as ''experts'' and so have impeded the finding of solutions. This new arena of forensic toxicology is being assembled piecemeal, as studies of individual clients aid population studies and vice versa. It would be preferable, obviously, if public funding could be found for it; but when such funding has been sought deliberately, its allocation has been too slow and frequently at odds with common sense and scientific and medical advice—and in any case it has rarely influenced or even impacted the effort to find what is actually going on with chemically exposed people. I hope that this commentary will help practitioners to understanding how problem-solving strategies might be improved.

It is clear that the Scandinavian system of holding a conference of the involved parties, including the injured and representatives of industry, labor, and biomedical science, usually expedites solutions. Other approaches are convoluted; and legal protections for corporations are both extensive and effective, trapping the unwary. My own first experience in industrial problem solving emulated the Nordic plan (as described in the Preface), with a partnership between the National Institute for Occupational Safety and Health (NIOSH), the North Carolina State Board of Health, and the environmental medicine program of the Duke University Medical Center in North Carolina, which I directed from 1969 to 1973. With the cooperation of and financial support from Burlington Industries, it resulted in the NIOSH recommendations for the U.S. Occupational Safety and Health Administration's cotton dust standard, followed by reduction of dust to 0.1 mg/m^3 in the textile mills and a cotton textile work environment that did not produce pulmonary disability, so that now known asthmatics work in this industry.

In spite of the inadequacy of monetary (legal) redress as applied to brain injury, it has been clearly shown that cash awards in the lawsuits, which drive up the costs of business insurance or make it unobtainable, can halt the use of dangerous technology. Before it was legally banned, asbestos was effectively removed from use in nearly all construction and consumer products by this process.

AUTHOR'S NOTE

Since 1992, I have seen and tested some 249 chemically exposed patients, including follow-up visits. I have given 66 depositions, and I gave testimony in trial for 9 patients. There were no apparent trends within the 5 years; 26.5% of those patients had my deposition taken in their legal cases, and 3.6% of them went to trial (13.6% of cases with my deposition).

Although almost all of the patients had neurobehavioral impairment, only about one quarter of them reached the legal discovery by deposition stage, and fewer than 4% of the cases were tried. If verdicts were split between plaintiffs and defendants, about 2% of the chemically injured had success by trial. It is unknown how many settled while in discovery or after deposition. The possibility is remote that the legal system benefits the chemically brain injured as a class. Even if most of the injured were compensated in dollars, that remedy for a damaged brain would be paltry. Only preventive measures are promising.

20

Social Changes Needed to Help Brains Survive

To offer the concept that most of the disease risks of the 1990s have chemical causes is as radical now as the theory that infectious agents cause disease was in the early nineteenth century.

—K. H. Kilburn

INTRODUCTION

How People and Society Must Change

Continued production and use of chemicals that are potentially harmful to human health will most certainly cause the destruction of society as we know it. Therefore, to protect the collective brains of humankind for our own and future generations, we as individuals must change our habits of consumption: from what we eat, and how we clean and keep up our homes and gardens, to how we clothe ourselves. These changes, plus others, must be reflected in precise and unequivocal instructions to industry to make human health its foremost priority. In this chapter we seek to identify those areas that people can change, individually and collectively. In a past era of industrial production or of grassroots activism we would have called this ''consumer action''; but now that term, which signifies destruction, is obsolete, and we substitute ''user'' for ''consumer.'' Here, then, the users are people acting for the protection and the conservation of their brains.

The methods used to implement change, arising from the individual and the community as well as through government and industry, are very different from each other. The government's role and response in social change are critical, but it is clear that user (formerly consumer) boycotts and changes in people's behavior will send powerful messages to the government, for stricter legislation, and to industry, which still regards profit as the key index of its activity.

Health Problems in Review

The following list shows where we stand with some major health problems:

1. *Chemical brain injury:* The dementias, the tragedies of life without recall or thought, are a silent epidemic emerging now.
2. *Cancer as a chemically caused epidemic:* The magnitude of the cancer problem is that it will kill 40 to 50% of Americans now alive.
3. *The attack on our hearts:* Heart disease now is the number two killer and is likely to remain so unless inhalation of chemicals in cigarette smoke is further curtailed.
4. *The new chemical plagues:* Arthritis and degenerative joint diseases will affect a third or more of Americans during their lifetime (80 million people).
5. *Beyond black lung:* The lung diseases have gone partially into remission as a national problem with a reduction in cigarette smoking by males.

Premature Brain Aging = Senility

A rapidly growing proportional of medical expenses and family resources, plus assets of Medicare and social security, go for care of the aged. As chemicals injure and age brains rapidly, functional brain age exceeds chronological age so that many demented people are sentenced to nursing homes or convalescent hospitals, euphemisms for storage bins for human beings, because their brains have been damaged by chemicals and they lack the capacity for self-care. It is a worse fate than most of us would dare imagine, to wander in mindlessness. Then, finally, technologically complex medical care succeeds in producing longevity with this incapacity, the epitome of what Oliver Wendell Holmes was fearful of as he wrote *Wonderful One Horse Shay* a hundred years ago (that one's parts would be exhausted piecemeal, and the whole human being would operate less well). To reverse this brain deterioration, we must dare to be novel, to make concern for the brain widespread, to move from individual to collective action to achieve this goal (perhaps even through the organization of a new political party dedicated to humankind instead of those for industry and profits). And, lastly, our approaches must be logical, well reasoned, and capable of making changes in present arrangements.

IMMEDIATE MEASURES FOR REVERSING THE DESCENT INTO DARKNESS

The steps for creating a safe world are clear, as the call to survive must overcome greed. First, a courageous few can show the way as they educate many people, helping them to understand that most degenerative diseases, particularly dementia, brain damage, premature aging, asthma, reproductive failure, and cancer, are caused by exposure to chemicals. The vanguard, the stewards of change, must include individuals with scientific and medical understanding. Second, we must make preserving the brains of humankind a prime social priority. Third, we must ban the use of dangerous chemicals—defined as those that damage humankind and the earth, our habitat—by enacting binding legislation (at the state level and, most important, the national level, as well as internationally) with prompt punishment for lawbreakers. We cannot afford to have these laws ignored. Finally, we must change industrial materials and production processes to closed cycles, outlaw open discharge, and make excessive waste obsolete by punishing polluters, major criminals in our world today.

These objectives can immediately be organized into stopgap measures that can be implemented swiftly, will function well in the short term, and will remove some of the most threatening hazards.

Cure Sick Buildings

An initial measure is to ban materials that outgas and create indoor disasters through sick buildings. The exposure of humans to construction materials and furnishings that release formaldehyde and other volatile organic chemicals that have been shown to cause brain damage should cease. These materials include wood products held together with phenolic resins and set with formaldehyde and other adhesives, glues, and mastics. Although these materials speed up assembly of buildings, the result is that the buildings become brain injury traps.

Stop Transportation of Toxic Chemicals

It is critical that we work as a community to prevent the inadvertent combination of toxic chemicals, a situation that occurs frequently and in its most rank form when materials are transported by rail. Often railroads carry chemicals in adjoining cars that produce dangerous combinations when mixed by accident (for example, carrying chlorine in a car next to one carrying creosote, the combination of which chemicals produces a deadly soup of chlorinated phenols that can cause brain damage, asthma, and sterility). Also, we must avoid the transportation through populated areas of toxic chemicals: petroleum products such as benzene, as well as tetraethyl lead and vinyl chloride monomer. These are such toxic materials that transporting them *at all* is a risk to our health and, in particular, our brains. We must provide an efficient mechanism for citizens not only to report but to initiate proceedings against the chemical culprits engaging in such transportation. These polluters need to be arrested and prosecuted for risking environmental contamination. Stiff criminal sanctions for breaking environmental rules and laws would make wrong doers desist, and would steer the social ship for the avoidance of brain-damaging exposures and those causing other degenerative diseases.

Enforce Criminal Prosecution of Polluters

Criminal prosecution for environmental misdeeds must become a reality in our society. As shown in Chapter 18, civil actions have had minor effects, which are late as well. The risk of wrist-tapping monetary fines will not force billion-dollar corporations to desist from making judgments (as made, for example, by a large automaker in the infamous rear-end collision fires) that they would rather pay insurance claims than reengineer for safety. Another proven incineration hazard is side-mounted so-called saddlebag gas tanks, which have been used in pickup trucks and even luxury automobiles. A corporation presenting such an obscene danger to the public, when unresponsive to civil action, must be administered criminal punishment.

Quarantine Toxic Technology Until It Is Replaced

We must clean up and remove sources of chemical catastrophes from urban areas to protect large numbers of people, whatever their socioeconomic situation. There is no excuse for having oil refineries in the midst of sizable populations, even if the refineries got there first. Yet because of nineteenth century ideas about transport and access, this has been allowed. Similarly, steel refining, aluminum re-refining, and many other activities that are judged essential but which generate noxious gases should be adequately isolated and quarantined to prevent even the wary from being exposed to their by products.

STRATEGIES FOR CHANGE

The major societal strategies, which could create a truly clean society, where chemical-related illness would be an aberration, must be based on widely disseminating information about the dangers of chemicals and educating the public. This raises the question of whether members of the public can comprehend the scientific information that should prove the threat to their health and sufficiently arouse the political and social activity necessary for change. I take hope from the success of consumer crusades and conservation efforts, which have often been successful in stopping the use of toxic technologies such as incinerators, strip-mining, and other destructive practices. Even if the entire citizenry does not fully understand these dangers and all their implications for humankind, our elected officials must be made to understand the seriousness of these issues.

Curtail Production of Unsafe Chemicals (Strategy 1)

There must be a drastic curtailment of chemical manufacture, which is producing or is in the course of producing substances that are toxic to the brains of workers and to people in surrounding areas. Otherwise, a projected fivefold increase in industrial (chemical) production by the year 2050 ensures catastrophe (1). These toxic materials are being identified at an increasing pace, and we already know that the use of many of them needs to be drastically limited (1, 2)—for example, hydrogen sulfide, chlorine, ammonia, vinyl chloride, chlorinated biphenyls, and many other commonly used pesticides (for no matter what their chemical makeup, if they are toxic to insects, they are toxic to humans and destructive to our brains). At least a century of experience shows that poisons, from arsenic to synthetic pyrethroids and the newest generation of organophosphates, are excessively toxic. Now is the time to quit using pesticides and examine our agricultural practices. On the basis of current scientific evidence, government must outlaw many of the surface coating practices (i.e., spraying, organic solvent paints, and vinyl chloride polymer coating on aluminum), now in use; and the production and use of solvents containing chlorine, methyl benzene, ethers, and a host of other synthetic chemicals must stop. In addition, carbon monoxide, phosgene, hydrogen chloride, sulfur dioxide, and the distillation products of fuels and a variety of other solvents must be regulated. Petroleum distillate fuels, which are a result of thermocatalytic cracking (i.e., gasoline and diesel fuel), must also be curtailed, or their production and use must be monitored and controlled.

Make Transforming Industry a Major Strategy (Strategy 2)

The closing of industrial manufacturing processes (7), making them ''closed loop,'' has been the subject of recent economic and technological investigation and discussion (3,4). It resembles the web of flow and reuse seen in natural (balanced) ecosystems. It applies nature's time-tested solution to humankind's problem (5). The idea is to eliminate waste and the production of hazardous materials (make waste an impossibility). By-products of industrial processes are to be contained and rerouted via the stream to the chemical engineer so that useful products emerge while processes are controlled and the feedstock continues to be enriched (1). In this way other products are derived, and a magic cauldron cycle ensues. There are extensive adaptations of this general idea, for example, in the recycling of plastics and in the steel, aluminum, glass, and wood and paper industries.

Figure 20.1 shows the intensity of materials use in some U.S. industries for most of the twentieth century.

Rational Use of Plastics

The production of plastics also needs to be strictly organized and regulated, according to the same rules and concepts of safety applicable to other hazardous materials. For the salvation of humankind and for minimal impact on the environment, we need maximum recyclability, without hazard and with vast curtailment of materials used. We live in a society of extreme overuse, exemplified by our overuse of plastic. In particular, overuse of disposable packaging is an issue we must address and that can be easily rectified. Informed decisions must be made about packaging, requiring changes in our current in consumer behavior, which poses even greater danger to society than do the products. A switch to safe and less wasteful (chemical-laden) packaging must be mandated.

A closed loop production process (in industry) is a system that accounts for all its products, as opposed to open-ended, wasteful toxic practices that harm the air, water, and soil. The production processes for plastics have fewer possible closed loop systems and thus far greater potential to cause continued harm than paper, metals, and glass production (see Table 20.1) (1, 6). We must develop, beginning with the source (usually petroleum), well-thought-out production–use–reuse procedures, by which products are all identified, used, and accounted for, and not allowed to escape to land, air, or water.

Steel Making and Reuse

A commonly used open system is the steel-making process, in which a hearth or Bessemer furnace is used. Iron ore, lime, and coal are burned together in the furnace; glassy slag floats and is skimmed from the surface; then iron is drained from the furnace, and all that remains goes up the stack and dissipates into the environment. Full accounting for the slag and the slag heap, for years ahead, takes into account its pollution of water downstream.

The various stages of the steel-making process that yield noxious products must be

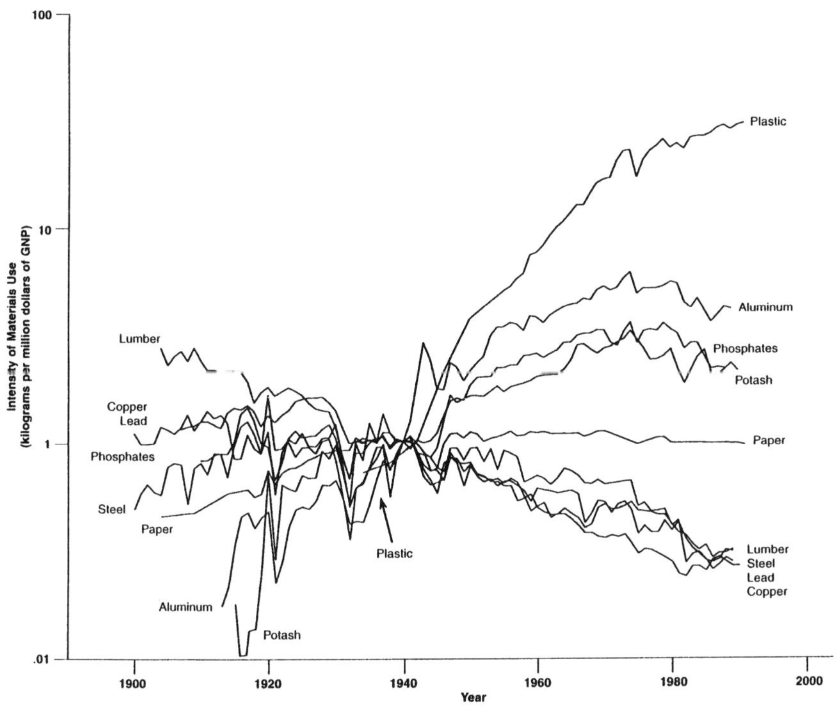

NOTE: Gross national product (GNP) is in 1982 dollars. All of the intensity ratios are normalized on 1940 (arbitrarily set equal to 1.0 in that year, with the values for other years adjusted accordingly) to facilitate comparison.

FIGURE 20.1. Intensity of materials use in the United States, 1900–90. (Reprinted with permission from *Technological Trajectories and the Human Environment.* Copyright © 1997 by the National Academy of Sciences. Courtesy of the National Academy Press, Washington, D.C.)

closed. For example, the stack must be scrubbed so that the small particles of carbon are saved for fuel; and the gases must be used to further oxidize these particles, resulting in efficient fuel use. The oxygen furnace now used for steel making exemplifies what has happened to steel production; the slag actually becomes a glassy product that can be used to make building boards for construction, to surface roads, and for other practical applications where glass-like materials are needed.

Aluminum Recycling That Is Nontoxic

Aluminum recycling is a popular example of a semi-closed loop production process; but many improvements still need to be made to the process to reduce toxicity and waste and to improve the purity of the recycled product (see Chapter 13). Aluminum recycling is a chemically contaminating process and exposes workers and people in surrounding areas to vinyl chloride monomer and other materials that are melted along with the aluminum. These contaminants are then openly removed (''burned off'') as in a primary refining process. Removal of polyvinyl chloride, other ''toxic when burned'' plastics, and metals such as lead, cadmium, and manganese earlier in the process would

TABLE 20.1 End use organic chemical products, U.S. production and sales, 1989, 1990 (1000 metric tons)

	Production		Sales	
	1989	1990	1989	1990
TOTAL		50338.8		39107.8
Dyes	174	117.0	146	104.0
Organic pigments	50	53.0	43	45.0
Medicinals	130	144.0	204	107.0
Flavor & perfume materials	64	60.0	38	37.0
Rubber processing chemicals	176	179.0	129	136.0
Pesticides	572	557.0	461	442.0
Thermosetting resins		4309.5		3177.0
Thermoplastic resins		25201.3		22093.9
Polymers for fibers		2358.5		1379.1
Polymers, water soluble		309.7		264.7
Elastomers		2233.1		1555.1
Plasticizers		890.7		826.5
Surfactants		5848.7		2718.1
Antifreeze	920	900.9		900.0
CFC's	417	308.3		300.0
Solvents				1200.0
Chelating agents		137.2		101.5
Fuel additives		4224.7		1935.6
Lube oil & grease additives		387.2		343.6
Textile chemicals (ex. surfactants)		22.4		19.8
Miscellaneous chemicals N.E.C.		2096.6		1421.9

Source: USITC 1992.

yield a cleaner final product and a safer workplace and environment. The amounts of manganese, chlorine, and fluorine (as cryolite) and of many other materials could also be altered, so as not to perpetuate the terrible conditions that exist as a result of effluents and wastes from aluminum remelt furnaces.

Glass Production and Reuse

Recycled glass can achieve near purity, the epitome of cleanliness, when glass intended for reuse is sorted by color. Unfortunately, as glass recycling has improved, the container industry has moved away from using glass, replacing it with plastic. This represents one of the worst choices with regard to potential for separation and recycling, mainly because at least ten different types of plastic are used in the production of containers. When recycled, the types must be separated, as they cannot be melted together to make useful products. The answer may be to reduce the number of materials used to one or two, easily recognizable types of plastic, just as we have done with three major metals: ferrous (iron) metals, aluminum, and copper.

Wood, Paper, and Substitutes

Forest products, which used to be considered highly safe, noninjurious, and "natural," are in fact treated with turpentine, naval stores, balsam, and derivative varnishes and coating materials—all substances that are hazardous to human health and the environment. Unfortunately, in the last 40 years as the demand for wood has outpaced supply, we have used up our grandchildren's trees. Public lands no longer have enough trees to meet the needs of the world's extraordinary consumption. Industry's response to meeting the insatiable demand for wood and preserving profits has led to the extremely ill-founded (as to their adverse effects) incorporation of highly toxic chemicals, such as phenyl formaldehyde, into the production processes for plywood, particle board, forest product (sawdust) board, and numerous other manufactured building materials—all of which are composed in part of wood and in part of chemicals. There must be alternatives to this solution.

Paper continues to be in high demand, and the magnitude of this industry has led to numerous toxic byproducts being caught in ponds and emitting hydrogen sulfide. The H_2S leaches into the environment, poisoning people and wildlife and delicate ecosystems. The bleaching process for the production of paper uses sulfur dioxide and/or chlorine, which in addition to producing whiter paper sheds toxic byproducts on people and the environment. These are only a few of the toxic chemicals in this industry; many others could be mentioned.

The paper reuse loop is mainly impeded now by poor organization and high transportation costs. These problems could be solved by miniaturizing and networking plants for recycling so that they could be near the sources of used paper and would require less energy for transportation. Increased recycling would save trees and would drastically reduce the toxic technology of paper making.

WHAT WE MUST DO IN SHAPING HUMAN ATTITUDES

A critical component of working toward a solution lies in human attitudes and in each individual's capacity to fight for survival. This book's message for change is stark and clean. Technology can only help to implement change and perhaps prevent further damage; it cannot actually bring about change or restore the earth to its once pristine state. As our examples show, there is not one answer but rather a series of answers. What must take place is a major reordering of the world's priorities and a drastic reduction in the industrial world's control over people's lives.

What Will Motivate Changes

The critical question is, what will motivate us to change our production processes as well as our consumer behavior? Victims of insidious chemical accidents and experiments on the public must march with medical and public health providers to save the collective human brain. This book presents a plan, for materials use cycles and industrial reordering to prevent brain injury, that must be put into practice. All of us must set aside trivial and fragmented concerns, personal issues, and egos to unite and form coalitions of the like-minded to fight against the chemical assault as one, to unite the public to save itself.

All of us, as participants in the use of resources and shapers of our own future, must do five things:

1. Give up adverse consumer habits.
2. Participate in user boycotts of harmful products that will make them economically unviable.
3. Vote for, and impress on our representatives, the need for making the key decisions

of the twenty-first century that will enable us to save our brains and other organs from chemical destruction.
4. Be vocal, and educate our fellow users about environmental health risks.
5. Heed the warning signs of adverse effects of chemicals, including headache, extreme fatigue, loss of recall, dizziness, red skin, shortness of breath, wheezing, and chest tightness or burning.

What to Do for Personal Safety

At the personal and family level there are ''consumer staples'' that need to be given up in order for us to live safely:

1. *Pesticides:* The use of pesticides in and about the home absolutely must stop. People must make peace with their insect coinhabitants of the earth and realize that the insects have natural predators. They also can be steered away from human dwellings by disconnecting their means of entry or by cutting back ivy and other foliage. Physical and electrical means can be used, and proven nontoxic chemicals such as boric acid can be used against ants and roaches indoors, to arrest or kill those that cannot be dealt within other ways. Bug lights are a good example of nonchemical pest control. A corollary is to demand organically grown produce from the grocer.
2. *Fat and sugar:* A superabundance of fat, fatty food, and products overly rich in calories must be avoided. Obesity is harmful to humans, and fat is a major problem; besides being a repository for excess calories, fat is used by the body for storage of many toxic organic chemicals. Note also that chemicals enter food from packaging materials, such as those for junk food, which must be tested for safety or not used. The motivation for overeating must be removed, and life must be structured such that there are satisfactions from exercising, participating in a variety of activities, and being creative. Then eating is not the only satisfaction. Food advertising and availability must be curtailed, with nutrition—not profit—the aim. The promotion of healthful lifestyles is crucial.
3. *Cleaning and sanitizing:* Detergents and cleaning agents must be chosen with care to avoid chlorine, ammonia, and some of the numerous other brain-violating chemicals. Again, picking clean ones, and boycotting those that smell of chlorine and other harmful chemicals, can bring about change.
4. *Cosmetics:* The same spirit of avoidance of harmful chemicals must be applied to cosmetics, many of which are totally unnecessary. Perhaps the most harmful cosmetics chemicals are the solvents in polishes for fingernails and toenails. These polishes and polish removers are extremely hazardous with their methyl ethyl ketone, acetone, and other brain solvents; so they must be forsworn and considered the worst of surface coatings.
5. *Surface coatings:* Paints, including a variety of surface coatings (epoxies, urethanes), have been engineered for greater safety. Southern California has already mandated that organic solvents be given up and has moved to water-based paint. We must be sure that the method of application is safe, reducing the enormous burdens of chemicals inhaled. This means that spray painting and even painting with the rollers that aerosolize vast amounts of paint must be given up for more direct application of paint systems. Many things could be painted in the factory in automated paint rooms, such as are used for refrigerators and aircraft.

Boycotts by Users

User boycotts of harmful products should arise out of the giving up of adverse products. If a united citizenry moves to forswear unsafe products, they have already boycotted them. Such boycotts should be directed first to pesticides, second to chlorinated cleaning agents and detergents, third to many paints, and fourth to fatty foods. As these products are boycotted, they will drop from sight and be replaced by alternatives, which after brief testing may or may not be certified as improvements.

We must move forward to a stable economy, producing materials for use that are of actual benefit to humankind rather than being empty parts of a profit-and-loss cycle. The benefits will include immediate waste reduction, with less need for waste disposal, particularly landfills and ocean dumping, which have spread chemically contamination all around us. With these conditions reversed, we can re-create a safer earth that is a friendlier place for us to live.

Redefining Government

We must take stock of and responsibility for our current chemical health crisis, and must develop pragmatic criteria for judging the effects of changes. Our options are to protect our own brains by individual action and to change social and economic (i.e., business) activity by governmental mandates, enforced either by the government or by our interactions with it.

Governments have a responsibility to their citizens; as Abraham Lincoln said, governments are constituted "to do for the people whatever they need done, but cannot do, at all, or cannot do so well in their own separate and individual capacities." Thus, we must define for our governments those problems that can be solved, as outlined above. The objectives are clear; this book focuses on the critical measurements of human brain function, and the societal problem of chemical brain injury. The problem can be solved. Governments and industry can develop the new technological engineering needed, working with informed citizens dedicated to collective human action.

Governmental Priorities

The following list ranks governmental priorities, beginning with the most important one.

Oil Refineries

Oil refining concerns manufacturing and distribution processes for primary products: natural gas, gasoline, diesel fuel, solvents, and lubricants. As an immediate (stopgap) measure, refineries need to be located where their leakage, fugitive emissions, explosions, and fire, which contaminate the earth and the atmosphere, will not occur. The refining process—which produces hydrogen sulfide and other deadly reduced sulfur gases, as well as benzene and other volatile organics, including toluene and xylene—will be of less concern as our transportation systems shift away from the use of petroleum products. They should be phased out so that their usage is minimized and possibly eliminated. This effort would include the strict regulation of diesel transportation, which, as pointed out in Chapter 14, appears to have undue health hazards for the human brain.

Manufacturing Sites

The next priority for government action has to do with the manufacturing sites for hazardous and unsafe materials and the workers who are handling such materials. These sites need to be isolated and quarantined until adequate solutions for safe storage and disposal can be developed. Perhaps even more important, a generation of safety and health provisions enacted to protect the workers need to be implemented and enforced. Political leaders responding to greed-motivated industry pressure gutted the regulations by withdrawal of funds. Now these funds must be not only restored but augmented so that industry will not regulate or police itself.

Transportation

A third area where change is needed is that of distribution or transportation. Remember the Exxon Valdez and Pudroe Sound. Both the routes used and the levels of safety with which materials are transported must be established and regulated. The unmonitored use of rail and truck routes through populated areas in the carrying (transportation) of hazardous chemicals is a recipe for disaster if an accident occurs. Least hazardous routes and times must be used.

Transportation, from the standpoint of both automobiles and highways, has issues of safety, fuel economy, and finally energy use that must be addressed (combined). This does not mean that new strategies will not present new hazards (such as hydrogen-powered vehicles); but with new technologies, we can design for safety and efficiency.

Agribusiness

Our concern here is the unreasonable hazards of agribusiness, mainly in the use of pesticides and herbicides. Causing human brain loss by pesticide use must be made a criminal offense at the corporate executive level. Reporting of such damage must be to the U.S. Environmental Protection Agency. Their investigation must be swift and the action of the Justice Department prompt.

Construction

Home construction and industrial and commercial construction are not greatly different in their use of hazardous materials. They both utilize formaldehyde, volatile organic chemicals, and other hazardous materials, including plastics, whose use must be diminished, if not eradicated completely. (Plastics use interfaces with manufacturing, waste reduction, and consumer concerns, and is discussed separately in an earlier section.)

Water Purification

Another important change is required in water purification systems, both for primary culinary use and for sewage treatment. Overshadowing much of this need is the issue of using a water priority system. Most important, however, is the need for a changeover from using chlorine to kill bacteria to using less hazardous on-site ozone generation and aeration.

This shift in priorities requires a reordering, a change in focus away from the issues that the media emphasizes, such as crime and illegal drug use, and toward the fundamental cause of most social ills, poverty. Issues of poverty and wealth must be addressed; and we can learn much from Sweden, Finland, Iceland, and Norway in this regard. A serious study of these issues will lead us to large corporations and their CEOs, producing unnecessary and harmful products as well as useful goods. We must learn to rein in the greed that permits the production of nonessential harmful chemicals.

GLOBAL ISSUES

Population Control as Top Global Concern

The final step for the new people, the post-consumers, is to reduce spaceship earth's human burden. Family size must decrease through control of births. Space is running out; the number of human participants on this spaceship threaten its *precarious life-supporting systems*. Overpopulation is reflected in other global concerns.

Other Global Concerns

Other major issues include:

1. *Global warming:* the oversupply of carbon dioxide (CO_2) from burning fossil fuel and CO_2's underutilization due to the disappearance of forests, with consequent global warming, including the loss of the ozone layer from the ascent of manufactured chlorine into the stratosphere.
2. *Loss of biodiversity:* species loss caused by habitat restrictions, due to an overwhelming influx of humans.
3. *Ocean contamination:* ocean exhaustion, particularly due to fishing industry depletion, including the loss of mammals, and the dumping of industrial and human wastes into the oceans.
4. *Devastated lands:* despoliation due to land depletion, deforestation, and the urbanization that has curtailed the agricultural use of many desirable parts of five continents.
5. *Pesticide and herbicide use:* The cause of the most direct and insidious brain damage due to environmental pollution is the myth, beginning with the use of DDT, that insects must die for humans to be fed and clothed. It implies that for humans to be content and secure, chemical warfare against insects is justified. As Rachel Carson observed, based on DDT, this whole myth is untrue and dangerous. Most chemical agents that kill insects harm human brains.

References

1. Ayres RU and Ayres LW: Chemical industry wastes: a materials balance analysis. INSEAD working paper.*
2. Duchin F and Lange GM: Strategies for environmentally sound economic development. In: *Investing Natural Capital: The Ecological Economics Approach to Sustainability,* AM Jansson, J Hammer, C Folke, and R Costanza (eds.). Washington, DC: Island Press, 1994.
3. Ayres RU: Economics, thermodynamics and process analysis. 94/11/EDS.*
4. Duchin F: Industrial input–output analysis: implication for industrial ecology. *Proc Natl Acad Sci* 1992;89:851–855.
5. Frosch RA: Industrial ecology: adapting technology for a sustainable world. *Environment* 1995;37:16–24, 34–37.
6. United States Trade Commission: *Synthetic Organic Chemicals 1992.* Washington DC: U.S. Government Printing Office, 1992.
7. Neutra RJ: *Survival through Design.* New York: Oxford University Press, 1969.
8. Wernick IK, Herman R, Govind S, and Ausubel JH: Materialization and dematerialization: measures and trends. In: *Technology Trajectories and the Human Environment.* Washington, DC: National Academy Press, 1997.

* INSEAD's Centre for the Management of Environmental Resources. An R & D partnership sponsored by Ciba-Geigy, Dan Foss, Otto Group, Royal Dutch/Shell, and Sandoz AG.

~~convert~~

forget :

see

actually - should

be periode, except

after Nov 17

publish, or, NY:

Suggested Reading

Arlien-Soborg, Peter: *Solvent Neurotoxicity.* Boca Raton, FL: CRC Press, 1992.

Ashford, Nicholas A. and Miller, Claudia S.: *Chemical Exposures: Low Levels and High Stakes.* New York: Van Nostrand Reinhold, 1991.

Breslin, Jimmy: *I Want to Thank My Brain for Remembering Me.* New York: Little, Brown and Co., 1996.

Carson, Rachel L.: *Silent Spring.* Boston: Houghton Mifflin Co., 1962.

Castleman, Barry I: *Asbestos: Medical and Legal Aspects* (4th ed.). Frederick, MD: Aspen Law and Business, 1996.

Coburn, Theo, Dumanoski, D., and Myers, J.P.: *Our Stolen Future.* New York: Dutton Penguin Books, 1996.

Damasio, Antonio R.: *Descarte's Error: Emotion, Reason and the Human Brain.* New York: Grosset/Putnam, 1994.

Earle, Sylvia C: *Sea Change: A Message of the Ocean.* New York: G. P. Putnam's Sons, 1994.

Edelman, Gerald M: *Bright Air, Brilliant Fire: On the Matters of the Mind.* New York: Basic Books, 1992.

Fagin, D., Lavelle, M., and Center for Public Integrity: *Toxic Deception: How the Chemical Industry Manipulates Science, Bends the Law and Endangers Your Health.* Secaucus, NJ: Birch Lane Press/Carol Publishing Group, 1997.

Fromm, Eric: *The Sane Society.* New York: Rinehart & Co. 1955.

Garrett, Laurie: *The Coming Plague.* New York: Farrar, Straus, & Giroux, 1994.

Harr, Jonathan: *A Civil Action.* New York: Random House, 1995.

Hartman, David E: *Neuropsychological Toxicology: Identification and Assessment of Human Neurotoxic Syndromes.* New York: Pergamon Press, 1988.

Hunter, Donald: *Diseases of Occupations* (4th ed.). Boston, MA: Little, Brown and Co., 1978.

Irvine, W: *Apes, Angels and Victorians: The Story of Darwin, Huxley and Evolution.* New York: McGraw-Hill Book Co., 1955.

James, William: *The Principles of Psychology* (1890). New York: Dover, 1950 (reprint).

Kohn, Howard: *Who Killed Karen Silkwood*? New York: Summit Books, 1981.

Kosslyn, Stephen M. and Kolnig, Oliver: *Wet Mind: The New Cognitive Neuroscience.* New York: Free Press, 1992.

London, Jack: *The Iron Heel.* New York: Sagamore Press, 1907/1957.

Matossian, Mary K: *Poisons of the Past: Molds, Epidemics, and History*. New Haven, CT: Yale University Press, 1989.

Neutra, Richard: *Survival through Design.* New York: Oxford University Press, 1954.

Packard, Vance: *The Waste Makers.* New York: David McKay Co., 1960.

Sacks, Oliver: *Awakenings.* New York: Summit Books, 1987.

Sacks, Oliver: *The Man Who Mistook His Wife for a Hat.* New York: Harper Collins, 1986.

Sinclair, Upton: *The Jungle.* New York: Bantam Books, 1906.

Stern, Gerald M: *The Buffalo Creek Disaster.* New York: Vintage Books, a Division of Random House, 1976.

Thompson, Tracy: *The Beast: A Reckoning with Depression.* New York: G. P. Putnam's Sons, 1995.

Udall, Stuart L: *The Myths of August.* New York: Cornelia and Michael Bessie Book, Pantheon Books, 1994.

Zinsser, Hans: *Rats, Lice and History.* Boston: Little, Brown and Company, 1963.

Index

Accidents
automobile, 316–318
mischance of exposure, 21
Adrenoleukodystrophy, 323
Adults
balance in, 38
differences between children and, 48
less testable, 51
Affective domain, 110–112
Affective states, altered, 348
Affective-symptomatic areas, testing for, 349
Age
coefficient suggestive increased, 51–52
interactions in prediction equations, 40–44
Aging
accelerated, 51–52
biomarkers needed, 53
changes in mice, chemical produced, 50
defined, 21
differential effects of, 51
exposure examined in context of, 22
longitudinal studies of brain, 50
perspective on dementia, 49–53
responses through, 36–37
tentative patterns, 42
Agribusiness, 374
Air monitoring data, 106–108
Alabama Reclamation aluminum remelt facility, 284–295
Alcoholism, studies of, 348
Aluminum recycling, 284–295
Alabama Reclamation aluminum remelt facility, 284–295
age coefficients, 288–290
cognitive function, 287
cohort comparison design, 285
discussion, 291–295
electrolytic aluminum refinery, 285
ex-worker complaints, 285
exposed and reference groups, 286
furnace fumes, 284
neurophysiological tests, 286
neurotoxicity of aluminum, 293
past diseases prevalences, 287
POMS scores, 287
pulmonary function impaired, 291
removal of dross, 284
results, 286–291
scrap dumped into metal shredder, 284

Aluminum recycling *(continued)*
sources of drinking water, 287
subjects, 285–286
testing of subjects, 285–291
workers and higher frequencies symptoms, 288
miscellaneous contaminants, 284–295
nontoxic, 369–370
vinyl chloride, 284–295
Alzheimer 2 cells, 323
American Rheumatism Association, 175, 201–202, 230
Amnesia, duration of post-traumatic, 317
Amplifiers, EMG, 25–26
Analysis
of covariance, 22
data, 31–44
Animal data, integrating human and, 50–51
ARA questionnaire, 160–162
Arsenic
adversely affects energy metabolism, 164
airborne, 152–165
ARA questionnaire, 160–162
and central nervous system effects, 163
confounding from occupational exposures, 162
damages or injures the brain questions, 163
discussion, 162–164
effects at Bryan/College Station, Texas, 152–165
exposure in six domains, 162
and exposure to neurotoxic chemicals, 163
impaired central nervous system function, 152
neurophysiological testing, 156–157
neuropsychological testing, 157–158
peripheral neuritis, 158
pulmonary functions, 160
residues measured in soil, 163
respiratory symptoms, 159
symptom frequencies, 158–159
water plume, 152
a carcinogen, 163–164
chronic poisoning, 164
protoplasmic poison, 163
testing of subjects, 153–162
methods, 153–155
results, 155–162
Asphyxiation, death by, 92
Astrocytes, 310, 322
Astroglia, 322–324
Atochem, 152–165
Atrophy, olivopontocerebellar, 321
Audiometry, hearing tested by, 81–82
Automobile accidents, 316–318

Balance
in adults, 38
as a detailed example, 37–40
function, 123–125
speed of sway, 24–25
Baselines, establishing, 338–339
Baton Rouge, Louisiana, 254–283
Bias, 113–114
litigation, 213
tester, 234
Biodiversity, loss of, 375
Biomarkers, 53
Birth defects, clusters of, 10, 14
Blink reflex latencies
children's, 46–47
long, 233
R-1, 25–26, 57
Boycotts by users, 373
Brain
aging, 50
distress signals of, 85–86
effects, 10–11
new chemical plagues of, 1–5
audience, 4
conclusions, 5
key points, 1–3
messages, 5
objectives, 4
premature aging, 365
processes that damage, 320–321
trauma, 339
Brain damage, 49–50, 88
Brain damage mechanisms from chemicals, 310–333

astrocytes, 310
astrocytic helper cells, 310
entry of chemicals into CNS, 311–316
lung to blood to blood-brain barrier route, 311
neurotoxicity, 310
speculative overview, 310–311
theories for chemical brain damage, 319–328
traumatic brain damage, 316–319
automobile accidents, 316–318
autopsy studies, 319
extracorporeal circulation, 318
follow-up physical evaluations, 318
and memory retraining methods, 317
and mnemonic techniques, 317
neurobehavioral impairment in patients, 317
neurological ill effects of open-heart surgery, 318–319
neurological and intellectual disturbances, 318
post-traumatic amnesia, 317
psychiatric interviews, 318
and psychosocial characterizations, 317
and Wechsler Adult Intelligence Scale (WAIS), 317
Brains, pervasiveness of impaired, 306–309
adverse affects of chemicals, 308
control groups, 306
study-by-study analyses, 306
Bryan, Texas, 152–165
Buildings, cure sick, 366
Business; *See* agribusiness

Cancer, clusters of, 14
Carbon monoxide, 321
Carcinogen, arsenic a, 163–164
Casper subjects, 114–123
Cautions in generalizing, 42
Central nervous system; *See* CNS (central nervous system)
Cerebroactive drugs, 343
Changes
in mice, 50
motivating, 371–372
people and society, 364–365
social, 364–376
Chelation, 341
Chemical brain damage, theories for
and adrenoleukodystrophy, 323
adverse metabolic effects on neurons, 320
and altered heme synthesis, 322
and Alzheimer 2 cells, 323
and astrocytes, 322
astroglia may have central role, 322–324
and calcium-binding proteins, 323
and carbon monoxide, 321
central nervous systems effects of chemicals, 319
diverse effects of chemicals, 319–322
enhanced emotional responses, 326
epilepsy from chemicals as limbic kindling, 326–328
excitotoxic nerve cell death, 321–322
and fear conditioning in rats, 325
and glial fibrillar acidic protein (GFAP) staining, 322–323
imitating spontaneous neurodegenerative diseases, 322
limbic system as target for chemicals, 324–326
linear regression analysis, 326
metabolism of 2,5-substituted hexacarbon solvents, 322
MPTP (N-methyl-4-phenyl-1,2,3,6-tetrahydropyridine), 321
and neurodegeneration, 321
olivopontocerebellar atrophy, 321
paroxysmal depolarizing shift (PDS), 328
polycystic ovarian syndrome, 328
processes that damage brain, 320–321
and progressive neuronal death, 321
receptors for N-methyl-D-aspartate (NMDA), 325
regeneration in adult mammalian central nervous system, 323
and seizures, 326
and solvents, 322

Chemical damage, seizures as signals of, 86–87
Chemical encephalopathy, 49–53, 334–340
Chemical exposures
  cumulative residential, 281
  effects of environmental, 9
  incidents of, 21
  relating effects to, 6–12
  transport-related, 16
Chemical injury, 339
Chemically produced aging changes in mice, 50
Chemicals
  causal hypotheses that downplay, 53
  curtail production of unsafe, 367–368
  focus of adverse effects from, 8–9
  hauling of hazardous, 16
  investigations of populations exposed to, 256
  specific patterns of impairment from particular, 71–74
  stop transportation of toxic, 366
  systems response to environmental, 10
  targets for
    brain, 11
    central nervous system, 11
  tests in people unexposed and exposed to, 21–61
Children, 59–61
  blink reflex latencies of, 46–47
  differences between adults and, 48
  exposed to TCE, 48
  prediction equations of, 44–48
  reciprocal of simple reaction time, 44
  recruitment of, 44
Chlordane
  a chlorinated cyclodiene insecticide, 176
  comparative prevalence of diseases, 174
  cyclodienes interaction with picrotoxin receptors, 177
  discussion, 176–178
  exposure still occurring, 178
  exposure to, 166
  frequency of 35 symptoms, 173
  neurobehavioral effects of residential, 166–179
  a neuropoison, 176–177
  and respiratory symptoms, 174
  testing of subjects, 167–176
    affective status, 171
    methods, 167
    results, 167–176
  used extensively as a termiticide, 166
Chlorine from a train derailment, 129–138
  adult abnormalities, 132
  comparison of subjects to regional unexposed subjects, 137–138
  discussion, 137–138
  effects on central nervous system, 137
  neurobehavioral impairment, 134–136
  neurobehavioral and pulmonary impairments, 133–134
  patients developed temporal lobe seizures, 137
  testing of subjects, 129–136
Civil law, 352
Cleaning and sanitizing, 372
Clinic patients, 64–69
CNS (central nervous system)
  entry of chemicals into the, 311–316
    cerebrospinal fluid, 311
    chemicals entering lungs, 314–315
    lipid-soluble materials, 311
    lung to blood to blood-brain barrier route, 311
    mechanisms of amplification, 314–315
    neural lesions, 315
    odor entry pathway, 312
    olfactory fibers discharge, 312
    olfactory route, 311–314
    quantitative measurements of performance, 315
    rate of damage determines effect, 315–316
    transmission of chemicals, 312
  regeneration in adult mammalian, 323
  understanding, 85–89
Coatings, surface, 372
Cognitive performance, 57
Color, 57
  discrimination, 27
  score equations, 47
Combustion Superfund site, 254–283

Comparisons
of predicted values to past normative values, 36
predicted values' utility for initial, 35–36
Confounding, 203, 233
factors, 112–113, 267, 279–280
from occupational exposures, 162
minimal, 211–213
occupational or personal exposures, 244
Construction, 374
Contamination, ocean, 375
Contrasts and uncertainties, 89
Cosmetics, 372
Covariance, analysis of, 22
Cresylate from a train derailment, 129–138
adult abnormalities, 132
testing of subjects, 129–136
Cross-sectional studies, 17
CRT (choice reaction time), 24

Damage, brain, 49–50
Data
air monitoring, 106–108
analysis, 31–44
age effect, 35
age interactions in prediction equations, 40–44
balance as a detailed example, 37–40
changing patterns of response through growth and aging, 36–37
comparison of predicted values to past normative values, 36
failure to model visual reproductions, 33–34
patterns of exposure, 40–44
predicted values' utility for initial comparisons, 35–36
profile of mood states, 33–34
stepwise multiple regression techniques, 31–32
validation of models, 32–33
integrating human and animal, 50–51
Death by asphyxiation, 92
Dementia
causal hypothesis, 53
organic, 52–53
causes, 52
prevalence unknown, 52–53
perspective on, 49–53
Diagnostic myths, 9
Diesel exhaust, 296–305
and adverse central nervous system effects, 296–297
air pollution from, 296
background, 296–297
and central nervous system (CNS), 303
chemicals impairing central nervous system, 304
discussion, 303–304
inhalation of petroleum combustion mists, 297
observed abnormalities, 304
risks to brain, 304
symptoms of, 296
testing of subjects, 297–303
and gasoline-diesel-fire-exposed subjects, 302
methods, 297–299
pulmonary function tests, 302–303
reaction times of subjects, 302
results, 299–303
Diet, 342
Discrimination, color, 27
Diseases
imitating spontaneous neurodegenerative, 322
multi-organ systemic, 11
Distress signals, brain's, 85–86
Divergent pattern, 42–44
Domain
affective, 110–112
neurophysiological, 108–109
neuropsychological, 109–110
perceptual motor, 47
Dose-response estimates, 14–15
Drugs, 343–344
Duration, exposure, 214
Dynamometers, 26–27
Dysfunction, progressive multi-system, 11–12

Electrolytic aluminum refinery, 285
EMG (electromyographic)
amplifiers, 25–26
recordings, 25
Emotional responses, enhanced, 326
Encephalopathy
chemical, 49–53
prognosis of chemical, 334–340
Environmental agencies, exposure driven, 6–7
Environmental chemicals, systems response to, 10
Environmental epidemiology, 214–216
Environmental Protection Agency, 166
Environmental toxicology, 12–16
transportation, 16
useful generalizations, 12–15
Epidemiology, 16–18
cross-sectional studies, 17
environmental, 214–216
exposure, 6–20
key steps, 18
longitudinal comparisons, 17
studying worst cases is economical, 17
Epilepsy, 326–328
Equations
age interactions in prediction, 40–44
children's prediction, 44–48
color score, 47
regression, 31
Errors
fingertip writing, 95–96
number writing, 82
Exhaust, diesel, 296–305
Experiments, human exposure to known toxins, 16–17
Exposures
confounding from occupational, 162
cumulative residential chemical, 281
duration of, 214
epidemiology of, 6–20
examined in context of aging, 22
and historical reconstruction or modeling, 12
incidents of chemical, 21
indices, 267–268
measuring doses of chemicals, 12
patterns of, 40–44
Extracorporeal circulation, 318

Fat and sugar, 372
Fear conditioning in rats, 325
Fields
tests correlated with visual, 80–81
visual, 27
Fingerprint effects, 89
Fingertip writing errors, 95–96
Forest products, 370–371
Frequencies, symptoms, 158–159, 201, 230, 267
Fumes, HCI, 139

Generalizing, cautions in, 42
GFAP (glial fibrillar acidic protein) staining, 322–323
Glass production and reuse, 370
Global issues, 375
Global warming, 375
Government, redefining, 373
Governmental priorities, 373–374
agribusiness, 374
construction, 374
manufacturing sites, 374
oil refineries, 373
transportation, 374
water purification, 374
Greed, overcoming, 365–371
Grip strength, 26–27
Groundwater
contamination, 217–227
treatment plant, 199
Groups, unexposed, 49
Growth, responses through, 36–37

Hazardous chemicals, hauling of, 16
HAZMAT (hazardous materials), 85, 140, 349
HCI (hydrochloric acid), 139–140
Head injury analogy, 339
Health
effects
adverse, 139–140
measuring or modeling exposures, 7–8
problems
appear after many years, 6
past exposures not measured, 7
risks, 12–13

Hearing, 27–29, 81–82
Heart; *See also* open-heart surgery
Heme synthesis, altered, 322
Herbicide use, 375
Houston subjects, 114–123
Humans
  and animal data, 50–51
  predicting risk, 13
  shaping attitudes, 371–374
HVOCs (halogenated volatile organic chemicals), 196
Hydrogen chloride
  adverse effects from, 139–151
  balance and reaction time functions, 148–149
  chronic neurobehavioral dysfunction, 150
  common industrial product, 150
  discussion, 145–150
  examination
    for confounding by exposure, 144
    of effect on balance, 145
  and exposed women, 142–143
  impaired neurobehavioral performance, 147
  and neurobehavioral examinations, 147–148
  proximity effect in balance function, 150
  reaction times delayed, 140–141
  release of, 140
  and respiratory symptoms, 144
  and symptom frequency, 143
  testing of subjects, 140–145
Hydrogen sulfide
  exposure, 92–128
    alternate explanations, 126
    attribution of effects, 127
    balance function, 123–125
    Casper subjects, 114–123
    death by asphyxiation, 92
    disastrous incident in Torrance, California, 96–104
    discussion, 125–127
    and exposed subjects, 95
    and fingertip writing errors, 95–96
    from refineries in cities, 92–128
    Houston subjects, 114–123
    impaired pulmonary function, 93
    inappropriate comparison group, 126–127
    induced unconsciousness, 92
    mechanisms, 127
    neurobehavioral dysfunction, 93
    neurobehavioral impairment, 92
    and neurobehavioral testing, 95
    and POMS score, 96
    reaction times, 123–125
    and refinery workers, 123–125
    16 patients, 93–96
    Unocal refinery exposure, 104–114
  no effect on memory, 71

Illnesses, physicians reject possible causes of, 70
Incidents of chemical exposure, 21
Independent variables, 35
Indices, exposure, 267–268
Industry, transforming, 368–371
Injury, chemical, 339
Insecticide, chlordane a chlorinated cyclodiene, 176

Lands, devastated, 375
Latencies, children's blink reflexes, 46–47
Latent periods, human health effects and long, 12
Legal proceedings, 352–363
  cases, 356–362
    Aiken et al. vs. Unocal, 357
    Alberton Citizens vs. Montana Rail Link, 361
    Alexander vs. Rust Engineering Company, 358
    Bell vs. Tenneco, 360
    Consolidated Texaco Refinery Litigation, 360
    Eura Charles et al. vs. Kings Park Apartments, 360
    Glen and Debra Hess vs. Texas Eastern Corporation, 359
    Gutierrez et al. vs. Electric Gin Co., 361
    Hill et al. vs. Lockheed-Marietta, 361

Legal proceedings *(continued)*
Janice Akin et al. vs. Big Three Industries et al., 359–360
Jarman et al. vs. Ford Motor Company, 358
Lillian Hayden et al. vs. Atochem NA, 358–359
Livingston Parish Police Jury vs. Arcadia Shipyard, 359
low effect cases, 361–362
McIntire vs. Motorola, Inc., 359
negative cases, 361–362
Norman Scott Albertson et al. vs. Dow Chemical Company, 357–358
Penny Newman et al. vs. J. B. Stringfellow, Jr., 356
Thomas vs. FAG Bearings, 358
Touchet vs. Baker-Hughes Chemical Company, 360
Valenzuela et al. vs. Hughes Aircraft, 357
civil law, 352
fugitive losses, 353
funding from plaintiffs' law firms, 352
health effects, 353
property damage, 353
redress of injury and disease, 353
spills, 353
Limbic connections and correlations, 87
Limbic system, 324–326
Litigation bias, 213
Lobelville, Tennessee, 181–194
Long-term memory tests, 47
Longitudinal comparisons, 17
Longitudinal studies of brain aging, 50

Manufacturing sites, 374
MCS (multiple chemical sensitivity), relationship to, 84–85
Memory, 59
hydrogen sulfide and effects on, 71
long-term tests, 47
retraining methods, 317
Metabolism, arsenic adversely affects energy, 164
Mice, aging changes in, 50
Mnemonic techniques, 317
Models, validation of, 32–33
Monitoring data, air, 106–108
Mood scores, 17–18
Motor domain, perceptual, 47
Motorola, 196–217
MPTP (N-methyl-4-phenyl-1,2,3,6-tetrahydropyridine), 321
MRC (Medical Research Council), 159
Muscle Shoals, AL, 284–295
Myths, diagnostic, 9

NBT (neurobehavioral test) scores, 218
Neoplastic diseases, latency of, 9–10
Nerve cell death, excitotoxic, 321–322
Neuritis, peripheral, 158
Neurobehavioral effects, 6–20
Neurobehavioral functions, methods for measuring, 21–61
blink, 57
children, 59–61
Bergholz-Steubenville, 60–61
Biloxi, 59–60
cognitive performance, 57
color, 57
deriving prediction equations for tests, 21–61
memory, 59
perceptual motor speed (PMS), 58
reaction time, 57
recall, 58
TCE effects on, 48
tests in people unexposed vs. those exposed to chemicals, 21–61
Neurobehavioral impairment in patients, 317
Neurobehavioral testing, 95
Neurodegeneration, 321
Neurodegenerative diseases, imitating spontaneous, 322
Neurological and intellectual disturbances, 318
Neuronal death, progressive, 321
Neurons, adverse metabolic effects on, 310
Neurophysiological domain, 108–109
Neurophysiological effects, toxic, 243–244

Neurophysiological functions, automatic, 348
Neurophysiological testing, 156–157, 200–201
Neurophysiological tests, 240, 263–264, 286, 336
Neuropoison, 176–177
Neuropsychological domain, 109–110
Neuropsychological testing, 157–158, 201
Neuropsychological tests, 29–31, 264–267
Neurotoxicology, future of
  and automatic neurophysiological functions, 348
  creating surrogates for levels of functions, 349
  needs and responsibilities, 347–351
  recommendations, 350–351
  standardizing descriptive language, 349
  testing for affective-symptomatic areas, 349
  testing issues, 347–350
    altered affective states, 348
    menu of measurements, 348
    studies of alcoholism, 348
Neutralization, 342
NMDA (N-methyl-D-aspartate), receptors for, 325
Nontoxic aluminum recycling, 369–370
Number writing errors, 82

Occupational exposures, 162, 233
Ocean contamination, 375
Oil refineries, 373
Olfactory-limbic system model, 324
Olivopontocerebellar atrophy, 321
Open-heart surgery, neurological ill effects of, 318–319
Organic dementia, 52–53
Ovarian syndrome, polycystic, 328

Pain, total body, 11
Paper, 370–371
Parallel difference patterns, 41
Patients
  clinic, 64–69
  consistency and patterns in restudied, 335
  neurobehavioral impairment in, 317
Patients, chemically exposed, 62–91
  associating patterns of dysfunction, 63–74
    assembling puzzle, 63
    attribution to chemicals, 70
    chemicals and patterns, 70–71
    clinical recognition, 70
    comparing patients to populations, 63–64
    exposures to chemical mixtures, 70
    group for clinic patients, 64–69
    patterns observed, 71–74
  new tests for miscellaneous functions, 78–85
    correlations with chemicals, 80
    frequency of symptoms, 82–84
    hearing tested by audiometry, 81–82
    number writing errors, 82
    POMS (profile of mood states) scores, 84–85
    relationship to multiple chemical sensitivity (MCS), 84–85
    tests correlated with visual fields, 80–81
    visual field defects, 80
  objectives, 62–63
  testing to detect impairment, 74–78
  understanding central nervous system (CNS), 85–89
    brain's distress signals, 85–86
    generalizations, 88–89
    interpretations of brain damage, 88
    limbic connections and correlations, 87
    mosaics to fingerprints, 89
    predictions, 88
    results of retesting across intervals, 87–88
    seizures as signals of chemical damage, 86–87
    uncertainties and contrasts, 89

Patterns
  changing, 36–37
  divergent, 42–44
  increasing difference, 42–44
  no effect of exposure, 40–41
  parallel difference, 41
  tentative aging, 42
PCBs (polychlorinated biphenyls)
  acne-like lesions, 193
  cause Yusho, 193
  children's measurements, 191
  contaminated water and soil, 180
  discussion, 187–194
  exposure, 181–182
  impact on brain function, 187
  pumping station use of, 193
  resembles effects of hydrogen sulfide exposure, 187
  testing of subjects, 182–187
    methods, 182
    results, 182–187
  35 symptom frequencies, 184
  visual field abnormalities, 184
  visual and neurobehavioral impairment associated with, 180–194
PDS (paroxysmal depolarizing shift), 328
Perceptual motor domain, 47
Performance
  cognitive, 57
  pre-exposure levels of, 18
Peripheral neuritis, 158
Personal safety, 372
Pesticides, 372, 375
Petroleum, 257
Physical evaluations, follow-up, 318
Physicians, reject possible causes of illnesses, 70
Physiological methods, 22–29
  balance, speed of sway, 24–25
  blink reflex latency R-1, 25–26
  color discrimination, 27
  grip strength, 26–27
  hearing, 27–29
  reaction time, 22–24
  spirometry, 29
  vibration, 26–27
  visual fields, 27
Physiological tests, 52
Picrotoxin receptors, 177
Plant, groundwater treatment, 199
Plastics, rational use of, 368
PMS (perceptual motor speed), 58
Poison, protoplasmic, 163
Polluters, criminal prosecution of, 366–367
POMS (profile of mood states), 9, 33–34, 180
POMS (profile of mood states) scores, 84–85, 96, 267, 287
Population control, 375
Predicted values, 35–36
Prediction equations, 49
  for children, 44–48
  deriving, 21–61
Problems, outside professional comfort zone, 9
Profile of mood states; *See* POMS (profile of mood states)
Prognosis and therapy, 334–346
  brain trauma and chemical injury, 339
  consistency and patterns in patients restudied, 333–336
  establishing baseline, 338–339
  groups show no improvement on retesting, 334–335
  head injury analogy, 339
  mechanisms of recovery, 339–340
  neurophysiological tests, 336
  prognosis of chemical encephalopathy, 334–340
  psychometric techniques, 336
  recall, 336–338
  retraining, 340
  test reproduction-stability, 336
Proteins, calcium-binding, 323
Psychiatric interviews, 318
Psychological tests, 52
Psychometric techniques, 336
Psychosocial characterizations, 317
Psychotherapy, 343–344
Public health agencies, 6–7
Pulmonary functions, 160, 302–303
Pulmonary status, 202

Questionnaire
  ARA, 160–162
  data, 239

Rats, fear conditioning in, 325
Reaction speeds, 22–23
Reaction times, 22–24, 57, 229
Recall, 47, 58, 336–338
Receptors, picrotoxin, 177
Recordings, electromyographic (EMG), 25
Recovery, mechanisms of, 339–340
Recruitment of children, 44
Refineries
  electrolytic aluminum, 285
  workers, 123–125
Regression
  equations, 31
  linear analysis, 326
  stepwise multiple techniques, 31–32
Rehabilitation, 343
Repeat testing 114; *See also* Testing
Respiratory symptoms, 159, 174, 230
Responses through
  aging, 36–37
  growth, 36–37
Retesting; *See also* Testing
  across intervals, 87–88
  groups showing no improvement on, 334–335
Retraining, 340
Rheumatic complaints, 230
Risk, predicting human, 13

Safety, personal, 372
Sanitizing and cleaning, 372
Scores
  profile of mood states (POMS) scores, 84–85, 96, 267, 287
  symptom frequency, 267
  test, 267–268
Seizures
  related to alterations of hippocampus, 326
  as signals of chemical damage, 86–87
Senescing defined, 21
Senility, 365
Sentinel profiles, 89
Signals
  brain's distress, 85–86
  of chemical damage, seizures as, 86–87
Social changes, 364–376
  cure sick buildings, 366
  enforce criminal prosecution of polluters, 366–367
  global issues, 375
    devastated lands, 375
    global warming, 375
    herbicide use, 375
    loss of biodiversity, 375
    ocean contamination, 375
    pesticide, 375
    population control, 375
  health problems in review, 365
  how people and society must change, 364–365
  introduction, 364–365
  needed to help brains survive, 364–376
  overcoming greed, 365–371
  premature brain aging, 365
  quarantine toxic technology until replaced, 367
  senility, 365
  shaping human attitudes, 371–374
    boycotts by users, 373
    governmental priorities, 373–374
    motivating changes, 371–372
    personal safety, 372
    redefining government, 373
  stop transportation of toxic chemicals, 366
  strategies, 367–371
    aluminum recycling that is nontoxic, 369–370
    curtail production of unsafe chemicals, 367–368
    forest products, 370–371
    glass production and reuse, 370
    rational use of plastics, 368
    steel making and reuse, 368–369
    transforming industry, 368–371
Solvents, 322
Speed of sway, 24–25, 37, 40
Speeds, reaction, 22–23
Spirometry, 29
SRT (simple reaction time), 23–24
Staining, glial fibrillar acidic protein (GFAP), 322–323
Steel making and reuse, 368–369

Stepwise multiple regression techniques, 31–32
Studies
of brain aging, 50
cross-sectional, 17
Subjects, sway speed, 40
Sugar and fat, 372
Surface coatings, 372
Sway speed, 24–25, 37, 40
Sweating, 341–342
Symptoms
frequencies, 82–84, 158–159, 201, 230
frequency scores, 267
respiratory, 159, 174, 230
Systemic diseases, multi-organ, 11

Tasks, performance on overlearned, 18
TCE (Trichloroethylene) exposures, 195–253
absorption and toxicology of, 195
children, 48
effects on neurobehavioral functions, 48
future considerations, 250–251
Muscle Shoals, Alabama community study, 235–247
affective status, 241
blunted affect scores, 245
confounding occupational or personal exposures, 244
discussion, 242–247
exposed population, 236–238
exposure surrogates and effects, 242
low scores on psychological tests, 245
neurophysiological tests, 240
questionnaire data, 239
rural unexposed scores, 245
testing of subjects, 238–242
toxic neurophysiological effects, 243–244
Northeastern Phoenix, Arizona community study, 196–217
comparisons with nonclients, 204–207
conclusions, 209–216
a critique of methods, 199
description of exposed subjects, 199–200
development of this study, 196–197
exposure estimates, 197–199
magnitude of disposal, 199
people investigated, 197
reasons for inconclusive past studies, 196
subjects in exposure zone since 1983, 207–209
residential and occupational, 195–253
Southwestern Tucson, Arizona community study, 217–227
environmental measurements, 220
exposed population, 218–219
eye closure latency, 221
groundwater contamination, 217–227
group comparisons, 220–225
mean speeds of sway, 221
neurobehavioral test scores, 224
no evidence of alcohol abuse, 224
profiles of mood states scores, 223
summary and conclusions, 225–227
unexposed subjects, 219–220
verbal recall, 223
visual reproduction, 223
summary and general conclusions, 247–251
testing of subjects, 200–204
American Rheumatism Association criteria, 201–202
confounding, 203
neurophysiological testing, 200–201
neuropsychological testing, 201
pulmonary status, 202
symptom frequencies, 201
Tinker Air Force Base and Environs study, 227–235
cognitive function tested by, 229
conclusion, 234–235
confounding, 233
discussion, 233–234
exposed population, 228–229
long blink reflex latencies, 233
occupational exposures, 233
profile of mood states scores, 230

respiratory symptoms, 230
rheumatic complaints, 230
simple and choice reaction times, 229
symptoms frequencies, 230
tester bias, 234
testing of subjects, 229–232
Tenneco, 181–194
Termiticide, chlordane used extensively as a, 166
Testable, adults perhaps less, 51
Tester bias, 234
Testing; *See also* Repeat testing; Retesting
neurobehavioral, 95
neurophysiological, 156–157, 200–201
neuropsychological, 157–158, 201
repeat, 114
standardizing the descriptive language, 349
Tests
and gender factors, 53
long-term memory, 47
neurophysiological, 240, 263–264, 286, 336
neuropsychological, 29–31, 264–267
in people exposed to chemicals, 21–61
in people unexposed to chemicals, 21–61
pulmonary function, 302–303
scores, 267–268
and socioeconomic factor, 53
and time factors, 53
TGPC (Tennessee Gas Pipeline Company), 181–194
Therapeutic interventions, possible, 340–344
avoidance, 340–341
cerebroactive drugs, 343
diet, 342
dietary possibilities, 341
drugs, 344
neutralization, 342
psychotherapy, 343–344
rehabilitation, 343
removal of toxicants, 341–342
chelation, 341
sweating, 341–342
Therapy and prognosis, 334–246
Time
key for tests, 53
reaction, 22–24, 57
Tinker Air Force Base (AFB), 227–235
Toluene-rich vapor exposures, 254–283
comparisons of mean test scores, 271
component of petroleum, 257
concentration of VOCs, 259
data analysis
combined dose surrogate, 273–275
direction, 272–273
distance, 271–272
duration, 273
discussion, 275–281
age-related differences, 278–279
bias by testers, 276
cognitive function, 278
confounding factors, 279–280
contamination effect zone, 277
cumulative residential chemical exposures, 281
effects based on inappropriate comparison, 275–276
exposure duration, 280
impairment of exposed subjects, 278
miscellaneous causal factors, 276–277
occupational exposures, 281
potential weaknesses, 277
reconstructing chemical exposures, 280–281
residential exposures, 281
self-selection, 279
subjects exposed to hydrogen sulfide, 277
surrogates for exposure, 280
exposure and exposure surrogates, 254–257
the subjects, 257
lead concentrations, 257
mean test scores, 269–270
populations exposed to chemicals, 256
reaction times, 270
regression models for scores, 269
subjects' recall of story, 265
testing of subjects, 257–275
confounding factors, 267

Toluene-rich vapor exposures *(continued)*
 data analysis, 268–275
 descriptive data, 260–268
 exposure indices, 267–268
 methods, 257–260
 neurophysiological tests, 263–264
 neuropsychological tests, 264–267
 profile of mood states, 267
 results, 260–268
 symptom frequency scores, 267
 test scores, 267–268
 unexposed cohort, 258
Torrance, California exposures, 96–104
Total body pain, 11
Toxic; *See also* Nontoxic aluminum recycling
Toxic chemicals, stop transportation of, 366
Toxic neurophysiological effects, 243–244
Toxic technology, enforce until replaced, 367
Toxicants, removal of, 341–342
Toxicology, environmental, 12–16
Toxins, human exposure to known, 16–17
Train derailment, chlorine and cresylate from, 129–138
Transportation, 374
Trauma, brain, 339

Uncertainties and contrasts, 89
Unexposed groups and prediction equations, 49
Unexposed subjects, sway speed with eyes closed of, 40
Unocal refinery exposure
 affective domain, 110–112
 air monitoring data, 106–108
 bias, 113–114
 confounding factors, 112–113
 exposure conditions, 106–108
 neurophysiological domain, 108–109
 neuropsychological domain, 109–110
 repeat testing, 114
 symptoms, 112
Users, boycotts by, 373

Validation of models, 32–33
Values, predicted, 35–36
Variables, independent, 35
Verbal recall, immediate, 47
Vibration, 26–27
Visual fields
 measurement of, 27
 tests correlated with, 80–81
Visual reproductions, 33–34
VOCs (volatile organic chemicals)
 analysis of water, 235
 concentration of, 259
Volunteers, exposed and unexposed, 17

WAIS (Wechsler adult intelligence scale), 18, 30, 49, 157, 241, 319, 348
Water purification, 374
Wechsler, David, 348
Wechsler stories, recall of, 170–171
Wood, 370–371
Workers
 healthy survivors, 15
 refinery, 123–125
Writing errors, fingertip, 95–96

Yusho, 193